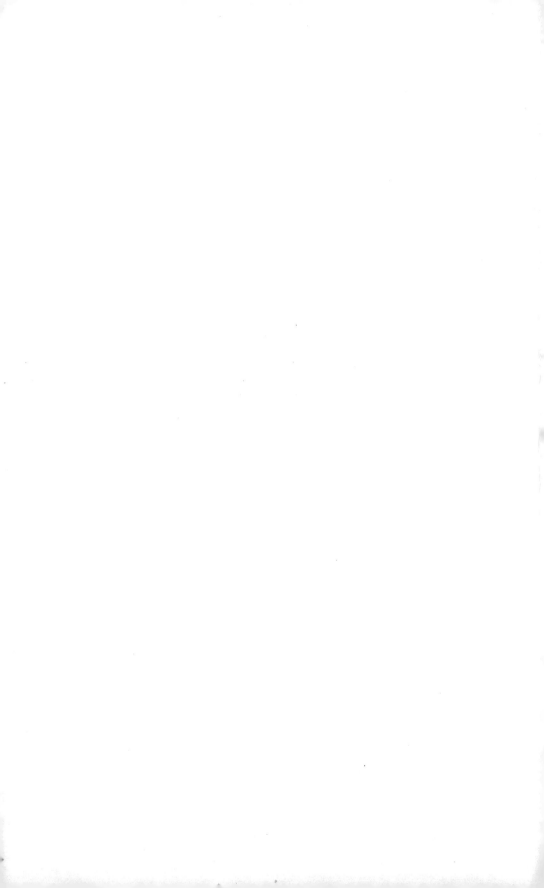

Cost-Effectiveness in Health and Medicine

Cost-Effectiveness in Health and Medicine

Second Edition

Edited by Peter J. Neumann
Tufts Medical Center
and
Gillian D. Sanders
Duke University

Louise B. Russell
Rutgers University

Joanna E. Siegel
Patient-Centered Outcomes Research Institute (PCORI)

Theodore G. Ganiats
University of California San Diego

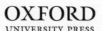

OXFORD
UNIVERSITY PRESS

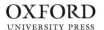

Oxford University Press is a department of the University of Oxford. It furthers
the University's objective of excellence in research, scholarship, and education
by publishing worldwide. Oxford is a registered trade mark of Oxford University
Press in the UK and certain other countries.

Published in the United States of America by Oxford University Press
198 Madison Avenue, New York, NY 10016, United States of America.

© Oxford University Press 2017

First Edition published in 1996

Catalog-in-Publication Data is on file with the Library of Congress
ISBN 978-0-19-049293-9

3 5 7 9 8 6 4 2

Printed by Sheridan Books, Inc., United States of America

Contents

Foreword

Harvey V. Fineberg

Four decades ago, Milton Weinstein and I led a group of colleagues in co-authoring a textbook, *Clinical Decision Analysis*, designed to help clinicians frame medical problems in a structured, systematic, and quantitative manner. The book emphasized that healthcare decisions typically involve considerations of health benefits, risks, and costs, many of which are uncertain at the time decisions have to be taken. We devoted a chapter to the consideration of economic costs and to the idea that cost-effectiveness analysis (CEA) could aid in the efficient allocation of limited resources. That chapter discussed issues such as the viewpoint or perspective from which a CEA can be conducted, how analysts could measure resource costs and health benefits, and how CEA could show the trade-offs involved in choosing among interventions. At the time, these concepts were relatively new to the medical community.

In the years since that book appeared, the field of CEA has advanced considerably to become a more familiar part of the American healthcare landscape. In the 1980s to the mid-1990s, the US Office of Technology Assessment sponsored a number of cost-effectiveness evaluations related to medical care. In 1996, the US Panel on Cost-Effectiveness in Health and Medicine produced a landmark report on the state of the art for conducting CEAs and offered recommendations for the field. A diverse group of scientists and scholars with backgrounds in medicine, economics, decision science, and ethics comprised that Panel. For a generation, their report served as a standard, widely cited reference.

Today, in the second decade of the twenty-first century, the landscape of healthcare has continued to change in major ways. Understanding of the molecular, behavioral, and social determinants of health has improved markedly. The organization and delivery of care have transformed dramatically, with health insurance exchanges, convenience clinics, accountable care organizations, value-based reimbursements, new patient databases, integrated delivery systems, and incentive-based wellness programs taking form or gaining new momentum. The past two decades have witnessed wondrous innovations in diagnostics and treatments for cancer, hepatitis C, arthritis, heart disease, and many other conditions.

Despite these advances—and because some of them create new, expensive possibilities—we continue to face the harsh reality that society cannot afford all of the healthcare from which people could possibly benefit. Explicitly or implicitly, we make choices about which programs to fund, which individuals and populations to screen, and which expensive new drugs to provide to which patients. Many system-wide inefficiencies persist. Health expenditures in the United States have risen to 18% of gross domestic product (GDP), far higher than those of other high-income countries, despite the fact that the nation underperforms on most population health metrics. Resources consumed in an unwieldy and inefficient healthcare system mean less money for education, infrastructure, environmental protection, and myriad other personal and social goods and investments.

The role of a CEA in informing decision makers on ways to take account of the array of costs and effects of different options is thus more compelling than ever. Fortunately, in this volume, a Second Panel on Cost-Effectiveness in Health and Medicine has produced a timely, comprehensive, and thoroughly updated guide. This book builds on the work of the original Panel by reviewing key concepts and analytic challenges in CEA. And the Second Panel provides a fresh examination of the field, departing in several key ways from the original Panel's work. Notably, the Second Panel revisits the original Panel's recommendation for a Reference Case, or standard set of method-ological practices that all CEAs should follow to improve quality and comparability. The Second Panel endorses the concept of a Reference Case, and supports the original Panel's recommendation that analysts take a broad societal perspective for Reference Case analyses. However, the Second Panel also recommends that analysts include a Reference Case from a narrower healthcare sector perspective, which the Panel notes is in line with the perspective that analysts have most commonly used over the last 20 years and that it believes will be most useful to many decision makers within the healthcare sector.

The Second Panel has revised the original Panel's work in many other ways, drawing on advances in empirical research, measurement techniques, database innovations, and the experience of health decision makers worldwide who have used CEA in numerous and diverse applications. This book contains three new chapters to capture a wealth of new research on modeling approaches, methods for evidence synthesis, and ethical considerations. It contains hundreds of updated references and examples. In Appendix A and Appendix B, it provides two worked examples to illustrate how to implement its updated recommendations.

The use of CEA raises a host of thorny ethical, social, economic, and policy questions. The Second Panel dives headlong into them. Like the original Panel, the Second Panel emphasizes that CEA is only one input into decisions and is not an exact science. At the same time, this work presents a strong case that CEA can be a useful tool to describe and characterize aspects of value that otherwise can be hard to take into account, in a format helpful for decision making.

This new edition deserves to find a receptive audience of new readers. The book should be of use to health policy makers, public and private payers, employers, health administrators, public health officials, and practicing physicians. It is especially timely given renewed emphasis on seeking ways to obtain better value for our nation's health spending. One hopes to see this work and the tools it describes used by health policy makers worldwide and in the education of future leaders in public health, management, policy, and medicine. Whether they are skeptics or proponents of CEA, readers will come away convinced that this Second Panel deliberated over the difficult questions that CEA provokes, wrestled mightily with them, and made a concerted attempt to consider both ideals and pragmatic solutions. This work sets a new standard for those who wish to make fully informed and well considered decisions about healthcare.

Harvey V. Fineberg
President of the Gordon and Betty Moore Foundation
and former President of the Institute of Medicine
(now National Academy of Medicine), 2002–2014.

Acknowledgments

This update to the 1996 report of the original Panel on Cost-Effectiveness in Health and Medicine has benefited from the contributions of many people. The book had its origins in discussions held by some of this book's editors with selected members of the original Panel, including Marthe Gold and Milton Weinstein. We appreciate their support, as well as that of other members of the original Panel, throughout the process of producing this update.

This project benefited enormously from generous funding from the Bill & Melinda Gates Foundation and the Robert Wood Johnson Foundation. We are especially grateful to Damian Walker of the Gates Foundation and Michael Painter of the Robert Wood Johnson Foundation for their help in securing the funding and overseeing the grants. The Second Panel received a small conference grant from the Agency for Healthcare Research and Quality (AHRQ), which funded a three-day in-person meeting in spring 2014, and parts of two subsequent meetings. We thank William Lawrence and Elisabeth Kato of AHRQ for their efforts in managing the process and helping with the meetings.

Jill Metcalf of the Society for Medical Decision Making (SMDM) was instrumental in providing the society's in-kind support for meeting space at two annual SMDM meetings. The University of California at San Diego Health Services Research Center sponsored part of the first in-person meeting of the Second Panel, supported the Leadership Group and the full Panel phone calls, and supported the public Web page.

We are grateful to Chad Zimmerman of Oxford University Press for all of his help shepherding this project into its final form. A huge thanks to Jeremy Goldhaber-Fiebert and John Nyman, who read the entire draft manuscript and provided many helpful comments on matters large and small.

We also thank David Kim of the University of Washington and Ba' Pham of the University of Toronto, the lead authors of the worked examples that appear in Appendices A and B, as well as David's coauthors, Gary Zarkin of RTI International and Sarah Duffy of the National Institute on Drug Abuse.

Numerous individuals worked hard behind the scenes. Julie Lannon of Tufts Medical Center provided logistical support for project meetings, grant funding, and countless other details. Sam Yang of Tufts Medical Center constructed the website for posting draft chapters for public comment. Beverly Perkins of Duke University scheduled dozens of teleconferences. We would also like the thank the following individuals for their help in conducting research, reviewing certain materials, or providing other behind-the-scenes support: Lusine Abrahamyan, Jordan Anderson, Chris Bojke, Jaime Caro,

James Chambers, Megan Chobot, Gerard de Pouvourville, Megan Farquhar, Kevin Frick, Justin Ingels, Isao Kamae, Kathryn Lallinger, Mackenzie Lowry, Petro Pechlivanoglou, John Richardson, Cayla Saret, Teja Thorat, and Simon Walker.

Finally, virtually every page of this book has profited from the careful editing of Rebecca Gray of Duke University, whose skill and attention to detail helped to bring clarity, consistency, and richness to the Second Panel's prose.

EXTERNAL REVIEWERS

The following individuals reviewed one or more chapters of the book: Paul Barnett, Andrew Briggs, Karl Claxton, Joshua T. Cohen, Phaedra Corso, Michael Drummond, Nir Eyal, Dennis Fryback, William Furlong, Afschin Gandjour, Louis Garrison, Marthe Gold, Dan Greenberg, Scott Grosse, James Hammitt, Neil Hawkins, Mark Helfand, Don Husereau, Emmett Keeler, Paul Krabbe, William Lawrence, Joseph Lipscomb, Daniel Mullins, Erik Nord, James O'Mahony, Donald Patrick, Mike Paulden, A. Simon Pickard, Michael Pignone, Daniel Polsky, K. V. Ramanath, Dennis Revicki, Mark Roberts, Lisa Robinson, Steven Teutsch, George Torrance, Joel Tsevat, Todd Wagner, Evelyn Whitlock, Milton Weinstein, John Wong, and Beth Woods. We are also grateful to several dozen individuals who commented on the publicly posted draft chapters in fall 2015.

Peter J. Neumann, Gillian D. Sanders, Anirban Basu, Dan W. Brock,
David Feeny, Murray Krahn, Karen M. Kuntz, David O. Meltzer,
Douglas K. Owens, Lisa A. Prosser, Joshua A. Salomon, Mark J. Sculpher,
Thomas A. Trikalinos, Louise B. Russell, Joanna E. Siegel, and Theodore G. Ganiats

About the Editors

Peter J. Neumann, ScD, is Director of the Center for the Evaluation of Value and Risk in Health, Institute for Clinical Research and Health Policy Studies, and Professor of Medicine, Tufts Medical Center and Tufts University.

Gillian D. Sanders, PhD, is Director of the Duke Evidence Synthesis Group and Professor of Medicine, Duke Clinical Research Institute and Duke University.

Louise B. Russell, PhD, is Distinguished Professor, Institute for Health and Department of Economics, Rutgers University.

Joanna E. Siegel, ScD, is Director of Dissemination and Implementation, Patient-Centered Outcomes Research Institute (PCORI).

Theodore G. Ganiats, MD, is Professor Emeritus, Health Services Research Center and Department of Family Medicine and Public Health, University of California, San Diego.

Second Panel on Cost-Effectiveness in Health and Medicine

Panel Members

Anirban Basu
University of Washington
Dan W. Brock
Harvard University Medical School
David Feeny
McMaster University
Murray Krahn
University of Toronto
Karen M. Kuntz
University of Minnesota
David O. Meltzer
University of Chicago
Peter J. Neumann (Co-Chair)
Tufts Medical Center
Douglas K. Owens
VA Palo Alto Health Care System and Stanford University
Lisa A. Prosser
University of Michigan
Joshua A. Salomon
Harvard T.H. Chan School of Public Health

Gillian D. Sanders (Co-Chair)
Duke University
Mark J. Sculpher
University of York
Thomas A. Trikalinos
Brown University

Leadership

Peter J. Neumann (Co-Chair)
Tufts Medical Center
Gillian D. Sanders (Co-Chair)
Duke University
Theodore G. Ganiats
University of California San Diego
Louise B. Russell
Rutgers University
Joanna E. Siegel
Patient-Centered Outcomes Research Institute (PCORI)

Technical Editor

Rebecca N. Gray
Duke University

First Panel on Cost-Effectiveness in Health and Medicine

Norman Daniels
Dennis G. Fryback
Alan M. Garber
David C. Hadorn
Mark S. Kamlet
Joseph Lipscomb
Bryan R. Luce
Jeanne S. Mandelblatt
Willard G. Manning, Jr.

Donald L. Patrick
Louise B. Russell (Co-chair)
George W. Torrance
Milton C. Weinstein (Co-chair)

US Public Health Service Staff
Marthe R. Gold
Kristine I. McCoy
Joanna E. Siegel

Introduction

Peter J. Neumann, Gillian D. Sanders, Louise B. Russell,
Joanna E. Siegel, and Theodore G. Ganiats

UPDATING THE WORK OF THE PANEL
ON COST-EFFECTIVENESS IN HEALTH
AND MEDICINE

By the early 1990s, the rising costs of healthcare and the need to prioritize resource allocation more rationally were firmly on the national agenda. The use of cost-effectiveness analysis (CEA) as a technique to inform healthcare decisions was beginning to gain traction. Increasingly, researchers were publishing CEAs in the medical literature. Public health officials, healthcare administrators, public and private payers, and other health policy makers were considering whether and how to incorporate the approach into their policy making processes.

For all of the interest, however, the field of CEA was characterized by substantial variation in methods and by disputes over a host of theoretical and practical issues. To address the matter, in 1993 the US Public Health Service convened a Panel of 13 non-government scientists and scholars with expertise in economics, clinical medicine, ethics, and statistics to review the state of the field and to provide recommendations for the use and conduct of CEAs in health and medicine. The primary goals were to improve the quality of CEAs and to promote comparability across studies.

In 1996 the Panel published its findings in a book and a series of papers. The work quickly became a standard, both in the United States and internationally; the book has sold more than 20,000 copies and has been cited more than 8,000 times. The Panel emphasized that the growing field of CEA provided an opportunity to rationalize health policy, but only if the technique and its application were well understood and implemented. Their report's introduction observed that the term "cost-effective" had come increasingly into common parlance, having been adopted by groups as disparate as the Congress, the business community, managed care organizations, the pharmaceutical industry, and the press. It further noted that the term was insufficiently precise to provide guidance to the many who might wish to use CEA to improve the quality and efficiency of the health system. This imprecision, the Panel argued, stemmed from various causes, including the fact that developers of the field of CEA and analysts who applied the methods came from different academic disciplines, including economics, medicine, operations research, psychology, public health, and ethics, each bringing their own particular concepts and language. Adding to the imprecision was the fact that CEA could be used to inform different kinds of decision makers, from purchasers of healthcare services to those who assess healthcare technology to advocates for particular illnesses or constituencies, all of whom might use the term "cost-effective" to garner resource investments. The Panel's report featured a recommendation that analysts present a "Reference Case" CEA, following a standard set of methods, to serve as a point of comparison across studies.

In the 20 years since publication of the Panel's book, the use of CEA has increased substantially. Moreover, the field has advanced in many ways—for example, in methods for evidence synthesis, in techniques for modeling, in the consideration of ethical issues surrounding use of CEA, and in standards for the reporting of results. Healthcare has also experienced dramatic changes, in terms of the organization, financing, and delivery of care, and in terms of technological progress, including the advent of "personalized" medicine and genomic approaches to care to scores of new drugs, devices, procedures, diagnostics, and public health programs, which raise new challenges and opportunities for CEA. In addition, the use of CEA by decision-making bodies around the world has advanced considerably. As one notable example, the creation of the United Kingdom's National Institute for Health and Care Excellence (NICE), perhaps the best known organization to apply CEA to inform healthcare decisions, was still several years in the future when the Panel's report was published. At the same time, the need to deliver healthcare efficiently, and the importance of using analytic techniques to understand clinical and economic consequences of strategies to improve health, have only increased. Healthcare spending in the United States comprised 13% of gross domestic product in 1995; by 2014, it was approaching 18%. For all of these reasons, this book provides a timely and long overdue update of the original Panel's work.

THE SECOND PANEL ON COST-EFFECTIVENESS IN HEALTH AND MEDICINE

In 2011 a group of leaders in the field of CEA in the United States, in consultation with members of the original Panel, began planning for an update to the 1996 book. Over the next several years, this group convened a new Panel and developed a process and structure for updating the original report.

Members of the Second Panel were invited by the leadership group of the Panel during the fall of 2012. Everyone who was invited accepted with enthusiasm, and all volunteered their time to participate in the initiative. The members of the Second Panel were selected on the basis of their experience in the field, and to provide broad expertise in the design and use of CEAs. The group met as a full Panel through regular teleconferences beginning in early 2013 and held five two- to three-day in-person meetings over the next several years to update and expand the recommendations of the original Panel. Chapter authors convened in separate teleconferences on a much more frequent basis. The Second Panel also benefited from the active participation of many members of the original Panel, as well as from external review by dozens of experts in the field.

Generous funding was provided by the Robert Wood Johnson Foundation and the Bill and Melinda Gates Foundation to support in-person meetings, the services of a medical editor, and research for two new worked examples. In addition, the Panel received a small conference grant from the Agency for Healthcare Research and Quality, which funded a three-day in-person meeting in spring 2014 and parts of two subsequent meetings; support from the University of California, San Diego Health Services Research Center, which funded part of the first in-person Panel meeting; and in-kind support from the Society for Medical Decision Making.

The objectives of the Second Panel on Cost-Effectiveness in Health and Medicine were similar to those of the original Panel: to review the state of the field and provide recommendations to improve the quality of CEAs and to promote their comparability. The intended audiences are also similar and include elected representatives, government policy makers, public health officials, healthcare administrators, payers, businesses, researchers, clinicians, patients, and consumers.

However, the Second Panel faced a very different landscape than the original Panel did, and the group was confronted by a new set of challenges. It is no longer accurate to call CEA a nascent or burgeoning field, nor is it realistic to explain variation in published studies by noting the newness of the concepts or the methods. The Second Panel had the advantage of drawing on two decades of methodological and policy advances, but it also had to deal with the challenge of sifting through and trying to make sense of diverse and sometimes contrasting opinions about, and experiences with, CEA.

INTRODUCTION TO THE SECOND EDITION

The book consists of 13 chapters, each of which addresses a different aspect of CEA: using CEA; theoretical foundations; the Panel's Reference Case recommendations; designing a CEA; modeling; identifying and quantifying consequences; identifying and valuing health outcomes; estimating costs; synthesizing evidence; discounting; reflecting uncertainty; ethics; and reporting. Following the precedent of the original report, this volume also contains two worked examples, one on alcohol use disorders (Appendix A) and one on end-of-life palliative care (Appendix B), which apply the Panel's recommendations.

This volume was conceived as an update of the original Panel's volume. The original book's structure and content provides the foundation. Nine of the 13 chapters are updates of similarly named chapters in the original book, though most have been substantially rewritten. There are four new chapters: on modeling, evidence synthesis, and ethics, and on the Second Panel's Reference Case recommendations. While material addressing modeling, evidence synthesis, and ethics was included in various places in the original volume, the Second Panel believed that dedicated chapters on these topics were warranted in this revision, given important developments and a wealth of new material in these areas.

This book also contains a dedicated chapter on the Second Panel's Reference Case recommendations (Chapter 3). As highlighted in that chapter, the Panel deliberated extensively on these core recommendations, which provide a foundation for many of the other recommendations throughout the book. One of the Second Panel's key recommendations—that analysts conducting CEAs present Reference Case analyses from both the healthcare sector and societal perspectives—represents a departure from the original Panel's recommendation. The rationale for this and other related recommendations are presented in Chapter 3.

As is in the original volume, the text here is directly primarily at those who conduct, or who direct the conduct, of CEAs. The book is not a "how-to-do-it" manual; rather, it provides an overview of the state of the field and a discussion of the component methods used in CEA in a manner that should be accessible to persons with some familiarity with CEA. Because CEAs have many different technical aspects, and correspondingly extensive theoretical and operational literature in the comprising disciplines, a number of issues cannot be dealt with in depth. Instead, references are provided so that the reader may pursue details elsewhere.

We hope the book will also prove useful to those, including decision makers, who wish to evaluate CEAs critically. While parts of the chapters provide relatively detailed discussion of technical areas, the book is designed to be accessible to people who wish simply to be sophisticated consumers of CEAs. We anticipate that it should be of use to health plans, insurers, health departments, and state and federal policy makers.

Cost-effectiveness analysis has become an important tool for decision making in diverse contexts. We have attempted to balance theoretical purity and the need for rigor with pragmatism and concerns about the burden on analysts. We have also been mindful that CEA has sometimes encountered resistance, particularly in the United States, among those who might use the technique. The Panel has tried to be clear-eyed about political realities and sensitive to factors other than CEA that are important in informing decisions.

The book includes applications to a range of contexts and settings. Examples interspersed throughout the text reflect interventions in public health and surgery, acute and chronic care, infectious disease and cancer, education programs, and genomics. While the Second Panel's work is focused primarily on US contexts, the book is intentionally international in its scope and intended impact. The report of the original Panel was influential around the world, with the work cited widely in CEAs across the globe and used in guidelines for coverage and reimbursement in numerous countries. The Second Panel included members from the United States, Canada, and the United Kingdom. It also included individuals whose work is focused on global health issues.

The Second Panel's members brought varying interests and experiences to this project. We strove to provide a balanced view on a wide variety of topics. It should be noted that David Feeny has a proprietary interest in Health Utilities Incorporated (HUInc.), Dundas, Ontario, Canada. HUInc. distributes copyrighted Health Utilities Index (HUI) materials and provides methodological advice on the use of the HUI.

No other Panel member reported a financial conflict of interest directly related to the topics in the book.

Cost-effectiveness analysis can help inform decisions about how to apply new tests and therapies so that they represent a judicious use of resources. It can help fill gaps in evidence about the estimated population-level public health impact of such interventions, and it can support decisions to disinvest in older interventions for which there are more effective and less costly alternatives. It provides a framework for comparing the relative value of different interventions, along with information that can help decision makers sort through alternatives and decide which ones best serve their programmatic and financial needs. The goal of this report is to promote the continued evolution of CEA and its use as a tool to support judicious, efficient, and fair decisions regarding the use of healthcare resources in the coming decades.

Overview of the Book

Peter J. Neumann, Gillian D. Sanders, Anirban Basu,
Dan W. Brock, David Feeny, Murray Krahn, Karen M. Kuntz,
David O. Meltzer, Douglas K. Owens, Lisa A. Prosser,
Joshua A. Salomon, Mark J. Sculpher, Thomas A. Trikalinos,
Louise B. Russell, Joanna E. Siegel, and Theodore G. Ganiats

In the 20 years since publication of the report of the original Panel on Cost-Effectiveness in Health and Medicine, researchers have advanced methods and applications of cost-effectiveness analysis (CEA), and policy makers have used the technique in various ways. Updating the original Panel's work provides an opportunity to reflect on the evolution of CEA and to provide guidance for the next generation of practitioners and consumers.

By estimating the magnitude of health outcomes and costs of interventions, CEA can show the trade-offs involved in choosing among interventions and thus contribute to better decisions. Chapter 1, *Using Cost-Effectiveness Analysis in Health and Medicine: Experiences since the Original Panel*, discusses the promise of CEA and the ways in which it has been applied. Since the original Panel's work, CEA has become a more common fixture on the public health and medical landscape. Researchers have investigated the cost-effectiveness of a wide range of interventions for diverse conditions and diseases. The number of CEAs published in journals has increased substantially. In the United States, public and private health organizations have funded and conducted CEAs.

Despite these trends, CEA has also encountered resistance. The US Medicare program is barred from using CEA in its coverage and reimbursement decisions, for example. The Patient Protection and Affordable Care Act of 2010 (42 U.S.C. § 18001 et seq.) prohibited the Patient-Centered Outcomes Research Institute (PCORI) from using cost per quality-adjusted life year (QALY) thresholds. In many ways, CEA has found a more welcome reception abroad, though the manner in which it has been applied has varied considerably. Decision makers involved in resource allocation decisions give the greatest weight and the deepest consideration to the clinical evidence. They have generally viewed CEA as one input, alongside other considerations—such as legal, ethical, cultural, and political concerns; patient expectations; and pragmatic issues of logistics and feasibility—to be considered in reaching decisions.

Chapter 2, *Theoretical Foundations of Cost-Effectiveness Analysis in Health and Medicine*, reviews the conceptual basis for CEA from varying perspectives, including actual decision makers who allocate resources from real budgets, and hypothetical decision makers who reflect some theoretically attractive decision-making perspective. The chapter considers CEA's foundations in terms of principles of constrained optimization, highlighting questions that this framework raises about what objectives should be maximized, what constraints should be considered, and what resources are to be consumed and what opportunities forgone. It also reviews welfare economic principles as the basis for evaluating the optimality of resource allocation in a social context.

The chapter points out that even among applications of CEA within health and medicine in which the objective is to maximize health, there are multiple questions to consider: how to measure and combine effects on survival and health-related quality of life; how to measure costs, including situations in which budget impacts may not reflect opportunity costs from a societal perspective; and how to treat effects that are uncertain or occur over time. Other topics covered include: theoretical issues that arise in the QALY model and their links to individual utility; metrics for valuing health consequences; differences between individual and social values; optimization with multiple budget constraints; measuring time costs; discounting; and research prioritization.

The book's first two chapters provide the foundation upon which the Panel makes its recommendations. Chapter 3, *Recommendations on Perspectives for the Reference Case,* considers issues involved in selecting a Reference Case. The original Panel recommended a Reference Case or set of standard methodological practices that all CEAs should follow to improve their quality and comparability. They further recommended that Reference Case analyses assume a societal perspective that reflects the perspective of a decision maker whose intention is to make decisions about the broad allocation of resources across the entire population. The original Panel also noted that in order to address specific decision contexts, analysts might also conduct CEAs from narrower perspectives, such as that of the healthcare sector, to reflect the view of a decision maker whose responsibility rests only within that sector.

The Second Panel endorses these concepts, but has also reconsidered and debated at length several conceptual and practical issues surrounding the question of what perspective or perspectives Reference Case analyses should assume. The Second Panel has observed that many, if not most, Reference Case analyses published over the years have *not* used a true societal perspective. Moreover, since publication of the original Panel's book, decision-making bodies have formally incorporated CEA into health technology assessment processes to inform coverage and reimbursement decisions, but generally have not adopted a societal perspective, preferring instead a narrower perspective.

Given this backdrop and various options, the Second Panel recommends that all studies report two Reference Case analyses: one based on a healthcare sector perspective and one based on a societal perspective. We also recommend that analysts summarize results of the Reference Case analyses in one of the conventional forms as an incremental cost-effectiveness ratio (ICER), net monetary benefit (NMB), or net health benefit (NHB). We recommend that the healthcare sector perspective include formal healthcare sector (medical) costs borne by third-party payers and paid for out-of-pocket by patients. Both types of medical costs include current and future costs, related and unrelated to the condition under consideration. The Panel agrees that it would be helpful to inform decision makers by summarizing the broader societal impacts as well. However, there are no widely agreed upon methods for quantifying and valuing some of these broader impacts in CEA. We therefore recommend that analysts present the items listed in the Impact Inventory in the form of disaggregated consequences across different sectors. We also recommend that analysts use one or more summary measures, such as an ICER, NMB, or NHB, that include some or all of the items listed in the Impact Inventory. Analysts should clearly identify which items are included and how they are measured and valued, and provide a rationale for their methodological decisions. We recommend that analysts clearly state the perspective of every analysis reported, and include other perspectives in addition to the two Reference Case perspectives, if relevant.

These recommendations are intended to provide a useful and pragmatic approach that will serve both producers and consumers of CEAs. They involve choices and compromises in the service of practicality, comparability, and flexibility. The intention is to highlight the societal and healthcare sector perspectives. Indeed, the main purpose of the Impact Inventory is to ensure that all consequences, including those outside of the formal healthcare sector, are considered regularly and comprehensively, as they have generally not been to date.

Chapter 4, *Designing a Cost-Effectiveness Analysis,* reiterates the original Panel's recommendation that before undertaking a CEA, analysts, in consultation with subject area experts and decision makers, must decide on an overall approach and on specific study design elements. The chapter highlights the importance of these early conceptualization and planning steps for focusing the study on relevant research questions, maintaining the focus as the study progresses, and avoiding analytical pitfalls midway through an analysis. A key departure from the work of the original Panel is in detailing how analysts should consider the two Reference Cases. Two other differences are noteworthy: recommending the use of an Impact Inventory, which, as described above, lists the consequences across sectors (e.g., healthcare, education, criminal justice system) affected by an intervention; and recommending that analysts develop a written protocol at the outset of an analysis that details key aspects of the CEA's design and conduct (e.g., the study objective; the intervention, comparator, and population under consideration; the time horizon; sources of data; a list of key assumptions). Analysts should update the protocol as the study progresses and note the changes from the original protocol.

The original Panel's report noted that the use of modeling is a valid mode of scientific inquiry for CEAs, but the group devoted relatively little attention to the practice. In contrast, the Second Panel has devoted an entire chapter to modeling (Chapter 5, *Decision Models in Cost-Effectiveness Analysis*), underscoring recent advances in the field and the appearance of recommendations on modeling in guidelines for conducting CEAs for health technology appraisals in several countries. The chapter emphasizes that analysts typically face a situation in which the data available to inform the costs and effects of different interventions come from disparate sources and often from studies for which analysts do not have access to primary data. Models fill in the gaps and help to structure analysts' thinking. They provide a framework for synthesizing data from disparate sources, allowing extrapolations beyond the time horizons of available data and to population subgroups and strategies not observed in studies. The chapter reviews the different types of decision models and their relative advantages and disadvantages. It also provides recommendations for model structure, output, evaluation of uncertainty, and validation.

Chapter 6, *Identifying and Quantifying the Consequences of Interventions*, considers the effects of different interventions or policies that are being compared. The chapter builds on the original Panel's chapter, "Assessing the Effectiveness of Health Interventions"; the new title reflects a broadened scope, with an emphasis on the applicability of CEA methods beyond clinical interventions, and it is consistent with the Second Panel's recommendation for an Impact Inventory as a key part of any CEA.

The chapter envisions two distinct phases for identifying and quantifying consequences: first, undertaking a broad and systematic accounting of relevant consequences of the decision being evaluated; and second, describing key data sources and measurement approaches that may be used. The chapter recommends that CEAs identify all significant consequences relating to health (survival and/or health status), as well as resource use in the formal and informal healthcare sectors and consequences in other sectors. The chapter considers various dimensions along which consequences may be distinguished, including the *sector* in which the consequences are realized (healthcare versus other sectors); groups with different degrees of proximity to the intervention (target population versus other affected groups); and different time points in relation to the intervention. The Impact Inventory provides a framework allowing analysts to list all consequences of an intervention, within and without the healthcare sector. This allows an opportunity to justify the omission of these elements and to consider whether inclusion of an item would likely alter the conclusions.

Chapter 7, *Valuing Health Outcomes*, follows the original Panel's conceptualization of health-related quality of life, incorporating the idea that health is a major determinant of overall well-being, while recognizing that factors other than health may also affect overall quality of life. The chapter examines preference-based and non-preference-based approaches to measuring health-related quality of life, discusses theoretical and practical issues in preference measurement, and provides guidance on how to select measures for use in CEAs. The chapter reviews the sizeable literature on preference measurement that has arisen since the original Panel's work, including issues pertaining to the validity, reliability, and responsiveness of different elicitation methods; the use of condition-specific preference-based measures; and whose preferences should be used in CEAs. The chapter also discusses special issues, such as states worse than dead; special populations, such as children; and spillover effects of the health of one family member on other family members.

The Second Panel retains many of original Panel's recommendations, for example, that Reference Case CEAs should measure health effects in terms of QALYs; that quality weights should be preference-based and interval-scaled; and that community preferences for health states are the most appropriate source of preferences for Reference Case analyses. The Second Panel also recommends the use of generic preference-based measures in order to enhance comparability across studies, though we emphasize that the instrument used should be fit for purpose in the sense that its measurement properties are adequate to measure the differences and changes in health across the interventions under consideration. Like the original Panel, the Second Panel has chosen not to endorse a particular generic preference-based measure. The recommendations also highlight the importance of sensitivity analyses that furnish information on the preferences of persons with specific conditions or characteristics, which in turn may affect cost-effectiveness ratios. Unlike the original Panel, the Second Panel observes that, in general, effects on productivity are unlikely to have been captured by most preference-based measures, and that evidence is not definitive that the effects of morbidity on leisure are necessarily reflected in the utility scores. It therefore recommends that financial consequences related to changes in health status be reflected in the numerator of cost-effectiveness ratios for Reference Case analyses conducted under the societal perspective.

Chapter 8, *Estimating Costs and Valuation of Non-Health Benefits in Cost-Effectiveness Analysis,* examines the process of identifying, quantifying, and valuing the resource costs associated with the use and consequences of healthcare interventions. The chapter categorizes the types of resources that most interventions require and describes how they are included in a CEA. A key departure from the work of the original Panel is the consideration of cost categories from the two Reference Case perspectives. The Second Panel recommends that some components (e.g., current and future medical costs and patients' out-of-pocket costs), should pertain to both sectors, while others (e.g., time costs for patients and caregivers, transportation costs, productivity benefits, consumption costs, and other sector costs) should be counted only for the societal Reference Case perspective.

Two other differences from the work of the original Panel are noteworthy. One pertains to the debate about whether productivity costs should be measured explicitly and incorporated with other resource costs, or whether these costs are already captured in QALYs so that their inclusion in the numerator would lead to "double counting." Unlike the original Panel, the Second Panel has concluded that productivity effects are not included in QALYs and therefore recommends that they be included in the numerator of the cost-effectiveness ratio, although the Panel recognizes the possibility that this could also lead to double counting. The Second Panel also differs from the original Panel on the issue of "future" costs—that is, whether related or unrelated (or both) healthcare costs should be accounted for during the additional life years produced by an intervention. The original Panel discussed the issue but did not reach consensus (noting that analysts could use their discretion) because of the lack of a developed theoretical basis for including future costs at the time of their report. Several papers since the original Panel have supported the inclusion of all future costs.

Thus, we recommend that analysts include all healthcare costs, related and unrelated, when an intervention extends life or when cost components cannot be readily identified as related to the target condition. Moreover, costs that are incurred due to differential survival of patients should net consumption costs from the measurements of productivity gains.

Chapter 9, *Evidence Synthesis for Informing Cost-Effectiveness Analysis*, is a new chapter, highlighting the importance of interpreting, adjusting, and synthesizing information in CEAs. The chapter emphasizes that, by maximizing use of available data, analysts can minimize bias and increase the likelihood of an optimal decision. The chapter goes beyond the original Panel's conception of evidence synthesis for CEAs by calling for analysts to undertake a *pre-analytical phase* (defining a question and identifying pertinent data from distinct sources), an *analytical phase* (positing and learning relationships across data from distinct sources), and a *post-analytical phase* (conjecturing on the implications of the learned relationships for the question at hand). The chapter draws from recent guidance on systematic reviews and meta-analyses. Among the Second Panel's recommendations are calls for analysts to provide a qualitative description and critique of the evidence base, to be explicit about whether and how bias in each study and across studies in the evidence base was handled, to produce bias-corrected estimates, and to be explicit about whether and how estimates were adjusted for transferability.

Chapter 10, *Discounting in Cost-Effectiveness Analysis*, updates the original Panel's chapter on time preferences. It follows the original Panel, as well as other economic evaluation guidelines, in recommending that analysts discount future outcomes and present cost-effectiveness ratios in present value terms. Only then will the interventions' cost-effectiveness ratios be appropriately adjusted for the differential timing of consequences so that decision makers can compare them from the same temporal baseline. The chapter updates the original Panel's discussion of rationales for discounting based on economic theory, as well as different approaches for selecting discount rates. It also reviews arguments for and against discounting health consequences and on whether analysts should use the same discount rate for health and costs. Finally, the chapter reviews alternative discounting methods, including hyperbolic discounting and declining discount rates.

The chapter follows the original Panel in recommending that in Reference Case analyses, costs and health effects should be discounted at the same rate. Further, given available data on real economic growth and corresponding estimates of the real consumption rate of interest, the Second Panel continues to recommend 3% as the most appropriate real discount rate for CEAs. The Panel also calls for sensitivity analyses, allowing for a reasonable range of rates, and allowing health and cost consequences to be discounted at different rates and conducted using different methods, and for more research on the topic of using different discount rates for health and cost outcomes in CEAs.

Chapter 11, *Reflecting Uncertainty in Cost-Effectiveness Analysis*, underscores that accounting for uncertainty in a manner consistent with the objectives and constraints of decision making is an essential part of any CEA. The characterization and reporting of uncertainty has evolved since the original Panel's report, and a range of analytical methods is now available to guide decisions about the adoption of interventions and the value of additional research. The chapter notes that conducting uncertainty analysis is important, in part because it can provide reassurance that models are working appropriately. Even more important, it can contribute to better decisions. In the context of decisions about the funding of new medical technologies, for example, uncertainty analysis can help inform options, such as whether to make an "accept" or "reject" decision now and whether to revisit that decision at some point in the future if additional evidence has emerged. The chapter reviews the pros and cons of deterministic sensitivity analysis and probabilistic sensitivity analysis (PSA), which characterizes uncertainty in all parameters simultaneously. It highlights structural (or model) uncertainty, which represents choices from what may be numerous plausible alternatives (e.g., how to model the effects of an intervention beyond the time horizon of the evidence source). It reviews the use of cost-effectiveness acceptability curves (CEACs), which present the probability of an intervention's being cost-effective for a range of different cost-effectiveness thresholds. The chapter also notes that assessments about the potential value of additional research (i.e., value-of-information analysis) can support decisions about funding health care interventions and research activities, including barriers to their implementation and potential solutions.

The Second Panel argues that the guiding principle in determining the best approach to uncertainty analysis should be how the analysis informs choices among policy options, including those relating to decisions for further research. The Panel notes that deterministic sensitivity analysis can provide useful insights into model behavior and validation but emphasizes that PSA provides stronger analytical support for decision making. The Panel urges that structural uncertainties be tested in analyses, that decision uncertainty be presented using probabilities for specified cost-effectiveness thresholds or CEACs, and that expected value-of-information analysis be used to guide decision making under uncertainty.

While material addressing ethical considerations was interspersed throughout the original Panel's report, this volume contains a standalone chapter on the topic (Chapter 12, *Ethical and Distributive Considerations*), reflecting substantial developments in the field. The chapter begins by underscoring that CEA—that is, the consideration of the opportunity cost of an intervention—is ethically justified. Without such consideration, we would not know if there were better uses of the resources at hand. The chapter also reaffirms the original Panel's principle that CEA is not by itself a sufficient decision-making standard and that it does not capture all relevant concerns. Maximizing the total quantity of health benefits will rarely be the only concern for decision makers. Who receives the benefits—the distributive concern—also matters. Most of the difficult issues in the use of CEAs are distributional issues arising when one is evaluating alternative interventions benefitting different groups of patients. They involve trade-offs between effects and costs for some patients versus different benefits and costs for other patients.

The chapter observes that the question of how to factor ethical concerns into CEAs is a normative one that raises complex and controversial issues, requiring attention by analysts and decision makers using CEA. It emphasizes that decision makers should have access to the best possible analyses of the ethical issues relevant to their decisions. For analysts conducting CEAs, issues include the following: How should states of health and disability be evaluated? Should all QALYs count equally? What costs and benefits should count in CEAs of health programs? Among the issues for those *using* CEA are these: whether priority should be given to the sickest or worst off; when large benefits to a small number of people should receive priority over small but greater aggregate benefits to a large number of people; the conflict between fair changes and best outcomes; whether use of CEA to set health priorities unjustly discriminates against disabled persons; the potential use of equity weights; and the use of cost per QALY thresholds. The chapter ends with several recommendations, emphasizing the importance of sensitivity analyses to illustrate the impact of alternative distributional choices.

In the final chapter (Chapter 13, *Reporting Cost-Effectiveness Analyses*), the Second Panel reiterates the original Panel's emphasis on the importance of presenting CEAs in a clear, organized, and complete fashion. Clarity and transparency in reporting enhances the accessibility and credibility of a CEA, as well as the degree to which research can be replicated or extended by other analysts and, ultimately, the likelihood that studies will influence decisions.

The chapter outlines information recommended for reporting in the "journal article," covering the design of the analysis; methods and data; results; and discussion. Like the original Panel, it also recommends inclusion of a technical appendix, which provides additional detail on methods and results (most journals now provide an option to publish supplementary material online). The chapter highlights several new areas that have emerged since the original Panel's report: the need for more clarity in identifying the perspective of the analysis; a structured abstract; reporting intermediate endpoints and disaggregated results; and updated guidance on disclosure of conflicts of interest. Finally, the chapter highlights the use of an Impact Inventory table intended to improve the clarity of the scope and boundaries of the analysis for both Reference Case perspectives.

Key areas for future research identified by the Second Panel include: the use of multi criteria decision analysis and group decision making; the use of CEA in value-based pricing; estimation of cost-effectiveness thresholds; the link between CEA and incentives for innovation; the role of CEA within health plans or guideline development; the impact of our two Reference Case perspectives on analyses and their findings; and the use of extended CEA to consider the financial risk protection benefits of interventions as well as the distributional consequences across households' wealth levels. The field would also benefit from further research on QALYs, including topics such as whether and to what extent respondents consider productivity effects in their valuations of health states, the relationship of community preferences to patient preferences for different health states, the elicitation of preference scores for path states, the sequence of states that patients experience, and methods for measuring health-related quality-of-life effects on family members of ill individuals ("family spillover effects"). This is not an all-inclusive list of topics for future research, but rather suggests topics that arose repeatedly during the deliberations of the Second Panel as areas where Panel members believed future research would prove fruitful.

In appendices to the book, two CEA "worked examples," one on alcohol use disorders (Appendix A) and one on end-of-life palliative care (Appendix B), highlight how the recommendations of the Second Panel, can be used in practice.

1

Using Cost-Effectiveness Analysis
in Health and Medicine
Experiences since the Original Panel

Peter J. Neumann, Louise B. Russell, Joanna E. Siegel,
Lisa A. Prosser, Murray Krahn, Jeanne S. Mandelblatt,
Norman Daniels, and Marthe R. Gold

1.1 INTRODUCTION

The original Panel on Cost-Effectiveness in Health and Medicine recommended the use of cost-effectiveness analysis (CEA) as an aid to decision making, recognizing that it does not, in and of itself, constitute a complete decision-making process. The Second Panel on Cost-Effectiveness in Health and Medicine has also recognized this reality and has sought, at the outset of its work, to understand the role CEA has played in real-world decisions. This chapter begins by introducing the concept of CEA and discussing how it can aid resource allocation decisions. The rest of the chapter describes experiences that have played an important role in shaping the recommendations of the Second Panel. It provides a brief overview of the original Panel's recommendations and describes how CEA has been used, in the United States and other countries, in the 20 years since the original Panel published its recommendations.

Cost-effectiveness analysis is a form of economic evaluation that assesses the health outcomes and costs of interventions designed to improve people's health. It has been used to assess a wide range of treatments and programs, from clinical interventions such as the pneumococcal vaccination for older adults (Smith et al. 2012), screening for colorectal cancer (Giorgi Rossi and Zappa 2008; Ness et al. 2000), and total knee arthroplasty (Losina et al. 2009), to community-based physical activity interventions (Roux

This chapter builds on concepts presented in Chapter 1 of the original Panel's book (Russell, L. B., J. E. Siegel, N. Daniels, M. R. Gold, B. R. Luce, and J. S. Mandelblatt. 1996. "Cost-Effectiveness Analysis as a Guide to Resource Allocation in Health: Roles and Limitations." In *Cost-Effectiveness in Health and Medicine*, edited by M. R. Gold, J. E. Siegel, L. B. Russell, and M. C. Weinstein, 3–24. New York: Oxford University Press).

et al. 2008) and bans on people using cellular phones while driving (Sperber, Shiell, and Fyie 2010). The results of an analysis are typically summarized in a series of incremental cost-effectiveness ratios (ICERs) that show, for one intervention compared with another, the cost of achieving an additional unit of health (see Table 1.1 for an example).

By estimating the magnitude of health outcomes and costs of interventions, and the uncertainty surrounding those estimates, CEA can make an important contribution

Table 1.1 Cost-effectiveness analysis: an example

	Vaccination strategy (in order of increasing effectiveness)		
	Strategy 1 vs no vaccination	Strategy 2 vs strategy 1	Strategy 3 vs strategy 2
Incremental cost per person, 2006 dollars	33	43	8
Incremental QALYs per person	0.00116	0.00094	0.00002
Incremental cost per QALY (ICER)	28,900	45,100	496,000

Strategy 1: PCV13 for high-risk adults at age 50 and all adults at age 65.

Strategy 2: PCV 13 for all adults at age 50 and again at age 65.

Strategy 3: PCV13 for all adults at age 50 and again at age 65, plus PPSV23 for all adults at age 75.

Abbreviations: ICER = incremental cost-effectiveness ratio; PCV13 = 13-valent pneumococcal conjugate vaccine; PPSV23 = 23-valent pneumococcal polysaccharide vaccine; QALY(s) = quality-adjusted life year(s).

Cost-effectiveness analysis (CEA) involves estimating the net, or "incremental," costs and effects of an intervention—its costs and health outcomes—compared with some alternative. The alternative might be the care that would be provided if the intervention were not used at all, or it might be a different intensity of the intervention, such as more (or less) frequent screening, or higher (or lower) doses of a medication. The "incremental cost-effectiveness ratio" (ICER) is calculated as the difference in costs between the two alternatives (net costs), divided by the difference in health outcomes (net effectiveness) and shows how much it costs to buy one more unit of health.

An evaluation of vaccination to prevent pneumococcal pneumonia and invasive pneumococcal disease in adults illustrates the main features of CEA (Smith et al. 2012). The study compared two vaccines, 13-valent pneumococcal conjugate vaccine (PCV13) and 23-valent pneumococcal polysaccharide vaccine (PPSV23). The two differ in the number of strains of the bacterium they cover. PPSV23 has been recommended for older adults since 1983; PCV13 was approved for use in adults in 2011. Although PPSV23 covers more strains of the pneumococcus, studies indicate that it is only effective against invasive disease, whereas PCV13 is effective against both invasive disease and the more common pneumonia.

Health outcomes were summarized as quality-adjusted life years (QALYs), a measure that adjusts length of life, in years, for good or poor health during those years. QALYs were estimated using a simulation model of the natural history of pneumococcal disease based on experts' estimates of the effectiveness of the two vaccines in adults and disease data from variety of sources, including the National Health Interview Survey and the Active Bacterial Core surveillance of the Centers for Disease Control and Prevention. Estimates took into account differences in risk of pneumococcal disease, response to the vaccine, and side effects of the vaccine.

to informing decisions about resource allocation. Many interventions are complex, involving numerous costs, and adverse as well as beneficial effects on health. Synthesizing the relevant information to arrive at overall estimates of an intervention's effects on health outcomes and costs can contribute to better decision making. In some cases, the decision is straightforward. If, for example, vaccination costs less than treating disease when it occurs, in addition to keeping people healthier, the choice is straightforward. Similarly, if one type of artificial hip is more expensive than another, and does not work as well for patients, the choice is again clear.

Decision making becomes more difficult when the choice is among interventions that produce better health but that also cost more than the alternatives. Decisions become more difficult still when options range across different types of interventions and patient populations, for example, not just vaccination versus no vaccination for one disease, or one type of hip prosthesis versus another, but decisions about the best mix of vaccinations, surgeries, medications, and public health interventions to promote the health of the population. Decision makers also sometimes face choices about whether to free up resources for expensive new technologies by adopting older technologies that cost less, but that are also less effective (Nelson et al. 2009). For example, a hospital unit may switch to an older, less expensive, and possibly less effective antibiotic to save room in the budget for expensive new agents for high-risk cases.

The broader the range of interventions, and the more the interventions differ from one another, the greater the need for ways of evaluating and summarizing information in a manner that facilitates comparisons among them. Health plans considering which services to cover, or advisory groups charged with providing guidance for the care of major health problems, often face such daunting choices.

Cost-effectiveness analysis has evolved to help fill that need. Cost-effectiveness studies can show the trade-offs involved in choosing among interventions. They help

---

Costs included the costs of the vaccine, its administration and side effects, and hospitalization to treat pneumococcal disease. These costs were estimated from published sources and from Healthcare Cost and Utilization Project data. Both costs and health outcomes were discounted at 3% per year to allow comparison of options with different costs and health outcomes over the lifetimes of older adults.

This table presents the estimated increases in costs and health (QALYs), per person, when three of these strategies are compared with no vaccination and with one another in order of increasing effectiveness. The first column compares strategy 1—vaccination with PCV13 following ACIP's age guidelines (high-risk adults at age 50, all adults at 65)—with no vaccination. On average, this option brings 0.00116 of a QALY per person, at a cost of $33 per person, which yields an ICER of $28,448 per QALY ($33/0.00116 QALYs); because the incremental costs and QALYs in the table are rounded, this ICER is slightly different from the published ICER of $28,900 per QALY.

The second column compares strategy 1 with a strategy that vaccinates all adults, not just high-risk adults, with PCV13 at age 50 and again at age 65 (strategy 2). This broader strategy yields still more good health, an increase of 0.00094 QALY per person, at a cost of $43; the cost per QALY is $45,100. The final column adds vaccination with PPSV23 at age 75 to those vaccinated with PCV13 at age 50 and age 65 (strategy 3) and compares that strategy with strategy 2. Although strategy 3 brings a little additional health (0.00002 QALY per person) at a small per-person cost ($8), the cost per QALY is $496,000.

define and illuminate the "opportunity cost" of each choice in terms of health: the health benefits lost when the next-best alternative is not selected. Table 1.2 illustrates the concept of opportunity cost using selected interventions. In addition to cost-effectiveness ratios, the table shows the number of healthy years of life that could be achieved if $1 million had been spent on the intervention in 2012 (column three). The third column thus expresses the results in terms that directly address the goal, improved health, and shows that interventions, and variants of an intervention, vary widely in the amount of health they can "buy" for $1 million.

The concept of opportunity cost in healthcare is based on the idea that if the goal is better health for the population, then it makes sense to choose interventions that bring the most health for the money until the money budgeted for healthcare runs out. The data in Table 1.2 suggest that one would choose smoking cessation programs, then total knee arthroplasty (TKA) for patients at low risk of operative complications, then aspirin to prevent heart disease in low-risk men (aspirin for high-risk men would be chosen immediately since it is cost-saving), and so on. If the PCV13 (Pneumococcal Conjugate Vaccine [13-valent]) vaccine were given to older adults, and no money was left to provide TKAs for low-risk people with advanced arthritis, the opportunity cost of PCV13 would be the additional 66 years of healthy life lost per $1 million spent (i.e., 84 years for low-risk TKA minus 18 for PCV13, third column of Table 1.2).

Table 1.2 is an example of a "league table." It arrays a variety of possible choices and allows the reader, or decision maker, to rank them on the basis of their cost-effectiveness, putting those that produce more health for the money ahead of those that produce less. In reality, decision makers do not have league tables to consult. It would be impossible to create a table that included a comparable CEA for every possible choice in health and medicine. Instead, decision makers who use CEAs can establish threshold cost-effectiveness ratios, which serve the same purpose: every intervention with a cost-effectiveness ratio below the threshold is selected, every intervention with a cost-effectiveness ratio above the threshold is not. In practice, the appropriate threshold is uncertain and never applied mechanically as part of decision making (see Section 1.3.3).

Regardless of the specific medical intervention or technology, CEA can be used as a "virtual laboratory" to compare alternative scenarios for the delivery of interventions (e.g., in different settings or populations), ideally ahead of investment in new approaches (Goddard et al. 2012; IOM [Institute of Medicine] 2012b). An analysis can show how results change as key assumptions or uncertain parameters vary over plausible ranges and help decision makers identify needs for further investment in empirical research (Claxton, Sculpher, and Drummond 2002; Hall et al. 2010; Wong et al. 2012).

1.2 THE ORIGINAL PANEL ON COST-EFFECTIVENESS IN HEALTH AND MEDICINE

1.2.1 The Charge to the Original Panel

The original Panel on Cost-Effectiveness in Health and Medicine was charged with "assessing the [then] current state-of-the science of the field and with providing

Table 1.2 Opportunity costs: Quality-adjusted life years gained for $1 million, selected interventions

	Additional cost per QALY gained (original year $)	Additional cost per QALY gained (2012 $)	QALYs gained per $1 million (2012 $)
Pneumococcal vaccine for older adults (Smith et al. 2012); see also Table 1.1			
PCV13 All at ages 50 and 65 vs high-risk at age 50 and all at age 65	45,100 (2006)	55,657	18
PCV13 for all at ages 50 and 65 + PPSV23 for all at age 75 vs PCV13 for all at ages 50 and 65	496,000 (2006)	612,107	2
Total knee arthroplasty (TKA) vs no TKA for advanced knee osteoarthritis (Losina et al. 2009)			
TKA, low risk of perioperative complications	9,700 (2006)	11,971	84
TKA, medium risk of complications	18,700 (2006)	23,077	43
TKA, high risk of complications	28,100 (2006)	34,678	29
Aspirin to prevent heart disease (Pignone et al. 2006)			
Men age 45, 10-year risk 2.5%	9,800 (2003)	13,686	73
Men age 45, 10-year risk 5.0% or higher	Cost-saving	Cost-saving	Cost-saving
Protease inhibitors (PIs) to treat chronic hepatitis C (Liu et al. 2012)			
Mild liver fibrosis			
Gene-assay-guided PIs plus PEG-INF + Rb vs PEG-INF + Rb	62,900 (2010)	67,192	15
Universal PIs vs gene-assay-guided use	102,600 (2010)	109,600	9
Advanced liver fibrosis			
Gene-assay-guided PIs plus PEG-INF + Rb vs PEG-INF + Rb	32,800 (2010)	35,038	29
Universal PIs vs gene-assay-guided use	51,500 (2010)	55,014	18
Screening once for HIV vs no screening (Paltiel et al. 2006)			
HIV prevalence = 1.0%	30,800 (2004)	41,209	24
HIV prevalence = 0.1%	60,700 (2004)	81,214	12
Diet/exercise to prevent diabetes (Eddy, Schlessinger, and Kahn 2005)			
For adults at high risk of diabetes	143,000 (2000)	227,495	4
For adults with diabetes	35,400 (2000)	56,317	18
Cardiac resynchronization to treat heart failure (Nichol et al. 2004)			
Cardiac resynchronization vs medical therapy	107,800 (2003)	150,543	7
Smoking cessation (Cromwell et al. 1997)			
15 programs weighted by % enrolled	1,915 (1995)	3,603	278

recommendations for conduct of studies in order to improve their quality and encourage their comparability" (Gold et al. 1996, xvii). As J. Michael McGinnis, Assistant Surgeon General (retired), explained in his Foreword to the 1996 book, "The overarching goal for this work has been to move the field forward so that over the next decade, state and federal decision makers will have access to robust information with respect to the true cost per health effect gained for the continuum of health-related interventions—be they preventive, palliative, curative, or rehabilitative" (Gold et al. 1996, vii).

The original Panel's charge directed its members to take a broad view and to consider how CEA could inform decisions across the entire range of health interventions. This charge had important implications for the nature of the recommendations: they needed to be tailored to suit decisions that could involve widely different kinds of people, health conditions, and interventions (Russell et al. 1996). With this broad focus the Panel noted that "comparability is essential if CEA is to help decision makers evaluate trade-offs" (Russell et al. 1996, 1173).

The Panel's recommendations were directed primarily at those who conduct, or who direct the conduct, of CEAs, but the Panel believed that those recommendations would also prove useful to professionals who wish to evaluate CEA critically, including health plans, health insurers, health departments, state and federal policy makers, and medical professional groups.

1.2.2 The Reference Case

To meet its charge the Panel's recommendations defined a "Reference Case" CEA, "a standard set of methods to serve as a point of comparison across studies" (Russell et al. 1996, abstract). The Reference Case was described in the book and three articles, all published in 1996. Russell et al. (1996) summarized its purpose and framework as follows: "To promote comparability of CEAs . . . , the panel proposes that studies include, either as the base case or in addition to it, a reference case. The reference case is defined by a standard set of methods and assumptions. It includes a set of standard results: the reference case results. While an investigator might also present results based on different methods and assumptions to serve the other purposes of the analysis, the reference case serves as a point of comparison across studies. *It should be included whenever the CEA is intended to contribute to decisions about the broad allocation of health care resources*" (Russell et al. 1996, 1173, emphasis added).

In explaining the need for the Reference Case the Panel observed that "a number of problems currently interfere with the broadest use of CEAs in informing larger health care resource allocation decisions. These difficulties are detailed throughout this book, but we note two at the outset because of their overarching importance": (1) the perspective of the analysis and (2) the measure of health outcome (Gold et al. 1996, xix). The Reference Case analysis is conducted from the societal perspective, which "accounts for benefits, harms, and costs to all parties" (Russell et al. 1996, abstract). Health outcomes in the Reference Case are summarized by quality-adjusted life years

(QALYs), a measure that allows improvements in health to be combined with improvements in the length of life.

1.2.3 The Societal Perspective

The original Panel chose the "societal" perspective for the Reference Case because it "represents the public interest rather than that of any group," and the Panel believed that the public interest was the most appropriate perspective for decisions about the broad allocation of health resources (Russell et al. 1996, 1174). The Panel continued: "The societal perspective is also a pragmatic choice, exactly because it does not represent the viewpoint of any particular group. Instead, it provides a benchmark against which to assess results from other perspectives. Only the societal perspective never counts as a gain what is another party's loss. If an employer adopts an intervention that reduces the employer's health insurance costs but increases costs for Medicare, or if a public health intervention improves the health of one group but causes unwanted side effects for another, the societal perspective includes both changes. No perspective has a stronger claim to be the basis for comparability across studies" (Russell et al. 1996, 1174).

The Panel recognized that specific decision makers—an insurer, a health plan, Medicare—may want to use its own perspectives in conducting a CEA. The Panel explicitly noted that "inclusion of a Reference Case in an analysis should not be construed as a requirement for performing a valid CEA" (Gold et al. 1996, xxi). Cost-effectiveness analyses done from these narrower perspectives are not, however, comparable with each other. If an analysis is intended to inform the broader allocation of health resources across diseases and interventions, comparability is "critical for this purpose [and] the analyst will want to include a Reference Case" (Gold et al. 1996, xxi). The use of a well-defined societal perspective can also highlight the inter-sectoral distribution of resources that are important to consider.

1.2.4 Defining Outcomes and Costs for the Societal Perspective

The original Panel made numerous recommendations about how to measure and value health outcomes and costs from the societal perspective (Gold et al. 1996, Appendix A). They viewed the use of QALYs to measure health outcomes as critical to evaluating interventions that targeted the full range of diseases and conditions: "For the reference case, the measure of health effect must be comparable across interventions and conditions and capable of capturing the impact of interventions with different effects. Life years gained, often used in CEAs done from the societal perspective, are an important metric, but give little credit to interventions that primarily improve quality of life (eg, cataract surgery) and fail to account for adverse effects" (Russell et al. 1996, 1174). The Panel proposed that health outcomes should be summarized as QALYs in the Reference Case and recommended properties necessary in a good QALY system (Gold et al. 1996, Appendix A).

1.3 EXPERIENCES WITH CEA

Since the 1990s the number of CEAs published in the peer-reviewed literature has grown rapidly. Figure 1.1 illustrates this for the subset of English-language studies that use cost per QALY as a summary metric, an approach sometimes termed "cost-utility analysis," or CUA.

The number of English-language CUAs published in the MEDLINE-indexed literature, for example, averaged 34 per year from 1990 to 1999 and 504 per year from 2010 to 2014 (Table 1.3) (Neumann et al. 2015). Studies have covered a wide range of interventions, diseases, and contexts (Table 1.3). As noted in Chapter 13, adherence to certain methodological and reporting practices has improved over time, which may reflect several factors, including greater availability of formal education on economic evaluation, stronger methodological requirements for CEAs in some jurisdictions, and perhaps an impact of the original Panel's recommendations (Neumann et al. 2005; Neumann et al. 2015; Phillips and Chen 2002).

Of particular importance for the Second Panel's deliberations, CEA is now used in decision making in some contexts in the United States, and more widely in many countries throughout the world, with still other countries developing plans to begin using it (Box 1.1 provides examples). The concept of a Reference Case has met an important need for using CEA, because comparability is central if decisions about the broad allocation of health resources are to be valid and acceptable to decision makers and the public. Public and private groups around the world have created their own guidelines to promote comparability for their own purposes, each in effect creating its own Reference Case. For example, as noted below, policy makers in the United Kingdom and Canada have published guidelines detailing how CEAs should be carried out if they are to be used to inform public decision making in those countries, and the Bill and Melinda Gates Foundation has developed guidelines for a CEA Reference Case

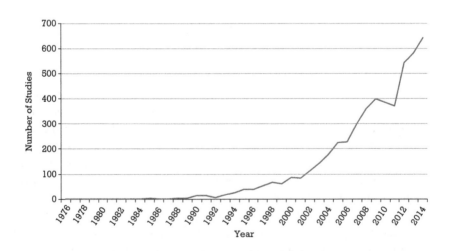

Figure 1.1 Growth in English-language published cost-per-QALY studies by year, 1976–2014.
Source: Tufts Medical Center Cost-Effectiveness Analysis (CEA) Registry (Center for the Evaluation of Value and Risk in Health n.d.).

Table 1.3 Growth and Characteristics of Published Cost-Utility Analyses (CUAs) from 1976 to 2014 (*n* = 5,000)

Characteristic	Number of CUAs	%
Year		
Pre-1990*	19	0.4
1990–1999	339	6.8
2000–2009	2,120	42.4
2010–2014	2,522	50.4
TOTALS	5,000	100.0
Country†		
United States	1,907	38.1
UK	898	18.0
Canada	383	7.7
Netherlands	361	7.2
Sweden	221	4.4
Germany	155	3.1
Other	1,426	28.5
Diseases		
Cardiovascular	870	17.4
Cancer	782	15.6
Infectious diseases	629	12.6
Musculoskeletal/rheumatological	469	9.4
Neuro-psychiatric and neurological conditions	471	9.1
Endocrine	337	6.7
Other	1,442	28.8
TOTALS	5,000	100.0
Intervention†		
Pharmaceutical	2,258	45.2
Surgical	675	13.5
Screening	591	11.8
Medical procedure	559	11.2
Care delivery	550	11.0
Health education/behavior	465	9.3
Medical device	378	7.6
Diagnostic	361	7.2
Immunization	329	6.6
Other	279	5.6

Source: Tufts Medical Center Cost-Effectiveness Analysis (CEA) Registry (Center for the Evaluation of Value and Risk in Health n.d.). Includes original cost-per-QALY estimates from articles published in English and indexed in MEDLINE.

*The first CUA in the Tufts CEA Registry was published in 1976.

†Categories are not mutually exclusive.

Box 1.1 Selected Milestones in Cost-Effective Analysis in Health and Medicine

United States

- 1977: One of the first cost-utility analysis (CUA) studies is published: "Public-health rounds at the Harvard School of Public Health. Allocation of resources to manage hypertension" (Stason and Weinstein 1977).
- 1980: Congress decides to make` the pneumococcal vaccination the first preventive service covered by Medicare based in part on a cost-effectiveness analysis (CEA) conducted by the Congressional Office of Technology Assessment (Act to amend title XVIII of the Social Security Act to provide for Medicare coverage of pneumococcal vaccine and its administration, Pub. Law No. 96-611, 94 Stat. 3566 [1980]).
- 1989: The Health Care Financing Administration (HCFA), later renamed the Centers for Medicare and Medicaid Services (CMS), issues proposed regulation to consider CEA in its coverage decisions (Medicare Program: Criteria and Procedures for Making Medical Services Coverage Decisions that Relate to Healthcare Technology. Federal Register Vol. 54, pp. 4302-4318 [1989]).
- 1990–1994: The Oregon Medicaid program issues ranked lists of the cost-effectiveness of various treatments. After intense public debate, the first list is modified into a second and then a third list that diminished the importance of cost-effectiveness in favor of expert judgment (Neumann 2005).
- 1992–1995: First published uses of the $50,000 per QALY threshold for cost-effectiveness (Grosse 2008).
- 1993–1996: Original Panel on Cost-Effectiveness in Health and Medicine convenes and releases recommendations for a Reference Case in an effort to standardize the comparison of health economic studies (Gold et al. 1996).
- 1996: The Centers for Disease Control (CDC) Community Preventive Services Task Force's "Community Guide" is created, with methods including the systematic review of the health impact and cost-effectiveness of services (Community Preventive Services Task Force 1996).
- 1997: The Balanced Budget Act of 1997 adds Medicare coverage for colorectal cancer screening and gives Medicare officials authority to examine expenditures and outcomes of strategies, a provision interpreted by the agency to allow it to use CEA in this context (Balanced Budget Act of 1997. Pub. Law No. 105-33 11 Stat. 251 [1997]).
- 1999: HCFA withdraws proposed regulation to consider CEA in its coverage decisions due to political opposition and legal challenges (Medicare Program; Procedures for Making National Coverage Decisions, Federal Registry, Vol. 64, No. 80, pp. 22619-22625 [1999]).
- 2000: The Academy of Managed Care Pharmacy (AMCP) publishes guidelines calling for health plans to request that drug companies submit economic evidence as well as clinical evidence for the review of drugs for formulary inclusion (Academy of Managed Care Pharmacy 2000).
- 2001: The US Preventive Services Task Force (USPSTF) considers a role for CEA in its recommendations (Saha et al. 2001), although ultimately CEA is rarely, if ever, used.

- 2003: The US Office of Management and Budget (OMB) establishes a requirement calling for formal cost–benefit analysis for new health or safety regulations with costs or benefits over $100 million (Office of Management and Budget 2003).
- 2004: Premera Blue Cross implements a policy under which cost-effectiveness is one of several criteria formally considered for pharmaceuticals undergoing review for formulary listing (Watkins, Minshall, and Sullivan 2006).
- 2006: The Institute of Medicine (IOM) report, *Valuing Health for Regulatory Cost-Effective Analysis,* is published, calling for a role for CEA, including cost per QALY, for analyses of regulations (Miller, Robinson, and Lawrence 2006).
- 2008: The Advisory Committee on Immunization Practices (ACIP) establishes guidelines for health economic evaluations for the CDC (Advisory Committee on Immunization Practices [ACIP] 2008).
- 2009: "Toward a Consensus on the QALY" is published (Drummond et al. 2009).
- 2010: The Patient Protection and Affordable Care Act (ACA) prohibits the newly created Patient-Centered Outcomes Research Institute (PCORI) from developing or using a cost-per-QALY threshold (Patient Protection and Affordable Care Act, 42 U.S.C. § 18001 et seq. [2010]).
- 2013–2016: Second Panel on Cost-Effectiveness Analysis in Health and Medicine is established and issues its report.

International Experiences

- 1987—Australia—An amendment to existing Australian law requires that cost and effectiveness must be accounted for in pharmaceutical reimbursement considerations (Australian Institute of Health and Welfare Act of 1987. Canberra, Australia).
- 1987—Sweden—Sweden creates the Council for Technology Assessment in Health Care (SBU; http://www.sbu.se/en/about-sbu) to critically review the scientific basis of methods used in healthcare and to evaluate their benefits, risks, and costs (Swedish Agency for Health Technology Assessment and Assessment of Social Services).
- 1992—Canada—Influential article proposes that Canada use a rough $20,000 to $100,000 ($Can) per QALY cost-effectiveness threshold (Grosse 2008; Laupacis et al. 1992).
- 1993—Australia—Australia becomes the first country to implement pharmacoeconomic guidelines to inform the newly created Pharmaceutical Benefits Advisory Committee (PBAC), which recommends pharmaceuticals to be placed on the publicly funded Pharmaceutical Benefits Scheme (PBS) (Edmonds et al. 1993).
- 1994—Canada—Canada's first set of national pharmaceutical guidelines is published (Canadian Coordinating Office for Health Technology Assessment [CCOHTA] 1994).
- 1998—Global—WHO establishes the WHO CHOICE project in order to provide information and strategic assistance for health decisions and resource allocation in 14 world regions (World Health Organization 2016).

- 1999—United Kingdom—UK establishes the National Institute for Clinical Excellence (NICE), now the National Institute for Health and Care Excellence, to create evidence-based guidelines for cost-effective medical care.
- 2001—Australia—Australia's PBAC rejects listing of Herceptin® (trastuzumab) for breast cancer after a CEA. In response, the government creates a "Herceptin Program" that would allow access to the drug (Birkett, Mitchell, and McManus 2001).
- 2002—Sweden—Swedish Parliament establishes the Dental and Pharmaceutical Benefits Board (TLV), which uses CEA to inform reimbursement decisions The New Pharmaceutical Benefits Reform, bill 2001/02:63, Swedish Parliament (2002).
- 2003—United Kingdom—NICE recommendations regarding health technology become mandatory (National Institute of Health and Clinical Excellence [NICE] 2003).
- 2004—United Kingdom—NICE adopts a Reference Case for health technology assessments (National Institute for Health and Care Excellence [NICE] 2004).
- 2004—Germany—Germany's Institute for Quality and Efficiency in Healthcare (IQWiG) is founded.
- 2005—Germany—A German court rules that the government must reimburse the treatment of a life-threatening disease when there is no alternative (Caro et al. 2010).
- 2005—France—The French National Authority for Health (Haute Autorité de Santé, HAS) is created to conduct health technology assessments (de Pouvourville 2013).
- 2005—Netherlands—The Netherlands incorporates mandatory cost-effectiveness data in national health decision making (Garattini, Cornago, and De Compadri 2007).
- 2006—South Korea—South Korea becomes the first country in Asia to include cost-effectiveness considerations formally in its reimbursement decisions by announcing reform legislation called the Positive List System (PLS) (Bae et al. 2013; Yang 2009).
- 2007—Germany—Germany implements healthcare reform that includes cost-effectiveness evaluation and a pharmaceutical ceiling price (Caro et al. 2010).
- 2007—Germany—IQWiG adopts an "efficiency frontier" approach (Klingler et al. 2013).
- 2008—France—France begins conducting economic assessments of care in addition to health technology assessments (de Pouvourville 2013).
- 2009—United Kingdom—NICE creates End-of-Life Guidelines that provide an exception for the NICE cost-per-QALY regulation in specific cases of end-of-life care when the treatment can extend life by at least 3 months (Rawlins, Barnett, and Stevens 2010).
- 2011–2012—France—The French HAS publishes a CEA guideline, and a subsequent law is enacted making CEA mandatory for determining pricing and reimbursement for new drugs and medical therapies (Haute Autorité de Santé 2012).
- 2012–2014—United Kingdom—UK debates the role of value-based pricing to supplement cost-effectiveness considerations and replaces the country's Pharmaceutical Price Regulation Scheme (Claxton, Sculpher, and Carroll 2011; Towse 2007).
- 2014—The Bill and Melinda Gates Foundation launches the Gates Reference Case, setting guidelines for reporting standards for international economic evaluations and priority setting in health and medicine (Bill and Melinda Gates Foundation Methods for Economic Evaluation Project [MEEP] 2014).

focusing on low and middle income countries (Bill and Melinda Gates Foundation Methods for Economic Evaluation Project [MEEP] 2014).

1.3.1 CEA in the United States

Cost-effectiveness analysis has received a mixed welcome in US healthcare settings over the years. On the one hand, CEAs have been published widely in the American medical literature, covering a diverse set of drugs, devices, and medical procedures (Neumann et al. 2015). Such analyses have shed light on the value of certain public health interventions, for example, strategies to address tobacco control, poor nutrition, obesity, and physical inactivity (Neumann et al. 2005). The results from these analyses have shown that certain environmental and policy-based strategies for curtailing smoking have been highly cost-effective (Levy et al. 2013; Levy et al. 2005; Ross et al. 2006); that seat belts and airbags have favorable cost-effectiveness ratios (Graham et al. 1997); and that state-funded nutritional education programs can save money (Dollahite, Kenkel, and Thompson 2008). Chokshi and Farley (2012) reviewed the cost-effectiveness of different approaches to disease prevention and found that nonclinical interventions focusing on environmental change, where behavior is influenced by social or physical environment, were most likely to be of good value or cost-saving compared with clinical, person-directed interventions (Chokshi and Farley 2012). Analyses have illustrated the cost-effectiveness of thousands of other interventions, including, more recently, genomic diagnostic tests and targeted therapies (Garrison et al. 2007; Hall et al. 2012; Kurian et al. 2007; Lyman et al. 2007; Vanderlaan et al. 2011).

Federal government agencies in the United States, such as the Agency for Healthcare Research and Quality, the Centers for Disease Control and Prevention (CDC), and the National Institutes of Health (NIH), have funded or conducted CEAs in selected areas (Neumann and Weinstein 2010; Siegel, Byron, and Lawrence 2005). Notable applications pertain to vaccination (Smith et al. 2010), newborn screening (Perrin et al. 2010), and cancer screening (Diaz et al. 2010).

The Advisory Committee for Immunization Practices (ACIP), which establishes national immunization policy recommendations on behalf of the CDC, has used CEA as part of its deliberations, though rarely, if ever, as the primary criterion in setting vaccine policy (Centers for Disease Control and Prevention [CDC] and Advisory Committee on Immunization Practices [ACIP] 2008; Smith 2010). Instead, ACIP considers CEA alongside other information, including reviews of epidemiology; vaccine efficacy, effectiveness, and safety; feasibility of program implementation; ethical, political, logistical, and budgetary concerns; and public comments (Smith and Metzger 2011; Stephens, Ahmed, and Orenstein 2014). For example, the influenza vaccination policy recommendation hinged on expectations that universal vaccination could potentially improve coverage rates in higher-risk subgroups, despite uncertainty about the cost-effectiveness (Fiore et al. 2008).

The Office of Technology Assessment (created and abolished by the US Congress in 1972 and 1995, respectively) conducted congressionally requested CEAs in the 1980s and early 1990s that were used to inform expansion of Medicare benefits to include screening for breast cancer (US Congress Office of Technology Assessment 1987), cervical cancer (US Congress Office of Technology Assessment 1990a), and colorectal cancer (US Congress Office of Technology Assessment 1990b). Pneumococcal vaccination was added to the Medicare benefit in 1981, for example, following a congressionally requested CEA that found vaccination to be cost-effective, including for individuals age 65 years and older (US Congress Office of Technology Assessment 1979). Cost-effectiveness analysis has been used on occasion to inform whether and how to add other preventive services (though not therapeutic or diagnostic services—see below) (Chambers, Cangelosi, and Neumann 2015). The Centers for Medicare and Medicaid Services (CMS) has reviewed cost-effectiveness evidence when covering certain preventive services, such as human immunodeficiency virus (HIV) screening (2010), screening and behavioral counseling for alcohol misuse (2011) (Chambers, Cangelosi, and Neumann 2015), as well as for lung cancer screening (2015) (Centers for Medicare & Medicaid Services 2015).

In addition, the Premera Blue Cross plan in the state of Washington has used cost-per-QALY estimates to inform its benefit design options, providing enrollees lower co-payments on drugs with favorable cost-effectiveness estimates and higher co-payment on those with less favorable estimates of value (Watkins, Minshall, and Sullivan 2006). The Academy of Managed Care Pharmacy has actively promoted its guidelines, which encourage health plans to request information on value and cost-effectiveness from pharmaceutical companies bringing new drugs to formulary committees for drug coverage (The AMCP Format Exeutive Committee 2016). The Department of Veterans Affairs and the Department of Defense have research groups that, among other things, perform CEAs of healthcare interventions. The Advisory Committee for Heritable Disorders in Newborns and Children considers economic evaluations in its evidence review process (Prosser et al. 2012). The CDC's Community Preventive Services Task Force conducts systematic reviews of CEAs and cost–benefit analyses for all recommended services (Community Preventive Services Task Force 2016). The Institute of Medicine (IOM) has recommended the use of cost- and comparative-effectiveness analysis to determine the net public health impact of new personalized approaches to care (IOM [Institute of Medicine] 2012b) as well as to establish the health and economic outcomes derived from investments in public health and prevention strategies (IOM [Institute of Medicine] 2012a). The American College of Physicians has endorsed the need for all healthcare payers, including Medicare, other government programs, private sector entities, and the individual healthcare consumer to consider comparative clinical effectiveness and cost-effectiveness information explicitly in their evaluation of clinical interventions (American College of Physicians 2008). The American College of Cardiology/American Heart Association (ACC/AHA) is integrating value considerations, including cost-per-QALY estimates, into its clinical guidelines (Anderson et al. 2014). The American Society of Clinical Oncology (ASCO) is considering how to incorporate formal considerations of value, based on considerations of clinical benefit, toxicity, and cost, into cancer treatment decisions (American Society of Clinical Oncology 2014). A nonprofit group, the Institute for Clinical and

Economic Research, has begun issuing widely discussed reports on the value of new drugs and other interventions, relying in part on cost-per-QALY analyses. A 2013 study reported that slightly more than half of the largest US physician societies consider costs in developing their clinical guidance documents, although many are vague about how they do this and whether and how they rely on formal CEAs (Schwartz and Pearson 2013).

State and federal policy makers have also selectively used cost–benefit analysis, which estimates an intervention's costs and effects, as does CEA, but summarizes both health and non-health benefits in monetary terms (see Chapter 2). For example, the US Environmental Protection Agency (EPA), like other US federal agencies, is required to conduct cost–benefit analyses of its "economically significant" regulations (Office of Management and Budget 2016). An EPA evaluation of the Clean Air Act, for example, valued reductions in mortality and illness as well as improvements in visibility at recreational sites and in residential areas, benefits to commercial timber, agricultural crops, and recreational fishing, and reduced materials damage (US Environmental Protection Agency Office of Air and Radiation 2011). For the year 2020, benefits are projected at almost $2 trillion, compared with costs of $65 billion (US Environmental Protection Agency Office of Air and Radiation 2011). In that calculation, mortality benefits make up 90% of the monetized benefits.

On the other hand, despite these and other developments, the application of CEA in the United States has also encountered resistance. The state of Oregon, for example, created a prioritized list of health interventions based on cost-effectiveness for its Medicaid program in the early 1990s in order to improve population health by better targeting resources. The program was criticized in many quarters, however, for explicitly rationing services for low-income individuals, and because the cost-effectiveness methodology prioritized some inexpensive treatments that produced small benefits for many people over life-saving but expensive treatments that produced critical benefits for few people (e.g., capping a tooth for exposed pulp was ranked above appendectomy for acute appendicitis) (see Chapter 12). Eventually, a revision of the list was published and used, but without information on cost-effectiveness, instead relying on clinical judgment (Hadorn 1991; Neumann 2005). No other state Medicaid program has proposed similar reforms based on the formal application of CEA.

The Medicare program has attempted to incorporate CEA into its decision-making processes for new technologies, but, except for certain preventive services, this use of CEA has been thwarted by legal and political obstacles (Neumann and Chambers 2012). The US Preventive Services Task Force (USPSTF) reviewed standards for CEA in the early 2000s (Pignone et al. 2002; Saha et al. 2001) but decided not to use these analyses in its recommendations, though the authorizing legislation for the task force does not prohibit it. Some US technology assessment efforts, such as those conducted by the Drug Effectiveness Review Project, have considered the strength of clinical evidence, but shied away from formal use of cost-effectiveness analysis (Neumann 2005). US health plans have adopted value-based insurance designs, tiered networks, and many other management tools aimed at constraining cost growth, but most have avoided explicit consideration of cost-effectiveness in coverage decisions about specific technologies (Neumann 2005).

Even where movements to advance CEA have emerged, they have sometimes been stymied or applied unevenly. In 2006, for example, the IOM published *Valuing Health for Regulatory Cost-Effectiveness Analysis* (Miller, Robinson, and Lawrence 2006), addressing the Office of Management and Budget's (OMB's) initiative for federal agencies to use CEA in addition to cost–benefit analysis (see Chapter 2 for a discussion of cost–benefit analysis) to measure the impact of major regulations (Miller, Robinson, and Lawrence 2006; Office of Management and Budget 2003). The report recommended using QALYs and other integrated measures of morbidity and mortality, and reporting cost-effectiveness ratios. However, the report's recommendations for CEA were never adopted or enforced by OMB. As a result, agencies vary greatly in the extent to which they report cost-effectiveness ratios for their regulations, as well as in the extent to which they follow the IOM recommendations (Lisa Robinson, personal communication).

Notably, the Patient Protection and Affordable Care Act (ACA) of 2010 (42 U.S.C. § 18001 et seq.) contained a provision stating that the newly created Patient-Centered Outcomes Research Institute (PCORI) "shall not develop or employ a dollars-per-quality adjusted life year (or similar measure that discounts the value of a life because of an individual's disability) as a threshold to establish what type of health care is cost effective or recommended," and that the "Secretary shall not utilize such an adjusted life year (or such a similar measure) as a threshold to determine coverage, reimbursement, or incentive programs under title XVIII." The language of the ACA suggests that use of QALYs in CEAs discriminates against people with disabilities—see Chapter 12 for a detailed discussion of the matter.

The ACA forbids the use of cost-per-QALY ratios "as a threshold." In a sense, this step does not reflect a departure from existing practices. The original Panel never recommended use of a threshold, and with some exceptions, such as the National Institute for Health and Care Excellence (NICE) (see below), organizations have generally not adopted explicit thresholds. However, the language of the ACA—and the mandate of the PCORI to focus on *clinical* comparative effectiveness research—suggests a de facto ban on the use of CEA—and PCORI has made it clear it does not review or fund CEAs (Neumann and Weinstein 2010).

The broader movement toward clinical comparative effectiveness analysis and "patient-centered" care also suggests an orientation away from explicit cost-effectiveness considerations. Researchers and funding agencies are emphasizing the importance of examining the clinical effectiveness of interventions, and how results vary across subgroups and different care strategies without explicit regard to the relative costs.

Reasons for the resistance to CEA are likely multifaceted and complex. Part of the explanation may be mistrust of the methods of CEA. Numerous studies have documented that methods can vary considerably and that evaluations of the same intervention can sometimes result in different conclusions (Neumann 2005). The reasons may also have to do with mistrust of the motives of those conducting CEAs. Studies have documented, for example, that CEAs funded by the pharmaceutical industry tend to report more favorable results (Bell et al. 2006; Friedberg et al. 1999). In contrast, authorities in other countries have developed processes to use CEAs, indicating that ways around these challenges can be found.

Some observers point to a desire on the part of many Americans to deny the underlying problem of resource scarcity and the need to explicitly ration care. The sentiment may be particularly acute in the United States, given the country's cultural and political traditions that emphasize personal and economic freedoms, as well as the practice of "defensive medicine," and providers' fears about lawsuits if they withhold effective, though costly, care (Neumann 2005). Others have countered that when members of the lay public are presented with cost-effectiveness information in a systematic way, they may be willing to use CEA to inform priorities for healthcare coverage (Gold et al. 2007). Still, substantial concern around the topic has been manifested by diverse stakeholders from product manufacturers and physician groups to patient advocates. Recent efforts to inform USPSTF decisions about breast (Mandelblatt et al. 2009; Mandelblatt et al. 2016) and colorectal cancer screening (Zauber et al. 2008), for example, used evidence from population-based models, but did not consider costs. Even so, a considerable backlash against these guidelines ensued, based in part on misconceptions that costs were being used to deny needed services (Partridge and Winer 2009).

The resistance to CEA might also reflect important and unresolved ethical questions, such as whether using CEA to set healthcare priorities unjustly discriminates against disabled persons, whether small benefits to a large number of persons receive priority over large benefits to a small number of persons, and whether priority should be provided to the sickest and worst off. These and other questions are explored in detail in Chapter 12.

Despite all of this, the growing number of CEAs published in American medical journals suggests that the technique may have an indirect influence on decisions even among organizations that claim they do not use it. For example, some research suggests that cost-effectiveness may play some role in Medicare decisions on coverage of new treatments and diagnostics, despite the agency's official stance that it does not consider such factors (Chambers, Neumann, and Buxton 2010). Furthermore, while many health plans use decision-making frameworks based on notions of "medical necessity," "standards of evidence," or whether an intervention is "experimental"—criteria commonly perceived to be free of value judgments and to exclude consideration of cost—in practice these criteria involve important value judgments, and costs often play a part without explicit acknowledgment.

1.3.2 CEA Outside the United States

Cost-effectiveness considerations have informed coverage and reimbursement processes in numerous other countries, and in some places they have found a more welcome reception than in the United States. By 2003, an article on the topic listed 21 different international guidelines for conducting CEA developed by government panels and specialty organizations, among others (Adam, Koopmanschap, and Evans 2003). The most frequent application is the requirement that pharmaceutical companies submit economic evaluations as a condition for achieving market access (Clement et al. 2009; Drummond 2013; Taylor et al. 2004). In this section we highlight selected examples of the use of CEA around the world.

1.3.2.1 *CEA in Canada*

Canadians have recognized the principle of "resource stewardship" as a key value of Canada's healthcare system, and they have enshrined it in health legislation (Excellent Care for All Act (2010) Ontario Pub. Law No. 46) and various health reform initiatives (Giacomini et al. 2012a; Giacomini et al. 2012b; Romanow 2002; Wagner et al. 2012). Cost-effectiveness analysis has played a role in health technology assessments and in decisions about drugs and non-drug interventions.

The link between CEA and policy has been most explicit for drug formulary decisions. In 1994, Ontario established cost-effectiveness guidelines for pharmaceuticals (Canadian Coordinating Office for Health Technology Assessment [CCOHTA] 1994). Subsequently, CEA assumed a larger role in formulary decisions across Canada, culminating in the establishment in 2002 of the national Common Drug Review (CDR), conducted by the Canadian Agency for Drugs and Technology in Health (CADTH) (McMahon, Morgan, and Mitton 2006). After receiving regulatory approval from Health Canada, drug manufacturers seeking market access usually submit a clinical and economic dossier to the CDR, which then evaluates the product based on submitted evidence. Provincial governments issue listing recommendations based on CDR guidance (Laupacis 2006; PausJenssen, Singer, and Detsky 2003).

The role of cost-effectiveness in decisions around non-drug technologies is often less clear, given the wide array of purchasers, including hospitals, long-term care facilities, clinics, individual clinicians, and others (Husereau et al. 2015). In 2011, CADTH launched the Health Technology Expert Review Panel to evaluate non-drug technologies (Canadian Agency for Drugs and Technologies in Health [CADTH] 2016). In Canada, as in most jurisdictions that use CEA, policy makers incorporate multiple factors into decisions. Canadian organizations give the greatest weight and deepest consideration to clinical evidence (PausJenssen, Singer, and Detsky 2003). Cost-effectiveness plays an important but supportive role, and typically it does not provide the central framework for decision makers. Rather, cost-effectiveness is one of several discrete factors considered alongside clinical and other evidence. There is no official cost-effectiveness threshold. Health technology assessments in Canada may also conclude that the evidence base is insufficient for decision making. In some jurisdictions there is a mechanism to commission primary research to address uncertainties—evaluations that are called variously "coverage with evidence development," "only-in-research," or "field evaluations" (Levin et al. 2011).

For example, the Pan-Canadian Oncology Drug Review considers drug effectiveness and safety, as well as patients' experiences and perspectives, in addition to cost-effectiveness (Walkinshaw 2011). Health Quality Ontario, which has the most developed model in Canada for evaluating non-drug technologies, considers cost-effectiveness alongside clinical evidence, social and ethical values, system feasibility (disruptiveness), and economic feasibility (affordability) (Johnson et al. 2009). This kind of multicriteria decision making is distinguished from multicriteria decision *analysis* (MCDA), in which weights are assigned explicitly to each criterion (Baltussen and Niessen 2006; Thokala and Duenas 2012), and the weighted attributes are integrated to calculate an overall score (Goetghebeur et al. 2010). Selected Canadian organizations have explored the use of MCDA (Tony et al. 2011).

Canadian organizations are also using CEA to evaluate technologies early in the development process, prior to regulatory approval. The MaRS-Excellence in Clinical Innovation Technology Evaluation (EXCITE) initiative (http://excite.marsdd.com/), for example, represents a joint government–industry exercise to gather clinical and economic evidence for regulatory and reimbursement approval simultaneously, in order to compress the time required for full evaluation. Review of economic evaluations and de novo CEAs are central activities of early health technology assessment. Economic modeling may inform clinical study design for new evaluations (Ijzerman and Steuten 2011).

1.3.2.2 *CEA in the United Kingdom*

The National Institute for Health and Care Excellence (NICE), formerly the National Institute for Clinical Excellence, has emerged as perhaps the most widely known health agency to use CEA. Established in 1999, in part to reduce regional variation in access to health services, NICE is a non-departmental public body serving England and Wales. It maintains a series of programs that cover guidance in areas including technology appraisal (pharmaceuticals, medical devices, and diagnostics), clinical guidelines, public health, social care, and staffing safety. The NICE advisory committees in all these areas are required to consider both effectiveness and cost-effectiveness information in developing their recommendations (Buxton 2006; Rawlins, Barnett, and Stevens 2010). In the context of technology appraisal, CEAs can also influence research undertaken in order to learn more about new technologies. "Only in Research" recommendations from NICE, which recommend coverage within the context of ongoing clinical research, are evolving to consider value-of-information (VOI) estimates derived directly from cost-effectiveness modeling (Claxton et al. 2012).

To improve the consistency and comparability of CEAs undertaken to inform its work, NICE adopted its own Reference Case, specifying a health decision maker's perspective (i.e., the goal is to maximize health gains within a limited budget), rather than the broader societal perspective recommended by the original US Panel (Langley 2004; National Institute for Health and Care Excellence [NICE] 2013). Its requirements include (1) the use of QALYs to measure health effects; (2) standardized descriptions of health states; (3) choice-based preference elicitation; and (4) the use of community preferences as weights for health states (see Chapter 7 for more details on these methods).

Although the use of cost-effectiveness information by NICE is now well-established, debates have continued about the appropriate ICER threshold to use to determine whether an intervention is cost-effective (see Section 1.3.3). On the one hand, NICE has asserted that its Appraisal Committee does not use a single fixed threshold and that use of such a threshold is inappropriate (Rawlins, Barnett, and Stevens 2010). However, NICE has also acknowledged the relevance of comparisons among treatments, consideration of opportunity costs in making recommendations, and use of a cost-effectiveness threshold within the range of £20,000 to £30,000 per QALY rather than a single threshold (Rawlins, Barnett, and Stevens 2010). Researchers have found the NICE recommendations to be correlated with cost-effectiveness results around this range (Buxton 2006; Dakin et al. 2015; Devlin and Parkin 2004; McCabe, Claxton, and Culyer 2008; National Institute for Health and Care Excellence [NICE] 2013; Rawlins, Barnett, and Stevens 2010). NICE has also explicitly noted categories of additional aspects of benefit (e.g., whether the technology meets "end-of-life" criteria, the innovative nature of the technology, and whether the assessment of change in health-related quality of life has been captured appropriately) that need to be shown in order to progress through the threshold range toward the upper bound (National Institute for Health and Care Excellence [NICE] 2013).

Under patient access schemes, there is scope for pharmaceutical manufacturers to negotiate (with the Department of Health rather than NICE) a lower price (that is not made public) for the National Health Service (NHS) rather than the list price, and for this price to be part of the CEA presented to NICE.

NICE has endeavored to incorporate the values of patients and the public in its decision-making processes. From the beginning, NICE convened a citizens' council comprised of 30 members representing a cross-section of the population of England and Wales to provide input on social values. Members participate for three years, and council deliberations occur over multiday sessions. The body has addressed questions such as the relevance of age in NICE treatment recommendations, reimbursement of orphan drugs to treat rare medical conditions, and the allocation of resources with the goal of narrowing inequalities (Littlejohns and Rawlins 2009; Rawlins 2005). Some exceptions to the cost-effectiveness threshold have come from citizen council recommendations, although NICE has not accepted all of the council's advice.

Policy discussions have also addressed the role of CEA in defining a "valued-based price" for individual pharmaceutical products. Following a report from the UK's Office of Fair Trading suggesting that drug prices often did not reflect their value, the government suggested value-based pricing (VBP) as a means of ensuring that the prices of individual products reflected their cost-effectiveness (Office of Fair Trading 2007). The government's vision, however, included a widening of the concept of cost-effectiveness to include factors not formally reflected in NICE methods or processes, including burden of disease and wider social effects (e.g., productivity and caregiver costs). A range of ideas was published for how VBP might be implemented, and NICE proposed a framework (Claxton 2007; Claxton, Sculpher, and Carroll 2011; Towse 2007); but in 2015 NICE officially abandoned its proposal following public consultation and instruction from the Department of Health (National Institute for Health and Care Excellence [NICE] 2014).

NICE continues to employ CEA, although debate continues. A new debate has been stirred by a study that measured the opportunity cost of adopting new technologies and concluded that a cost-effectiveness threshold of £13,000 per QALY is a more appropriate figure for the NHS (see Section 1.3.3) (Claxton et al. 2015). Moreover, while NICE has emerged as the model for how a national health system can use CEA, observers point out that NICE is not responsible for the vast majority of healthcare decisions in the UK, most of which are made by local commissioners, primary care organizations, and hospitals whose judgments about priorities are unclear and whose use of CEA is limited.

1.3.2.3 *CEA in Other Countries*

Policy makers have used CEA in varying degrees in other countries. Australia, for example, pioneered the use of cost-effectiveness requirements for pharmaceuticals in the early 1990s and has been an active producer and consumer of analyses over the years (Birkett, Mitchell, and McManus 2001). In Europe, government agencies in countries including Belgium, Finland, Hungary, the Netherlands, Norway, Poland, Portugal, and Sweden have established guidelines or requirements for CEA to accompany assessments of prescription drugs for reimbursement purposes (Carlsson 2004; Drummond 2013; Garattini, Cornago, and De Compadri 2007; Iglesias et al. 2005; Kaló et al. 2013). These countries vary in the prescriptiveness of their guidelines in terms of the perspective and in the extent to which they recommend or require QALYs. For example, health authorities in Sweden, an early leader in health technology assessment and economic evaluation, have used cost-utility analyses and, unlike some other jurisdictions, have emphasized a broad societal perspective (Drummond 2014). Thus, in analyses to inform drug reimbursement decisions, the Swedish Dental and Pharmaceutical Benefits Board (TLV) accounts for additional costs and burden of disease outside of medical expenditures. In some countries—for example, Italy and Spain—CEAs have not been mandatory, though they can be included voluntarily in submissions by pharmaceutical companies to health authorities (Drummond 2013; Garattini, Cornago, and De Compadri 2007).

Germany's system has focused on estimating benefits and costs of interventions compared to clinical alternatives within a disease category, rather than across diseases (Caro et al. 2010; Klingler et al. 2013). Within Germany, the use of cost-per-QALY ratios has been considered discriminatory on ethical grounds (see Chapter 12 for a discussion of the topic) (Caro et al. 2010). In 2007, the German Institute for Quality and Efficiency in Health Care (IQWiG) adopted an "efficiency frontier" approach, which identifies the most efficient interventions for a given medical condition by plotting available interventions for the condition on a "benefit versus cost" plane, and selecting those that offer the highest benefit-per-cost, where benefits are typically measured in disease-specific terms (Klingler et al. 2013). If the efficiency of the new intervention is equal to or better than alternatives, it is deemed efficient and the requested price is accepted as reimbursable (Klingler et al. 2013).

The process changed in 2010 when policy reforms modified the price-setting process of new drugs to address effectiveness before considerations of efficiency (Klingler et al. 2013). The reimbursable price is based on the degree to which the new intervention's effectiveness exceeds that of existing treatments. An efficiency assessment became a rare tool employed in cases where neither the initial proposed price nor the price emerging from arbitration was acceptable to the reimbursement authorities and drug companies (Klingler et al. 2013). In those cases, either side may request an efficiency frontier assessment and must accept the price threshold that emerges. Proponents of the approach have argued that it provides a minimum reimbursement level and leaves overall prioritization decisions to policy makers, allowing them to incorporate elements (e.g., sensitivity toward expensive treatments for rare diseases) other than cost-effectiveness into their decisions (Caro et al. 2010; Dintsios and Gerber 2010). The drawback is that unlike the cost-per-QALY approach, the narrowly defined efficiency frontier may result in inefficient resource allocation across diseases or therapeutic areas, because it does not allow for comparisons across them (Caro et al. 2010; Drummond and Rutten n.d.; Gandjour, Gafni, and Schlander 2014; Klingler et al. 2013; Sculpher and Claxton 2010).

French health authorities, with input from their scientific advisory board, the Haute Autorité de Santé (HAS), have also shied away from CEA over the years, emphasizing instead rankings of drugs based on comparative clinical value (as well as factors such as the severity of the disease and size of the target population) to inform coverage and reimbursement (de Pouvourville 2013; Drummond et al. 2014). The evaluation involves ranking new drugs relative to existing therapies on a five-point scale from (1) major therapeutic advance to (5) no therapeutic progress. The findings are then used in price negotiations between manufacturers and the government pricing agency (Drummond et al. 2014). However, in 2012, HAS published a CEA guideline, after which a law was enacted requiring CEA for determining the pricing for new drugs and medical therapies (Haute Autorité de Santé 2012). These guidelines highlight cost-utility analysis—as well as other considerations, such as public health benefits and ethical issues—and thus suggest a desire for a more objective measure of efficiency to inform the process (de Pouvourville 2013). Still, the precise role of CEA and key questions such as how the information will relate to the evaluation of clinical value and what threshold to use in France are, as of 2014, unanswered (de Pouvourville 2013).

In Asia, CEA is gradually making its way into the healthcare systems of several countries, including South Korea, Thailand, and Taiwan. In 2006, South Korea was the first country in the region to incorporate formally the use of economic evidence in drug reimbursement decisions (Bae et al. 2013; Yang 2009). Thailand and Taiwan are developing policies to use economic evidence in health technology assessment. The government of Japan has announced a plan to make evidence of cost-effectiveness a requirement for determining prices for drugs and medical devices, and it is expecting to introduce a pilot system in 2016 (Kamae 2014). Other countries around the world, such as Argentina, Brazil, China, Indonesia, Malaysia, Mexico, the Philippines, and Singapore have shown varying degrees of interest (Drummond 2013; Elsisi et al. 2013; Iglesias et al. 2005; Kamae 2010; Yang 2009). In many low and middle income countries interest is high, but the number and quality of studies remains low and is hampered by lack of expertise (Odame 2013). Although still small compared with CUAs in high income countries, the number of CUAs focused on low and middle income countries has risen steadily from 26 during 2000–2006 to 135 from 2007–2012 (Neumann et al. 2015).

The World Health Organization (WHO) has promoted the use of CEA in healthcare through its CHOICE (*CHO*osing *I*nterventions that are *C*ost-*E*ffective) project, initiated in 1998 to encourage the use of economic evaluation for health decisions in 14 regions around the world (World Health Organization 2013). The program provides analytic tools to help policy makers prioritize health interventions for leading causes of disease (Ha and Chisholm 2011; Hutubessy, Chisholm, and Edejer 2003; Patel et al. 2011; Salomon et al. 2012). The World Health Organization has suggested that an appropriate cost-effectiveness threshold in terms of resources per disability-adjusted life years (DALYs) is roughly one to three times a country's gross domestic product (GDP) per capita, although, like other commonly used thresholds, its rationale has been questioned (Neumann, Cohen, and Weinstein 2014; WHO Commission on Macroeconomics and Health 2001), and WHO has been reviewing alternative threshold estimation methods (Centre for Health Economics 2015). As noted elsewhere in this volume (Chapter 7), QALYs and DALYs are metrics used to measure population health, and both integrate morbidity and mortality, though there are some differences in how they are constructed, and DALYs have been used more extensively in global health analyses. In 2014, the Bill and Melinda Gates Foundation, a major funder of health initiatives in low and middle income countries, published the "Gates Reference Case," a set of economic principles, methodological specifications, and reporting standards using cost per DALY estimates (Bill and Melinda Gates Foundation Methods for Economic Evaluation Project [MEEP] 2014). By creating international guidelines for CEAs, the Gates Reference Case is designed to help decision makers in low and middle income countries when conducting economic comparisons of health interventions.

1.3.3 Use of Cost-Effectiveness Thresholds

To support decision making, CEA requires some idea of the maximum ICER that is consistent with an intervention's being cost-effective—the "cost-effectiveness threshold." However, use of such thresholds for decision-making purposes has varied across time and context and has been the subject of considerable debate. Over the years, researchers in the United States have most often cited $50,000 per QALY as a "reasonable" benchmark, though more recently $100,000 per QALY has also been cited (Neumann, Cohen, and Weinstein 2014). The $50,000-per-QALY standard is sometimes attributed to the US government decision to mandate Medicare coverage for patients with end-stage renal disease in the 1970s. Because the cost-effectiveness of dialysis at the time was roughly $50,000 per QALY, it is said that the government's decision implicitly endorsed that threshold (Grosse 2008; Neumann, Cohen, and Weinstein 2014). However, the link to the dialysis decision is tenuous, and the $50,000-per-QALY standard did not gain widespread use until the mid-1990s, when a series of articles began referencing it as a benchmark even though there seemed little theoretical or empirical basis for the claim.

During the past 20 years, researchers in the United States and elsewhere have attempted to deduce what constitutes a reasonable threshold (Culyer et al. 2007; Grosse 2008; Neumann, Cohen, and Weinstein 2014). On the basis of assumptions about people's willingness to pay for health gains and attitudes toward risk, some investigators have supported a threshold of roughly double per capita annual income (Garber and Phelps 1997; WHO Commission on Macroeconomics and Health 2001), although, as noted, the WHO, which had supported such estimates, has been reviewing alternative threshold estimation methods. Others have inferred a threshold of $200,000 to $300,000 per QALY based on trends in healthcare spending and population health gains, or on contingent valuation surveys or preferences revealed in marketplace transactions (Braithwaite et al. 2008; Hirth et al. 2000). The US Environmental Protection Agency (EPA) has used a value for a statistical life of $7.4 million (in 2006 dollars) in its cost–benefit analyses of regulations (US Environmental Protection Agency National Center for Environmental Economics 2016); this suggests that a QALY is worth almost $300,000, assuming that each life saved gains 35 QALYs and a discount rate of 3%.

An important question is how relevant "value of health" or "demand side" evidence—that is, the willingness-to-pay data described in the preceding paragraph—is to estimating the cost-effectiveness threshold and allocating healthcare resources. Some investigators have argued that demand side considerations are secondary to the "supply side" constraints on resources available to deliver healthcare (McCabe, Claxton, and Culyer 2008; Woods et al. 2015). That is, in principle, the cost-effectiveness threshold should depend on the available budget and the costs and benefits of alternative uses for that budget (Neumann, Cohen, and Weinstein 2014). The supply side approach focuses on the health outcomes of the marginal intervention (with the highest ICER) that must be given up in order to provide resources for a particular intervention (Drummond et al. 2015). Hence, the cost-effectiveness threshold can be thought of as a measure of opportunity cost in terms of health: if additional costs are imposed by a new intervention, what other health-enhancing activities are made unavailable to other patients? If other outcomes are relevant to the decision (e.g., productivity effects), these would also be included in the measure of opportunity costs (Claxton et al. 2015). As discussed in Chapter 2, this type of threshold is consistent with the shadow price of the budget constraint (Stinnett and Paltiel 1996).

Researchers in the UK have recently attempted to measure the health opportunity cost threshold in that country. Using data to estimate the relationship between changes in spending and mortality in the UK, along with other sources and assumptions, they estimated a threshold of £12,936 per QALY (Martin, Rice, and Smith 2008). There is ongoing debate as to whether such an empirically measured threshold reflects the shadow price of the budget constraint. For example, changes in spending that are brought about by budget cuts could potentially displace not just the marginal intervention but other interventions with lower ICERs. However, estimating the actual services displaced and consequent health forgone, and comparing this with the estimated health generated by the new investment, may be more relevant for decision making (Eckermann and Pekarsky 2014; Paulden, McCabe, and Karnon 2014).

In an important sense, all health system funding is constrained, in that expenditures cannot increase automatically to accommodate all expensive new interventions, and opportunity costs are often imposed in the United States through higher premiums and/or co-payments, which in turn influence treatment use and health outcomes. However, some decision makers, such as those at the US Medicare program, do not face rigidly fixed budgets. In these settings, the opportunity cost associated with an intervention extends to the basket of goods and services outside the healthcare sector.

From a societal perspective, one might consider numerous areas of constrained expenditure in different sectors and conclude that there are many cost-effectiveness thresholds reflecting supply side considerations. In contrast, in the United States, most sectors do not have constrained expenditures in a practical sense, although there is an overall budget constraint. A demand side concept of a cost-effectiveness threshold from a societal perspective would involve quantifying trade-offs between all sources of social value, so any definition of the threshold would depend on which social welfare function is adopted. Although defining an explicit social welfare function is challenging, a demand side threshold for health from a societal perspective might be based on public willingness to pay. For example, average willingness-to-pay estimates could be interpreted as informing what people perceive to be a fair exchange between the QALY they are "purchasing" within the healthcare sector and what they must give up from expenditures outside that sector.

Decisions makers in most jurisdictions, including those in the United States, do not employ strict cost-effectiveness thresholds, and CEA is only one of many inputs into decisions. Because a wide range of settings may best be characterized as a hybrid between the two archetypes described in the preceding paragraphs (a demand side and a supply side concept of thresholds), a range of cost-effectiveness threshold values may be appropriate, depending on how new technology is funded. However a CEA threshold is estimated, its inference from empirical information is problematic because of data limitations and, therefore, the assumptions that become necessary. Debate about appropriate thresholds and methods to estimate them is a key area for future research (Woods et al. 2015).

1.4 CONCLUSIONS

1.4.1 CEA Illustrates Trade-offs Involved in Choosing Among Health Interventions

Cost-effectiveness anaylsis evaluates the health outcomes and costs of interventions designed to improve health. Studies show the trade-offs involved in choosing among interventions and thus help to define and illuminate the opportunity cost of each choice: the health benefits lost when the best alternative is not selected.

The concept of opportunity cost in health is premised on the notion that if the goal is better health, then it makes sense to choose interventions that produce the most health for the money. If the same measure of health outcome, such as healthy years of life gained (QALYs), is used to evaluate all the alternatives, they can be ranked by their cost-effectiveness ratios. Even when decision makers consider the additional goal of distributing societal health fairly, which may sometimes diverge from the goal of producing the most health for the money, CEA can help illuminate the trade-offs involved in deciding to give up some gains in population health in order to reduce some identified health inequalities.

1.4.2 The Reference Case Provides a Standard Set of Methods to Promote the Comparability of CEAs

Comparability is highly desirable if CEA is to help decision makers evaluate trade-offs. Decision makers around the world have recognized the importance of conducting CEAs in ways that are consistent across diseases and interventions. Inclusion of standardized components, as well as standardization of methods within a perspective, is intended to enhance consistency and comparability across studies. The Second Panel's specific recommendations about the Reference Case analysis are given in Chapter 3.

1.4.3 The Use of CEA in Healthcare Has Increased Over Time

The number of published CEAs has increased dramatically over the years, with applications to diverse interventions (i.e., clinical as well as policy and population-based), diseases, and contexts. Adherence to methodological and reporting practices in published CUAs has improved somewhat over time. Policy makers have used CEA in various ways. Notable applications in the United States pertain to public health programs and clinical guidelines. Cost-effectiveness analysis has played an important role in the adoption of drugs and other technologies in numerous countries around the world. In some countries, pharmaceutical companies are required to submit economic evidence as a condition of achieving market access. In addition, cost-effectiveness analysis has been used to inform decisions about non-drug technologies and clinical guidelines; to influence the funding and design of research studies; and to evaluate technologies early in the development process, prior to regulatory approval.

1.4.4 The Use of CEA Has also Encountered Resistance

Despite this progress, the application of CEA has also encountered opposition. Some agencies that might be expected to embrace the approach have relegated it to a secondary role or ignored it entirely. Because of the sensitivity associated with imposing limits on healthcare, some organizations have policies that require them to avoid any consideration—or appearance of consideration—of cost, even when CEA would inform strategies for delivering or targeting care. Some of the resistance may reflect ethical concerns, but it also comes from political pressures to provide care that has efficacy regardless of costs. Where parties have used cost-effectiveness information as part of evidence reviews, they have tended not to use explicit cost-effectiveness thresholds. Rather they have used CEA to illustrate trade-offs between costs and health outcomes, and to inform recommendation for target populations or subgroups.

1.4.5 The Usefulness of CEA Varies with Setting and Context

Experience has shown that context and setting play a role in whether and how CEA is used. In some countries, such as the UK, Canada, and Australia, where there is a centralized decision-making process for the reimbursement of pharmaceuticals or other technologies, there is a longer history of using CEA, and its application is more formal and extensive. Nonetheless CEA is not applied exactly the same way in all situations. For example, the UK gives special consideration to specific circumstances or conditions, including end-of-life treatments and treatments for children or disadvantaged populations. Some organizations, including NICE, have established procedures to incorporate the values of patients and the public. The composition and interactions of the decision group (e.g., clinicians, policy makers, methodologists, industry representatives, and patient representatives) is also important.

1.4.6 CEA Is an Aid to Decision Making

Experience shows that where policy makers have incorporated CEA into decision-making processes, they have not applied it as the sole decision criterion. In practice, multiple factors are brought to bear on resource allocation decisions. Cost-effectiveness is only one element among many, including patient's expectations; legal, ethical, cultural, and political concerns; and pragmatic issues of logistics and feasibility. Most health organizations involved in resource allocation decisions seem to give the greatest weight and the deepest consideration to the clinical evidence. Cost-effectiveness can play an important role, but typically it does not provide the central framework for decision makers.

1.5 REFERENCES

Academy of Managed Care Pharmacy. 2000. Principles of a Sound Drug Formulary System. October 2002. Accessed http://www.amcp.org/WorkArea/DownloadAsset.aspx?id=9280.

Adam, T., M. A. Koopmanschap, and D. B. Evans. 2003. Cost-effectiveness analysis: can we reduce variability in costing methods? *Int J Technol Assess Health Care* 19 (2):407–420.

Advisory Committee on Immunization Practices (ACIP). 2008. "ACIP: Guidance for Health Economics Studies. Guidance for Health Economics Studies Presented to the ACIP." Accessed May 22, 2015. http://www.cdc.gov/vaccines/acip/committee/guidance/economic-studies.html.

The AMCP Format Executive Committee. 2016. The AMCP Format for Formulary Submissions: Welcome to Version 4.0. *J Manag Care Spec Pharm* 22 (5):444–446.

American College of Physicians. 2008. Information on cost-effectiveness: an essential product of a national comparative effectiveness program. *Ann Intern Med* 148 (12):956–961.

American Society of Clinical Oncology. 2014. ASCO Value Framework Fact Sheet. www.asco.org/sites/www.asco.org/files/asco_value_fact_sheet_final_10_09_14.pdf.

Anderson, J. L., P. A. Heidenreich, P. G. Barnett, M. A. Creager, G. C. Fonarow, R. J. Gibbons, J. L. Halperin, M. A. Hlatky, A. K. Jacobs, D. B. Mark, F. A. Masoudi, E. D. Peterson, and L. J. Shaw. 2014. ACC/AHA statement on cost/value methodology in clinical practice guidelines and performance measures: a report of the American College of Cardiology/American Heart Association Task Force on Performance Measures and Task Force on Practice Guidelines. *J Am Coll Cardiol* 63 (21):2304–2322.

Australian Institute of Health and Welfare Act of 1987. Canberra, Australia. https://www.legislation.gov.au/Details/C2014C00481/Html/Text#

Bae, S., S. Lee, E. Y. Bae, and S. Jang. 2013. Korean guidelines for pharmacoeconomic evaluation (second and updated version): consensus and compromise. *Pharmacoeconomics* 31 (4):257–267.

Baltussen, R., and L. Niessen. 2006. Priority setting of health interventions: the need for multi-criteria decision analysis. *Cost Eff Resour Alloc* 4:14.

Bell, C. M., D. R. Urbach, J. G. Ray, A. Bayoumi, A. B. Rosen, D. Greenberg, and P. J. Neumann. 2006. Bias in published cost effectiveness studies: systematic review. *BMJ* 332 (7543): 699–703.

Bill and Melinda Gates Foundation Methods for Economic Evaluation Project (MEEP). 2014. The Gates Reference Case: What It Is, Why It's Important, and How to Use It. London: NICE International. http://www.nice.org.uk/Media/Default/About/what-we-do/NICE-International/projects/Gates-Reference-case-what-it-is-how-to-use-it.pdf.

Birkett, D. J., A. S. Mitchell, and P. McManus. 2001. A cost-effectiveness approach to drug subsidy and pricing in Australia. *Health Aff (Millwood)* 20 (3):104–114.

Braithwaite, R. S., D. O. Meltzer, J. T. King, Jr., D. Leslie, and M. S. Roberts. 2008. What does the value of modern medicine say about the $50,000 per quality-adjusted life-year decision rule? *Med Care* 46 (4):349–356.

Buxton, M. J. 2006. Economic evaluation and decision making in the UK. *Pharmacoeconomics* 24 (11):1133–1142.

Canadian Agency for Drugs and Technologies in Health (CADTH). 2016. "Health Technology Expert Review Panel." Accessed January 6. https://www.cadth.ca/collaboration-and-outreach/advisory-bodies/health-technology-expert-review-panel.

Canadian Coordinating Office for Health Technology Assessment (CCOHTA). 1994. *Guidelines for Economic Evaluation of Pharmaceuticals: Canada*. 1st ed. November 1994. Ottawa: CCOHTA.

Carlsson, P. 2004. Health technology assessment and priority setting for health policy in Sweden. *Int J Technol Assess Health Care* 20 (1):44–54.

Caro, J. J., E. Nord, U. Siebert, A. McGuire, M. McGregor, D. Henry, G. de Pouvourville, V. Atella, and P. Kolominsky-Rabas. 2010. The efficiency frontier approach to economic evaluation of health-care interventions. *Health Econ* 19 (10):1117–1127.

Center for the Evaluation of Value and Risk in Health. n.d. The Cost-Effectiveness Analysis Registry [Internet]. Institute for Clinical Research and Health Policy Studies, Tufts Medical Center, Boston. Available from: www.cearegistry.org.

Centers for Disease Control and Prevention (CDC), and Advisory Committee on Immunization Practices (ACIP). 2008. Update: recommendations from the Advisory Committee on Immunization Practices (ACIP) regarding administration of combination MMRV vaccine. *MMWR Morb Mortal Wkly Rep* 57 (10):258–260.

Centers for Medicare & Medicaid Services. 2015. Decision Memo for Screening for Lung Cancer with Low Dose Computed Tomography (LDCT) (CAG-00439N). February 5, 2015. www.cms.gov/medicare-coverage-database/details/nca-decision-memo.aspx?NCAId=274.

Centre for Health Economics. 2015. iDSI Workshop on Cost-Effectiveness Thresholds: Conceptualisation and Estimation. 26 June 2015—London, UK. Summary Report. York, UK: Centre for Health Economics, University of York. http://www.york.ac.uk/media/che/images/news/iDSI_Summary_Report-FINAL.pdf.

Chambers, J. D., M. J. Cangelosi, and P. J. Neumann. 2015. Medicare's use of cost-effectiveness analysis for prevention (but not for treatment). *Health Policy* 119 (2):156–163.

Chambers, J. D., P. J. Neumann, and M. J. Buxton. 2010. Does Medicare have an implicit cost-effectiveness threshold? *Med Decis Making* 30 (4):E14–E27.

Chokshi, D. A., and T. A. Farley. 2012. The cost-effectiveness of environmental approaches to disease prevention. *N Engl J Med* 367 (4):295–297.

Claxton, K. 2007. OFT, VBP: QED? *Health Econ* 16 (6):545–558.

Claxton, K., S. Palmer, L. Longworth, L. Bojke, S. Griffin, C. McKenna, M. Soares, E. Spackman, and J. Youn. 2012. Informing a decision framework for when NICE should recommend the use of health technologies only in the context of an appropriately designed programme of evidence development. *Health Technol Assess* 16 (46):1–323.

Claxton, K., M. Sculpher, and S. Carroll. 2011. *Value-Based Pricing for Pharmaceuticals: Its Role, Specification and Prospects in a Newly Devolved NHS. CHE Research Paper 60.* York, UK: Centre for Health Economics, University of York. https://www.york.ac.uk/media/che/documents/papers/researchpapers/CHERP60_value_based_pricing_for_pharmaceuticals.pdf.

Claxton, K., M. Sculpher, and M. Drummond. 2002. A rational framework for decision making by the National Institute For Clinical Excellence (NICE). *Lancet* 360 (9334):711–715.

Claxton, K., M. Sculpher, S. Palmer, and A. J. Culyer. 2015. Causes for concern: is NICE failing to uphold its responsibilities to all NHS patients? *Health Econ* 24 (1):1–7.

Clement, F. M., A. Harris, J. J. Li, K. Yong, K. M. Lee, and B. J. Manns. 2009. Using effectiveness and cost-effectiveness to make drug coverage decisions: a comparison of Britain, Australia, and Canada. *JAMA* 302 (13):1437–1443.

Community Preventive Services Task Force. 1996. The Guide to Community Preventive Services.

Community Preventive Services Task Force. 2016. "The Guide to Community Preventive Services." Accessed January 8. www.thecommunityguide.org/index.html.

Cromwell, J., W. J. Bartosch, M. C. Fiore, V. Hasselblad, and T. Baker. 1997. Cost-effectiveness of the clinical practice recommendations in the AHCPR guideline for smoking cessation. Agency for Health Care Policy and Research. *JAMA* 278 (21):1759–1766.

Culyer, A., C. McCabe, A. Briggs, K. Claxton, M. Buxton, R. Akehurst, M. Sculpher, and J. Brazier. 2007. Searching for a threshold, not setting one: the role of the National Institute for Health and Clinical Excellence. *J Health Serv Res Policy* 12 (1):56–58.

Dakin, H., N. Devlin, Y. Feng, N. Rice, P. O'Neill, and D. Parkin. 2015. The influence of cost-effectiveness and other factors on NICE decisions. DOI: 10.1002/hec.3086. *Health Econ* 24 (10):1256–1271 de Pouvourville, G. 2013. HAS to be NICE? *Eur J Health Econ* 14 (3):363–366.

Devlin, N., and D. Parkin. 2004. Does NICE have a cost-effectiveness threshold and what other factors influence its decisions? A binary choice analysis. *Health Econ* 13 (5):437–452.

Diaz, M., S. de Sanjose, J. Ortendahl, M. O'Shea, S. J. Goldie, F. X. Bosch, and J. J. Kim. 2010. Cost-effectiveness of human papillomavirus vaccination and screening in Spain. *Eur J Cancer* 46 (16):2973–2985.

Dintsios, C. M., and A. Gerber. 2010. Some essential clarifications: IQWiG comments on two critiques of the efficiency frontier approach. *Health Econ* 19 (10):1139–1141.

Dollahite, J., D. Kenkel, and C. S. Thompson. 2008. An economic evaluation of the expanded food and nutrition education program. *J Nutr Educ Behav* 40 (3):134–143.

Drummond, M. 2013. Twenty years of using economic evaluations for drug reimbursement decisions: what has been achieved? *J Health Polit Policy Law* 38 (6):1081–1102.

Drummond, M. 2014. "Why has Sweden Been so Prominent in Health Economics?" In *Portrait of a Health Economist: Essays by Colleagues and Friends of Bengt Jönsson*, edited by A. J. Culyer and G. Kobelt, 39–44. Lund, Sweden: Swedish Institute for Health Economics.

Drummond, M., D. Brixner, M. Gold, P. Kind, A. McGuire, E. Nord, and the Consensus Development Group. 2009. Toward a consensus on the QALY. *Value Health* 12 Suppl 1:S31–S35.

Drummond, M., G. de Pouvourville, E. Jones, J. Haig, G. Saba, and H. Cawston. 2014. A comparative analysis of two contrasting European approaches for rewarding the value added by drugs for cancer: England versus France. *Pharmacoeconomics* 32 (5):509–520.

Drummond, M., and F. Rutten. n.d. The IQWiG methodology paper version 1.0. www.vfa.de/embed/stellungnahme-iqwig-methodenentwurf-drummond-rutten.pdf.

Drummond, M. F., M. J. Sculpher, K. Claxton, G. W. Torrance, and G. L. Stoddart. 2015. *Methods for the Economic Evaluation of Health Care Programmes*. 4th ed. Oxford: Oxford University Press.

Eckermann, S., and B. Pekarsky. 2014. Can the real opportunity cost stand up: displaced services, the straw man outside the room. *Pharmacoeconomics* 32 (4):319–325.

Eddy, D. M., L. Schlessinger, and R. Kahn. 2005. Clinical outcomes and cost-effectiveness of strategies for managing people at high risk for diabetes. *Ann Intern Med* 143 (4):251–264.

Edmonds, D. J., D. M. Dumbrell, J. G. Primrose, P. McManus, D. J. Birkett, and V. Demirian. 1993. Development of an Australian Drug Utilisation Database: A Report from the Drug Utilization Subcommittee of the Pharmaceutical Benefits Advisory Committee. *Pharmacoeconomics* 3 (6):427–432.

Elsisi, G. H., Z. Kaló, R. Eldessouki, M. D. Elmahdawy, A. Saad, S. Ragab, A. M. Elshalakani, and S. Abaza. 2013. Recommendations for reporting pharmacoeconomic evaluations in Egypt. *Value Health Reg Issues* 2 (2):319–327.

Fiore, A. E., D. K. Shay, K. Broder, J. K. Iskander, T. M. Uyeki, G. Mootrey, J. S. Bresee, N. S. Cox, Centers for Disease Control and Prevention (CDC), and Advisory Committee on Immunization Practices (ACIP). 2008. Prevention and control of influenza: recommendations of the Advisory Committee on Immunization Practices (ACIP), 2008. *MMWR Recomm Rep* 57 (RR-7):1–60.

Friedberg, M., B. Saffran, T. J. Stinson, W. Nelson, and C. L. Bennett. 1999. Evaluation of conflict of interest in economic analyses of new drugs used in oncology. *JAMA* 282 (15):1453–1457.

Gandjour, A., A. Gafni, and M. Schlander. 2014. Determining the price for pharmaceuticals in Germany: comparing a shortcut for IQWiG's efficiency frontier method with the price set by the manufacturer for ticagrelor. *Expert Rev Pharmacoecon Outcomes Res* 14 (1):123–129.

Garattini, L., D. Cornago, and P. De Compadri. 2007. Pricing and reimbursement of in-patent drugs in seven European countries: a comparative analysis. *Health Policy* 82 (3):330–339.

Garber, A. M., and C. E. Phelps. 1997. Economic foundations of cost-effectiveness analysis. *J Health Econ* 16 (1):1–31.

Garrison, L. P., Jr., D. Lubeck, D. Lalla, V. Paton, A. Dueck, and E. A. Perez. 2007. Cost-effectiveness analysis of trastuzumab in the adjuvant setting for treatment of HER2-positive breast cancer. *Cancer* 110 (3):489–498.

Giacomini, M., F. Wagner, M. Krahn, J. Abelson, N. Sikich, and K. Kaulback. 2012a. "Social and Ethical Values for Health Technology Assessment in Ontario." Health Quality Transformation Ontario 2012 (www.hqontario.ca/Events/Health-Quality-Transformation-2012), Ontario, October 2012.

Giacomini, M., F. Wagner, M. Krahn, J. Abelson, N. Sikich, K. Kaulback, and D. Simeonov. 2012b. "Addressing Social and Ethical Issues in HTA: Developments at the Ontario Health Technology Advisory Committee (OHTAC)." Canadian Bioethics Society Meeting, Montreal, Canada; June 2012.

Giorgi Rossi, P., and M. Zappa. 2008. Re: Cost-effectiveness of cervical cancer screening with human papillomavirus DNA testing and HPV-16,18 vaccination. *J Natl Cancer Inst* 100 (22):1654; author reply 1654–1655.

Goddard, K. A., W. A. Knaus, E. Whitlock, G. H. Lyman, H. S. Feigelson, S. D. Schully, S. Ramsey, S. Tunis, A. N. Freedman, M. J. Khoury, and D. L. Veenstra. 2012. Building the evidence base for decision making in cancer genomic medicine using comparative effectiveness research. *Genet Med* 14 (7):633–642.

Goetghebeur, M. M., M. Wagner, H. Khoury, D. Rindress, J. P. Gregoire, and C. Deal. 2010. Combining multicriteria decision analysis, ethics and health technology assessment: applying the EVIDEM decision-making framework to growth hormone for Turner syndrome patients. *Cost Eff Resour Alloc* 8:4.

Gold, M. R., P. Franks, T. Siegelberg, and S. Sofaer. 2007. Does providing cost-effectiveness information change coverage priorities for citizens acting as social decision makers? *Health Policy* 83 (1):65–72.

Gold, M. R., J. E. Siegel, L. B. Russell, and M. C. Weinstein, eds. 1996. *Cost-Effectiveness in Health and Medicine*. New York: Oxford University Press.

Graham, J. D., K. M. Thompson, S. J. Goldie, M. Segui-Gomez, and M. C. Weinstein. 1997. The cost-effectiveness of air bags by seating position. *JAMA* 278 (17):1418–1425.

Grosse, S. D. 2008. Assessing cost-effectiveness in healthcare: history of the $50,000 per QALY threshold. *Expert Rev Pharmacoecon Outcomes Res* 8 (2):165–178.

Ha, D. A., and D. Chisholm. 2011. Cost-effectiveness analysis of interventions to prevent cardiovascular disease in Vietnam. *Health Policy Plan* 26 (3):210–222.

Hadorn, D. C. 1991. Setting health care priorities in Oregon. Cost-effectiveness meets the rule of rescue. *JAMA* 265 (17):2218–2225.

Hall, P. S., C. McCabe, J. M. Brown, and D. A. Cameron. 2010. Health economics in drug development: efficient research to inform healthcare funding decisions. *Eur J Cancer* 46 (15):2674–2680.

Hall, P. S., C. McCabe, R. C. Stein, and D. Cameron. 2012. Economic evaluation of genomic test-directed chemotherapy for early-stage lymph node-positive breast cancer. *J Natl Cancer Inst* 104 (1):56–66.

Haute Autorité de Santé. 2012. Choices for Methods for Economic Evaluation. Saint-Denis La Plaine, France. www.has-sante.fr/portail/upload/docs/application/pdf/2012-10/choices_in_methods_for_economic_evaluation.pdf.

Hirth, R. A., M. E. Chernew, E. Miller, A. M. Fendrick, and W. G. Weissert. 2000. Willingness to pay for a quality-adjusted life year: in search of a standard. *Med Decis Making* 20 (3):332–342.

Husereau, D., A. J. Culyer, P. Neumann, and P. Jacobs. 2015. How do economic evaluations inform health policy decisions for treatment and prevention in Canada and the United States? *Appl Health Econ Health Policy* 13 (3):273–279.

Hutubessy, R., D. Chisholm, and T. T. Edejer. 2003. Generalized cost-effectiveness analysis for national-level priority-setting in the health sector. *Cost Eff Resour Alloc* 1 (1):8.

Iglesias, C. P., M. F. Drummond, J. Rovira, for the NEVALAT Project Group. 2005. Health-care decision-making processes in Latin America: problems and prospects for the use of economic evaluation. *Int J Technol Assess Health Care* 21 (1):1–14.

Ijzerman, M. J., and L. M. Steuten. 2011. Early assessment of medical technologies to inform product development and market access: a review of methods and applications. *Appl Health Econ Health Policy* 9 (5):331–347.

IOM (Institute of Medicine). 2012a. *For the Public's Health: Investing in a Healthier Future.* Washington, DC: The National Academies Press.

IOM (Institute of Medicine). 2012b. *Integrating Large-Scale Genomic Information into Clinical Practice: Workshop Summary.* Washington, DC: The National Academies Press.

Johnson, A. P., N. J. Sikich, G. Evans, W. Evans, M. Giacomini, M. Glendining, M. Krahn, L. Levin, P. Oh, and C. Perera. 2009. Health technology assessment: a comprehensive framework for evidence-based recommendations in Ontario. *Int J Technol Assess Health Care* 25 (2):141–150.

Kaló, Z., J. Bodrogi, I. Boncz, C. Dózsa, G. Jóna, R. Kövi, and B. Sinkovits. 2013. Capacity building for HTA implementation in middle-income countries: The case of Hungary. *Value Health Reg Issues* 2 (2):264–266.

Kamae, I. 2010. Value-based approaches to healthcare systems and pharmacoeconomics requirements in Asia: South Korea, Taiwan, Thailand and Japan. *Pharmacoeconomics* 28 (10):831–838.

Kamae, I. 2014. "A Japanese-Style Approach to Value-Based Pricing: Scientific Basis and Theoretical Potential." In *Portrait of a Health Economist: Essays by Colleagues and Friends of Bengt Jönsson*, edited by A.J. Culyer and G. Kobelt, 73–80. Lund, Sweden: Swedish Institute for Health Economics.

Klingler, C., S. M. Shah, A. J. Barron, and J. S. Wright. 2013. Regulatory space and the contextual mediation of common functional pressures: analyzing the factors that led to the German Efficiency Frontier approach. *Health Policy* 109 (3):270–280.

Kurian, A. W., R. N. Thompson, A. F. Gaw, S. Arai, R. Ortiz, and A. M. Garber. 2007. A cost-effectiveness analysis of adjuvant trastuzumab regimens in early HER2/neu-positive breast cancer. *J Clin Oncol* 25 (6):634–641.

Langley, P. C. 2004. The NICE reference case requirement: implications for drug manufacturers and health systems. *Pharmacoeconomics* 22 (4):267–271.

Laupacis, A. 2006. Economic evaluations in the Canadian Common Drug Review. *Pharmacoeconomics* 24 (11):1157–1162.

Laupacis, A., D. Feeny, A. S. Detsky, and P. X. Tugwell. 1992. How attractive does a new technology have to be to warrant adoption and utilization? Tentative guidelines for using clinical and economic evaluations. *CMAJ* 146 (4):473–481.

Levin, L., R. Goeree, M. Levine, M. Krahn, T. Easty, A. Brown, and D. Henry. 2011. Coverage with evidence development: the Ontario experience. *Int J Technol Assess Health Care* 27 (2):159–168.

Levy, D. T., J. A. Ellis, D. Mays, and A. T. Huang. 2013. Smoking-related deaths averted due to three years of policy progress. *Bull World Health Organ* 91 (7):509–518.

Levy, D. T., L. Nikolayev, E. Mumford, and C. Compton. 2005. The Healthy People 2010 smoking prevalence and tobacco control objectives: results from the SimSmoke tobacco control policy simulation model (United States). *Cancer Causes Control* 16 (4):359–371.

Littlejohns, P., and M. Rawlins, eds. 2009. *Patients, the Public and Priorities in Healthcare.* Abingdon (UK): Radcliffe Publishing.

Liu, S., L. E. Cipriano, M. Holodniy, D. K. Owens, and J. D. Goldhaber-Fiebert. 2012. New protease inhibitors for the treatment of chronic hepatitis C: a cost-effectiveness analysis. *Ann Intern Med* 156 (4):279–290.

Losina, E., R. P. Walensky, C. L. Kessler, P. S. Emrani, W. M. Reichmann, E. A. Wright, H. L. Holt, D. H. Solomon, E. Yelin, A. D. Paltiel, and J. N. Katz. 2009. Cost-effectiveness of total knee arthroplasty in the United States: patient risk and hospital volume. *Arch Intern Med* 169 (12):1113–1121; discussion 1121–1122.

Lyman, G. H., L. E. Cosler, N. M. Kuderer, and J. Hornberger. 2007. Impact of a 21-gene RT-PCR assay on treatment decisions in early-stage breast cancer: an economic analysis based on prognostic and predictive validation studies. *Cancer* 109 (6):1011–1018.

Mandelblatt, J. S., K. A. Cronin, S. Bailey, D. A. Berry, H. J. de Koning, G. Draisma, H. Huang, S. J. Lee, M. Munsell, S. K. Plevritis, P. Ravdin, C. B. Schechter, B. Sigal, M. A. Stoto, N. K. Stout, N. T. van Ravesteyn, J. Venier, M. Zelen, E. J. Feuer, and the Breast Cancer Working Group of the Cancer Intervention and Surveillance Modeling Network (CISNET). 2009. Effects of mammography screening under different screening schedules: model estimates of potential benefits and harms. *Ann Intern Med* 151 (10):738–747.

Mandelblatt, J. S., N. K. Stout, C. B. Schechter, J. J. van den Broek, D. L. Miglioretti, M. Krapcho, A. Trentham-Dietz, D. Munoz, S. J. Lee, D. A. Berry, N. T. van Ravesteyn, O. Alagoz, K. Kerlikowske, A. N. Tosteson, A. M. Near, A. Hoeffken, Y. Chang, E. A. Heijnsdijk, G. Chisholm, X. Huang, H. Huang, M. A. Ergun, R. Gangnon, B. L. Sprague, S. Plevritis, E. Feuer, H. J. de Koning, and K. A. Cronin. 2016. Collaborative modeling of the benefits and harms associated with different U.S. breast cancer screening strategies. *Ann Intern Med* 164 (4):215–225.

Martin, S., N. Rice, and P. C. Smith. 2008. Does health care spending improve health outcomes? Evidence from English programme budgeting data. *J Health Econ* 27 (4):826–842.

McCabe, C., K. Claxton, and A. J. Culyer. 2008. The NICE cost-effectiveness threshold: what it is and what that means. *Pharmacoeconomics* 26 (9):733–744.

McMahon, M., S. Morgan, and C. Mitton. 2006. The Common Drug Review: a NICE start for Canada? *Health Policy* 77 (3):339–351.

Miller, W., L. A. Robinson, and R. S. Lawrence, eds. 2006. *Valuing Health for Regulatory Cost-Effectiveness Analysis.* Washington, DC: The National Academies Press. http://www.nap.edu/openbook.php?record_id=11534.

National Institute for Health and Care Excellence (NICE). 2003. *Technology Appraisal Guidance [archived].* London: NICE.

National Institute for Health and Care Excellence (NICE). 2004. *Technology Appraisal Guidance [archived].* London: NICE.

National Institute for Health and Care Excellence (NICE). 2013. *Guide to the Methods of Technology Appraisal 2013. NICE article [PMG9].* London: NICE. http://publications.nice.org.uk/pmg9.

National Institute for Health and Care Excellence (NICE). 2014. Value Based Assessment. See Item 4 at: http://www.nice.org.uk/media/default/Get-involved/Meetings-In-Public/Public-board-meetings/Agenda-Papers-September-2014-Public-Board-Meeting-1.pdf.

Nelson, A. L., J. T. Cohen, D. Greenberg, and D. M. Kent. 2009. Much cheaper, almost as good: decrementally cost-effective medical innovation. *Ann Intern Med* 151 (9):662–667.

Ness, R. M., A. M. Holmes, R. Klein, and R. Dittus. 2000. Cost-utility of one-time colonoscopic screening for colorectal cancer at various ages. *Am J Gastroenterol* 95 (7):1800–1811.

Neumann, P. J. 2005. *Using Cost-Effectiveness Analysis to Improve Health Care: Opportunities and Barriers.* New York: Oxford University Press.

Neumann, P. J., and J. D. Chambers. 2012. Medicare's enduring struggle to define "reasonable and necessary" care. *N Engl J Med* 367 (19):1775–1777.

Neumann, P. J., J. T. Cohen, and M. C. Weinstein. 2014. Updating cost-effectiveness—the curious resilience of the $50,000-per-QALY threshold. *N Engl J Med* 371 (9):796–797.

Neumann, P. J., A. B. Rosen, D. Greenberg, N. V. Olchanski, R. Pande, R. H. Chapman, P. W. Stone, S. Ondategui-Parra, J. Nadai, J. E. Siegel, and M. C. Weinstein. 2005. Can we better prioritize resources for cost-utility research? *Med Decis Making* 25 (4):429–436.

Neumann, P. J., T. Thorat, J. Shi, C. J. Saret, and J. T. Cohen. 2015. The changing face of the cost-utility literature, 1990-2012. *Value Health* 18 (2):271–277.

Neumann, P. J., and M. C. Weinstein. 2010. Legislating against use of cost-effectiveness information. *N Engl J Med* 363 (16):1495–1497.

Nichol, G., P. Kaul, E. Huszti, and J. F. Bridges. 2004. Cost-effectiveness of cardiac resynchronization therapy in patients with symptomatic heart failure. *Ann Intern Med* 141 (5):343–351.

Odame, E. A. 2013. Systematic Review of Economic Evaluation Literature in Ghana: Is Health Technology Assessment the Future? *Value Health Reg Issues* 2 (2):279–283.

Office of Fair Trading. 2007. The Pharmaceutical Price Regulation Scheme. An OFT Market Study. OFT. London, England. http://webarchive.nationalarchives.gov.uk/20140402155108/ http://www.oft.gov.uk/shared_oft/reports/comp_policy/oft885.pdf.

Office of Management and Budget. 2003. Informing Regulatory Decisions: 2003 Report to Congress on the Costs and Benefits of Federal Regulations and Unfunded Mandates on State, Local, and Tribal Entities. https://www.whitehouse.gov/sites/default/files/omb/assets/ omb/inforeg/2003_cost-ben_final_rpt.pdf.

Office of Management and Budget. 2016. "Frequently Asked Questions." Accessed January 8. www.reginfo.gov/public/jsp/Utilities/faq.jsp.

Paltiel, A. D., R. P. Walensky, B. R. Schackman, G. R. Seage, 3rd, L. M. Mercincavage, M. C. Weinstein, and K. A. Freedberg. 2006. Expanded HIV screening in the United States: effect on clinical outcomes, HIV transmission, and costs. *Ann Intern Med* 145 (11):797–806.

Partridge, A. H., and E. P. Winer. 2009. On mammography—more agreement than disagreement. *N Engl J Med* 361 (26):2499–2501.

Patel, V., S. Chatterji, D. Chisholm, S. Ebrahim, G. Gopalakrishna, C. Mathers, V. Mohan, D. Prabhakaran, R. D. Ravindran, and K. S. Reddy. 2011. Chronic diseases and injuries in India. *Lancet* 377 (9763):413–428.

Paulden, M., C. McCabe, and J. Karnon. 2014. Achieving allocative efficiency in healthcare: nice in theory, not so NICE in Practice? *Pharmacoeconomics* 32 (4):315–318.

PausJenssen, A. M., P. A. Singer, and A. S. Detsky. 2003. Ontario's formulary committee: how recommendations are made. *Pharmacoeconomics* 21 (4):285–294.

Perrin, J. M., A. A. Knapp, M. F. Browning, A. M. Comeau, N. S. Green, E. A. Lipstein, D. R. Metterville, L. Prosser, D. Queally, and A. R. Kemper. 2010. An evidence development process for newborn screening. *Genet Med* 12 (3):131–134.

Phillips, K. A., and J. L. Chen. 2002. Impact of the U.S. panel on cost-effectiveness in health and medicine. *Am J Prev Med* 22 (2):98–105.

Pignone, M., S. Earnshaw, J. A. Tice, and M. J. Pletcher. 2006. Aspirin, statins, or both drugs for the primary prevention of coronary heart disease events in men: a cost-utility analysis. [Summary for patients in *Ann Intern Med.* 2006 Mar 7;144 (5):I29; PMID: 16520469]. *Ann Intern Med* 144 (5):326–336.

Pignone, M., S. Saha, T. Hoerger, and J. Mandelblatt. 2002. Cost-effectiveness analyses of colorectal cancer screening: a systematic review for the U.S. Preventive Services Task Force. *Ann Intern Med* 137 (2):96–104.

Prosser, L. A., S. D. Grosse, A. R. Kemper, B. A. Tarini, and J. M. Perrin. 2012. Decision analysis, economic evaluation, and newborn screening: challenges and opportunities. *Genet Med* 14 (8):703–712. DOI: 10.1038/gim.2012.24

Rawlins, M., D. Barnett, and A. Stevens. 2010. Pharmacoeconomics: NICE's approach to decision-making. *Br J Clin Pharmacol* 70 (3):346–349.

Rawlins, M. D. 2005. Pharmacopolitics and deliberative democracy. *Clin Med (Northfield Il)* 5 (5):471–475.

Romanow, R. J. 2002. Building on Values: The Future of Health Care in Canada—Final Report. Commission on the Future of Health Care in Canada. http://publications.gc.ca/collections/Collection/CP32-85-2002E.pdf.

Ross, H., L. M. Powell, J. E. Bauer, D. T. Levy, R. M. Peck, and H. R. Lee. 2006. Community-based youth tobacco control interventions: cost effectiveness of the Full Court Press project. *Appl Health Econ Health Policy* 5 (3):167–176.

Roux, L., M. Pratt, T. O. Tengs, M. M. Yore, T. L. Yanagawa, J. Van Den Bos, C. Rutt, R. C. Brownson, K. E. Powell, G. Heath, H. W. Kohl, 3rd, S. Teutsch, J. Cawley, I. M. Lee, L. West, and D. M. Buchner. 2008. Cost effectiveness of community-based physical activity interventions. *Am J Prev Med* 35 (6):578–588.

Russell, L. B., M. R. Gold, J. E. Siegel, N. Daniels, and M. C. Weinstein. 1996. The role of cost-effectiveness analysis in health and medicine. Panel on Cost-Effectiveness in Health and Medicine. *JAMA* 276 (14):1172–1177.

Saha, S., T. J. Hoerger, M. P. Pignone, S. M. Teutsch, M. Helfand, J. S. Mandelblatt, and T.U.S.P.S.T.F. Cost Work Group. 2001. The art and science of incorporating cost effectiveness into evidence-based recommendations for clinical preventive services. *Am J Prev Med* 20 (3 Suppl):36–43.

Salomon, J. A., N. Carvalho, C. Gutierrez-Delgado, R. Orozco, A. Mancuso, D. R. Hogan, D. Lee, Y. Murakami, L. Sridharan, M. E. Medina-Mora, and E. Gonzalez-Pier. 2012. Intervention strategies to reduce the burden of non-communicable diseases in Mexico: cost effectiveness analysis. *BMJ* 344:e355.

Schwartz, J. A., and S. D. Pearson. 2013. Cost consideration in the clinical guidance documents of physician specialty societies in the United States. *JAMA Intern Med* 173 (12): 1091–1097.

Sculpher, M., and K. Claxton. 2010. Sins of omission and obfuscation: IQWIG's guidelines on economic evaluation methods. *Health Econ* 19 (10):1132–1136.

Siegel, J. E., S. C. Byron, and W. F. Lawrence. 2005. Federal sponsorship of cost-effectiveness and related research in health care: 1997-2001. *Value Health* 8 (3):223–236.

Smith, J. C. 2010. The structure, role, and procedures of the U.S. Advisory Committee on Immunization Practices (ACIP). *Vaccine* 28 Suppl 1:A68–A75.

Smith, J. G., and N. L. Metzger. 2011. Evaluation of pneumococcal vaccination rates after vaccine protocol changes and nurse education in a tertiary care teaching hospital. *J Manag Care Pharm* 17 (9):701–708.

Smith, K. J., B. Y. Lee, M. P. Nowalk, M. Raymund, and R. K. Zimmerman. 2010. Cost-effectiveness of dual influenza and pneumococcal vaccination in 50-year-olds. *Vaccine* 28 (48):7620–7625.

Smith, K. J., A. R. Wateska, M. P. Nowalk, M. Raymund, J. P. Nuorti, and R. K. Zimmerman. 2012. Cost-effectiveness of adult vaccination strategies using pneumococcal conjugate vaccine compared with pneumococcal polysaccharide vaccine. *JAMA* 307 (8):804–812.

Sperber, D., A. Shiell, and K. Fyie. 2010. The cost-effectiveness of a law banning the use of cellular phones by drivers. *Health Econ* 19 (10):1212–1225.

Stason, W. B., and M. C. Weinstein. 1977. Public-health rounds at the Harvard School of Public Health. Allocation of resources to manage hypertension. *N Engl J Med* 296 (13):732–739.

Stephens, D. S., R. Ahmed, and W. A. Orenstein. 2014. Vaccines at what price? *Vaccine* 32 (9):1029–1030.

Stinnett, A. A., and A. D. Paltiel. 1996. Mathematical programming for the efficient allocation of health care resources. *J Health Econ* 15 (5):641–653.

Swedish Agency for Health Technology Assessment and Assessment of Social Services. http://www.sbu.se/en/about-sbu/

Taylor, R. S., M. F. Drummond, G. Salkeld, and S. D. Sullivan. 2004. Inclusion of cost effectiveness in licensing requirements of new drugs: the fourth hurdle. *BMJ* 329 (7472):972–975.

Thokala, P., and A. Duenas. 2012. Multiple criteria decision analysis for health technology assessment. *Value Health* 15 (8):1172–1181.

Tony, M., M. Wagner, H. Khoury, D. Rindress, T. Papastavros, P. Oh, and M. M. Goetghebeur. 2011. Bridging health technology assessment (HTA) with multicriteria decision analyses (MCDA): field testing of the EVIDEM framework for coverage decisions by a public payer in Canada. *BMC Health Serv Res* 11:329.

Towse, A. 2007. If it ain't broke, don't price fix it: the OFT and the PPRS. *Health Econ* 16 (7): 653–665.

US Congress Office of Technology Assessment. 1979. A Review of Selected Federal Vaccine and Immunization Policies, Based on Case Studies of Pneumococcal Vaccine. September 1979. Washington, DC: US Government Printing Office. https://www.princeton.edu/~ota/disk3/1979/7915/7915.PDF.

US Congress Office of Technology Assessment. 1987. Breast Cancer Screening for Medicare Beneficiaries: Effectiveness, Costs to Medicare and Medical Resources Required. Washington, DC: US Government Printing Office. http://catalog.hathitrust.org/Record/002976847.

US Congress Office of Technology Assessment. 1990a. The Costs and Effectiveness of Screening for Cervical Cancer in Elderly Women-Background Paper. OTA-BP-H-65. Washington, DC: US Government Printing Office.

US Congress Office of Technology Assessment. 1990b. The Costs and Effectiveness of Colorectal Cancer Screening in the Elderly-Background Paper. OTA-BP-H-74. Washington, DC: US Government Printing Office.

US Environmental Protection Agency National Center for Environmental Economics. 2016. "Frequently Asked Questions on Mortality Risk Valuation." Accessed January 6. http://yosemite.epa.gov/EE%5Cepa%5Ceed.nsf/webpages/MortalityRiskValuation.html.

US Environmental Protection Agency Office of Air and Radiation. 2011. The Benefits and Costs of the Clean Air Act from 1990 to 2020: Summary Report. March 2011. www.epa.gov/cleanairactbenefits/feb11/summaryreport.pdf.

Vanderlaan, B. F., M. S. Broder, E. Y. Chang, R. Oratz, and T. G. Bentley. 2011. Cost-effectiveness of 21-gene assay in node-positive, early-stage breast cancer. *Am J Manag Care* 17 (7):455–464.

Wagner, F., M. Giacomini, M. Krahn, J. Abelson, N. Sikich, and K. Kaulback. 2012. "Ethics as Evidence: Identifying Social and Ethical Values in Heath Technology Assessment." Annual Meeting of the American Society for Bioethics and Humanities, Washington, D.C.

Walkinshaw, E. 2011. National assessment of cancer drugs commences. *CMAJ* 183 (13):E985–E986.

Watkins, J. B., M. E. Minshall, and S. D. Sullivan. 2006. Application of economic analyses in U.S. managed care formulary decisions: a private payer's experience. *J Manag Care Pharm* 12 (9):726–735.

WHO Commission on Macroeconomics and Health. 2001. *Macroeconomics and Health: Investing in Health for Economic Development. Report of the Commission on Macroeconomics and Health.* Geneva: World Health Organization. http://www1.worldbank.org/publicsector/pe/PEAMMarch2005/CMHReport.pdf.

Wong, W. B., S. D. Ramsey, W. E. Barlow, L. P. Garrison, Jr., and D. L. Veenstra. 2012. The value of comparative effectiveness research: projected return on investment of the RxPONDER trial (SWOG S1007). *Contemp Clin Trials* 33 (6):1117–1123.

Woods, B., P. Revill, M. Sculpher, and K. Claxton. 2015. *Country-Level Cost-Effectiveness Thresholds: Initial Estimates and the Need for Further Research. CHE Research Paper 109.* York, UK: Centre for Health Economics, University of York. https://www.york.ac.uk/media/che/documents/papers/researchpapers/CHERP109_cost-effectiveness_threshold_LMICs.pdf.

World Health Organization. 2013. Launch of the World Health Report 2013: Research for Universal Health Coverage. WHO. www.who.int/dg/speeches/2013/whr_20130815/en/.

World Health Organization. 2016. "Cost Effectiveness and Strategic Planning (WHO-CHOICE)." Accessed January 8. http://www.who.int/choice/cost-effectiveness/en/.

Yang, B. M. 2009. The future of health technology assessment in healthcare decision making in Asia. *Pharmacoeconomics* 27 (11):891–901.

Zauber, A. G., I. Lansdorp-Vogelaar, A. B. Knudsen, J. Wilschut, M. van Ballegooijen, and K. M. Kuntz. 2008. Evaluating test strategies for colorectal cancer screening: a decision analysis for the U.S. Preventive Services Task Force. *Ann Intern Med* 149 (9):659–669.

2

Theoretical Foundations
of Cost-Effectiveness Analysis
in Health and Medicine

David O. Meltzer, Anirban Basu, and Mark J. Sculpher

2.1 INTRODUCTION

Cost-effectiveness analysis (CEA) is intended to provide guidance as to how to make decisions to maximize desired outcomes given constraints, most commonly financial constraints. Economic theory suggests that guidance concerning decision making may be especially useful when decision makers do not fully understand or experience the benefits and costs of their decisions, or are unable to make decisions in their own interest, because decisions made under those circumstances may not lead to maximizing desired outcomes, such as the well-being (utility) of individual decision makers, given available resources.

There are many reasons to believe that guidance to support decision making may be especially useful in health and medicine. For example, in public health, or in situations in which healthcare is financed by public or private insurance, spending decisions are generally not tied to individuals' valuations of interventions because individuals typically do not bear the full costs of decisions about those interventions. To address the potential inefficiencies created by the gap between the cost of care and what patients pay for it, efficient resource allocation in health typically requires that payers and other public and private decision makers decide whether and how to cover services based on the costs and benefits of those services. Even when individuals bear all the benefits and costs of interventions, CEA may help individuals make better decisions by providing summary measures of benefits and costs and by integrating them into a coherent framework to maximize desired outcomes given available resources.

This chapter builds on concepts presented in Chapter 2 of the original Panel's book (Garber, A. M., M. C. Weinstein, G. W. Torrance, and M. S. Kamlet. 1996. "Theoretical Foundations of Cost-Effectiveness Analysis." In *Cost-Effectiveness in Health and Medicine*, edited by M. R. Gold, J. E. Siegel, L. B. Russell, and M. C. Weinstein, 25–53. New York: Oxford University Press).

While the theoretical foundations of CEA have been an area of active debate for as long as the field has been in existence, there is broad agreement that CEA is intended to provide information on how to maximize some objective or set of objectives subject to some constraint or set of constraints. This agreement is important because some of the most important ideas in CEA stem directly from principles of constrained optimization.

However, recognition that CEA arises out of the desire to maximize one or more objectives subject to one or more constraints raises important questions about what objectives should be maximized and what constraints exist and need to be considered. What objectives are to be valued? What resources are to be consumed and what opportunities will be foregone as a result? Without good answers to such questions, CEA cannot provide reliable guidance as to how to maximize desired objectives given available resources. However, such questions about how to define and measure benefits and costs are often difficult to answer in any given context and may be difficult to compare across contexts. Answering such questions involves both normative exercises (e.g., what values and constraints should we consider?) and positive exercises (e.g., how can we measure the values and constraints we wish to consider, and how do we best determine how to allocate resources to maximize some objective given a set of resource constraints?). Economic theory has much to contribute to answering such questions, but it is not sufficient to answer them fully.

Moreover, even among applications of CEA within health and medicine, where the objective is taken to be to maximize health or some objective function that includes health, there are multiple contexts in which decision makers may ask such questions. This may be particularly true in health systems (such as the US system) in which multiple levels and components of government influence health policy, and in which substantial decision making about resource allocation is delegated to private entities. Additional challenges are added by the growing use of CEA methods to inform not just the allocation of medical interventions, but coverage policies and even research priorities (see Chapter 1). Healthcare systems—often viewed from the perspective of single national payers or local healthcare authorities with defined budgets, such as those in some European countries—have played an important role in shaping perspectives on what costs to include in CEA. A perspective that is rationally taken by a decision maker in one context may not be appropriate in another context. For example, costs that result from a decision, but are not borne by the decision maker, may be seen as irrelevant by that decision maker.

Variations in perspective or methods that reflect differences in context also create challenges if one hopes to compare CEAs of different interventions to one another. The desire for comparability led the original Panel on Cost-Effectiveness in Health and Medicine and others to seek standardization in the conduct and reporting of CEAs through the creation of "Reference Cases." A Reference Case may specify how benefits or costs are to be measured or combined into measures of value, such as cost-effectiveness or net benefit. Myriad issues arise in such discussions, including how to define the objective function to be maximized (e.g., in terms of measures of health, the utility of individuals, or measures of social value); how to measure costs, including when the impact of a decision on the budget of one entity (e.g., individual, employer) may not reflect the full opportunity cost of a decision for all entities (i.e., opportunity costs from a societal perspective); and how to treat effects that are uncertain or that occur over time). How best to answer such questions will vary across decision makers according to the perspective they take. Differences between so-called welfarist views of CEA and extra-welfarist views discussed later in this chapter (see Section 2.4) often reflect differences in how benefits and costs are measured and valued. Pragmatic concerns, such as how decision makers in publicly financed healthcare systems may view budget impact, may also shape the choice of perspective and selection of one or more Reference Cases. Choices of Reference Cases are consequential because comparisons of results based on one Reference Case may not carry over to other perspectives.

Recommendations about the appropriate perspectives for the Reference Case analyses are taken up in Chapter 3. In the present chapter we discuss concepts that have provided a foundation for CEA methods and their application in various contexts. Accordingly, this chapter explores the theoretical basis of CEA with an emphasis on the perspectives that could be taken by various decision makers. In some cases, the perspective examined is one that does not reflect that of any actual decision maker but some theoretically attractive decision-making perspective, such as that of a representative consumer. In other cases, the perspective examined is that of actual decision makers, such as a national health authority. Actual decision makers may apply normative frameworks that cause them to neglect certain effects and costs of policies because they are not of direct concern to those decision makers or within their scope of interest or authority and responsibilities, even if they are of concern to others. For example, a national health authority might choose to make spending decisions to maximize health subject to its own budget, but neglect effects on other private or public budgets (e.g., patient costs due to co-payments or costs to pensions due to changes in survival). Decisions made based on such limited definitions of benefits or costs, generally fail to meet a critical criterion of optimal decision making if viewed from a broader perspective. The importance of a broader perspective motivated the original Panel to recommend that CEAs be carried out from a "societal" perspective, attempting to measure all benefits and costs, regardless of to whom they accrue. However, the concept of optimal decision making from a societal perspective also raises a number of challenges, such as how the objectives and constraints of individual decision-making entities (e.g., public sector organizations, private companies, and individual consumers) can all be appropriately reflected; and whether and how consensus can be reached with regard to how to define social value.

Economic theory describes one theoretically attractive standard for evaluating the optimality of resource allocation in a social context, which is that the standard makes it impossible to make any entity better off without making another worse off. This concept of "Pareto optimality" suggests the potential to measure benefits and costs from a societal perspective that is derived from measures of benefits (and costs) that accrue to individual decision makers (Pareto 2014). Economic theory suggests that voluntary, fully informed exchange between individuals is always Pareto improving in the sense that both parties must benefit from the exchange.

However, in considering policy decisions, it is generally not the case that no one is made worse off. To address this, the concept of Pareto optimality has been extended to support decisions based on *potential* Pareto improvements, which assess whether the benefits accruing to individuals are large enough that those persons could potentially transfer enough of those benefits to others who would otherwise be harmed so that everyone could potentially benefit. This is also known as the Kaldor-Hicks Criterion (Hicks 1939; Kaldor 1939). Because such transfers often do not occur in practice, this concept is critical in justifying the use of cost–benefit analysis (CBA), which is widely used to inform governmental decisions. The concept of potential Pareto improvement is also relevant in justifying the use of CEA. In the context of CEA, strong assumptions are required to assess whether potential Pareto improvement could occur because decisions can affect multiple individuals so that an approach is needed to compare the value of those effects across individuals. For example, when a decision positively affects the health or utility of some individuals and negatively affects the health or utility of others, assessing potential Pareto improvement requires accepting the validity of interpersonal comparisons of health or utility. Thus, accepting the recommendation of the original Panel for a "societal perspective" Reference Case that seeks to include all benefits and costs regardless of to whom they accrue requires a willingness to accept these strong assumptions. However, the need for such assumptions is not unique to the societal perspective; taking a "healthcare sector" perspective that maximizes health subject to a budget constraint also requires an assumption that the value of changes in health can be compared across individuals.

This chapter focuses on constrained optimization as the core principle underlying CEA and provides insights into important theoretical issues that are relevant in applying CEA, such as how to measure benefits and costs. These issues are critical to understanding the original Panel's efforts to articulate a societal perspective as a Reference Case, and the potential for other perspectives to be valuable Reference Cases, especially that of the healthcare sector. Accepting that any perspective will have important limits, our analysis highlights strategies that can be used to understand those limits and perform additional analysis to address them when possible. In addition to discussing Reference Case analyses, we also consider CEAs that reflect the perspectives of one or more critical stakeholders.

Following this introduction, this chapter proceeds with a discussion of the derivation of the concept of cost-effectiveness from principles of constrained optimization (Section 2.2). It then proceeds to discuss the valuation of effectiveness at the individual level (Section 2.3) and the population level (Section 2.4). Section 2.5 then discusses a number of specific areas that have been subjects of theoretical controversy, including with respect to the measurement of costs of time and costs projected to occur in the future. Section 2.6 covers a few newer theoretical issues that arise in using CEA to inform policy decisions in the context of heterogeneous populations in which individuals make choices and to use CEA to inform research priorities. Conclusions are summarized in Section 2.7.

2.2 COST-EFFECTIVENESS AS CONSTRAINED OPTIMIZATION

Constrained optimization is the process of identifying how to achieve the largest amount of some desired outcome or outcomes given one or more constraints. Such a process can be viewed as having multiple steps:

1. Define the set of possible intervention choices;
2. Identify the desired outcome or outcomes;
3. Identify the relevant constrained resource or resources;
4. Identify the outcomes (effects) and resources consequences (costs) associated with each of the possible choices;
5. Eliminate dominated choices;
6. Describe the trade-offs associated with all the possible choices and identify choices that are optimal given these trade-offs.

We address these six steps in order, focusing on major principles and areas of theoretical controversy. Although we describe these as steps, they can almost never be executed in a purely linear fashion because the completion of any one step may force re-examination of earlier steps.

2.2.1 Defining the Set of Possible Intervention Choices

The importance of defining the set of possible intervention choices is not an area of theoretical controversy. However, as discussed in Chapter 4, it is an essential first step in any CEA because it is not possible to determine whether any choice will produce the greatest level of benefits given available resources unless it has been compared to all other relevant potential choices.

Failure to consider all relevant options is far easier than it may appear. Alternative treatment options or medical interventions can easily be neglected. Analysts may miss the fact that an intervention can be applied in different populations or subpopulations. The timing of interventions (e.g., screening tests) can be varied with respect to start dates, frequency, or stopping dates. Some options may be neglected if they are not relevant because they are infeasible or are clearly dominated by alternatives. Additional concerns arise when interventions may be combined with each other and interact in terms of benefits or costs. When such interactions are substantial, comparisons are best made between alternative combinations of interventions.

Comparison of one intervention (or combination of interventions) to another that omits relevant alternatives cannot identify either alternative as producing the greatest benefit with limited resources; however, such a comparison may be useful in identifying cases in which one intervention (or combination of interventions) is preferred over another even if neither is best (as long as the limits to this simple comparison are understood).

2.2.2 Identifying the Desired Outcome or Outcomes

The identification of outcome or outcomes to be considered in a CEA is the subject of Chapter 6. If the interventions being considered have the potential to affect multiple outcomes that are valued, each must typically be measured. To develop measures of cost-effectiveness that provide clear guidance for decision making, it is useful to combine outcomes into a common metric. For example, effects on one or more health conditions or other determinants of well-being can be mapped into a measure of quality of life; survival to different ages can be combined to calculate life expectancy; and quality of life and survival can be combined into quality-adjusted life years (QALYs).

All such composite measures require assumptions, and these assumptions may have theoretical foundations that carry implications for how a CEA should be performed and its results interpreted. For example, if it is desired that a composite outcome measure be a measure of welfare, and outcomes are uncertain, then it may be valuable to refer to expected utility theory, which posits that the value of a set of uncertain outcomes equals the expected value of that set of outcomes. If these composite measures are used to inform decision making, it is important to understand the value judgments implicit in the assumptions required to justify these composite measures.

Because QALYs are the most commonly used composite measure of health outcomes in CEA in health and medicine, the theoretical basis of QALYs is of particular importance. Many analysts view QALYs as a measure of health and see the problem addressed by CEA as being to maximize health subject to relevant constraints, most commonly budget constraints. In contrast, other analysts view QALYs as a measure of utility or welfare and see the problem addressed by CEA as maximizing welfare subject to some budget constraint. This difference is important because if an analyst is comfortable providing guidance for policy decisions based only on health effects, then CEA results can immediately translate into policy decisions. In contrast, as discussed below, if analysts wish to make decisions in order to maximize welfare they must either find a way to reflect all relevant aspects of welfare in the CEA ratio or combine CEA with other approaches.

While the choice among such alternative assumptions may sometimes be driven largely by the intended meaning and use of the analysis, some assumptions may also be amenable to empirical assessment. For example, the key empirical findings supporting prospect theory (Kahneman and Tversky 1979) argue that individuals often do not make choices consistent with expected utility theory but instead value losses and gains differently and use heuristics in considering probabilities. If one believes that such choices reflect rational self-interest rather than cognitive errors, then such empirical evidence might imply that outcomes measures (such as QALYs) that specify composite outcomes by assuming that expected utility reflects patient value may be flawed.

Theoretical frameworks also sometimes present uncomfortable challenges. For example, if a QALY is viewed as reflecting individual utility in the sense in which the term *utility* is used within the context of neoclassical economic theory, then Arrow's Impossibility Theorem (Arrow 1950) has proved that is not possible to develop a single measure of the welfare of a population of persons that meets a set of basic assumptions about measuring welfare. Because a single outcome measure is typically needed to assess cost-effectiveness, this presents a challenge if the goal is to determine how to maximize welfare. When presented with such challenging implications of a theoretical framework, an analyst may respond in a number of ways. One is to reject the validity of approaches that violate these assumptions, but this leaves the analyst without an approach to address the original question posed. Another is to accept deviations from a welfare economic framework and argue that violation of the assumptions of the framework does not invalidate a set of conclusions. For example, one can assume that measures of utility are cardinal and can be compared and aggregated across individuals into measures of welfare at the population level. A final approach is to adopt an alternative theoretical framework. For example, an alternative perspective to the view that QALYs are a measure of utility is that QALYs are a measure of health. Depending on which of these perspectives one takes, the use of QALYs to support decision making could be viewed as maximizing either health or some (likely imperfect) measure of welfare at the population level subject to a budget constraint.

Whatever the measure of benefit chosen for CEA, it is important that the assumptions, value judgments, and limitations of CEA be understood and appropriately reflected as its results are used to inform decision making. This may be particularly important when the effects of an intervention on an important outcome are not well captured by the measure of benefit used. One example is when an intervention has effects on other individuals or on sectors (e.g., education, crime) that may not be well captured by QALYs. In such cases, delineating all the consequences of the intervention and the extent to which they are captured in the CEA framework and valuing them, when possible, is especially important if one wishes to use the analysis to guide decisions using a broader perspective, such as a societal one that seeks to incorporate effects on all affected parties. One approach to delineating consequences in this manner is the "Impact Inventory" recommended in this volume (see Chapter 4).

Although QALYs are most widely used in CEAs for interventions that affect both length and quality of life, there is also a long history of valuing the benefits of health interventions using other metrics. In CBA, the method of economic evaluation commonly used outside of healthcare, willingness to pay is used to combine different outcomes into a single metric that is measured in monetary terms (Office of Management and Budget 2003). Cost–benefit analysis is often favored by economists because of its connection to the Pareto principle or the potential Pareto improvement principle described above; if one person is—or would be—willing to pay another person an amount that that person is willing to accept in some transaction, that transaction must make both better off and therefore be Pareto improving, or potentially Pareto improving. In areas where exchanges occur in competitive markets, an additional advantage of CBA is that prices can often be used to infer value. In healthcare, because of insurance, the provision of care in the absence of ability to pay, and the provision of care through complex bundles, market-based transactions that meet the requirements for competitive markets and efficient market outcomes are the exception. This diminishes the attractiveness of willingness to pay as a measure of value in healthcare to some degree. Nevertheless, as an alternative, contingent valuation approaches may be used to survey individuals to ask their potential willingness to pay for specific interventions. While such approaches may be criticized for the hypothetical nature of the answers they provide, their results have been shown to correlate with actual decisions, and they are commonly used in economic evaluation (Brookshire, Coursey, and Schulze 1987).

Another, and probably more important, reason that many people—both patients and medical providers—may be reluctant to use CBA in healthcare is that they have an intrinsic reluctance to put an explicit monetary value on health, including survival. It is worth noting, however, that CEA does not avoid this in the sense that a cost-effectiveness threshold has to be defined to decide whether an intervention is cost-effective. As described below, principles of constrained maximization imply that the threshold should reflect the marginal benefit forgone by the existence of a constraint, for example, the marginal change in health outcomes associated with imposing additional cost on a budget constraint (often called the "shadow price" of the constraint). However, CEA differs from CBA in that it does not require that the actual value of a unit of health benefit be explicitly defined to identify an intervention as cost-effective. Instead, CEA requires only that one determine that the threshold is above the level of the cost-effectiveness ratio of the intervention being considered in order to assess whether the intervention is cost-effective.

Another reason that willingness to pay is often criticized is the likelihood that individuals with lower incomes will not be willing to pay as much to achieve an improved outcome as individuals with higher incomes, so that allocations based on willingness to pay would tend to allocate greater resources to more affluent persons. Though the strength of empirical evidence of greater valuation of health among wealthier persons is not clear (Viscusi and Aldy 2003), this is an often-cited reason that CEA has been more widely used than CBA.

These concerns with CBA must also be viewed within the context of distributional issues that arise with models that seek to maximize QALYs. How one thinks about the problem is fundamentally tied to the view one takes about the goals of decision makers and the organizations in which they operate, as well as how it is intended that CEA be used to achieve those goals. Such views could include that the objective of decision making and/or the use of CEA is to maximize some measure of social welfare tied as closely as possible to individual measures of utility (e.g., potential Pareto improvements), or that the goal is to maximize total QALYs, or that there is some other objective that is not based in classic welfare economics. For example, a distributional concern can be viewed as an equity constraint that effectively implies that a higher value be placed on outcomes for certain groups (Epstein et al. 2007). The implications of these alternative normative bases are discussed further below, and related considerations are explored in depth in Chapter 12.

2.2.3 Identifying the Relevant Constrained Resource or Resources

The constrained resource or resources that are relevant for a given CEA generally depend on the perspective or perspectives selected. Although constraints sometimes reflect limits on the quantity of a specific resource (e.g., livers available for transplantation or a finite supply of skilled clinical staff), resource constraints are most often reflected in budget constraints defined in monetary terms. Defining budget constraints typically requires identifying the amount of money available, all of the services consumed, and their associated prices. In a competitive market, such prices may equal costs, which is of particular interest when a CEA is performed from a societal perspective. However, prices are less likely to equal costs in the healthcare sector, where prices are often not set by competitive markets. Moreover, when CEA is performed from some perspectives, neglecting whole classes of costs may be appropriate. For example, a CEA conducted from the perspective of a payer might consider only costs borne by that payer, neglecting costs borne by the patient through co-payments or costs expected to occur after affected individuals are no longer insured by that payer. In contrast, a CEA performed from a patient perspective might not be concerned with costs borne by the insurer, unless those costs would eventually be passed on to patients, whereas co-payments or patient time costs would be valued. The narrow scope of such analyses may be considered a limitation for policy making, as it would ignore any costs covered by insurance. Similarly, a perspective that neglected patient costs would favor interventions even when they placed prohibitive costs on patients. Examples such as these illustrate why the original Panel argued that a Reference Case CEA should include all costs and benefits, regardless of to whom they accrue. This makes it possible to assess the potential for a decision to be Pareto improving by having individuals who pay the costs of health be compensated by those who are benefitting from the intervention.

An alternative view is that budget constraints reflect institutional arrangements established to balance conflicting and contradictory claims on resources. For example, the democratic process that exists in many countries can be viewed as establishing a socially legitimate "higher authority" that has shaped a series of decentralized decision-making institutions with broad responsibilities and associated budgets (Drummond et al. 2015). Under this view, the role of CEA is to inform decision makers in a way that understands their objectives and respects their constraints (including their budgets). A key element of CEA within this framework is to quantify the opportunity costs resulting from the budget constraint—that is, outcomes forgone when constrained resources are used in one way rather than another. Such opportunity costs can be quantified and reflected as the cost-effectiveness threshold, against which the incremental benefits of an option that imposes additional cost over that of a comparator can be assessed (i.e., comparing an ICER with a threshold) (Claxton et al. 2015).

In this context, a broader societal perspective can be viewed as ensuring that costs that fall on other budgets or effects that are outside the decision maker's set of objectives are also identified and quantified. The Impact Inventory recommended in this volume (see Chapter 4), can inform a broader debate and potentially influence the higher authority, for example, in setting the responsibilities and budgets of the decision-making institutions. Aggregation of costs and outcomes across sectors into a single metric indicating overall social value can be a guide to policy. However, to achieve this aggregation while also reflecting each sector's legitimate responsibilities and constraints is challenging methodologically; approaches exist, but they need further development (Claxton et al. 2010).

2.2.4 Identifying the Outcomes (Effects) and Resources Consequences (Costs) Associated with Each of the Possible Choices

Once the desired outcome(s) and constrained resource(s) have been identified, the effects of each of the possible choices on them must be delineated. Chapter 6, describes methods for estimating these effects. Chapter 8 focuses on issues in the measurement of costs.

2.2.5 Eliminating Dominated Choices

In comparing alternative interventions, some choices may be strictly dominated by—that is, be worse in both outcomes and costs than—one or more other choices. This is more likely to happen when outcomes are measured in terms of estimated means (expected value) and can be measured in a single dimension, such as relief of a single symptom, than when multiple outcomes are relevant. More typically, alternative choices improve some outcomes and worsen others. In such cases, aggregate measures of outcome, such as QALYs, may be used to suggest that the net effect of a choice on outcomes dominates the net effect of another choice. A related idea is extended dominance, which is illustrated in Figure 2.1. Extended dominance exists when the outcome of a choice (D) is dominated by a linear combination of two other choices (A, C), as represented by the line between A and C in Figure 2.1. Some investigators may find that the concept of extended dominance is better explained as being relevant when, in addition to the choice being examined (e.g., B vs A) there is an alternative option (C), which is more effective and has a lower ICER than D relative to A. Given a threshold, that option (D) can never be cost-effective.

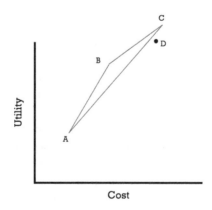

Figure 2.1 Illustration of extended dominance.

2.2.6 Describing the Trade-offs Associated with All Possible Choices and Identifying Choices That Are Optimal Given These Trade-offs

The core insight of CEA in health and medicine is that, in the absence of strictly dominated options, an optimal allocation of resources is defined by whether the ratio of changes in costs divided by changes in benefits is less than a cost-effectiveness threshold that represents the benefits forgone elsewhere as a result of committing constrained resources to the most effective set of options available given the overall level of available resources.

In any context, benefits and costs may be defined as appropriate to that context through the choice of the objective function and budget constraint. Specifying these correctly can be complicated. For that reason, it is useful to illustrate the basic principles using a more stylized framework of a representative consumer for whom benefits are defined by a utility function $U(c, m_1, m_2)$ that is a function of consumption, c, and two medical interventions, m_1 and m_2, where the goal is to maximize that individual's utility subject to a budget constraint defined by $p_c c + p_1 m_1 + p_2 m_2 = I$, where the p_c, p_1, and p_2 are the prices of consumption and goods 1 and 2, and I is income. These principles of constrained maximization can be presented in various ways, depending on the relevant objectives and constraints. Here a utility maximization framework is used reflecting conventional welfare economics. Other perspectives could be used (such as that of a national health agency) for defining benefits and costs. Many conclusions of constrained maximization, such as the importance of comparing marginal changes in benefits relative to costs, transcend the definitions of benefits and costs selected.

Taking this utility maximization perspective, the conditions for maximizing this utility function subject to the budget constraint can be derived by defining a Lagrange multiplier problem to maximize $L = U(c, m_1, m_2) + \lambda^*(I - p_c c - p_1 m_1 - p_2 m_2)$ by choosing levels c, m_1, and m_2. This is accomplished by maximizing L with respect to c, m_1, m_2, and λ. In Lagrange multiplier problems, λ has the interpretation of the increase in the objective function that arises with relaxation of the constraint, which is sometimes called the shadow price of the budget constraint, and also defines the cost-effectiveness threshold. In this case, in which the objective function is the utility function, λ is the marginal gain in utility per increased dollar of income, and it can also be interpreted as the shadow price of the budget constraint, which defines the cost-effectiveness threshold.

Maximizing L implies that an optimal allocation of c, m_1, and m_2 exists when:

$$p_1 / (\partial U / \partial m_1) = 1 / \lambda$$

$$p_2 / (\partial U / \partial m_2) = 1 / \lambda$$

$$p_c / (\partial U / \partial c) = 1 / \lambda, \text{ which together imply}$$

$$p_1 / (\partial U / \partial m_1) = p_2 / (\partial U / \partial m_2) = p_c / (\partial U / \partial c) = 1 / \lambda$$

and $I - p_c c - p_1 m_1 - p_2 m_2 = 0$

The conditions described by these equations can be interpreted in several related frameworks (Phelps and Mushlin 1991), including CEA, net health benefit (NHB), and net monetary benefit (NMB, more often called CBA). We shall consider each of these frameworks briefly, concluding with a brief discussion of decision rules.

2.2.6.1 *Cost-Effectiveness Analysis (CEA)*

The first two elements in the equations above are both ratios of costs (prices) divided by effectiveness (represented here as gains in utility with increases in use of medical interventions). The third term is the ratio of the cost of consumption to the utility gain that comes from consumption. All three of these terms take the general form of changes in costs (medical expenditure or consumption) per unit of resource use divided by the change in utility per unit of resource use. Thus, the ratios measure the cost per unit of effectiveness. Cost-effectiveness ratios emerge from optimization as the relevant statistic for determining optimal spending levels. Indeed, the last term $(1/\lambda)$ reflects the dollar value of a gain in utility. Equivalently, λ can be understood as the utility gain from an increase of one dollar in available resources.

The equality of all these ratios at the point of optimization implies that the cost of a gain in utility from spending on consumption and on each of the medical interventions should be equal. This provides the theoretical basis for the cost-effectiveness ratio. Since the incremental benefits of interventions generally decline as the quantity of intervention increases, spending more on consumption or a medical intervention than these optimal levels has smaller incremental benefits (i.e., $dU/\partial m$ is low) and therefore a higher cost-effectiveness ratio. In contrast, spending that is below optimal levels has greater incremental benefits (i.e., $\partial U/\partial m$ is high), and therefore a lower cost-effectiveness ratio. Thus, the decision rule of CEA is to pursue interventions for which the cost-effectiveness ratio is less than the dollar value of a gain in utility $(1/\lambda)$, which is often called the cost-effectiveness threshold.

2.2.6.2 *Net Health Benefit (NHB)*

Among the most widely cited innovations in CEA since publication of the original Panel's report is the concept of net health benefit (NHB) (Stinnett and Mullahy 1998), which describes the gain in health that comes from an intervention net of the opportunity cost in forgone health due to the resource required by that intervention. The term "net health benefit" is easiest to relate to CEA if CEA is viewed as maximizing health subject to a budget constraint. In this case, the utility function would depend only on health. However, the idea can be generalized to measure the gain in any measure of utility net of forgone utility due to resource costs. To see this, one can take the above equalities and multiply them by λ throughout to give them a form such as $\partial U/\partial m - \lambda p_m = 0$. The first term here is the utility gain from the medical intervention. Since λ is the utility that could be gained from added resources, and since p_m is the resources needed for that intervention, the second term is the utility forgone due to the resources required for the intervention. Thus, the equation describes the net benefit of the intervention after its costs are considered. At the optimum, the marginal net benefit should be zero. However, at levels below that margin, and when interventions are discrete, benefits will typically exceed costs so that intervention will have a net health benefit. In a net health benefit framework, all interventions with a positive net health benefit should be pursued.

2.2.6.3 *Net Monetary Benefit (NMB)*

If, instead of multiplying by λ, the above equalities are divided by λ and rearranged, they take the form $\partial U / \partial m / \lambda - p_m = 0$. In this case, the first term is the utility gain per unit of the intervention divided by the utility gain per dollar in added resources, which implies that the ratio is the dollar value of the gain in utility per unit of the intervention. Subtracting the cost of the intervention causes the expression to describe the net monetary benefit of the intervention (valued in dollars). As with the net health benefit this should be zero at the margin, but for suboptimal levels of utilization or interventions that are not continuous, the net monetary benefit will be positive.

2.2.6.4 *Decision Rules*

Whether using ICERs to perform traditional CEA, or using the NHB or NMB frameworks, CEA has the same fundamental grounding in constrained optimization, and in some sense the decision rules associated with all three frameworks are the same: interventions should be pursued if and only if their ICER is less than the cost-effectiveness threshold, which is the same as having a positive NHB or positive NMB. Below we discuss issues that may arise with any of these frameworks and cases in which their application in any given situation may make one or the other them preferable. It is worth noting, however, that several common practices in the use of CEA are not well supported by theory. For example, it is often said that an intervention is "highly cost-effective" when its cost-effectiveness ratio is far below an established cost-effectiveness threshold, or that one intervention is "more cost-effective" than another because it has a lower cost-effectiveness ratio. Neither statement is well grounded in theory. In each case, an intervention could have a very low cost-effectiveness ratio but a very small benefit and offer a smaller net benefit than other interventions with higher cost-effectiveness ratios. Cost-effectiveness theory based on constrained maximization implies that all interventions below a specified threshold should be implemented. As a result, it may be harmful for decision makers to prioritize interventions that appear "highly cost-effective" over other interventions with cost-effectiveness ratios that are higher but still below the established threshold for cost-effectiveness. As noted above, the broad use of insurance within healthcare to shield patients from financial risk makes the application of CEA particularly important because patients cannot be expected to take cost into account in their purchasing decisions. This presses payers— whether government or private—to think about costs and benefits of their purchasing decisions on behalf of patients. Within this context, private and public payers may have perspectives that differ from one another and that do not reflect the broader costs and benefits of their decisions. For example, a private payer with high turnover of enrolled patients may not be interested in longer term effects on costs of the patients they are responsible for. Even public decision makers may have very narrow perspectives if, for example, their budgeting process requires them to account only for costs that occur in the near term.

2.3 VALUING EFFECTIVENESS

The effects of health interventions are almost always highly multidimensional. At a basic level, these effects can be conceptualized as changes in the likelihood of a series of states of health, and perhaps other dimensions of well-being, occurring at various points in time over an individual's lifetime. The primary task of valuation is to determine how to assign values to these probability distributions of health states occurring over time. As discussed below, uncertainty is often addressed by reliance on expected utility theory to calculate the expected or average outcome. The distribution of outcomes over time is often addressed by adding up outcomes over time, while discounting future outcomes. Below and in Chapter 10, we discuss the rationale for discounting health outcomes over time, which is typically justified based on the idea that utility in the present is more valuable than utility in the future, but this has been an area of continuing controversy (see also Chapter 12).

Perhaps the most challenging and controversial aspect of valuing health outcomes is the assignment of value to specific health states. Health states include whether an individual is alive or dead, and an essentially infinite number of possible combinations of specific health outcomes among the living. The vast number of potential outcomes implies that one health intervention will rarely dominate another in all ways and motivates efforts to combine outcomes into a common metric of value. Chapter 7 provides an in-depth discussion of approaches to assessing the valuation of these health states in a common metric, focusing on QALYs. QALYs are the sum of the number of years lived (or expected to be lived), weighting each year by a quality of life weight between 0 and 1, where 0 is equal to dead and 1 is equal to perfect health, and intermediate states are valued between 0 and 1 using a range of techniques with a basis in economics, psychology, and decision science. The possibility of negative values representing states worse than death is discussed in Chapter 7.

Most CEA analysts consider QALYs measures of health. Others may see them as measures of utility and/or wish to connect them to underlying principles of welfare economics. The rationale for thinking of QALYs as a measure of health is primarily that QALYs are calculated by combining survival probabilities and quality-of-life measures, and most quality-of-life measures used to define health states for QALYs are defined only by health status. The primary rationale for thinking of QALYs as a measure of utility or welfare is that maximizing welfare may be seen as a more general objective for decision making than maximizing health, because health is clearly not the sole determinant of welfare. For example, consumption of other goods clearly affects well-being and may do so in ways that interact with health in complex ways.

For those who aspire to connect QALYs and utility theory, a number of important issues must be addressed. Key early contributions by Pliskin, Shepard, and Weinstein (1980) and Johannesson, Pliskin, and Weinstein (1993) described a set of non-trivial conditions about preferences with respect to length and quality of life that are required for QALYs to be consistent with utility theory that implicitly or explicitly view these measures as a comprehensive measure of welfare. Bleichrodt and Quiggin (1999) demonstrate that if individuals' utility functions are multiplicative in health-related quality of life and consumption, and they are willing to trade off length of life for quality of life at a constant rate, and they are risk neutral, then maximizing QALYs will maximize utility. Hammitt (2013) generalizes this finding while also pointing out that even a minimal set of assumptions needed to derive QALYs may not be plausible. Indeed, a number of assumptions made in estimating QALYs may be problematic. For example, the standard gamble approach to utility assessment asks individuals to consider alternative gambles over combinations of the probability of survival and quality of life. As a result, the valuation of these gambles is likely to be affected by risk aversion, producing bias in estimates of valuations of risk-free health states.

Given the uncertainty in future health states, expected utility theory (Raiffa 1968; von Neumann and Morgenstern 1944) is often used to combine a probability distribution of outcomes into an "expected value" that reflects the average of outcomes. The classic treatment of expected utility theory takes an axiomatic approach to deriving expected utility from a set of core principles and tends to view expected utility maximization as a "normative" behavior, deviations from which may be considered to be errors. In some cases, potential deviations from the assumptions of the standard expected utility framework have been shown to be capable of being incorporated into the expected utility framework (Arrow 1965; Machina 1982; Pratt 1964) with only minimal assumptions. In other cases, critiques are more fundamental. For example, Kahneman and Tversky (1979) describe specific patterns by which actual decisions deviate from those predicted by expected utility theory. The replicability of such patterns suggests that, although they could be considered cognitive errors, they might also reflect ways in which expected utility theory fails to capture preferences in the context of uncertainty (Abdellaoui, Bleichrodt, and Paraschiv 2007). This said, there is also evidence to suggest that elements of expected utility theory (e.g., probabilities, health state valuations) have the ability to predict choices of individuals, suggesting that the construct possesses at least some level of predictive validity. If one takes the perspective that the ability to predict behaviors, as opposed to having a basis in logical axioms, should form the basis of theoretical foundation for valuation, it follows that the predictive power of alternative theories (i.e., expected utility theory, prospect theory) should determine the choice of methods (Friedman 1953). Alternatively, if decisions that are not consistent with expected utility theory are viewed as errors, such findings are of less concern.

2.4 FROM INDIVIDUALS TO POPULATIONS

While CEA can be applied at the level of a single individual, and key principles of CEA can be derived from maximization models described at the individual level, CEA is typically applied at the population level. The extension of CEA from individuals to populations raises a range of issues depending on the underlying theoretical framework being considered.

When CEA is viewed as maximizing health or some other measure of benefit other than individual utility (e.g., Culyer [1991] and Williams [1993]), it is often not a controversial step to extend the concept of maximizing the health of an individual (measured, e.g., by life expectancy or quality-adjusted life expectancy) to maximizing the health of a population [measured using the same metric(s)]. This is not to say that alternative approaches do not exist; analysts typically weight the life expectancy of all persons equally, but arguments have been made on grounds of equity to weight the outcomes of individuals differently, for example, putting the most weight on those individuals who are worse off (Bleichrodt, Diecidue, and Quiggin 2004). Recognizing the potential for differences in preferences among individuals also raises questions about whose preferences to use in performing CEA. It has been argued by some that average preferences in society should be measured because society often bears the costs of the interventions; alternatively, it has been argued that the preferences of individuals should be used, as they are the ones who will experience the health states.

When CEA is viewed as seeking to maximize welfare, the challenges of moving from models of welfare maximization at the individual level to models of welfare maximization at the population level become even more complex. Indeed, attempts to characterize the welfare of populations run throughout the history of utilitarian thought. In the case of strict utilitarianism, building from the welfare of individuals to the welfare of populations occurs by adding the utilities in some way. Approaches to welfare economics that build on individual preferences are both in keeping with the traditions of welfare economics and consistent with current concepts of patient-centered outcomes research that recognize and seek to tailor medical decisions to individuals based on their attributes, including preferences. Strict aggregation of individual utilities, in which utilities are defined as cardinal measures of individual welfare, has long been recognized (and criticized) as inherently subjective. Accordingly, there has been an emphasis on ordinal measures of utility as the basis of welfare economics. However, it was not until the seminal contributions of Arrow (1963) that it was appreciated that there is no aggregation of individual preferences into a social welfare function that can satisfy a minimal set of foundational principles (unrestricted domain, non-dictatorship, Pareto efficiency, and independence of irrelevant alternatives). Normative frameworks that justify maximizing QALYs as a measure of population welfare have been derived based on conditions in which individuals make decisions about social resource allocation behind a "veil of ignorance," where they may be aware of the possible outcomes and their likelihood but are unaware of which outcomes they themselves will experience (Harsanyi 1953, 1955, 1975; Kamlet 1992; Keeney 1976; Keeney and Kirkwood 1975; Rawls 1971).

Welfare economic foundations have also been criticized for not recognizing that social values may differ from individual values so that societal measures of welfare cannot be derived solely from individual measures of welfare. Such "extra-welfarist" (Williams 1993) views argue that CEA should not be concerned about whether its approaches are rooted in welfare economics. For example, while welfare economics might be used to argue that a change in allocation of resources should be preferred when it produces a potential Pareto improvement, an extra-welfarist perspective could argue that meeting such a compensation test criterion is not adequate to ensure that welfare increases because society has preferences over the distribution of welfare among individuals. Some normative frameworks (e.g., that of Rawls [1971]) argue that social well-being is defined by the worst-off member of society and reject the QALY framework. Accepting that argument would require a rejection of the Pareto principle, because changes in welfare at the individual level would imply improved social welfare only if they improve the welfare of the worst-off member of society with no weight given to changes in the welfare of others. It is not surprising that such pure Rawlsian principles have not been found highly useful in forming the theoretical foundations of CEA even when distributional concerns are widely recognized as important. Even when approaches to equity concerns are less extreme, however, their impact on CEA has been greatly limited by lack of agreement on whether and how individual preferences should be aggregated to best reflect aggregate social welfare under various patterns of resource allocation (Sen, 1995).

This is not to say, however, that distributional or altruistic concerns have had no place in the development of CEA. Indeed, practices such as the one mentioned above, in which average wages rather than individual wages are used to value time, reflect such concerns. Similarly, even those theorists who rely heavily on welfare economics as a framework for CEA have explored how altruistic concerns among individuals (e.g., in the family) that cause benefits and costs of medical interventions to "spill over" onto others may be incorporated into CEA (Basu and Meltzer 2005). Health may also be considered by some to be a "merit" good, an economic term that refers to a good that is valued by other persons independent of how it is valued by the individual whose health is affected. Distributional concerns have also played a role in shaping methodological debates about issues such as discounting health benefits; if costs are discounted at a different rate than benefits, then it may make sense for current generations either to consume all resources or to push as much consumption as possible infinitely far into the future (Gold et al. 1996, 219–221) unless there are countervailing forces, such as changes over time in the value of health (Claxton et al. 2011; Gold et al. 1996, 219–221; van Hout 1998). Discounting is discussed further below and in Chapter 10. More recent work has also examined distributional issues related to the financial effects of healthcare programs for individuals and groups (Asaria et al. 2015; Verguet, Laxminarayan, and Jamison 2015).

The lack of agreement on an extra-welfarist framework for social decision making, and Arrow's work establishing the impossibility of developing a ranking system that satisfies even a basic set of apparently reasonable requirements of a pure welfare-economic framework, suggest the need for caution in applying any single framework to develop an approach to CEA in health and medicine. Instead, these models can be reasonably understood as tools to approximate what might be more ideal representations of value (Garber and Phelps 1997; Arrow, personal communication). From this perspective, welfare economic principles may not be able to provide satisfying answers to some methodological questions but may still be highly informative for others. The critical challenge is to understand, for any given question, whether welfare economics provides insight into the question, under what conditions, and what the advantages and disadvantages are of translating those insights into practice.

For example, economic theory implies clearly that the value people place on an hour of their leisure time can be inferred from their hourly wage (net of taxes). Accordingly, an analyst could decide to value time in a CEA at individuals' wages. However, some decision makers might reasonably find the distributional consequences of decisions based on such a valuation unacceptable and choose to use average wages to value time in all instances. From a welfare-economic perspective, such decisions carry costs in terms of lost welfare. However, there has not been research to establish that a more detailed accounting of variation in the value of time across individuals would produce a substantially different pattern of resource allocation. In the absence of such data, it is not unreasonable to adopt assumptions such as these that may be more attractive from a normative perspective.

This is also consistent with what has been described as the social decision-making approach to economic analysis (Sugden and Williams 1978). This argues that, given the impossibility of a consensual definition of social welfare (whether based on individual preferences or an extra-welfarist range of considerations), CEA provides a partial means of informing decisions. From this perspective, decision-making institutions can be seen as representing an (imperfect) expression of social preferences, and the objectives they are held accountable for and the constraints under which they operate should be the starting point for analysis to guide resource allocation. Thus, under a social decision-making framework, CEA is a means of presenting the potential gains in relevant benefits (defined by decision makers' objectives) of alternative options and opportunity costs (implied by their budget and other constraints). Analysts may also seek to provide information on costs and effects that fall outside of the decision maker's immediate purview, as this can inform a wider debate about resource allocation and policy.

Conclusions like these are consonant with the idea that CEA methods are designed to provide useful data to inform decisions (rather than to dictate them). A theoretical assumption that seems to prevent CEA from being useful will typically be reexamined and adjusted. This interplay between theory and practical application is among the most challenging issues in exploring the theoretical foundations of CEA.

2.5 SPECIFIC AREAS OF THEORETICAL CONTROVERSY

2.5.1 Optimization with Multiple Budget Constraints

The maximization problem described above, in which there is a single objective function and a single budget constraint, is generally viewed as the classic problem of constrained optimization in economics and yields the intuitive result that the last dollar of spending for each use of funds should yield the same amount of incremental benefit. However, in some situations, budgets may not be mutable across purposes. For example, a government might have a fixed healthcare budget and a fixed budget for non-healthcare expenditures. In such cases, the maximization problem for a decision maker might be to spend money in each category to maximize the objective function subject to these two budget constraints. In the example cited earlier, in which there is a single budget constraint (Maximize $L = U(c, m_1, m_2) + \lambda^*(I - p_c c - p_1 m_1 - p_2 m_2)$ over c, m_1, m_2 and λ) might become $L = U(c, m_1, m_2) + \lambda_{NonHealth}^*(I_{NonHealth} - p_c c) - \lambda_{Health}^*(I_{Health} - p_1 m_1 - p_2 m_2)$ over c, m_1, m_2, $\lambda_{NonHealth}$ and λ_{Health}. In this case the choice of c is trivial because any part of the budget not spent on health goes to consumption, but there is a choice about how much to spend on medical interventions 1 and 2 (m_1 and m_2); the amounts selected would generally not be the same as if a single budget constraint applied to both. Moreover, the incremental benefit of spending on medical care and consumption would not generally be equal, so that λ_c and λ_m would not be equal. An example such as this could be extended to the more realistic case of multiple sectors with separate budgets: for example, healthcare, public health, education, and criminal justice. The different valuations of spending in these sectors (in terms of individuals' willingness to forgo consumption to experience those outcomes) in turn might have implications for the welfare implications of "spillovers" across sectors. For example, with two budget-constrained sectors—say, public health and education—it would be possible to maximize sector-specific benefits using CEA and a cost-effectiveness threshold based on the shadow price of the budget constraint (λ_m). Public health may be considered underfunded if the value of a marginal dollar spent (in terms of individuals' consumption) on public health exceeds the value of a marginal dollar spent in other sectors (e.g., education).

Reallocation of resources across sectors would seem to be an obvious solution in such cases. However, whether a higher authority (e.g., the US federal government) would consider this a basis for a reallocation of resources between the sectors is unclear because there may be reasons why individuals' valuations of the outcomes of different sectors (in terms of their willingness to forgo consumption) should not reflected in the cost-effectiveness thresholds/shadow prices of those specific budget allocations (Drummond et al. 2015). First, there may be differential costs associated with the process of raising funds for collectively funded activities like healthcare and public education, so it may be quite appropriate not to allocate funding to the point where the cost-effectiveness thresholds equal the consumption values of the outcomes. Second, individuals' willingness to forgo consumption to enjoy the benefits of these budget-constrained sectors is not the same as cost-effectiveness thresholds. The latter reflects how much society is willing to devote to these activities given the range of social objectives, relevant constraints, and other claims on pooled resources. Therefore, the consumption value of outcomes from budget-constrained sectors will equal the cost-effectiveness thresholds of those sectors only under several strong assumptions: that governments seek to allocate budgets to collectively funded activities such as healthcare and education on the basis of individuals' preferences; that these preferences are reflected completely through social decision making and political processes; and that there are not differential costs involved in raising funding across these sectors.

These issues represent an important challenge in implementing a societal perspective in CEA because of the need to reflect the constraints that operate in each sector and the implied cost-effectiveness thresholds associated with those constraints, and the associated need to provide a definition of social welfare (social welfare function). In this context, a disaggregated approach to presenting the range of costs and effects falling in the different budget-constrained sectors, on consumption, and on the wider economy may be helpful. The Impact Inventory discussed in Chapter 4 is an example of such an approach.

2.5.2 Measuring Time Costs

The valuation of time is a common concern in CEA from a societal perspective. Time may be valued in several different contexts, including in the workplace and at home, and it is important to identify the right approach for any given context. For example, when an intervention extends length of life, time is typically valued through QALYs. When an intervention has effects on the amount of leisure time a patient or family member has, time may also sometimes be viewed as being valued through a change in QALYs, but as a dimension of quality of life. The extent to which this is an appropriate assumption depends on the extent to which the quality-of-life measure reflects that leisure time. This is partially an empirical matter related to the context of the health state for which quality of life is affected and how utility is assessed. Complex issues in accounting for time also arise because health status (and even consumption) is often produced using time in addition to market inputs (Becker 1965; Feeny 2000). For example, quality of life could be assessed for a home dialysis regimen that requires 10 minutes of set-up per day vs one that requires 1 hour of set-up per day. If the health states are clearly defined, then it is plausible that the value of time would be well assessed in the context of quality-of-life measurement. In such a case, it would be double counting to explicitly account for the cost of time again in some other way. In contrast, imagine a comparison of two one-time treatments in which one took 10 min and the other took an hour. In such a context, it is unlikely that any quality-of-life measure could be meaningfully applied to assess the value of that single event. Based on this example, a direct valuation of the cost of time would be indicated. Another example in which direct measurement of the cost of time would be appropriate would be if the health state was not viewed as reflecting differences in leisure time. Using the dialysis example above, this might happen, for instance, if a generic quality-of-life measure was collected among people with a given condition (e.g., end-stage renal disease) but did not reflect differences in leisure time depending on treatment modality.

When a direct valuation of the cost of time is indicated because it is not reflected in quality-of-life measures, the appropriate concept of opportunity cost should be used. An example is when an intervention causes an hour of leisure time to be lost.

Economic theory suggests that if someone is not working, then the value to them of an hour of their leisure should be worth at least as much to them as they could earn by working. In economic terms, this would equal their after-tax wage rate. This would typically be calculated as their hourly wage rate multiplied by (1— their marginal tax rate). Note that this valuation of time would be a lower bound on the value of leisure, as leisure must be worth at least this much to explain the decision not to work. As a result, it is generally assumed that a small incremental amount of leisure would not be worth more than the wage rate if taxes were not an issue, because the added leisure is assumed to be happening at the margin, and thus to be just worth the forgone earnings. Thus, the value of leisure would often be assumed to equal the after-tax wage rate. This assumption may be less valid for large changes in leisure or for persons who choose not to work, because the value of leisure may differ greatly from the wage rate in those contexts. Nevertheless, average wage rates and taxes are often used for convenience. Average wage and tax rates may also sometimes be used for ethical reasons. Ethical concerns might arise if an affected group's actual wage rate were used if the group affected by an intervention had a very low hourly wage, so that saving their leisure time would be viewed as having no value. An example might be a severely mentally disabled group who could not maintain any employment. Strategies to consider in cases such are discussed further in Chapter 12.

A related issue arises when an intervention is viewed as reducing time spent working. Economic theory again provides some insight; if employers are paying workers a wage to work and also paying their fringe benefits, then the output those workers produce must (at the margin) be equal to their wages plus the cost of their benefits. Such a "loaded" wage rate would be an appropriate one to use in valuing lost productivity. Some investigators might argue that even this estimate of the opportunity cost of time is too low if the productivity of co-workers is adversely affected by someone's absence. Again, seeking specific evidence for such effects would be appropriate.

A final case worth considering is one in which a medical intervention requires time, but it is not clear whether that time would result in reduced leisure or reduced hours worked. Because the marginal value of leisure time is below wage rates after taxes and above wage rates after including the cost of fringe benefits, these two estimates might provide a range of estimates of the value of time that might be examined.

2.5.3 Multi-period Decision Making

The above model of cost-effectiveness describes a simple one-period model, but because health can affect survival, it is usual to examine the cost-effectiveness of health and medical interventions in a multi-period framework that reflects the effects of health interventions over time, including effects on both survival and health outcomes over time, as well as related effects on costs. From a welfarist perspective, such a multi-period perspective is naturally modeled as part of a lifetime utility maximization problem. However, essentially the same issues may arise in other multi-period maximization problems, such as a healthcare system trying to determine how to allocate healthcare budgets over time to maximize health outcomes.

To address such problems, it is necessary to make some assumptions about how to consider uncertainty in outcomes (especially survival) at the individual and population levels. To move from the individual level to the population level, the uncertainty inherent in survival at the individual level can be modeled either as the expected utility of a representative individual or of a population of individuals. Claxton (1999) and Meltzer (2001) have shown that the average outcomes and costs provide sufficient statistics for decision making if the objective is to maximize expected outcomes net of costs or that risks are small or readily diversifiable and hence can be neglected. This is not true if decision makers are risk averse, if that risk aversion is a legitimate consideration in analyses supporting decision making, and if the risks being considered are large. Because maximizing the expected utility for a representative individual is analytically easier than maximizing the welfare of a population of individuals, we use the former to develop a framework for CEA.

Thus, similar to the framework used in Meltzer (1997) and Garber and Phelps (1997), lifetime utility can be viewed as a discounted sum of the expected utility of health outcomes. Utility in any given period can be viewed as depending on consumption of goods in that period and health in that period $U_t(C, H_t)$. While both survival and health conditional on survival could be treated as uncertain, from an expositional perspective it is easier to treat health given survival as deterministic. Let S_t be the probability of surviving to age t. In addition, utility in future periods is assumed to matter less than utility in current periods, typically following a discounting function β^t where $\beta < 1$. Combining these, the expected lifetime utility of a representative individual is the probability-weighted sum over all potential time periods of the utility at each time $S_t U_t(C_t, H_t)$. Using these principles, similar to Meltzer (1997), it is possible to set out a model for the individual's lifetime consumption of healthcare, funded from that individual's own income stream. Health expenditure $m_i(t)$ on technology i at time t is chosen so as to maximize lifetime utility as follows:

$$\max_{\{m_{i(t)}\}_{i=1}^n} EU = \sum_{t=0}^{T} \beta^t S(t)U(t)$$

where

$U(t) = U(C(t), H(t))$

$S(t) = S(m(j): j = 0,1,\ldots,t-1)$ is probability of survival to period t

$$m(j) = \sum_{i=1}^{n} m_i(j)$$

$H(t) = H(m(j): j = 0,1,\ldots,t-1)$ is health status at period t

$H(0) = H_0$

With income in period t of $I(t)$, the associated lifetime budget constraint is:

$$\sum_{t=0}^{T}\left(\frac{1}{1+r}\right)^{t} S(t)\left(C(t)+\sum_{i=1}^{n}m_{i}(t)\right)=\sum_{t=0}^{T}\left(\frac{1}{1+r}\right)^{t} S(t)I(t)$$

where

$I(t)$ is income in period t

$C(t)$ is non-health consumption n in period t

yielding the set of first-order conditions for $m_{i}(t)$:

$$\frac{\left(\frac{1}{1+r}\right)^{t} S(t)+\sum_{\tau=T}^{T}\left(\frac{1}{1+r}\right)^{\tau}\frac{\partial S(\tau)}{\partial m_{i}(\tau)}\left(C(\tau)+\sum_{j=1}^{n}m_{j}(\tau)-I(\tau)\right)}{\sum_{\tau=t}^{T}\beta^{t}\left[\frac{\partial S(\tau)}{\partial m_{i}(t)}U(\tau)+S(\tau)\frac{\partial U(\tau)}{\partial m_{i}(t)}\right]}=\frac{1}{\lambda}=\mu$$

where λ is the shadow price of lifetime income. The parameter μ indicates the threshold level that determines the quantity of each treatment, reflecting the opportunity cost of medical care in the form of forgone lifetime consumption opportunities.

These equations provide the theoretical basis for CEA applied to an individual's consumption of health services, in which the benefits of healthcare to the individual are balanced against the opportunity costs, expressed in the consumption opportunities forgone by the individual. The denominator represents the benefits accruing from the intervention, expressed in terms of the increased duration and quality of life. The numerator represents the expected increased costs associated with the planned use of the intervention at time t; the first term is the discounted expected cost of spending at time t, whereas the second term is the change in expected future costs beyond time t because of the changes in survival to different ages due to that spending, multiplied by net resource use at that age. It is this second term that is the basis for the need to include future costs in CEAs if they are to be performed from a societal perspective. Though an early analysis by Garber and Phelps (1997) suggested such future costs could be neglected without changing the ranking of medical interventions, that result holds only when net resource use (consumption + medical expenditure – earnings) is zero at all ages, which is clearly not the case. In contrast, failing to include future costs will bias analyses to favor interventions that extend life over interventions that improve the quality of life, at least among older persons, where net resource use is positive.

Multi-period CEA also raises issues in a QALY framework about changes over time in the consumption value of health, that is, how changes in health (QALYs) translate into changes in utility. To see this, it is useful to rewrite the above equation invoking the necessary condition for the derivation of QALYs noted above; namely, that utility functions are multiplicative in health-related quality of life and consumption (Bleichrodt and Quiggin 1999).

$$\frac{\left(\dfrac{1}{1+r}\right)^t S(t) + \displaystyle\sum_{\tau=T}^{T}\left(\dfrac{1}{1+r}\right)^\tau \dfrac{\partial S(\tau)}{\partial m_i(\tau)}\left(C(\tau) + \displaystyle\sum_{j=1}^{n} m_j(\tau) - I(\tau)\right)}{\displaystyle\sum_{\tau=t}^{T}\beta^t\left[\dfrac{\partial S(\tau)}{\partial m_i(t)}U(c(\tau))H(\tau) + S(\tau)U(c(\tau))\dfrac{\partial H(\tau)}{\partial m_i(t)}\right]} = \frac{1}{\lambda} = \mu$$

This equation illustrates that variation in the utility of consumption over time will change the value of improvements in health, making the translation of improvements in health into improvements in utility a complex calculation. Hammitt (2013) describes the conditions one must place on the structure of the utility function for changes in QALYs to be able to reflect changes in utility, and Claxton et al. (2011) discuss how changes in the consumption value of health over time might affect how the value of future benefits might be discounted, as well as associated thresholds for determining cost-effectiveness. This is discussed further in Chapter 10. Note that if the utility of consumption is constant over time, then it can be taken out of the denominator and multiplied to the threshold λ. Therefore, even with the multi-period framework and accounting for future costs, QALY maximization is equivalent to utility maximization (Bleichrodt and Quiggin 1999).

2.6 METHODS FOR SPECIFIC DECISION-MAKING PERSPECTIVES

2.6.1 Policy Making, Heterogeneity, and Choice

Many CEAs pertain to whether it is better that one or another approach to health-care be applied in specific clinical situations. The specificity of a given clinical situation can be defined based on any number of patient or clinical character-istics, which could include both objective attributes (e.g., age) and subjective attributes (e.g., preferences). However, even when analyses and resulting recom-mendations are quite specific, most policy decisions informed by CEAs do not mandate that one or the other approach be followed. Instead, decision makers (patients, clinicians, healthcare institutions) make choices based on those analy-ses, and those choices, in turn, affect outcomes. This distinction is important because those choices will vary among decision makers in ways that are likely to be systematically related to attributes of the decision maker that can affect outcomes. For example, a patient who prefers one approach to another may be more likely to choose that approach, or a provider (e.g., a surgeon) who is better at applying one approach may be more likely to use that approach. In modeling studies, these choices imply that use of average patient attributes to model out-comes of policies may be biased. They also suggest that approaches that incor-porate variation in patient preferences into models of decision making and value may be more accurate predictors of the effects of policies (Basu and Meltzer 2007; Meltzer et al. 2005).

2.6.2 Research Prioritization

Value-of-information (VOI) analysis is another example of where policy makers may use cost-effectiveness methods to inform policy making. This is addressed in greater detail in Chapter 11, but it essentially seeks to estimate the expected value of research by comparing the expected value of the best decision that can be made in the absence of research to the expected value of the best decision that can be made in the presence of research. A major challenge in these analyses is obtaining information on a priori and a posteriori probabilities that describe the likelihood of various outcomes both before and after research is performed. A range of techniques have arisen to try to bound VOI estimates in the context of limited information. These are discussed in Chapter 11.

2.7 CONCLUSIONS

Stemming from principles of constrained optimization, CEA in health and medicine seeks to maximize health outcomes given finite resources. Economic models, including ones rooted in welfare economics, can provide valuable insights into methods for CEA, although such models do not always provide straightforward guidance for many practical applications of CEA. Clarity concerning the objectives of CEA is critical in deciding when theoretical foundations are used to inform practice.

2.8 REFERENCES

Abdellaoui, M., H. Bleichrodt, and C. Paraschiv. 2007. Loss aversion under prospect theory: a parameter-free measurement. *Manage Sci* 53 (10):1659–1674.

Arrow, K. J. 1950. A difficulty in the concept of social welfare. *J Polit Economy* 58 (4):328–346.

Arrow, K. J. 1963. *Social Choice and Individual Values*. 2nd ed. New Haven: Yale University Press.

Arrow, K. J. 1965. *Aspects of the Theory of Risk Bearing*. Helsinki: Yrjö Jahnssonin Säätiö.

Asaria, M., S. Griffin, R. Cookson, S. Whyte, and P. Tappenden. 2015. Distributional cost-effectiveness analysis of health care programmes—a methodological case study of the UK Bowel Cancer Screening Programme. *Health Econ* 24 (6):742–754.

Basu, A., and D. Meltzer. 2005. Implications of spillover effects within the family for medical cost-effectiveness analysis. *J Health Econ* 24 (4):751–773.

Basu, A., and D. Meltzer. 2007. Value of information on preference heterogeneity and individualized care. *Med Decis Making* 27 (2):112–127.

Becker, G. S. 1965. A theory of the allocation of time. *Econ J* 75 (299):493–517.

Bleichrodt, H., E. Diecidue, and J. Quiggin. 2004. Equity weights in the allocation of health care: the rank-dependent QALY model. *J Health Econ* 23 (1):157–171.

Bleichrodt, H., and J. Quiggin. 1999. Life-cycle preferences over consumption and health: when is cost-effectiveness analysis equivalent to cost-benefit analysis? *J Health Econ* 18 (6):681–708.

Brookshire, D. S., D. L. Coursey, and W. D. Schulze. 1987. The external validity of experimental economics techniques: analysis of demand behavior. *Econ Inq* 25 (2):239–250.

Claxton, K. 1999. The irrelevance of inference: a decision-making approach to the stochastic evaluation of health care technologies. *J Health Econ* 18 (3):341–364.

Claxton, K., S. Martin, M. Soares, N. Rice, E. Spackman, S. Hinde, N. Devlin, P. Smith, and M. Sculpher. 2015. Methods for the estimation of the National Institute for Health and Care Excellence cost-effectiveness threshold. *Health Technol Assess* 19 (14) 1–503.

Claxton, K., M. Paulden, H. Gravelle, W. Brouwer, and A. J. Culyer. 2011. Discounting and decision making in the economic evaluation of health-care technologies. *Health Econ* 20 (1):2–15.

Claxton, K., S. Walker, S. Palmer, and M. Sculpher. 2010. *Appropriate Perspectives for Health Care Decisions. CHE Research Paper 54.* York, UK: Centre for Health Economics, University of York. http://www.york.ac.uk/media/che/documents/papers/researchpapers/rp54_appropriate_perspectives_for_health_care_decisions.pdf.

Culyer, A. J. 1991. "The Normative Economics of Health Care Finance and Provision." In *Providing Health Care: The Economics of Alternative Systems of Finance and Delivery*, edited by S. McGuire, P. Fenn, and K. Mayhew. New York: Oxford University Press.

Drummond, M. F., M. J. Sculpher, K. Claxton, G. W. Torrance, and G. L. Stoddart. 2015. *Methods for the Economic Evaluation of Health Care Programmes.* 4th ed. Oxford: Oxford University Press.

Epstein, D. M., Z. Chalabi, K. Claxton, and M. Sculpher. 2007. Efficiency, equity, and budgetary policies: informing decisions using mathematical programming. *Med Decis Making* 27 (2):128–137.

Feeny, D. 2000. Response to Lenert and Kaplan: a utility approach to the assessment of health-related quality of life. *Med Care* 38 (Supplement II 9):II-151–II-154.

Friedman, M. 1953. "The Methodology of Positive Economics." In *Essays in Positive Economics*, 3–43. Chicago: University of Chicago Press.

Garber, A. M., and C. E. Phelps. 1997. Economic foundations of cost-effectiveness analysis. *J Health Econ* 16 (1):1–31.

Gold, M. R., J. E. Siegel, L. B. Russell, and M. C. Weinstein, eds. 1996. *Cost-Effectiveness in Health and Medicine.* New York: Oxford University Press.

Hammitt, J. K. 2013. Admissible utility functions for health, longevity, and wealth: integrating monetary and life-year measures. *J Risk Uncertain* 47 (3):311–325.

Harsanyi, J. C. 1953. Cardinal utility in welfare economics and in the theory of risk-taking. *J Polit Economy* 61 (5):434–435.

Harsanyi, J. C. 1955. Cardinal welfare, individualistic ethics, and interpersonal comparisons of utility. *J Polit Economy* 63 (4):309–321.

Harsanyi, J. C. 1975. Can the Maximin Principle serve as a basis for morality? A critique of John Rawls's theory. *Amer Polit Sci Rev* 69 (2):594–606.

Hicks, J. R. 1939. The foundations of welfare economics. *Econ J (London)* 49 (196):696–712.

Johannesson, M., J. S. Pliskin, and M. C. Weinstein. 1993. Are healthy-years equivalents an improvement over quality-adjusted life years? *Med Decis Making* 13 (4):281–286.

Kahneman, D., and A. Tversky. 1979. Prospect theory: an analysis of decision under risk. *Econometrica* 47 (2):263–291.

Kaldor, N. 1939. Welfare propositions of economics and interpersonal comparisons of utility. *Econ J (London)* 49 (195):549–552.

Kamlet, M. S. 1992. *The Comparative Benefits Modeling Project: A Framework for Cost-Utility Analysis of Government Health Care Programs.* Bethesda, MD: US Department of Health and Human Services, Public Health Service.

Keeney, R. L. 1976. A group preference axiomatization with cardinal utility. *Manage Sci* 23 (2):140–145.

Keeney, R. L., and C. W. Kirkwood. 1975. Group decision making using cardinal social welfare functions. *Manage Sci* 22 (4):430–437.

Machina, M. J. 1982. Expected utility analysis without the independence axiom. *Econometrica* 50 (2):277–323.

Meltzer, D. 1997. Accounting for future costs in medical cost-effectiveness analysis. *J Health Econ* 16 (1):33–64.

Meltzer, D. 2001. Addressing uncertainty in medical cost-effectiveness analysis implications of expected utility maximization for methods to perform sensitivity analysis and the use of cost-effectiveness analysis to set priorities for medical research. *J Health Econ* 20 (1):109–129.

Meltzer, D. O., E. S. Huang, S. E. S. Brown, and Q. Zhang. 2005. "Effects of patient self-selection on cost-effectiveness: implications for intensive therapy for diabetes [poster presentation]." 27th Annual Meeting of the Society for Medical Decision Making, San Francisco, October 21–24, 2005. https://smdm.confex.com/smdm/2005ca/techprogram/ P2361.HTM.

Office of Management and Budget. 2003. "Circular A-4." September 17, 2003. Subject: Regulatory Analysis. https://www.whitehouse.gov/omb/circulars_a004_a-4/.

Pareto, V. 2014. *Manual of Political Economy: A Critical and Variorum Edition.* Oxford: Oxford University Press.

Phelps, C. E., and A. I. Mushlin. 1991. On the (near) equivalence of cost-effectiveness and cost-benefit analyses. *Int J Technol Assess Health Care* 7 (1):12–21.

Pliskin, J. S., D. S. Shepard, and M. C. Weinstein. 1980. Utility functions for life years and health status. *Oper Res* 28:206–224.

Pratt, J. W. 1964. Risk aversion in the small and in the large. *Econometrica* 32 (1-2):122–136.

Raiffa, H. 1968. *Decision Analysis: Introductory Lectures on Choices under Uncertainty.* Reading, MA: Addison-Wesley.

Rawls, J. 1971. *A Theory of Justice.* Cambridge, MA: Harvard University Press.

Sen, A. 1995. Rationality and social choice. *Am Econ Rev* 85 (1):1–24

Stinnett, A. A., and J. Mullahy. 1998. Net health benefits: a new framework for the analysis of uncertainty in cost-effectiveness analysis. *Med Decis Making* 18 (2 Suppl):S68–S80.

Sugden, R., and A. H. Williams. 1978. *The Principles of Practical Cost-Benefit Analysis.* Oxford: Oxford University Press.

van Hout, B. A. 1998. Discounting costs and effects: a reconsideration. *Health Econ* 7 (7): 581–594.

Verguet, S., R. Laxminarayan, and D. T. Jamison. 2015. Universal public finance of tuberculosis treatment in India: an extended cost-effectiveness analysis. *Health Econ* 24 (3):318–332.

Viscusi, W. K., and J. E. Aldy. 2003. The value of a statistical life: a critical review of market estimates throughout the world. *J Risk Uncertainty* 27 (1):5–76.

von Neumann, J., and O. Morgenstern. 1944. *Theory of Games and Economic Behavior.* Princeton: Princeton University Press.

Williams, A. 1993. Priorities and research strategy in health economics for the 1990s. *Health Econ* 2 (4):295–302.

3

Recommendations on Perspectives
for the Reference Case

Peter J. Neumann, Gillian D. Sanders, Anirban Basu,
Dan W. Brock, David Feeny, Murray Krahn, Karen M. Kuntz,
David O. Meltzer, Douglas K. Owens, Lisa A. Prosser,
Joshua A. Salomon, Mark J. Sculpher, Thomas A. Trikalinos,
Louise B. Russell, Joanna E. Siegel, and Theodore G. Ganiats

3.1 THE ORIGINAL PANEL'S REFERENCE CASE

The original Panel on Cost-Effectiveness in Health and Medicine recommended a "Reference Case," a set of standard methodological practices that all cost-effectiveness analyses (CEAs) should follow to improve comparability and quality (Gold et al. 1996). They recommended that Reference Case analyses assume a societal perspective that reflects the perspective of a decision maker whose intention is to make decisions about the broad allocation of resources across the entire population. In a CEA conducted from a societal perspective, the analyst considers all parties affected by the intervention and counts all significant outcomes and costs that flow from it, regardless of who experiences the outcomes or costs. The original Panel also noted that, to address specific decision contexts, analysts might also conduct CEAs from narrower perspectives, such as that of the healthcare sector, to reflect the view of a decision maker whose responsibility rests only within that sector.

The Second Panel endorses the Reference Case concept for the purposes originally intended: providing guidance to improve the quality of CEAs and to promote comparability across studies. However, the Second Panel reconsidered and debated at length the issue of what perspective the Reference Case should take. Although the Panel recognized the merits of a societal perspective for a Reference Case, we also grappled with several issues related to its use.

3.2 THE SOCIETAL PERSPECTIVE: EXPERIENCE SINCE THE ORIGINAL PANEL

Since publication of the original Panel's recommendations in 1996, there has been an explosion of CEAs in the literature, and many, if not most, have *not* used the societal perspective (Daigle et al. 2012; Diaby et al. 2015; Garrison et al. 2010; Neumann 2009). Even when analysts state that they have used a societal perspective, they have often omitted important elements, so that the perspective of the analysis is essentially a narrower one (Brettschneider et al. 2015; Kokorowski, Routh, and Nelson 2013; Neumann 2009; Stone et al. 2000). Most analyses are limited to treated patients and not extended to family members or others. In many if not most cases, time costs involved in receiving an intervention and for self-management, recommended for inclusion in the societal perspective analysis, have not been considered. Analysts have infrequently identified and quantified consequences outside the healthcare sector, despite the fact that the original Panel recommended that such effects be considered if they are important. Some analysts may have considered such elements in the course of conducting their CEAs, but ultimately judged that their inclusion would not materially affect results. In practice, however, it seems that analysts have seldom given such elements serious consideration, and adoption of a societal perspective in CEA has been uncommon. Moreover, since publication of the original panel's book, decision-making bodies—primarily in Europe, Australia, and Canada—have formally incorporated CEA into health technology assessment processes to inform coverage and reimbursement decisions, but generally have not adopted a societal perspective, preferring instead a more focused view (see Chapter 1).

3.3 THE SECOND PANEL'S CONSIDERATIONS REGARDING PERSPECTIVE

Although analysts presumably will always consider the perspective related to the decision context they wish to inform (e.g., that of a particular payer), there are important questions concerning general recommendations for the Reference Case. One option for the Second Panel was to continue to recommend a societal perspective for the Reference Case—and indeed to reiterate the original Panel's commitment to the importance of such a perspective. The societal perspective has the advantages of capturing the full consequences of investments in interventions designed to improve health and of reflecting the broad public interest, two elements that are useful for decision makers, even if they are making decisions from another perspective. There are concerns, however, about the practicality of the societal perspective—both in terms of the burden it places on analysts and its relevance for decision makers faced with budget allocation decisions, as suggested by the fact that few analysts or decision makers have taken this perspective. Moreover, one could argue that there is no single "societal perspective," but numerous ones depending on what elements are considered to represent social value, and how those elements are valued. By emphasizing the societal perspective, the Second Panel might be seen as disregarding the revealed preference of practitioners as it has evolved over the past 20 years, and providing advice that is not closely tied to any particular decision maker or budget holder.

Another option in establishing the Reference Case was to recommend a narrow healthcare payer or health system perspective for that would align more closely with many decision makers' viewpoints and reflect existing practice. A disadvantage of this approach is that it would potentially ignore many important consequences of healthcare investment decisions. That is, one could argue that elected officials and administrators of public programs and others who are responsible for population health (e.g., officials at the Medicare program or the Centers for Disease Control and Prevention [CDC]), should consider the full consequences of their choices and recommendations.

Yet another option was to recommend that analysts present multiple perspectives, for example, a healthcare sector perspective and a societal perspective, in addition to any specific perspective an analyst wishes to inform (e.g., that of a particular payer). This option would have the advantage of illustrating the consequences of decisions from different viewpoints, and of allowing analysts to include the perspective they deem most closely related to the decision problem at hand. The disadvantage would be the potential burden that conducting analyses from multiple perspectives places on analysts.

With these issues, options, and considerations in mind, the Second Panel has made the following recommendations to promote quality and comparability, while recognizing the different preferences, needs, and authorities of decision makers, and the importance of preserving flexibility for analysts in accommodating those factors. The Panel has also cited as important the value that stems from illustrating the consequences of making decisions from different viewpoints.

3.4 RECOMMENDATIONS

3.4.1 Recommendation 1: Reference Cases and Reference Case Perspectives

We recommend that all studies report a Reference Case analysis based on a healthcare sector perspective and another Reference Case analysis based on a societal perspective. The Reference Cases are defined by recommendations for components to consider for evaluation, methods to use, and elements for reporting. We recommend that Reference Case analyses measure health effects in terms of QALYs. Standardizing methods and components within a perspective is intended to enhance consistency and comparability across studies.

3.4.2 Recommendation 2: Healthcare Sector Reference Case

We recommend that the results of the healthcare sector Reference Case analysis be summarized in the conventional form, as an incremental cost-effectiveness ratio (ICER). Net monetary benefit (NMB) or net health benefit (NHB) may also be reported, and a range of cost-effectiveness thresholds should be considered. We recommend that the healthcare sector perspective include formal healthcare sector (medical) costs borne by third-party payers or paid for out-of-pocket by patients. Both types of medical costs include current and future costs, related and unrelated to the condition under consideration.

3.4.3 Recommendation 3: Societal Reference Case: The Impact Inventory and Summary and Disaggregated Measures

3.4.3.1 *Recommendation 3.A. Inclusion of an Impact Inventory*

The Second Panel continues to strongly support evaluation of the broader impacts of interventions designed to improve health. We recommend that the societal Reference Case analysis include medical costs (current and future, related and unrelated) borne by third-party payers or paid for out-of-pocket by patients, time costs of patients in seeking and receiving care, time costs of informal (unpaid) caregivers, transportation costs, effects on future productivity and consumption, and other costs and effects outside the healthcare sector. To make this evaluation more explicit and transparent, we recommend inclusion of an "Impact Inventory" that lists the health and non-health impacts of an intervention that should be considered in a societal Reference Case analysis (described in more detail in Chapters 6 and 13). The main purpose of the Impact Inventory is to ensure that all consequences, including those outside the formal healthcare sector, are considered regularly and comprehensively, as they have generally not been to date.

3.4.3.2 *Recommendation 3.B. Quantifying and Valuing Non-Health Components in the Impact Inventory*

We recommend that analysts attempt to quantify and value non-health consequences in the Impact Inventory, unless those consequences are likely to have a negligible effect on the results of the analysis.

3.4.3.3 *Recommendation 3.C. Summary and Disaggregated Measures*

The Second Panel agrees that it would be helpful to inform decision makers through the quantification and valuation of all health and non-health impacts of interventions, and to summarize those impacts in a single quantitative measure such as an ICER, NMB, or NHB. However, there are no widely agreed upon methods for quantifying and valuing some of these broader impacts in CEA. We therefore recommend that analysts present the items listed in the Impact Inventory in the form of disaggregated consequences across different sectors. We also recommend that analysts use one or more summary measures, such as an ICER, NMB, or NHB, that include some or all of the items listed in the Impact Inventory. Analysts should clearly identify which items are included and how they are measured and valued, and provide a rationale for their methodological decisions.

3.4.4 Recommendation 4: Reporting the Reference Cases and Other Perspectives

3.4.4.1 *Recommendation 4.A. Stating the Perspective*

We recommend that analysts clearly state the perspective of every analysis reported.

3.4.4.2 *Recommendation 4.B. Presenting Other Perspectives*

Where specific decision makers have been identified, such as a particular public or private payer, analysts may wish to present results from that decision maker's perspective in addition to the Reference Case perspectives. In these cases, we recommend that analysts clearly state the primary decision maker(s) whose deliberations are intended to be informed by the analysis.

3.4.4.3 *Recommendation 4.C. The Importance of Transparency and Sensitivity Analysis*

The items included in a CEA and the manner in which they are valued involve numerous choices. We recommend that analysts be transparent about how they have conducted analyses, and that they convey how results change with alternative assumptions. Sensitivity analysis should describe as clearly as possible the assumptions to which the results for different perspectives are sensitive.

3.5 THE REFERENCE CASE RECOMMENDATIONS IN CONTEXT

The Second Panel intends its recommendations to provide a useful and pragmatic approach that will serve both producers and consumers of CEAs. Given the varied contexts for healthcare decision making, there is no perfect solution for Reference Case analyses; our recommendations involve choices and compromises in the service of practicality, comparability, and flexibility.

In considering our options, a key question was how prescriptive to be in making recommendations—that is, what level of detail the recommendations should contain. In the interest of promoting comparability across studies, we advocate that specific components be included in CEAs and, in the remainder of this book we provide guidance on their valuation for purposes of constructing an ICER. At the same time, we recognize that being overly prescriptive has drawbacks. It may place undue burdens on analysts. It may promote an approach that analysts who have specific decision makers and budget holders in mind may find irrelevant to their own contexts. Moreover, prescribing certain choices—for example, how to value a person's time—has distributional implications that raise challenging ethical questions.

We recommend the healthcare sector perspective for Reference Case analyses because it is closely tied to resource implications considered by many decision makers in the US healthcare sector. However, we recognize that, as with the societal perspective, decisions about precisely which items to include in the healthcare sector perspective are at some level arbitrary. For example, consider our recommendation to include patients' out-of-pocket costs in the healthcare sector perspective while excluding patient and informal caregiver time costs. One might argue that out-of-pocket costs, such as copayments, should be included only in the societal perspective, thus leaving the healthcare sector perspective to focus on medical costs falling directly on health payer budgets. At the same time, one could argue that patient and informal caregiver time costs should be included in the healthcare sector perspective, as they reflect genuine resources used in the healthcare sector.

Our reasoning for including out-of-pocket costs in the healthcare sector perspective is that excluding them would reduce this perspective to a payer perspective—a narrower and qualitatively different point of view. For public decision makers, such as Medicare officials, who may wish to consider a healthcare sector perspective, to exclude patients' out-of-pocket costs seems inappropriate and inconsistent with their missions to improve population health. In contrast, exclusion of time costs from the healthcare sector perspective follows conventional practice, which generally omits such costs, and relates more closely to the decision makers' perspective. We acknowledge that this choice is somewhat arbitrary but emphasize that there is no choice that would satisfy the goals of practicality, feasibility, and comparability, as well as theoretical consistency from all points of view.

Further, we continue to recommend inclusion of a Reference Case analysis from a societal perspective because of the importance of capturing the broad consequences of health interventions, including consequences outside the healthcare sector (e.g., in education, the legal system, and public health). All of these effects should be enumerated and, to the extent possible, valued and summarized in the societal Reference Case analysis. The societal perspective we recommend includes patient and informal caregiver time costs, transportation costs, effects on future productivity and consumption in added years of life, and other costs and effects outside the healthcare sector. The intention is to account for—and capture as fully as possible—all non-trivial impacts of an intervention. Indeed, our intention is to go beyond the original Panel's recommendation for the societal perspective, moving the field toward explicit enumeration of all of these effects in an Impact Inventory and toward fuller accounting of these impacts in all societal perspective CEAs.

We have developed the healthcare sector Reference Case perspective, which is in line with the perspective analysts have most commonly used over the last 20 years, to be useful to a broad range of decision makers within the healthcare sector. At the same time, we recommend the societal perspective to provide all decision makers the added benefit of a broader view and to provide a case that will be valuable to a wider array of stakeholders. In the worked examples (Appendix A and Appendix B), we demonstrate the feasibility and value of conducting Reference Case analyses from both perspectives. We also emphasize that when a parameter estimate or an element of the analysis is unlikely to have an appreciable effect on the result, the analyst can feel free to use shortcuts to obtain such elements or to exclude them from the analysis altogether. We further underscore the importance of analysts being as transparent as possible in documenting their methods, providing the rationale for choices made, and conducting sensitivity analysis to explore how results change with different assumptions.

We believe that differentiating between the healthcare sector perspective and the societal perspective will provide more clarity to consumers of CEAs than has been the case in years past. The common practice of presenting an analysis from the healthcare sector perspective, and labeling it a societal perspective, has created the impression that such analyses are the same when they are not. We extend our emphasis on clarity of perspective by recommending that analysts identify any specific decision maker whose decisions are intended to be influenced by the analysis, and conduct additional analyses from perspectives specific to that decision maker if they will provide useful information. The appropriate cost-effectiveness threshold to apply to inform decisions (see Chapter 1) may depend on the perspective taken. If one takes a healthcare sector perspective, and the additional costs falls entirely on the health system budget, the threshold can be expressed in terms of health opportunity costs. If these costs fall on other individuals or sectors outside the healthcare sector, then opportunity costs cannot be quantified in health terms alone, and a different threshold may be appropriate. Finally, we acknowledge that there remain many challenging issues, such as valuation of effects outside the healthcare sector and coordination with other methods already used to evaluate those effects. Addressing these challenges will continue to provide opportunities to advance the field of CEA.

3.6 REFERENCES

Brettschneider, C., H. Djadran, M. Härter, B. Lowe, S. Riedel-Heller, and H. H. König. 2015. Cost-utility analyses of cognitive-behavioural therapy of depression: a systematic review. *Psychother Psychosom* 84 (1):6–21.

Daigle, M. E., A. M. Weinstein, J. N. Katz, and E. Losina. 2012. The cost-effectiveness of total joint arthroplasty: a systematic review of published literature. *Best Pract Res Clin Rheumatol* 26 (5):649–658.

Diaby, V., R. Tawk, V. Sanogo, H. Xiao, and A. J. Montero. 2015. A review of systematic reviews of the cost-effectiveness of hormone therapy, chemotherapy, and targeted therapy for breast cancer. *Breast Cancer Res Treat* 151 (1):27–40.

Garrison, L. P., Jr., E. C. Mansley, T. A. Abbott, 3rd, B. W. Bresnahan, J. W. Hay, and J. Smeeding. 2010. Good research practices for measuring drug costs in cost-effectiveness analyses: a societal perspective: the ISPOR Drug Cost Task Force report—Part II. *Value Health* 13 (1): 8–13.

Gold, M. R., J. E. Siegel, L. B. Russell, and M. C. Weinstein, eds. 1996. *Cost-Effectiveness in Health and Medicine.* New York: Oxford University Press.

Kokorowski, P. J., J. C. Routh, and C. P. Nelson. 2013. Quality assessment of economic analyses in pediatric urology. *Urology* 81 (2):263–267.

Neumann, P. J. 2009. Costing and perspective in published cost-effectiveness analysis. *Med Care* 47 (7 Suppl 1):S28–S32.

Stone, P. W., R. H. Chapman, E. A. Sandberg, B. Liljas, and P. J. Neumann. 2000. Measuring costs in cost-utility analyses. Variations in the literature. *Int J Technol Assess Health Care* 16 (1):111–124.

4

Designing a Cost-Effectiveness Analysis

Douglas K. Owens, Joanna E. Siegel, Mark J. Sculpher, and Joshua A. Salomon

Before undertaking a cost-effectiveness analysis (CEA), the analyst, in consultation with subject area experts and decision makers, must decide on an overall approach and on specific aspects of the study design. These early conceptualization and planning steps are essential for focusing the study on relevant research questions, maintaining the focus as the study progresses, and avoiding analytical pitfalls midway through an analysis. We refer to this process as *designing* the CEA. In designing the analysis, the analyst should consider the following items, each of which is discussed in this chapter: the objectives of the CEA, the audience, the type of economic evaluation to be undertaken (such as cost-effectiveness or cost–benefit analysis), the perspective of the analysis, the definition of the interventions, the target population, the comparators, the scope of the study, the time horizon, the analysis plan, a conceptual model for the study, the type of data required, and how the data will be collected. In section 4.15 at the end of this chapter, we provide recommendations about these important aspects of the design of economic analyses. Those recommendations are also cited parenthetically where they will enhance the discussion.

The major change to the recommendations from the original Panel, as noted in Chapter 3, is that we now recommend two Reference Case analyses, one conducted from a healthcare sector perspective and the other from a societal perspective. As part of the societal Reference Case analysis, we recommend the use of an "Impact Inventory," which lists the consequences—including health and non-health consequences—across

---

This chapter builds on concepts presented in Chapter 3 of the original Panel's book (Torrance, G.W., J.E. Siegel, and B.R. Luce. 1996. "Framing and Designing the Cost-Effectiveness Analysis." In *Cost-Effectiveness in Health and Medicine*, edited by M.R. Gold, J.E. Siegel, L.B. Russell and M.C. Weinstein, 54–81. New York: Oxford University Press).

all of the sectors (e.g., healthcare, education, criminal justice system) affected by an intervention. The Impact Inventory provides a framework both for thinking about consequences during the design stage of a CEA and for presenting these consequences when reporting results.

To assess the impact of an intervention, CEA describes and contrasts the costs and outcomes that would be expected to occur with the intervention and the costs and outcomes of one or more comparators that do not include the intervention. This general approach has many variations: More intensive forms of an intervention can be compared with less intensive forms (with the less intensive form serving as the comparator); different types of prevention or treatment can be compared for the same health problem; prevention of a problem can be compared to treating it. Although many interventions studied with CEA are clinical in nature, we recognize the importance of a broader set, such as public health interventions, or interventions in non-healthcare sectors (for example, transportation) that have important influences on health.

Analysts, working together with subject and policy experts, approach a cost-effectiveness study with a general conception or question about the cost of an intervention and its impact on relevant outcomes. To move from this general idea to the concrete details necessary to assess cost-effectiveness, the analyst addresses a series of decisions that constitute the study design.

4.1 OBJECTIVES OF THE CEA

Broadly speaking, the goal of CEA, as discussed in Chapter 1, is to inform policy makers or others involved in healthcare decisions about the degree to which alternative interventions improve health, given their costs. For a specific study to be relevant, it must take into account the policy context and the controversies that relate to decisions about the use of an option. It must address an appropriate audience, and it must be conducted from one or more perspectives, including ones that are relevant to that audience. Before beginning a study, it is thus essential to assess the decision-making process related to the intervention and to have an idea about how the study will contribute to this process. Examination of the decision context allows the analyst, with appropriate input from decision makers, to clarify the objectives of a particular study.

A number of questions should be considered: Is there a specific decision motivating the analysis, or is the analysis intended to contribute to a general policy discussion? Are the costs and effects of a health intervention confined to the healthcare sector or do they extend to other sectors (e.g., education, the criminal justice system, the environment)? Who will make decisions regarding the alternative options? Will the decision makers help inform or participate in the analysis? What groups will influence the decision, either by providing information directly to decision makers or by developing their own recommendations? What issues are of concern to these parties?

For example, an analyst considering a study about breast cancer screening in the United States might predict that decisions about screening for breast cancer will be constrained by the benefit packages offered by public or private payers. Her purpose might be to assess the cost-effectiveness of options in terms of screening strategies based on the latest evidence of screening and treatment effectiveness to inform benefits policy. Alternatively, and as we recommend, the analyst would also consider the question from the broader societal perspective. She would note that decisions about screening have traditionally been made by individual physicians and patients based on the recommendations of groups such as the US Preventive Services Task Force, the American Cancer Society, and the American College of Physicians. New policies may draw on existing recommendations, and the analyst could evaluate screening policies from the broad societal perspective, as well as from the perspective of public or private payers.

Understanding the decision context will guide the choice of audience and the perspective of the study. These choices will, in turn, affect many of the other decisions made in designing the study. As noted in Chapter 3, we recommend that studies intended to inform resource allocation decisions (or to be comparable with those that do) report both a healthcare sector perspective Reference Case and a societal perspective Reference Case. A specific decision context should not induce the analyst to undertake an inappropriately narrow analysis. However, as noted in Chapter 3 the objectives of an analysis may prompt the inclusion of other perspectives as well. In addition, the decision context may affect the alternatives assessed or the comparisons made within an analysis.

As the breast cancer screening example demonstrates, CEAs often address emerging issues and often are intended to supply information for future debates. In such cases, just as when an analysis pertains to a current and identifiable policy debate, envisioning how the study will be used and establishing its objectives in advance of undertaking the analysis serve to define and focus the study.

For the analysis of both emerging issues and existing interventions or practices, CEAs can be either "what-is" studies or "what-if" studies, depending on the data available for the analysis and its quality. Much of this chapter is directed at the "what-is" type of study, where reasonably good data on costs and outcomes can be obtained or estimated (see, e.g., Paltiel et al. [2006], Sanders et al. [2005], and Sanders, Hlatky, and Owens [2005]). However, some studies must be undertaken well before good data are available if they are to address relevant policy questions in a timely manner. "What-if" studies can investigate the magnitude of costs that an intervention can generate and/or the level of effects necessary for the intervention to meet acceptable standards of cost-effectiveness (Long, Brandeau, and Owens 2009; Sanders et al. 2001). Such a study determines the thresholds with regard to costs and effects that the intervention must achieve to be acceptable. For both "what-is" and "what-if" studies, representing uncertainty is important (see Chapter 11). For example, a decision analysis using value-of-information analysis can extend the "what-if" analysis by including all relevant existing evidence, being explicit about its uncertainty, putting a value on future research, and indicating the type of research that is of highest priority (Soares et al. 2013). It should be noted that "what-if" studies can be done according to most Reference Case recommendations, but analysts should take special care to highlight the uncertainty about effectiveness and the corresponding uncertainty about cost-effectiveness, and what this implies about research priorities. In addition, "what-if" studies can evaluate interventions, such as screening, as applied to different target groups or to different age cutoffs for beginning and ending an intervention when there is no direct evidence about the intervention in those groups or age ranges (de Koning et al. 2014). Finally, CEA can be used to understand the factors that contribute to the overall costs and outcomes of an intervention, which may help decision makers adapt interventions to their needs (Teutsch and Murray 1999).

4.2 AUDIENCE

Who is the target audience for the study? When specific decision makers are responsible for a decision, these individuals will normally be the primary audience to whom the study is addressed. Some decision makers will have specific requirements or formats for studies to be submitted to them. For example, many countries have guidelines for the listing of new pharmaceuticals in government formularies (See Chapter 1). These guidelines specify such features as the comparison intervention and the perspective the study should adopt.

Often, there is no single identifiable decision maker. A CEA may be intended to influence opinion on a subject or simply to add to the weight of information on an intervention. For example, in the United States, medical specialty societies such as the American College of Physicians frequently issue practice guidelines; these guidelines may be influenced by information in a CEA. A CEA may be intended to inform the recommending groups and/or the relevant medical practitioners directly.

Primary audiences for a CEA may include health plans, government entities, the US Public Health Service, or state health departments, as well as individual healthcare providers. Often there are additional decision makers who can use the same or similar information. Such secondary audiences may be groups who are not decision makers, but have an interest in the study results, such as patient advocacy groups, the press, the research community in the public and private sectors, or the general public.

In designing a CEA, it is important to determine the audience for the study before the analysis is begun. A CEA on a new treatment for hepatitis C virus infection might have payers, providers, advocacy groups, patients, and policy makers as potential audiences. The identification of the audiences will affect the analyst's strategy and methodological choices. In this example, the analyst, relevant decision makers, and subject experts would consider the debates occurring in each of these groups and the data cited in these debates. Consideration of the audience will also affect the issues highlighted in the report of the CEA.

4.3 TYPES OF ANALYSIS

Before undertaking an analysis, the analyst, in consultation with relevant decision makers, should determine the type of analysis or analyses that will best illuminate the subject of the study. Many different forms of information can contribute to a decision. These may include a set of cost-effectiveness and related studies. Cost-effectiveness analysis can be distinguished from other related types of economic analysis. Not all of these approaches are widely used, but we outline them here because they are complementary forms of analysis (**Recommendation 1; see section 4.15**). They are return-on-investment analysis, cost-minimization analysis, cost-consequence analysis, and cost–benefit analysis. Establishing which type of economic analysis is most useful depends on the objectives and scope of the analysis and the intervention under consideration.

4.3.1 Return-on-Investment Analysis

Return-on-investment (ROI) analyses aim to evaluate the financial return from investment in an intervention. They typically assess the timing and quantity of financial returns relative to the timing and quantity of costs. The ROI for an intervention depends on the time horizon for which the ROI is estimated; thus, the ROI often changes for different time horizons. As usually conducted, an ROI analysis considers costs and cost savings. This approach creates an important limitation when applied to health interventions because the analysis does not include the health effects. For this reason, we recommend the use of other analytic approaches that capture health benefits (or harms) and costs and cost savings.

4.3.2 Cost-Minimization Analysis

Cost-minimization analysis is an economic analysis in which the effectiveness of the intervention and the comparator are presumed to be equal. In this case, the decision simply revolves around the costs. Although the effectiveness of alternative interventions is rarely exactly equal, this assumption may be a reasonable approximation in some cases. For example, when a generic version of a pharmaceutical becomes available, it may be reasonable to assume equivalent outcomes to the branded version. However, the analyst should only make such an assumption if there is evidence or a clear rationale to support equivalent effectiveness. The uncertainty associated with any evidence that seems to suggest equivalent outcomes needs to carefully assessed (Briggs and O'Brien 2001).

4.3.3 Cost-Consequence Analysis

Cost-consequence analysis is a disaggregated type of study that makes few assumptions and puts a relatively greater burden on the consumer of the analysis. (In this context, "consequence" refers specifically to health outcomes. This contrasts with the usage in the present book, especially in Chapter 6, where "consequences" is used to refer to all outcomes considered in a CEA, including costs.) The costs and health outcomes of the intervention compared to one or more relevant alternatives are computed separately and listed. The analysis itself does not combine these components, for example, by totaling across different types of health effects (cases, disability, deaths), costs, and savings (such as medical costs, patient out-of-pocket costs, and costs of patient time), nor does it indicate the relative importance of the various outcomes. This assessment is left to the user of the study.

Cost-consequence analysis is based on the premise that users of the study can and should make the value judgment trade-offs necessary to integrate a disparate list of pros and cons (costs and health outcomes) of the various alternatives and reach a final decision. One concern is whether these individuals—whether clinicians, elected officials, health services managers, or others—are the right source of values across outcomes. An additional practical issue is whether decision makers can cope with the cognitive burden of making all the necessary value judgments and trade-offs. Cost-consequence analysis can be a useful starting point for a CEA, however, by presenting the various costs and health outcomes in a disaggregated form, which can aid transparency prior to further analysis to assess trade-offs. As such, cost-consequence analysis may be considered similar to the Impact Inventory discussed in Chapters 3, 6 and 13.

4.3.4 Cost-Effectiveness Analysis (CEA)

In CEA, the differential costs and health outcomes associated with an option are used to calculate the incremental cost-effectiveness ratio (ICER) relative to non-dominated comparators (Box 4.1). Health outcomes can range from intermediate outcomes, such as reduction in blood pressure measured in millimeters of mercury or disability days averted, to more distal outcomes, such as lives saved, life years gained or quality-adjusted life years (QALYs) gained. The QALY (or analogous measure) is a comprehensive measure of outcome used in CEA, incorporating both health-related quality of life and survival. However, QALYs do not capture non-healthcare sector effects, which may be very important for some interventions.

The particular type of CEA that uses QALYs is often referred to as cost-utility analysis and is sometimes included under the rubric of CEA. We will use the latter convention, describing these analyses as CEAs with QALYs as the measure of effectiveness (Greenberg et al. 2010).

4.3.5 Cost–Benefit Analysis

In cost–benefit analysis (CBA) all incremental consequences are valued in monetary units (e.g., dollars), so the overall analysis of an intervention's costs and effects can be conducted entirely in these units. This monetary valuation of outcomes is usually seen as the distinguishing feature of CBA. However, to inform decisions using CEA, a cost-effectiveness threshold needs to be defined, and this threshold can be used to translate an ICER into a measure of net monetary benefit (NMB), so that outcomes are effectively expressed in monetary units. There is a literature on the theoretical links between CBA and CEA (see Chapter 2).

At a practical level, the methods of monetary valuation of outcomes differ between CEA and CBA. For CBA, the focus is on valuing the consequences of interventions using the preferences or utilities of the gainers and losers. In CBA, preferences, represented by willingness-to-pay, are taken as being reflected in market prices where markets exist or inferred using other methods. Willingness-to-pay is used to assess the value of a statistical life, which can be assessed directly by survey, using approaches

Box 4.1 Calculation of the Incremental Cost-Effectiveness Ratio, Healthcare Sector Perspective*

Let:

IC = incremental cost

IE = incremental health outcome (e.g., QALYs)

$ICER$ = incremental cost-effectiveness ratio

TC_1 = total costs, present value, for intervention

TC_2 = total costs, present value, for comparator

E_1 = total health outcomes, present value, for intervention

E_2 = total health outcomes, present value, for comparator

$C1_1$ = total payer costs, present value, for intervention

$C1_2$ = total payer costs, present value, for comparator

$C2_1$ = total patient out-of-pocket costs, present value, for intervention

$C2_2$ = total patient out-of-pocket costs, present value, for comparator

$C3_1$ = future medical costs, other conditions, present value, for intervention

$C3_2$ = future medical costs, other conditions, present value, for comparator

$$TC_1 = C1_1 + C2_1 + C3_1$$

$$TC_2 = C1_2 + C2_2 + C3_2$$

Then:

$$IC = TC_1 - TC_2$$

$$IE = E_1 - E_2$$

$$ICER = IC / IE$$

*This box illustrates how to calculate the incremental cost-effectiveness ratio (ICER) for the healthcare sector perspective. Total health outcomes (effects) from the intervention and comparator are represented by E_1 and E_2. Costs are broken into components representing payer costs, patient out-of-pocket costs, and future related and unrelated payer and patient medical costs. The ICER is calculated as the incremental cost divided by the incremental health outcome.

---

such as *contingent valuation* or *conjoint analysis,* or inferred from decisions actually made by individuals that involve trade-offs between risks to life and money (Russell 2014). A CBA determines the net social benefit of the intervention: the incremental benefit of the intervention less the incremental costs, all measured in dollars. A positive net social benefit indicates that from the CBA perspective, the intervention is worthwhile, although decisions to implement it are likely to be subject to budget constraints.

Because CBA entails valuing all outcomes in monetary terms, in principle it allows for comparisons across healthcare and other sectors, such as the environment, education, and defense spending. For example, a local government could use CBA to inform a decision about whether to use tax dollars for a road improvement program that saved commuting time, reduced pollution, and improved access to recreational facilities versus a health initiative offering free vaccinations and other programs to promote child health and welfare. However, where constraints exist (e.g., relating to specific budgets in each sector), the opportunity costs associated with those constraints need to be reflected, and this is true of both CEA and CBA (Sculpher and Claxton 2012).

Cost-consequence analysis, CEA, and CBA are not mutually exclusive. Cost-consequence analysis is a precursor to both CEA and CBA, and much of the information obtained for a CEA can be used in a CBA. For interventions with substantial non-healthcare sector benefits, CBA may be more appropriate than CEA. In many cases the effort required at the margin to add an additional analytic technique is small. We therefore recommend that, for the societal Reference Case analysis, analysts present the items listed in the Impact Inventory in the form of disaggregated consequences across different sectors. We also recommend that analysts use one or more summary measures, such as an ICER, NMB, or net health benefit (NHB), that include some or all of the items listed in the Impact Inventory. Analysts should clearly identify which items are included and how they are measured, and they should provide a rationale for their methodological decisions (see **Recommendations 4–5**, and Chapter 3). We encourage analysts to be explicit about the assumptions and value judgments in each summary measure they report.

In any of these types of analyses, a useful tool is *scenario analysis,* a type of "what-if" analysis in which the analyst can examine different scenarios that may be of special interest to decision makers. In scenario analysis, the analyst may assess effects for which there is sparse or no evidence, combinations of circumstances that exist in the real world but that differ significantly from the base-case analysis, or factors that may be subject to variation, such as the price of the intervention. Scenario analyses can also assess variation in circumstances or settings that may influence the intervention alternatives or how the intervention is delivered. For example, the comparators may be different in rural settings compared to major medical centers.

4.4 PERSPECTIVES

Cost-effectiveness analyses can be undertaken from a number of different perspectives. The choice of the study perspective is an important methodological decision because it determines which costs and effects to count and how to value them. The appropriate perspective depends on the objective of the study, the context, and the relevant decision makers.

As indicated above, we recommend that analysts conduct Reference Case analyses from both the healthcare sector and societal perspectives (**Recommendations 2–5**). Other perspectives may, however, be relevant for specific decision makers. To illustrate, we briefly consider four perspectives potentially relevant to the analysis of health interventions: the payer perspective, the healthcare sector Reference Case perspective, the healthcare sector with time cost perspective, and the societal Reference Case perspective. Although we note two additional perspectives here, the remainder of this book will focus on the healthcare sector and societal Reference Case perspectives.

The *payer perspective* includes the consequences that a specific payer considers relevant. This perspective will be more or less narrow depending on whether the payer is private or public. For a US private commercial payer (insurer), for example, costs might include reimbursement for medical care paid for by the insurer and consequences for patients covered by the insurer. In the United States, this perspective would omit costs (both monetary and time) borne by patients. In non-US settings with single public payers, such as the United Kingdom, Canada, and many European countries, the payer perspective may be the most relevant for healthcare decisions and would typically include a broader array of medical costs, benefits, and harms.

As noted above, the US private payer perspective omits an important proportion of medical costs borne by patients, namely, out-of-pocket costs (co-payments and deductibles), as well as time costs incurred by patients and informal (unpaid) caregivers and their transportation costs. In the United States, we call the perspective that includes medical costs borne by both payers and patients the *healthcare sector perspective*. This is one of two Reference Case analyses recommended here (**Recommendations 2–3**).

Because some interventions also impose significant time costs on patients and informal caregivers, analysts or decision makers may wish to include these costs as well, a perspective we call the *healthcare sector with time cost perspective*. Quantifying time costs may be relatively straightforward for some interventions but more challenging for others (Russell 2009).

Some interventions to improve health may have important consequences outside of the healthcare sector. For example, a successful intervention to treat substance abuse might reduce costs in the criminal justice system. A successful intervention for autism may positively affect educational attainment. Public health interventions may have particularly broad consequences across non-healthcare sectors, including the environment and the criminal justice system. For interventions that have important non-healthcare sector consequences, we recommend that the analyst include such consequences when feasible. We call the perspective that includes all consequences across sectors the *societal perspective* (**Recommendation 4**). Thus, the societal perspective is the broadest and most comprehensive perspective, and incorporates all costs and all effects regardless of who incurs the costs and who obtains the effects, and regardless of whether they are health or non-health costs or effects. It includes time costs, transportation costs, and changes in productivity and consumption, as well as other effects in non-healthcare sectors. The societal perspective may be defined by the jurisdiction of the decision maker and the applicability of the decision. Often, it is delimited by national borders; however, the societal perspective should not be confused with a "governmental" perspective, which may include only a subset of costs and effects.

Although our recommendations are consistent with the original Panel's definition of the societal perspective, the cross-sector consequences have seldom been modeled in practice. Our emphasis on including such consequences is an important feature of the new Reference Case recommendations.

We recommend that the societal perspective include changes in productivity and consumption. The reason is that health interventions that improve (or decrease) health-related quality of life or that increase length of life may have important effects on the ability of people to participate in the labor force, engage in unpaid volunteer work, or participate in productive work within the household. And because an increase in length of life is accompanied by an increase in consumption in terms of what people spend to live, healthcare interventions may result in changes in both productivity and consumption (**Recommendation 4**). Productivity is usually measured in terms of wages, and consumption is measured in annual expenditures by age. Analysts should be aware that inclusion of productivity measured by wages reflects a value judgment that productivity is an important and relevant byproduct of health interventions, and may advantage interventions that affect groups of people who can participate in either paid or unpaid work (see Chapter 2). This value judgment raises important ethical questions. For example, children and the elderly who are not working will not be valued the same as people in the workforce; women may not be valued equally to men. Inclusion of productivity and consumption may result in resource allocations that some observers may consider discriminatory. These are important limitations that analysts and decision makers need to consider carefully. More generally, as an analysis moves from the narrower healthcare sector perspective to the broader societal perspective, more social value judgments of this sort will need to be made.

To summarize our Reference Case recommendations in somewhat greater detail, we suggest that analysts include Reference Case analyses from both the healthcare sector perspective and the societal perspective (see Chapter 3 and **Recommendations 2–5**). Table 4.1 summarizes the cost components included in these two perspectives.

The healthcare sector Reference Case includes formal healthcare sector (medical) costs borne by third-party payers plus patients' out-of-pocket medical costs. Both types of medical expenditures include current and future costs that are related and unrelated to the condition under consideration. We recommend that the results of the healthcare sector Reference Case analysis be summarized in the conventional form, as an ICER. The net monetary benefit (NMB) or net health benefit (NHB) may also be reported, and a range of cost-effectiveness thresholds should be considered.

We also recommend that analysts include a Reference Case analysis from a societal perspective (**Recommendation 4**). A societal perspective is particularly important when interventions are likely to have important effects on sectors of the economy outside of the formal healthcare sector, and when there is a need or desire to understand the wide range of costs and effects. A societal perspective includes medical costs (current and future, related and unrelated) borne by third-party payers and paid for out-of-pocket by patients, time costs of patients in seeking and receiving care, time costs of informal caregivers, transportation costs, effects on future productivity and consumption, and other costs and effects outside the healthcare sector. Because there are no widely agreed methods for quantifying and valuing some of these broader impacts in economic evaluation, we recommend that analysts present the items listed in the

Table 4.1 Cost components included in the two Reference
Case perspectives

Cost component	Reference Case perspective	
	Healthcare	Societal
Formal healthcare sector:*		
Paid for by third-party payers	✓	✓
Paid for by patients out-of-pocket	✓	✓
Informal healthcare sector:		
Patient time	–	✓
Unpaid caregiver time	–	✓
Transportation costs	–	✓
Non-healthcare sectors:		
Productivity	–	✓
Consumption	–	✓
Social services	–	✓
Legal or criminal justice	–	✓
Education	–	✓
Housing	–	✓
Environment	–	✓
Other (e.g., friction costs)	–	✓

*Includes current and future costs, related and unrelated to the condition
under consideration.

Impact Inventory in the form of disaggregated consequences across different sectors. We also recommend that analysts use one or more summary measures, such as an ICER, NMB, or NHB, that include some or all of the items in the Impact Inventory. If using a summary measure, such as an ICER, the analyst should consider presenting that measure in various ways that reflect alternative judgments and assumptions about valuation. The analyst should also consider the constraints that exist in delivering an intervention and how to reflect those constraints from both narrow and broad perspectives. Perhaps most notably, budget constraints exist in many sectors of the economy (e.g., those that are publicly funded), which means that opportunity costs are incurred when new programs or interventions impose additional costs. In CEA, these opportunity costs can be reflected in terms of cost-effectiveness thresholds (McCabe, Claxton, and Culyer 2008), but when costs fall on different sectors of the economy, some with their own budget constraints, a summary measure would need to reflect the implications for opportunity costs (Claxton et al. 2010).

The decision to use a societal perspective has important methodological ramifications. It means that all costs and all effects should be considered no matter who pays the costs or experiences the effects. For example, if an intervention has an effect on the number of children with learning disabilities, costs or benefits to the educational system are counted. It means that all types of resources of value to society should be considered;

thus, patients' time costs (lost work time, lost leisure time) are counted, as discussed earlier and in Chapter 8. It means that opportunity costs associated with any constraints (e.g., limited budgets) need to be reflected appropriately (see Chapter 2). Assessing opportunity costs, however, may be challenging. It also means that, because societal resources are being allocated, the general public (the source of the societal resources) is typically the appropriate source of preferences for health outcomes (see Chapter 7 for a full discussion, including alternative approaches such as using patients' preferences).

Finally, we note that there are interventions designed to improve health whose costs may fall primarily outside of the healthcare sector. For example, interventions aimed at reducing pollution will have important health effects, but the costs of the intervention may occur primarily in manufacturing, transportation, or other sectors. Public health interventions such as provision of housing may have healthcare sector consequences (reduced emergency room visits), but the bulk of the intervention costs are outside of the healthcare sector. In these examples, the healthcare sector perspective would fail to capture important consequences, and thus analysis from a societal perspective is appropriate.

Decision makers dealing with choices affecting organizations or specific interest groups may wish to conduct CEA from the narrower perspective of the entity of interest. Fortunately, doing a CEA from one perspective does not preclude using other perspectives as well. The preferred approach when a specific perspective is needed (such as that of a healthcare organization or the patient and family) is to conduct the CEA and present results both from the healthcare sector and societal Reference Case perspectives, and from the narrower perspective relating to the particular interests of that decision maker. (See Box 4.2 for a note on the potential burden on analysts from the inclusion of two Reference Case analyses.)

Box 4.2 A Note on Potential Analyst Burden

As we note throughout this volume, the Second Panel has deliberated extensively about how prescriptive to be in its recommendations, recognizing the potential for placing an undue burden on analysts. We anticipate that our recommendations to provide Reference Case analyses from both a healthcare sector perspective and a societal perspective, and to include all of the recommended detail for each perspective, could provoke an objection from some readers concerned about burden. We also recognize that analysts can provide only so much information in a 3,000 word journal article (see Chapter 13). However, as noted in Chapter 3, the Second Panel believes its recommendations, particularly the inclusion of an Impact Inventory table either within the main article or in a technical appendix, will provide a useful and pragmatic approach that will promote comparability and quality in analyses and serve varied contexts. We emphasize that analysts should exercise judgment. When a parameter estimate or an element of the analysis is unlikely to have an appreciable effect on the result, the analyst can feel free to use shortcuts to obtain them or to exclude them from the analysis altogether. Ultimately, the purpose of CEAs is to inform decision makers. Striking an appropriate balance between the development of rigorous, high-quality CEAs and the need to provide timely and useful information will be part of ongoing research and dialogue.

4.5 DEFINING THE INTERVENTION

The intervention to be analyzed in the CEA must be clearly specified (**Recommendation 6**). The intervention may consist of clinical interventions (lung cancer screening), programs, policies, or even system changes (e.g., teams to enhance quality or coordinate care). The intervention may include a large number of variations—for example, variations in the frequency of the intervention, in the ages and types of patients involved, or in the presence of comorbidities or risk factors. Screening for breast cancer, for example, can consist of self-examination, clinical examination, and mammography, in various combinations, and screening can be conducted at different frequencies—every year, every 2 years, or less often. In addition to distinctions in interventions or comparators, the analyst should consider how to assess relevant subgroups and heterogeneity of benefits, harms, or costs. For example, breast cancer screening strategies can vary for women in different age groups (ages 40–49 versus ages 50–65) and for different risk groups within age groups. Thus, many strategies may be evaluated across a range of different subgroups. This is entirely appropriate, as one of the strengths of CEA is its ability to demonstrate the relative cost-effectiveness of interventions given a wide range and variety of options and ways in which cost-effectiveness may vary across subgroups. However, it is essential in designing the study to define precisely what interventions and variations are to be included.

In general, the components of the intervention should be well enough specified so that the audience of the study can compare the subject of the CEA to other specific, real-world interventions and know whether their cost-effectiveness is likely to be similar or very different. For example, a smoking cessation intervention could be based in a community center or hospital outpatient clinic; it could utilize counselors or physicians; it could consist of a single counseling session or weeks of group meetings. Only if the analyst specifies these components can the consumers of the CEA know the extent to which the results apply to, for example, the smoking cessation program run within their own local hospital clinic.

The types of intervention characteristics that will be important depend on the analysis. Some aspects of the intervention that the analyst should consider are these: the specific technologies used, the type of personnel delivering the intervention, the site of delivery, whether the intervention is bundled with other services, the timing of the intervention, and the healthcare system and country in which the intervention is delivered. The target population, discussed immediately below, is another critical aspect of the intervention definition.

4.6 TARGET POPULATION

The target population is the population for whom the intervention is intended (see **Recommendations 7–8**). Depending on the intervention, this may consist of individuals of a given age and sex, individuals living in a particular region, those with a specific disease, those with a certain risk profile, or groups defined by combinations of these characteristics. The target population can have a dramatic effect on the cost-effectiveness of an intervention because both the costs and effects of an intervention can vary substantially across groups. We also note that, for some interventions, consequences may extend to individuals outside of the population that receives the intervention. For example, smoking cessation may have benefits beyond those that accrue to the person who quits smoking through reduction in second-hand smoke exposure to nonsmokers. And a screening program for HIV will have effects beyond those to the person screened because treatment of HIV results in reduced transmission, thus providing a broader community benefit (Long, Brandeau, and Owens 2009; Sanders, Hlatky, and Owens 2005).

The choice of target population will generally depend on the context of the analysis. For example, an analysis of public health programs designed to screen and treat medically underserved populations for high cholesterol in a defined geographic location would have a much different target population than an analysis focusing on alternative treatments for persons already identified with high cholesterol.

A target population can be divided into effectiveness subgroups, identifiable groups that would be expected, on the basis of previous research, to experience a different level of effectiveness from the intervention. For example, screening women over age 60 years will yield a greater number of breast cancer cases detected compared to screening younger women (Nelson et al. 2009). Although the elderly have a lower life expectancy, the cost per QALY gained could be lower (more favorable) for this subpopulation than for other groups—a possibility that the analyst would likely wish to explore by dividing a broad target population into the relevant age subgroups for analysis.

The target population may also differ in baseline risk. When such differences exist, an intervention may provide different absolute changes in outcomes even when relative risk reductions are stable across risk groups.

There may also be "cost subgroups" within a target population. A cost subgroup is a particular subgroup that would be expected to have different resource consumption or savings as a result of the intervention. As a result of economies of scale, a smoking cessation program for pregnant women conducted in an urban setting might cost less per person than the same program in a rural area where there were fewer pregnant women, and, as a result, fewer participants attending the program. In this example, the differences may raise important questions of equity and fairness, and analysts should make the assumptions and their implications clear to decision makers (see Chapter 12 for a more detailed discussion).

Heterogeneity in effectiveness or costs can generate subgroups (see **Recommendation 8**) that will, in general, have differential cost-effectiveness. It is important in designing the study to identify such subgroups and to determine the extent to which subgroup analyses will be undertaken. To ignore these in CEA can result in forgone health benefits or wasted resources (Coyle, Buxton, and O'Brien 2003; Sculpher 2008). Subgroup analyses may also be of interest to the decision maker if they address groups of particular importance, but this advantage must be balanced against the decreased precision when smaller subgroups are considered based on available data. For example, many clinical trials may suggest heterogeneity of intervention effects but do not have sufficient power to provide strong evidence on the differential effectiveness of an intervention in various subgroups. Often, statistical or simulation modeling is needed to infer the effects of interventions in subgroups. As noted previously, subgroup analyses may raise important questions of equity, and the analysis should make these considerations apparent to decision makers (see Chapter 12).

The target population may also contain preference subgroups, that is, groups that have significantly different preferences for the relevant outcomes (Basu and Meltzer 2007). For example, breast cancer screening in women ages 40 to 49 provides modest reductions in breast cancer mortality, but it involves risks of false-positive mammograms and overdiagnosis (diagnosis of breast cancer that, left untreated, would not affect a woman's health). Some women may be particularly averse to the health-related quality-of-life decrements associated with the diagnostic cascade that occurs after a false-positive mammogram, whereas others might have stronger concerns about breast cancer mortality (Qaseem et al. 2007). When these preferences are reflected in the health utility measure in a CEA, they may lead to differences in the cost-per-QALY result for the subgroups. The analysis might demonstrate that a particular program is more cost-effective for individuals with certain preferences than for those with different preferences. Thus, it may be important to include preference subgroups within the target population in the analysis.

4.7 COMPARATORS

Selection of one or more appropriate comparator interventions is crucial in a CEA (**Recommendations 9–10**). In theory, if study resources were unlimited, the ideal approach would be to identify all possible intervention variations applicable to the particular problem and all possible comparator interventions and their variations, including a "do-nothing" option. Costs and effects would be gathered on all of these interventions. Incremental cost-effectiveness would be used to analyze the results and to present the findings to the decision makers (see Chapter 13).

In reality, resources for undertaking CEAs are limited, and studies may not be able to assess all possible interventions and comparators. However, as a rule and at a minimum, Reference Case analyses from the healthcare sector and societal perspectives should compare the intervention to relevant alternatives and to the existing practice for addressing the health problem (the status quo), which may itself be variable between locations, healthcare settings, and clinicians. The question being addressed is, "What is the cost-effectiveness of replacing existing practice with the new intervention or relevant alternatives?" If the comparators included in the analysis do not include existing practice, the results can be deceptive. For example, if a new drug treatment for hypertension is compared to "no treatment," or to an expensive and not very effective alternative, the analysis will overstate the new drug's cost-effectiveness. That is, the comparison would not reflect the true value of an incremental change in practice.

Using the status quo as a primary comparator raises the problem of defining it. The status quo is often not a single intervention but a mixture of different approaches. For example, current pharmacologic treatment of type II diabetes involves over 20 therapeutic options.

When the status quo is a mixture of different interventions, there are two possible approaches to selecting the comparator(s) for the analysis. One approach, which we recommend, is to select each intervention, or at least the main ones, as comparators in the analysis. This has the advantage of identifying the cost-effectiveness of all the interventions and enables users of the CEA to assess how the new intervention compares with specific existing practices. However, it also requires data on each intervention, and it presupposes that the interventions are truly alternatives, in the sense that any of them can be given to any of the patients.

The alternative approach is to use the status quo mixture of interventions as a single comparator. The two approaches address different questions. The first addresses the question, "Assuming that patients could receive any of the current interventions of the status quo, or the new intervention under study, which would be recommended using CEA?" The second addresses the question, "What is the ICER of a shift in practice from the current mixed status quo approach to the new intervention under study?" The second approach has the disadvantage that current practice may not be optimal, and may have limited generalizability if practice patterns for the status quo differ across settings. This approach is appropriate only if the status quo mixture cannot be separated into individual interventions.

Comparing a new intervention with current practice is useful for evaluating the impact of replacing an existing intervention with an alternative, which is often the goal of a CEA. However, if existing practice is relatively cost-ineffective, the new intervention can appear better than it would if compared to other real options. In essence, the new intervention is being compared to a "straw man," rather than to truly desirable choices. Unfortunately, we may not know whether or not the status quo is cost-effective in its own right, since, more often than not, existing practice has not been subjected to careful evaluation.

To circumvent the problem that existing practice may not be the most suitable comparator, an analysis should investigate a range of other alternatives. These may include the best available alternative (as defined by evidence-based clinical guidelines or some appropriate authority), and particularly any viable low-cost alternatives. A "do-nothing" option (an option defined in a relative sense as not doing the type of intervention in question, as opposed to the absence of any care—for example, treatment of disease when it occurs is often the "do-nothing" approach for a preventive intervention) may be important to consider. In some cases, the do-nothing approach will be existing practice, but in others it will be a distinct option—one that provides a comparator for the status quo option as well as the new intervention. In general, and specifically for the Reference Case analyses, we recommend that analysts consider the full range of available and feasible options, including existing practice (the status quo) and a do-nothing option, as appropriate (**Recommendation 9**).

4.8 COMPARATORS FOR INTERVENTIONS OF VARYING INTENSITY OR DURATION

Interventions often vary in intensity, defined by frequency of screening, dosage of treatment, or positivity criteria applied to a screening test. When there are variations in the intensity of an intervention, each variation in the intervention that is more intense is compared to the next less intense option being considered. That is, it is important to use the next less intense option as the comparator in order to calculate the incremental cost-effectiveness of the option. For example, annual screening with mammography for breast cancer should be compared to biennial screening (every 2 years), which in turn should be compared to screening every 3 years. If a biennial option is available, it is the cost-effectiveness of one additional screening in a 2-year period that is at issue. If annual screening were instead compared to no screening, the resulting cost-effectiveness ratio would credit the annual program with benefits that could have been obtained by the less intensive biennial screening plan.

In interventions of varying intensity, the analyst is also faced with specifying the intervention options—which, in reality, are part of a continuum of options—that will be compared. In the mammography example above, a CEA could compare mammography every 1, 2, or 3 years, or it could compare mammography every 1, 3, or 5 years. The options selected (or developed) for inclusion may have a significant effect on the results. Annual screening will appear more cost-effective when it is compared to screening every 3 years than when it is compared to screening every 2 years. Moreover, if screening every 2 years is an option, the comparison against every 3 years is incorrect and misleading.

We recommend that the analyst use the principle of including in the analysis all frequencies (or levels of intensity in other dimensions) that are genuinely feasible and likely to be considered by decision makers. This determination will be a matter of judgment. For example, if an annual screening program is an option, should screening every 6 months also be included? What is the least intensive version of the intervention to be considered in the analysis—that is, the one to be compared to "no intervention?" Should it be screening every 5 years, every 7, or once in a lifetime? The analyst will have to decide at what point comparisons are no longer realistic and when programs differ little enough in their effect that finer distinctions will not offer much additional insight.

In summary, a CEA should consider the full range of available and feasible options, including existing practice (the status quo) and a do-nothing option, as appropriate. This approach will ensure that the most cost-effective policy and the appropriate comparators for estimation of ICERs are included in the analysis. Omission of relevant comparators may result in the estimation of ICERs that are overly favorable or otherwise misleading (Cantor and Ganiats 1999). Analysts should therefore carefully justify exclusion of any alternative from the comparator set.

4.9 SCOPE

In designing a CEA, the analyst and relevant decision makers must consider the boundaries, or scope, of the study (**Recommendation 7**). Spillover effects ripple out from every intervention designed to improve health. The question is how far to follow such ripples. A smoking cessation program for pregnant women potentially affects both the women's health and that of their infants, as smoking during pregnancy can cause low birthweight, respiratory distress syndrome, and other problems for infants. The smoking cessation program would clearly affect the health of the mother, and a

CEA presumably would include effects on the mother's probability of developing lung cancer, heart disease, and other smoking-related illness. However, the scope of the study could be broader still. For other children in the family, the risks associated with the mother's second-hand smoke will be eliminated if she quits smoking. Should the analyst track down these impacts or not? In theory, they are all relevant, but part of designing the study involves drawing practical limits around the analysis.

Three aspects of scope can be differentiated. The first concerns the groups of people to be considered in the analysis. A childhood illness or disability will likely require parents to spend time away from work, paid or unpaid. Infectious diseases, such as HIV, tuberculosis, and measles, are transmitted across populations and, over time, a single case can ultimately affect very large numbers of individuals. Many interventions will have their greatest effect on the health of the index patient but will also affect the well-being of the family, other relatives, friends and neighbors.

The analysis should generally encompass all populations where effects are notable. However, if the effects on a particular group are small relative to the major costs and outcomes considered in the analysis—that is, if they would have a negligible effect on the study results—they can reasonably be excluded. As part of the definition of the boundaries of the study, the analyst should clearly delineate the groups of people included in the analysis and explain the exclusion of other affected groups.

Although the societal perspective prescribes that consequences for all affected persons be included in the analysis, in practice many analyses have not included health-related quality-of-life effects on persons other than the individuals directly affected by the intervention. Thus, in an analysis of an intervention for Alzheimer's disease, an analyst might have included the costs of caretaking provided by a spouse or children and the health-related quality-of-life impact on the individual suffering from the disease, but not the effects of the illness on the health-related quality of life of family members (Neumann et al. 1999). Excluding such benefits will lead to an estimate of cost-effectiveness for an intervention that is less favorable than would an analysis that included these costs and benefits.

Research on health-related quality-of-life effects for family members is somewhat limited. However, as the research base continues to develop, we encourage analysts to think broadly about the people affected by an intervention and to begin to include health-related quality-of-life effects of these individuals in sensitivity analyses when it is thought they may be important. We also note that public health and environmental interventions may have broad health effects, and analysts should reflect such effects to the extent possible.

A second aspect of scope involves the types of health outcomes to be counted. A study may focus primarily on life years gained, or it may also incorporate health-related quality of life. Health-related quality of life itself can incorporate many domains of health, including physical, mental, and emotional health. We recommend the use of QALYs, which encompass changes in both length of life and health-related quality of life, to capture outcomes (see Chapter 7). In designing the analysis, the analyst should decide which of these types of health outcomes are most appropriate for inclusion in the study.

Third, non-health effects can also be important. For example, an intervention that provides treatment for substance use disorders might also cause reductions in expenditures in the criminal justice system if the program reduced crime related to substance use (see the worked example, Appendix A). An environmental cleanup might have effects on property values as well as health effects.

In a significant change from the original Panel's recommendation, the Second Panel recommends that all analyses at least enumerate in an Impact Inventory the costs and effects of an intervention across all relevant sectors (**Recommendation 5**). Thus, if an intervention has effects on sectors beyond healthcare, such as education, the environment, or the criminal justice system, the analyst would, at a minimum, list such effects in the Impact Inventory (see Chapter 13). We also encourage analysts to quantify and value such outcomes. This change recognizes the intent of the original Panel to include all such effects, along with the reality that few analyses have done so. For some interventions, particularly in public health, non-healthcare sector consequences may be very important.

Analysts can reasonably exclude from the analysis consequences that have little impact on cost-effectiveness, but we recommend listing these consequences in the Impact Inventory and justifying their exclusion (**Recommendation 11**).

Defining the boundaries of a study can be thought of as drawing a circle around the study to contain its scope. In circumscribing the study, the analyst must attempt to balance the need to capture all significant costs and effects of the intervention that will be relevant to the decision maker with the need to contain the study to the form of a manageable and feasible project. Considering the elements of the Impact Inventory when defining the scope of the analysis can help significantly with these tasks by elucidating the healthcare and non-healthcare sector effects to be included and measured in the analysis, while also identifying effects up front that may be difficult to measure quantitatively but should be acknowledged in the analysis.

4.10 TIME HORIZON

The time horizon of the CEA should extend far enough into the future to capture important differences in consequences—both intended and unintended (**Recommendation 12**). As a result, some analyses follow patients for the duration of their lives. For certain interventions, such as the removal of environmental toxins, the intervention effects may run even longer, requiring a time horizon that extends for generations. In contrast, an intervention for which all consequences occur over a short time horizon can be evaluated without use of a lifetime time horizon.

Frequently, the appropriate time horizon extends beyond the availability of primary data, and the analyst will need to extrapolate to longer time horizons using modeling. It is often useful to analyze the data using different time horizons: for example, a short-term horizon that includes only primary data and a long-term horizon that also incorporates modeled data. An analysis of smoking cessation programs for pregnant women that used a short time horizon, for example, could focus on the success of these programs in helping mothers quit smoking for the duration of their pregnancy. The study would focus on the health outcomes for the infant. A longer time horizon would be able to incorporate the health benefits for the mother as well. However, this analysis would need to model the long-term success of these programs and the effects on the health of the mother of having stopped smoking for short and long periods of time. Analysts should recognize that using a time horizon that does not encompass all consequences can provide a misleading estimate of the cost-effectiveness of an intervention (Sanders et al. 2005).

It is particularly important to extend the analysis far enough into the future to capture important health effects. For example, consider an analysis of a cholesterol-lowering program based on a clinical trial with a 5-year follow-up period. If only years of life within the 5 years were included, then any differential between programs in survival beyond the 5-year period would be lost. The gain in life years for the group with the higher 5-year survival would be grossly underestimated. Hence, at a minimum, modeling should be used to estimate gains in life expectancy due to differential survival. As noted, the time horizon should also be sufficient to capture relevant costs. Chapter 5 further discusses recommendations for the appropriate time horizon.

When a positive discount rate is used, as is recommended for Reference Case analyses (Chapter 3), the time horizon of the study will in many cases be effectively limited by the discount rate. That is, costs and effects occurring far in the future will change the cost-effectiveness ratio very little. Analysts should explore the impact of varying the discount rate (the rate at which future benefits and costs are discounted), particularly for interventions that have benefits far in the future (e.g., preventive interventions that may have benefits many decades in the future) as noted in Chapter 10.

4.11 THE ANALYSIS PLAN

Designing the data collection and analysis plan for the CEA involves three basic steps. First, the analyst, in consultation with subject experts and decision makers, must develop a conceptual model describing the intervention and its effects on health and non-health outcomes. Essentially, the model describes the course of events with the intervention versus without the intervention. Second, the analyst must determine how to collect the data on costs, health effects, non-health effects, and preferences for health effects for the intervention and the relevant comparators from the perspectives selected. The tasks required for this step vary greatly depending on whether, and to what extent, the analysis will collect primary data (e.g., collecting cost data as part of a clinical trial), use existing data (e.g., performing secondary analyses on data from administrative databases or published reports), or estimate parameters using mathematical models. The key principle is that the analyst should use all relevant evidence (Chapter 9). Finally, the analyst must develop the analytic methods to combine the information appropriately into a CEA.

We recommend that analysts develop a written protocol for the design and conduct of the study (**Recommendation 13**). Such a protocol will help the analysts scope the problem appropriately, summarize the analysis plan, and will make design decisions transparent to stakeholders interested in the conduct and results of the study. The protocol should describe, at a minimum, the objectives of the study, including the research questions; the type of economic evaluation to be conducted; the perspective of the analysis; the intervention and comparator; the population under consideration; the time horizon for the study; sources of data; a list of key assumptions; and an analysis plan, including the outcomes the analysis will assess. The analysts should update the protocol as the study progresses, and should note the changes from the original protocol.

4.12 THE CONCEPTUAL MODEL

The conceptual (or schematic) model serves as a guide to the conduct of a CEA. In concrete and well-defined steps, the conceptual model outlines an "event pathway" stemming from the use of the intervention or comparators, and linking them to health and non-health outcomes. It reflects the analyst's conception of how the intervention is used and the manner in which it affects the course of the disease of interest, its treatment, and the health status of the target population and other affected individuals. Graphical representations of the conceptual model are useful both for designing the analyses and for communicating about the model to the users of the analysis. An example is provided in Figure 4.1.

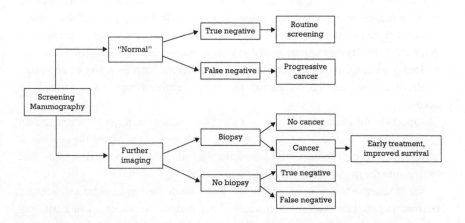

Figure 4.1 A simplified schematic of a conceptual model for breast cancer screening. Initial mammography leads to either a "normal" mammogram, which can be a true-negative or false-negative result, or to further imaging. Further imaging can lead to a biopsy, or if the initial mammogram were a false-positive, no biopsy. Biopsy can lead to an early cancer diagnosis. A more realistic conceptual model would include substantial additional detail. The comparator (not shown) is no screening.

The conceptual model includes all relevant effects—positive and negative, intended and unintended—of the intervention being considered and the alternatives to it. For example, a conceptual model of a breast cancer screening intervention would allow for false-positive and false-negative results, as well as correct results of screening, and would identify the possible events following each of these results (Figure 4.1). The model would outline disease-related and clinical events in the screened population (stages of cancer, surgery, medical treatments) within the bounds of the scope, time horizon, and other aspects of the study design, and would also include harms from the intervention, including overdiagnosis (diagnosis of a "cancer" that would not become apparent in a woman's lifetime) and other adverse events associated with diagnosis or therapy. Similarly, a conceptual model of a bicycle helmet program would trace the possible types of bicycle accidents, the potential range of injuries with and without the protection of a helmet, and the lifetime consequences of these injuries.

While the event pathway is generally constructed to represent health effects, depicting health states and events that have an impact on health, it also reflects the cascade of cost implications resulting from an intervention. The same events that cause changes in the health state of an individual generally trigger costs. The screening intervention that uncovers disease, for example, requires a visit to a clinician or other screening site, expends the patient's time, and uses healthcare resources including a clinician's time and laboratory tests. When costs arise from an event that is not explicit in a "clinical" event pathway—such as when a person moves from an acute care facility to a rehabilitation hospital without a change in health status—it may be useful to represent the change as a separate step or "state" in the pathway.

Decision trees or probability trees may be used to represent schematically the conceptual model (Chapter 5). The intervention and each comparator can be represented by main branches in the tree, and subsequent events, including probabilistic events, can be depicted by the further branches of the tree. Decision trees are a convenient graphic for displaying the probability of various outcomes, the costs associated with various clinical events, and preferences for the different outcomes. Some conceptual models will have enough complexity that other graphical representations will be needed.

Aspects of the conceptual model will affect the analyst's range of choice regarding the inputs to the CEA and, to some extent, the methods for conducting the analysis. It is useful to consider these aspects of the conceptual model as it is being designed—and to structure the model to support a workable study.

The manner in which events and health states are defined in an event pathway has far-reaching implications for the conduct of the analysis, because the event pathway specifies the types of data to be used. For example, if a model of a smoking cessation program links smoking history states to ultimate survival, the data requirements will be different from a model linking smoking history to cardiac events and cancer, and then linking these events to survival.

The time periods during which movement along the event pathway occurs are also part of the conceptualization of the analysis. The appropriate time period—that is, the size of a unit of time in the model, as distinct from the time horizon of the analysis—depends on the intervention under study and the conditions it affects. For some conditions, the unit of 1 year provides sufficient detail. For other conditions, however, important changes in a patient's condition, including his or her chances of survival, may occur in just a few days, weeks, or months. In these cases, the time period used will generally be shorter. For still other conditions, a mixture may be necessary: Events in the immediate aftermath of the condition and its treatment may require short periods of time to define health states and their probabilities, whereas later events may be adequately represented by probabilities that change from one year to the next (see Chapter 5).

The definition of health outcomes in the conceptual model has an important effect on the types of preference weights that can be used to assign health-related quality-of-life values in the study. If the analyst intends to use existing preference weights from the literature to calculate QALYs—as will often be the case—the model must use health states for which utility scores are already available. For example, if the model has an average weight for "kidney failure," it would only be necessary to know the impact of an intervention on that state. But if the model had weights for different health states associated with kidney failure, it would be necessary to know the distribution of those health states for a population with kidney failure (see Chapter 7). Analysts should also consider non-health consequences for those interventions that have important effects outside of health.

The conceptual model, as noted above, outlines the full range of events stemming from the intervention. Because it will guide the analysis, it should be considered in great detail, including costs and effects at all levels of importance. However, in most CEAs it is not efficient, nor would it be feasible, to measure and include every relevant effect and cost in the analysis itself. Costs or effects that are not important in the context of the analysis may be excluded. However, it is often difficult to identify such costs and effects in advance. After constructing the conceptual model, therefore, the analyst—perhaps in consultation with subject matter experts and decision makers—should consider the importance of components of the analysis to determine whether an element should be included, excluded, or investigated further to determine its importance.

The process of designing a study is generally an iterative one. As the analyst learns more about the details of the analysis, the conceptual model can be reevaluated and refined. The feasibility of gathering primary data and the availability of secondary data on event probabilities, health outcomes, and resource use all affect the ultimate form of the analysis. For example, the types of data on survival, healthcare utilization, and cost available for smokers might determine the choice of conceptual models in the smoking cessation example discussed earlier.

In most analyses, the conceptual model developed at this early stage of the study will later be incorporated into a mathematical or simulation model for use in actually calculating net cost and net effectiveness for the population, subgroup, or individual undergoing the intervention (see Chapter 5). In developing the conceptual model, therefore, it is useful to consider the technical form of the analysis so that the steps can be readily translated into this operational form.

4.13 COLLECTING THE DATA

As part of the design of the CEA, the analyst must decide what types of data to include in the analysis. The analyst can collect primary data (e.g., as part of a clinical trial) on costs, effects, health states, and non-health consequences. Secondary data—obtained from studies in the literature, administrative databases, or other sources of existing data—can be used instead of, or in addition to, primary data. Decision models can be used to combine primary and secondary data in various ways to generate estimates of consequences. Finally, collecting data on health-related quality of life raises special issues, which are discussed briefly below.

The estimates of costs and effects of relevance for the analysis are those for the population or group that is actually affected by the health intervention, with the exception that community preferences for health states are most appropriate for the Reference Case analyses. Methods for identifying and valuing the consequences of an intervention are discussed in much greater detail in later chapters (see Chapters 6, 7, and 8).

As discussed later, when subgroup estimates are used in an analysis, the results may diverge from what they would have been for a broader population in ways that the researcher believes to be ethically controversial. So, for example, while many analysts would not consider the difference in life expectancy between adults and children a source of discrimination against adults, assigning different time costs to employed and unemployed individuals is much more controversial. In these cases, the analyst may want to conduct sensitivity analyses to demonstrate the effect of group-specific estimates. Sensitivity analyses systematically vary the value of a variable to assess its impact on the important outcomes of the analysis. In planning data collection, the analyst will want to consider whether ethically sensitive issues will arise and be prepared to collect both group-specific data and data for a broader population (see recommendations about using sensitivity analysis to inform ethical issues in Chapter 12).

We now discuss two approaches to collecting and integrating the evidence on which the analysis is based. In some analyses, much or all of the data are collected as part of a clinical trial. These *trial-based analyses* collect data on health outcomes and costs in the same population. Because most interventions are not studied in clinical trials that assess both effectiveness and costs, a more common approach is *model-based CEA*. Many analyses use a hybrid of these two approaches—for example, a study may be based primarily on trial data, but use a model to extrapolate results beyond the trial period.

4.13.1 Trial-Based CEA

There are many examples of CEAs that have been conducted using primary data on costs and outcomes collected for individual patients in a clinical trial, either a randomized controlled trial (RCT) or some form of observational study (Neumann et al. 2015; Ramsey et al. 2015). In these trial-based CEAs, estimates of mean costs and outcomes are generated for the alternatives being compared in the clinical trial. In such studies, data on healthcare utilization are collected during, and sometimes after, the trial. Utilization information includes, for example, the number of hospital admissions and lengths of stay, tests and procedures, physician visits, and drugs prescribed. Patients are often surveyed to estimate time costs, and health-related quality-of-life information can be assessed prospectively via questionnaire or computer-based interview (Joyce et al. 2009). In the case of CEAs conducted in the context of an RCT, the randomized, double-blinded, and controlled nature of the primary study is often seen as having high internal validity, minimal bias, and tight protocol control.

Clinical trials that collect data on both health and economic outcomes can provide an important input to guide decision making, and a range of methodological and practical enhancements have been made to them over recent years (Glick et al. 2014). However, such trials can have a number of limitations and may rarely be entirely suitable given the principles of CEA (Sculpher 2015). For example, a clinical trial cannot serve as the sole source of data for a CEA unless the trial includes all of the options available to manage a particular set of patients, includes all patient groups that are candidates for the intervention, incorporates all relevant evidence, and has a time horizon long enough to capture all relevant health impacts and costs. It would be an uncommon occurrence for a trial to satisfy all these criteria. In addition, if the intervention has costs and effects that fall outside the healthcare sector, these must be included in the societal perspective Reference Case, but, again, it would be unusual for a trial to capture all such effects. Thus, the circumstances in which a single clinical trial will provide sufficient data to perform a Reference Case analysis from either a healthcare sector or societal perspective will be limited.

4.13.2 Model-Based CEA

Given the above-described limitations of trial-based CEA, CEA is most frequently conducted using decision models as the primary feature of the analysis (see Chapter 5). A model-based CEA generally uses estimates of costs and effects from a variety of sources, including RCTs, observational studies, administrative databases, and meta-analyses. Often, data on costs and effects or event probabilities have to be obtained from multiple different sources. The advantages and disadvantages of each type of data source from the perspective of CEA are discussed in Chapter 6 (for effectiveness data) and in Chapter 8 (for designs commonly used to assess resource utilization).

Decision models provide a framework for decision making under uncertainty (Sox, Higgins, and Owens 2013). In the context of CEA, such models are useful, and often essential for (1) extrapolating beyond the time horizon of available data; (2) extrapolating from intermediate outcomes (for example, blood pressure or cholesterol level) to outcomes such as length of life and health-related quality of life; (3) extrapolating to other population subgroups not directly observed in studies; (4) extrapolating to interventions that either were not studied in the same trial or have not been studied; (5) weighing benefits, harms, and costs; and (6) assessing the implications of evidential and other forms of uncertainty for decisions (see Chapters 5 and 11 for fuller discussions). The models offer a means to combine data from disparate sources to depict the cascade of events resulting from an intervention. They are useful for scenario building and for exploring the future implications of alternative policies.

Because few clinical trials will capture all of the relevant interventions and populations, or have a sufficient time horizon, the vast majority of CEAs will require modeling. To address the limitations of trials, an increasingly common design for CEA is to combine a clinical trial with a decision model. Often, these designs begin with primary data—for example, from a clinical trial. These data may be sufficient to make circumscribed inferences regarding health and cost consequences, but a model is required to extend the analysis beyond the original setting and time frame to estimate ultimate patient outcomes and cost-effectiveness.

4.13.3 Data on Health-Related Quality of Life

Many CEAs assess interventions that affect health-related quality of life. The analysis will therefore require data on the quality of life of relevant health states and the impact of the intervention on quality of life of the health states. These data can be obtained from primary or secondary sources (see Chapter 7).

Preference weights are assessments of the health-related quality of life associated with health states. They can be obtained along with cost and effectiveness data from subjects in a clinical trial. In this case, patients can give preference weights for their own health states and for other states relevant to the study but hypothetical to the patient at the time of the interview. Analysts can also obtain preference weights for a cost-effectiveness study from existing studies that have collected data on preferences for health states (see, e.g., Joyce et al. [2009]).

Another option that is being widely used in clinical trials involves gathering primary prospective data on the health status of patients in the trial using a generic preference-based measure of health-related quality of life that already has preference weights available (e.g., the Quality of Well-Being Index or the Health Utilities Index; see Chapter 7). The actual health status of the patients can then be scored with the pre-established preference weights, eliminating the need to undertake primary measurement of preferences.

4.14 CONCLUSIONS

Designing the CEA is a critical first step that is often given inadequate attention. The conceptualization and planning steps involved are essential for focusing the study on relevant research questions, defining its methodology, maintaining the focus as the study progresses, and avoiding analytical pitfalls midway through an analysis. The study design should be informed by consultation with subject area experts and decision makers, and by the policy choices being evaluated, and its design should be documented in a written protocol that is updated as the study proceeds.

4.15 RECOMMENDATIONS

1. Cost-effectiveness analysis (CEA), return-on-investment analysis, cost-minimization analysis, cost-consequence analysis, and cost–benefit analysis are alternative forms of analysis. The use of one does not preclude the use of the others.

2. We recommend that all studies report a Reference Case analysis based on a healthcare sector perspective and a Reference Case analysis based on a societal perspective. The Reference Cases include recommended methods, elements for reporting, and recommendations concerning what to include in the healthcare sector and societal perspectives. Inclusion of standardized components and standardization of methods within a perspective are intended to enhance consistency and comparability across studies.

3. We recommend that the results of the healthcare sector Reference Case be summarized in the conventional form, as an incremental cost-effectiveness ratio (ICER). The net monetary benefit (NMB) or net health benefit (NHB) may also be reported, and a range of cost-effectiveness thresholds should be considered. We recommend that the healthcare sector perspective analysis include all formal healthcare (medical) costs—current and future, and related and unrelated—regardless of who bears the costs.

4. The Second Panel strongly supports evaluation of the broader impacts of health interventions. Thus, we recommend that analysts include a societal perspective Reference Case analysis. The societal perspective is essential whenever interventions are likely to have important effects on sectors of the economy outside of healthcare, and when there is a need or desire to understand all costs and effects regardless of to whom they accrue. The societal perspective includes medical costs (current and future, related and unrelated) borne by third-party payers or paid for out-of-pocket by patients, time costs of patients in seeking and receiving care, time costs of informal caregivers, transportation costs, effects on future productivity and consumption in added years of life, and other costs and effects outside the healthcare sector. The Second Panel agrees that it would be helpful to inform decision makers through the quantification and valuation of all health and non-health consequences of interventions, and to summarize those consequences in a single quantitative measure. However, there are no widely agreed upon methods for quantifying and valuing some of these broader impacts in CEA. We therefore recommend that analysts present the items listed in the Impact Inventory in the form of disaggregated consequences across different sectors. We also recommend that analysts use one or more summary measures, such as an ICER, NMB, or NHB, that include some or all of the items listed in the Impact Inventory. Analysts should clearly identify which items are included and how they are measured, and provide a rationale for their methodological decisions.

5. To help make the evaluation more explicit and transparent, we recommend inclusion of an Impact Inventory in every societal Reference Case analysis, even if the analyst does not quantify or value effects beyond the healthcare sector. The Impact Inventory lists the health and non-health impacts of an intervention that the analyst should consider in a societal Reference Case analysis.

6. All aspects of the interventions that may affect their cost or effectiveness should be defined for the analysis. These will include the target population and features such as the specific technologies used, the type of personnel delivering the intervention, the site of delivery, whether the service is "bundled" with other services, the frequency of the intervention, and its timing.

7. The scope of a study should be defined broadly enough to encompass the full range of groups of people affected by the intervention and all important consequences. For example, if an intervention affects both mother and child, the analyst should include the health impacts and costs to each.

8. When there is heterogeneity in estimates of cost-effectiveness between different subpopulations, the analyst should present these differences as subgroup analyses. The analyst should be aware that subgroup analyses may raise ethical issues and questions of equity as outlined in Chapter 12, which provides a framework for consideration of ethical questions that may be important to the analyst, decision makers, and stakeholders.

9. Both Reference Case analyses should consider the full range of available and feasible options, including existing practice (the status quo) and a do-nothing option, as appropriate.

10. Options being compared may include more than specific interventions, extending, for example, to therapeutic strategies, alternative treatment starting and/or stopping rules, joint or sequential diagnostic test strategies, alternative levels of intensity of an intervention, and public health interventions. In all cases, these should be specified as mutually exclusive options and be compared using incremental CEA.

11. Costs and outcomes that have little impact on the estimate of cost-effectiveness or the likelihood of an intervention being cost-effective, and therefore little impact on the relevant decisions, can reasonably be excluded from an analysis. Their magnitude should be indicated in the Impact Inventory, clarifying the decision to exclude them.

12. The time horizon adopted in a CEA should be long enough to capture all differences between options in relevant costs and effects.

13. We recommend that analysts develop a written protocol for the design and conduct of the CEA. The protocol should describe, at a minimum, the objectives of the study, including the research questions; the type of economic evaluation to be conducted; the perspective of the analysis; the intervention and comparators; the population under consideration; the time horizon for the study; sources of data; a list of key assumptions; and an analysis plan, including the outcomes the analysis will assess. The analysts should update the protocol as the study progresses and note any changes from the original protocol.

4.16 REFERENCES

Basu, A., and D. Meltzer. 2007. Value of information on preference heterogeneity and individualized care. *Med Decis Making* 27 (2):112–127.

Briggs, A. H., and B. J. O'Brien. 2001. The death of cost-minimization analysis? *Health Econ* 10 (2):179–184.

Cantor, S. B., and T. G. Ganiats. 1999. Incremental cost-effectiveness analysis: the optimal strategy depends on the strategy set. *J Clin Epidemiol* 52 (6):517–522.

Claxton, K., S. Walker, S. Palmer, and M. Sculpher. 2010. *Appropriate Perspectives for Health Care Decisions. CHE Research Paper 54*. York, UK: Centre for Health Economics, University of York. http://www.york.ac.uk/media/che/documents/papers/researchpapers/rp54_appropriate_perspectives_for_health_care_decisions.pdf.

Coyle, D., M. J. Buxton, and B. J. O'Brien. 2003. Stratified cost-effectiveness analysis: a framework for establishing efficient limited use criteria. *Health Econ* 12 (5):421–427.

de Koning, H. J., R. Meza, S. K. Plevritis, K. ten Haaf, V. N. Munshi, J. Jeon, S. A. Erdogan, C. Y. Kong, S. S. Han, J. van Rosmalen, S. E. Choi, P. F. Pinsky, A. Berrington de Gonzalez, C. D. Berg, W. C. Black, M. C. Tammemagi, W. D. Hazelton, E. J. Feuer, and P. M. McMahon. 2014. Benefits and harms of computed tomography lung cancer screening strategies: a comparative modeling study for the U.S. Preventive Services Task Force. *Ann Intern Med* 160 (5):311–320.

Glick, H. A., J. A. Doshi, S. S. Sonnad, and D. Polsky. 2014. *Economic Evaluation in Clinical Trials*. 2nd ed. Oxford: Oxford University Press.

Greenberg, D., C. Earle, C. H. Fang, A. Eldar-Lissai, and P. J. Neumann. 2010. When is cancer care cost-effective? A systematic overview of cost-utility analyses in oncology. *J Natl Cancer Inst* 102 (2):82–88.

Joyce, V. R., P. G. Barnett, A. M. Bayoumi, S. C. Griffin, T. C. Kyriakides, W. Yu, V. Sundaram, M. Holodniy, S. T. Brown, W. Cameron, M. Youle, M. Sculpher, A. H. Anis, and D. K. Owens. 2009. Health-related quality of life in a randomized trial of antiretroviral therapy for advanced HIV disease. *J Acquir Immune Defic Syndr* 50 (1):27–36.

Long, E. F., M. L. Brandeau, and D. K. Owens. 2009. Potential population health outcomes and expenditures of HIV vaccination strategies in the United States. *Vaccine* 27 (39):5402–5410.

McCabe, C., K. Claxton, and A. J. Culyer. 2008. The NICE cost-effectiveness threshold: what it is and what that means. *Pharmacoeconomics* 26 (9):733–744.

Nelson, H. D., K. Tyne, A. Naik, C. Bougatsos, B. K. Chan, and L. Humphrey. 2009. Screening for breast cancer: an update for the U.S. Preventive Services Task Force. *Ann Intern Med* 151 (10):727–737, W237–W742.

Neumann, P. J., R. C. Hermann, K. M. Kuntz, S. S. Araki, S. B. Duff, J. Leon, P. A. Berenbaum, P. A. Goldman, L. W. Williams, and M. C. Weinstein. 1999. Cost-effectiveness of donepezil in the treatment of mild or moderate Alzheimer's disease. *Neurology* 52 (6):1138–1145.

Neumann, P. J., T. Thorat, J. Shi, C. J. Saret, and J. T. Cohen. 2015. The changing face of the cost-utility literature, 1990-2012. *Value Health* 18 (2):271–277.

Paltiel, A. D., R. P. Walensky, B. R. Schackman, G. R. Seage, 3rd, L. M. Mercincavage, M. C. Weinstein, and K. A. Freedberg. 2006. Expanded HIV screening in the United States: effect on clinical outcomes, HIV transmission, and costs. *Ann Intern Med* 145 (11):797–806.

Qaseem, A., V. Snow, K. Sherif, M. Aronson, K. B. Weiss, D. K. Owens, and the Clinical Efficacy Assessment Subcommittee of the American College of Physicians. 2007. Screening mammography for women 40 to 49 years of age: a clinical practice guideline from the American College of Physicians. *Ann Intern Med* 146 (7):511–515.

Ramsey, S. D., R. J. Willke, H. Glick, S. D. Reed, F. Augustovski, B. Jonsson, A. Briggs, and S. D. Sullivan. 2015. Cost-effectiveness analysis alongside clinical trials II—An ISPOR Good Research Practices Task Force report. *Value Health* 18 (2):161–172.

Russell, L. B. 2009. Completing costs: patients' time. *Med Care* 47 (7 Suppl 1): S89-93.

Russell, L. B. 2014. Do we really value identified lives more highly than statistical lives? *Med Decis Making* 34 (5):556–559.

Sanders, G. D., A. M. Bayoumi, V. Sundaram, S. P. Bilir, C. P. Neukermans, C. E. Rydzak, L. R. Douglass, L. C. Lazzeroni, M. Holodniy, and D. K. Owens. 2005. Cost-effectiveness of screening for HIV in the era of highly active antiretroviral therapy. *N Engl J Med* 352 (6):570–585.

Sanders, G. D., M. A. Hlatky, N. R. Every, K. M. McDonald, P. A. Heidenreich, L. S. Parsons, and D. K. Owens. 2001. Potential cost-effectiveness of prophylactic use of the implantable cardioverter defibrillator or amiodarone after myocardial infarction. *Ann Intern Med* 135 (10):870–883.

Sanders, G. D., M. A. Hlatky, and D. K. Owens. 2005. Cost-effectiveness of implantable cardioverter-defibrillators. *N Engl J Med* 353 (14):1471–1480.

Sculpher, M. 2008. Subgroups and heterogeneity in cost-effectiveness analysis. *Pharmacoeconomics* 26 (9):799–806.

Sculpher, M. 2015. Clinical trials provide essential evidence, but rarely offer a vehicle for cost-effectiveness analysis. *Value Health* 18 (2):141–142.

Sculpher, M., and K. Claxton. 2012. Real economics needs to reflect real decisions: a response to Johnson. *Pharmacoeconomics* 30 (2):133–136.

Soares, M. O., J. C. Dumville, R. L. Ashby, C. P. Iglesias, L. Bojke, U. Adderley, E. McGinnis, N. Stubbs, D. J. Torgerson, K. Claxton, and N. Cullum. 2013. Methods to assess cost-effectiveness and value of further research when data are sparse: negative-pressure wound therapy for severe pressure ulcers. *Med Decis Making* 33 (3):415–436.

Sox, H. C., M. C. Higgins, and D. K. Owens. 2013. *Medical Decision Making*. 2nd ed. Chichester: John Wiley & Sons Ltd.

Teutsch, S. M., and J. F. Murray. 1999. Dissecting cost-effectiveness analysis for preventive interventions: a guide for decision makers. *Am J Manag Care* 5 (3):301–305.

5

Decision Models in Cost-Effectiveness Analysis

Karen M. Kuntz, Louise B. Russell, Douglas K. Owens,
Gillian D. Sanders, Thomas A. Trikalinos,
and Joshua A. Salomon

5.1 OVERVIEW

Cost-effectiveness analysis (CEA) in health and medicine involves estimating the expected costs and health effects of competing alternatives over a relevant time horizon. The purpose is to derive estimates of the incremental costs and effects of one alternative compared to another in the form of an incremental cost-effectiveness ratio (ICER), net monetary benefit (NMB), or net health benefit (NHB). If a single clinical study, whether a randomized controlled trial (RCT) or an observational study, collected data on costs (resource utilization) and health effects over the relevant time horizon, then one could use data-analytic techniques to calculate an ICER or NHB (O'Brien et al. 1994; Willan and Briggs 2006). It is often the case, however, that the data available to inform the costs and effects of different interventions come from disparate sources and often from studies for which analysts do not have access to primary data. In addition, basing a CEA on a single data set has several limitations in that a single study excludes evidence from other data sources and may only address a limited number of alternative interventions that pertain to the decision problem (Sculpher et al. 2006). Because of these limitations it is common practice to use a decision model to derive estimates for CEAs.

Decision models provide a framework for decision making under uncertainty (Hunink et al. 2014; Raiffa 1968; Sox, Higgins, and Owens 2013). They help structure the analysts' thinking and facilitate the communication of assumptions. Decision models not only provide a structural framework for synthesizing data from disparate sources but also allow for extrapolations that are often required to reflect the decision context appropriately. The types of extrapolations most relevant for CEAs include (1) extrapolating beyond the time horizon of available data; (2) extrapolating from intermediate outcomes to long-term outcomes such as length and health-related quality of life; (3) extrapolating to population subgroups not observed in studies; (4) extrapolating long-term outcomes associated with diagnostic test strategies; and (5) extrapolating to strategies that have not been studied in a head-to-head trial. The structure of a decision model provides the means with which empirical observations from different data sources and different study populations are used to inform the relevant measures for CEA. The process of linking observed data (at the individual participant or aggregate level) to mean estimates of costs and effects via a model structure requires assumptions and extrapolations, which should be made with intent and transparency.

Decision modeling was a well-established method of conducting CEAs by the mid-1990s; however, the original Panel devoted little attention to it and made only one recommendation specific to modeling: "Where direct primary or secondary empirical evaluation of effectiveness is not possible (e.g., in important subpopulations or in differing time frames), the use of modeling to estimate effectiveness is a valid mode of scientific inquiry for CEAs" (Gold et al. 1996, 309).

At its outset, the Second Panel recognized the importance of decision modeling in the conduct of CEAs and chose to devote an entire chapter to provide guidance on the development and implementation of decision models. This decision was driven in part by the inclusion of recommendations for developing decision-analytic models in several country-specific guidelines for conducting CEAs for health technology appraisals, including those developed in the United Kingdom (National Institute for Health and Care Excellence [NICE] 2013), Canada (Canadian Agency for Drugs and Technologies in Health [CADTH] 2006), and Australia (Australian Government Department of Health 2013). Those guidelines recognize the importance of using decision models to synthesize evidence from multiple sources and to extrapolate to decision-relevant outcomes. In addition, the Good Research Practices in Modeling Task Force—a collaboration between the International Society for Pharmacoeconomics and Outcomes Research (ISPOR) and the Society for Medical Decision Making (SMDM)—published best practice recommendations for several types of modeling approaches in 2012 (Briggs et al. 2012; Caro et al. 2012; Eddy et al. 2012; Karnon et al. 2012; Pitman et al. 2012; Roberts et al. 2012; Siebert et al. 2012). In this chapter, we draw upon these sources to inform our recommendations.

We first discuss modeling in the context of conceptualizing the CEA, which draws on guidance provided in Chapter 4. Our position is that a decision model would be informative and necessary in most CEAs, and we present and review several benefits of modeling. We also review the different types of decision models available and their relative advantages and disadvantages, and we discuss different ways for analysts to simulate populations and the implications for CEAs. We provide recommendations for the development of decision models related to model structure, data sources (drawing on guidance from Chapter 9), model output (drawing on guidance from Chapter 13), model uncertainty (drawing on guidance from Chapter 11), and model validation.

5.2 CONCEPTUALIZING THE DECISION PROBLEM

Prior to undertaking a CEA the analyst must develop a broad conceptualization of the decision problem with input from clinical and policy experts (see **Recommendation 1** in section 5.11) (Roberts et al. 2012). Broadly speaking, the conceptualization process involves defining the objectives of the analysis, the population(s) of interest, the intended audience, the interventions and comparators, the type of analysis (cost-minimization, cost-consequence, cost-effectiveness, or cost–benefit analysis), the perspective and its boundaries, the duration of the intervention, the time horizon, and the outcomes of interests.

Chapter 4 provides detailed guidance on determining the scope of the CEA. Briefly, the analyst should delineate the groups of people who will be affected by the intervention. In addition to those directly affected by the intervention, there may be effects on caregivers or other persons to consider in some cases. When modeling an infectious disease the analyst should be clear about the bounds of the population at risk of becoming infected. The types of outcomes that will be generated by the model should be clearly specified during model development; this is especially important when the outcomes of interest range beyond the typical outcomes of life expectancy, quality-adjusted life expectancy, and lifetime costs. For example, when evaluating colorectal cancer screening, the decision maker may also wish to know about cancer incidence reduction, or the additional number of colonoscopies required over a lifetime. Finally, the analyst should consider whether there are costs or effects beyond the health care sector that are important to include.

The initial conceptualization process is a critical prerequisite to the development of any decision model. The process should include both individuals with expertise in modeling and content experts for the particular problem, and it should be conducted independent of the data identification phase (**Recommendation 2**). The conceptualization informs the choice of model type, the type of population simulation (e.g., single cohort, whole population), the structure of the model (e.g., characterization of the disease and care processes), and the types of evidence needed to inform model parameters. Categories of data typically required for model parameterization describe the progression of the disease process in the absence of intervention or with usual care (often referred to as natural history) and include health state or event descriptions, changes in health over time, health-related quality-of-life weights (i.e., utilities), and costs associated with various health states or events. Interventions modify the natural history of the disease process. Interventions also impose harms and resource costs for which data are needed (see, e.g., Chapter 6).

The conceptualization of the decision problem will help the analyst choose among alternative approaches for developing the decision model. We describe the types of models later in this chapter (section 5.5); they include simple decision trees, state-transition cohort models, microsimulations, dynamic transmission models, and dynamic systems models. Different types of models have different strengths and limitations, and the choice will in large part depend on the conceptualization of the problem and the analyst's expertise. For many problems, more than one type of model could be appropriate.

5.3 NEED FOR A DECISION MODEL

A CEA should compare all interventions that are relevant for a particular decision problem (within reason). As noted above, RCTs generally compare a limited number of interventions. A CEA should also adopt a time horizon that is long enough to capture all relevant consequences, which is typically longer than the follow-up time in an RCT. For CEAs that evaluate interventions that affect survival, a lifetime time horizon should be used to estimate the total gains in life expectancy of the intervention relative to its comparator. Finally, an RCT typically represents only a portion of the information about evidence and uncertainty that pertains to a decision problem. Sculpher et al. recommend the "use of decision-analytic models, coupled with full evidence synthesis, as the only framework that has the potential to meet all requirements for economic evaluation for decision making" (Sculpher et al. 2006, 682). We agree that a decision model informed by a full review of the evidence will be necessary for most, if not all, CEAs. An important first step when conducting a CEA should be a consideration of the need for a decision model (**Recommendation 3**). If a decision model is not being used, the analyst should justify the reasons.

A decision model structures the sequences and likelihoods of events and states of nature that can occur over time under alternative interventions (strategies). By simulating a virtual target population, the model projects the costs and health outcomes associated with alternative interventions, incorporating all of the evidence deemed relevant for the purpose. A decision model often incorporates mathematical functions that represent knowledge about the disease—for example, the relationships between risk factors and disease, or between the disease and clinical outcomes. While there are different types of models, all provide a systematic and explicit way to examine a decision process and to estimate costs and health outcomes over a specified time horizon. Evidence that informs parameters may be available from multiple sources, and a single study may contribute to the estimation of more than one model parameter (or functional combinations of parameters). Modeling provides the mathematical tools for synthesizing all evidence and facilitating assessments of consistency across sources. Modeling also makes it possible to evaluate the uncertainty of model parameters and assumptions.

5.4 DECISION MODEL PROJECTIONS

As already noted, there are several situations that arise in the conduct of CEAs that require extrapolation: (1) extrapolating beyond the time horizon of available data; (2) extrapolating from intermediate (surrogate) outcomes to long-term outcomes such as life expectancy and quality-adjusted life expectancy; (3) extrapolating to population subgroups not observed in studies; (4) extrapolating long-term outcomes associated with diagnostic test strategies; and (5) extrapolating to strategies that have not been studied in head-to-head comparisons (**Recommendation 3**). Below we describe the most common types of extrapolations used in modeling and provide some examples.

For this chapter we distinguish between two situations: (1) trial or observational data are sufficient and individual-level data are available to the analyst; and (2) trial data are not sufficient or individual-level data are not available to the analyst. We refer to the former as trial-based CEAs and the latter as model-based CEAs. We make this distinction because there are statistical methods available that would be appropriate only in cases where individual-level data are available (Glick et al. 2014).

5.4.1 Extrapolation Beyond the Time Horizon of Available Data

The original Panel recommended that "[t]he time horizon adopted in a CEA should be long enough to capture all relevant future effects of a health intervention"(Gold et al. 1996, 305). When the interventions affect survival, it will be necessary to project health outcomes and costs over the remaining lifetimes of patients to capture all relevant future effects. The Second Panel reaffirms this recommendation (see Chapter 4), which is also common in the guidelines of national health technology assessment agencies (Australian Government Department of Health 2013; Canadian Agency for Drugs and Technologies in Health [CADTH] 2006; National Institute for Health and Care Excellence [NICE] 2013).

To extrapolate a CEA beyond the time horizon of the data, it is generally desirable to decompose the natural history of the disease or condition being studied. Using "usual care" or "standard care" to represent natural history may be preferred because it allows the analyst to use current outcome data.

For trial-based CEAs, primary data on the control (or usual care) group can be used to model survival, disease-free survival, or costs directly using statistical methods. When extrapolation is necessary, analysts typically fit parametric survival functions to the trial data (Guyot et al. 2011; Latimer 2013). Parametric functions make it possible to project costs, life years, or quality-adjusted life years (QALYs) beyond the time period covered by the data. Using the fitted function or functions, analysts can extrapolate survival to estimate outcomes in each year after the trial's end and over the remainder of the CEA's time horizon. Analysts typically fit separate functions to the control group and then apply a hazard ratio from the trial to estimate outcomes for the intervention group(s) (Guyot et al. 2011; Latimer 2013). Although using survival analysis methods allows analysts to project a survival curve beyond the time horizon of the data, it may not adequately capture changes in the health-related quality of life for the cohort. For this the analyst may adopt statistical methods to incorporate health-related quality of life effects into the analysis (Gelber et al. 1995).

For model-based CEAs, analysts typically use epidemiological studies, disease registries, and vital statistics data to model the natural history of the disease over patients' lifetimes. For these situations the modeler will need to develop a model structure that describes the disease process, estimate the natural history parameters from available data taken from multiple sources, and specify the necessary assumptions required for extrapolations. The health states or events described in the model should allow different costs (resource use), health-related quality-of-life weights (utilities), and intervention effects (benefits, costs, and risks) to be assigned.

An almost universal outcome in CEA for health interventions is mortality. Even if the intervention does not have a direct effect on mortality, if the time horizon is long enough it is generally not good to assume that no deaths occur during that time. Country-specific life tables are available and report the overall mortality rate for a population for each age (by sex and race), which reflects the rate of dying from any cause for that year (e.g., the rate at which 52-year-old women in the population of interest would be expected to die in their 53rd year of life). Typically, analysts incorporate age-, sex-, and race-specific mortality rates from life tables to represent other-cause mortality—that is, deaths from causes not related to the disease being modeled. If the disease of interest represents an appreciable proportion of all-cause mortality, then the analyst should subtract this cause from the life-table rates. Disease-specific mortality (related to the disease of interest) can be estimated from clinical studies and be combined with non-disease-specific mortality (e.g., other-cause mortality). There are several ways to combine these two rates of death, depending on the amount of age-specific data available for disease-specific causes of death. Two alternative basic assumptions that are available when there are no age-specific data are these: (1) the disease-specific mortality rate is additive with the age-dependent other-cause mortality rates or (2) the disease-specific mortality is represented as a multiplicative factor with other-cause mortality (Kuntz and Weinstein 1995). If life-table mortality is not provided to a sufficiently old age, the analysis will need to extrapolate age-dependent other-cause mortality rates for older ages.

The analyst may need to make assumptions about how the disease-specific mortality rate changes over time, ideally with input from clinical experts. It is often assumed that, given no change in a person's disease status, the disease-specific component of all-cause mortality (whether additive, multiplicative, or age-specific) persists for a lifetime. For cancer patients, however, a common assumption is that disease-specific mortality returns to that of a cancer-free person after a period of time (e.g., 10 years).

In a similar manner, if changes in health status can be estimated by age (e.g., the chance of progressing from mild angina to moderate angina), then as the cohort ages these age-specific rates apply, although typically the analyst must make assumptions about how rates might change when people age beyond the ages observed in clinical studies (typically informed by the age-specific pattern among the observed age range).

5.4.2 Projecting Efficacy Beyond the Trial Data

A measure of relative risk, drawn from effectiveness studies and often based on clinical trials or, preferably, a meta-analysis of those trials, can be applied to the natural history parameters to estimate the difference in the disease trajectory owing to the intervention over the time horizon of the CEA. The efficacy of interventions is often measured in RCTs, which can last a few months or a few years. For some conditions, such as advanced cancer, a short trial may be long enough to allow a CEA to base estimates of health outcomes and costs on the trial data, and only the trial data (Latimer 2013). Also, in cases where mortality is not affected by the intervention (either as a benefit or a harm), such as nonsteroidal anti-inflammatory therapy for patients with osteo-arthritis, it may be reasonable to adopt a time horizon that is shorter than a lifetime if all costs and effects are captured with the shorter period. For many interventions, however, such as screening for breast cancer (Mandelblatt et al. 2009), administration of statins for elevated cholesterol (Prosser et al. 2000), or management of a chronic condition such as diabetes (CDC Diabetes Cost-effectiveness Group 2002), the health outcomes and costs may continue for decades beyond the first screening or prescription or diagnosis, and far beyond the time period covered by any trial.

Regardless of how the natural history component of the model is developed (i.e., whether trial-based or model-based), the bigger issue in extrapolating beyond available data concerns what to assume about the effectiveness of the intervention after the time horizon of the trial. Will the intervention continue to be as effective beyond the trial period? Will its benefits increase or decrease? Might the intervention even turn out to be harmful over the longer term? Projecting intervention effectiveness is key to a CEA because effectiveness determines the *differences* in mortality and morbidity benefits attributed to the intervention each year over the time horizon of the analysis. Those differences determine the denominator—the net difference in QALYs—of an ICER.

Typically, the efficacy of an intervention is expressed in the form of a hazard ratio (HR) when trial outcomes are measured as time to an event (e.g., myocardial infarction, recurrence, death, composite outcome). Often, published RCTs refer to the HR as a relative risk, but it is in fact a ratio of rates (hazards) and not probabilities (risks). The hazard ratio usually assumes that the relative effect of the intervention is proportionally the same over the duration of the trial, which is called a "proportional hazards assumption." Analysts may choose therefore to project over patients' lifetimes the same effectiveness observed in clinical trials.

Analysts need to explore the accuracy of this, or any other, assumption about the intervention's effect. The original Panel suggested: "It is often useful to analyze the data using several time horizons: a short-term horizon that includes only primary data and a long-term horizon that also incorporates modeled data" (Gold et al. 1996, 68). The Canadian Agency for Drugs and Technologies in Health (CADTH) (2006) makes the same recommendation using virtually the same words. In contrast, NICE recommends routinely exploring alternative scenarios: ". . . for duration of treatment effects, scenarios might include when the treatment benefit in the extrapolated phase is: (i) nil; (ii) the same as during the treatment phase and continues at the same level; or (iii) diminishes in the long term" (National Institute for Health and Care Excellence [NICE] 2013, 51).

The Second Panel agrees with the NICE recommendations and finds the recommendation from the original Panel and CADTH to be inconsistent with the recommendation that the time horizon should be long enough to capture all benefits, costs, and harms of the intervention. A shortened time horizon should be used in a sensitivity analysis only if the analyst believes there is a need to show the impact of extrapolations beyond the time horizon of the data; in such cases, the limitations of the shorter horizon should be stressed. For example, Hlatky, Owens, and Sanders (2006) reported the differences in ICERs between a within-trial analysis (i.e., using the time horizon of the trial) and a lifetime analysis for implantable cardioverter defibrillators (ICDs). Using data from one clinical trial they found an ICER of $299,100 per QALY for the 3-year time horizon of the trial, whereas the ICER was $141,200 per QALY for a lifetime time horizon with conservative assumptions about the benefit after 3 years (Table 5.1).

Figure 5.1 illustrates three possible assumptions the analyst can make to extrapolate intervention effects beyond a hypothetical trial with a follow-up time of 5 years. For each of the three alternative scenarios noted, we illustrate the annual hazard rate as a function

Table 5.1 Effect of time horizon on marginal cost-effectiveness of ICD compared with drug therapy

Clinical trial	Within-trial analysis (years of follow-up)				Lifetime time horizon		
	1	2	3	4	Convergent survival[†]	Parallel survival	Divergent survival
			CIDS (O'Brien et al. 2001)				
$/LY	2,175,800	476,800	231,500	—	105,400	58,000	40,200
$/QALY	2,441,000	598,900	299,100	—	141,200	78,400	54,700
			AVID (Larsen et al. 2002)				
$/LY	629,100	211,400	117,200	—	60,400	34,000	23,500
$/QALY	796,500	275,400	154,300	—	79,300	46,000	32,000
			CASH (Kuck et al. 2000)				
$/LY	603,700	182,800	—	—	70,300	33,200	18,900
$/QALY	765,800	239,000	—	—	91,500	44,900	25,700
			MADIT (Mushlin et al. 1998)				
$/LY	339,600	107,200	58,900	40,700	27,600	17,400	15,200
$/QALY	440,400	141,700	78,400	54,400	36,900	23,600	20,700

Source: Table 1 in Hlatky, Owens, and Sanders (2006).

[†] Convergent survival assumes that the survival of the ICD cohort and the drug therapy cohort converge over 5 years after the end of the trial and then are equal to the drug therapy arm.

Abbreviations: AVID = Antiarrhythmics Versus Implantable Defibrillators; CASH = Cardiac Arrest Study Hamburg; CIDS = Canadian Implantable Defibrillator Study; ICD = implantable cardioverter defibrillator; LY = life year; MADIT = Multicenter Automatic Defibrillator Implantation Trial; QALY = quality-adjusted life year.

of time (i.e., model input) and the corresponding implications for the survival curves. The area between the two survival curves represents life years gained with intervention. The area to the left of the 5-year mark represents the benefit observed in the trial; the area to the right of 5 years represents benefit derived with extrapolation. Note that even if the analyst assumes that the HR falls to 1 (i.e., nil effect) after a certain time, the intervention group continues to accrue benefit. If the analyst chooses to limit the time horizon of the analysis to the time horizon of the trial, then the benefit would be just that to the left of the 5-year mark. An analysis with a time horizon equal to the trial period assumes, in effect, that if a life were saved during the study the person would die instantly at the end of the 5-year trial period, which we do not find to be a reasonable assumption.

5.4.3 Linking Intermediate Outcomes to Long-term Outcomes

Often clinical studies use intermediate (surrogate) outcomes (e.g., blood pressure control) because they are more likely to occur and/or more likely to occur much sooner

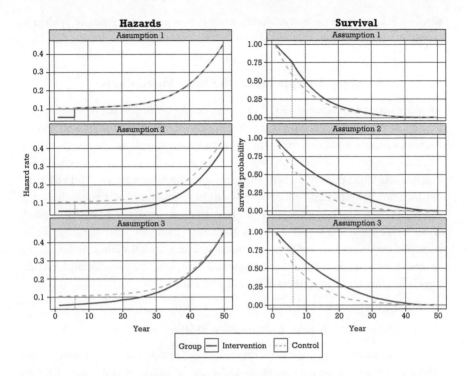

Figure 5.1 Extrapolation assumptions for intervention effect.

than the final outcome of interest (e.g., disease-specific mortality), thus allowing for studies with shorter time frames and smaller sample sizes. However, both patients and decision makers may also be interested in longer-term outcomes. For example, trials that evaluate interventions for patients with insulin-dependent diabetes may use intermediate outcomes such as retinopathy and neuropathy, whereas patients and decision makers are more interested in preventing blindness and amputation. Decision models can provide information on these longer-term outcomes by incorporating epidemiological data on the relationship between intermediate and long-term outcomes. Direct evidence on interventions and long-term outcomes remains preferable, but in its absence decision models contribute valuable information.

A good example of how the use of decision models has been shown to work well for extrapolating intermediate trial outcomes to longer-term outcomes is the case of cholesterol-lowering therapy. Many of the early RCTs of cholesterol-lowering drugs showed only that the drugs reduced cholesterol levels and did not demonstrate a reduction in cardiac events, such as myocardial infarction or cardiac death, or overall mortality. Early CEAs of cholesterol-lowering drugs—for example, the study by Goldman et al. (1991)—used the Framingham 10-year risk equations to translate the reductions in cholesterol levels to reduction in cardiac mortality. The Scandinavian Simvastatin Survival Study was the first RCT of a cholesterol-lowering drug to use overall death as the primary outcome and demonstrated a significant reduction in overall mortality (Scandinavian Simvastatin Survival Study Group 1994). The CEA performed alongside that trial, which incorporated modeling to project to a lifetime horizon, reported similar CEA results to the earlier studies using the surrogate outcome and epidemiological risk model (Johannesson et al. 1997).

5.4.4 Extrapolating to Other Populations

Intervention studies (especially RCTs) are often conducted in selected populations and may exclude, for example, older individuals or those with comorbidities; however, a decision maker is usually interested in assessing interventions in these groups as well. The analyst must define the target population for whom the program is intended. For example, the target population could be narrowly defined to represent 55- to 64-year-old men newly diagnosed with acute myocardial infarction (AMI) but without any significant comorbid conditions. For this population the evidence base may be good. Other target populations, such as 75- to 84-year-old men with AMI and a significant comorbid condition, may not be represented in existing clinical studies. In these cases, analysts must make assumptions about how to derive parameters specifically for a subpopulation that is underrepresented in clinical studies.

5.4.4.1 *Extrapolating to Other Ages*

The natural history of disease often depends on a person's age. In addition, health-related quality-of-life weights (utilities) and costs for similar health states or events may differ by age. For CEAs conducted for a particular age range of patients, and for which the disease of interest affects mortality, it is important to try to distinguish mortality components attributable to the disease versus nondisease (other) causes. This allows the analyst to use age-specific mortality from country-specific life tables to represent other causes of death and to derive a disease-specific component that may not depend on age.

If the intervention effect parameter is derived from an RCT, it likely will pertain only to a select subpopulation based on the inclusion criteria in the trial. Unless the trial reports efficacy by age, it is not possible to know if efficacy differs by age. Analysts typically assume that the intervention has the same effect across age groups and they evaluate this assumption in sensitivity analysis.

5.4.4.2 *Extrapolating to Different Comorbidity Levels*

The presence of one or more comorbidities will likely have an effect on mortality, health-related quality of life, costs, and possibly treatment effectiveness. The analyst should consider whether there are certain high-risk groups for which the intervention may have different cost-effectiveness compared with average-risk groups. For example, Sisk et al. (2003) evaluated the cost-effectiveness of vaccination against invasive pneumococcal disease among high-risk patients (based on comorbid conditions and race) and found that for certain high-risk groups vaccination was cost saving.

People with comorbidities are often excluded from clinical trials. In these cases analysts will need to make reasonable assumptions about whether or not the effectiveness of the intervention is similar across different groups of patients defined by baseline risk. Sometimes, the (independent) effect of comorbidities is to increase other-cause mortality rates in some predictable way (e.g., by a multiplying factor), with no impact on the disease prognosis. Some comorbid conditions, however, may affect other-cause mortality and the natural history of disease, or adherence to treatment. For example, co-infection with hepatitis C virus and HIV may accelerate the course of HIV disease compared to mono-infected individuals, and HIV may increase cardiovascular mortality through mechanisms that are not completely understood.

5.4.4.3 *Extrapolating to Different Assumptions about Adherence*

By using an efficacy estimate directly from an RCT, the analyst assumes that the adherence to the intervention or strategy observed in the trial is the same as would be observed in practice. It has been shown that the "efficacy" that is estimated from an RCT is often different from the "effectiveness" that would be observed in practice, with adherence being one of the reasons for this difference (Revicki and Frank 1999; Singal, Higgins, and Waljee 2014). It may be desirable for the analyst to consider more realistic scenarios about adherence to estimate costs and effects of interventions (Gandjour 2011). Modelers may explicitly incorporate non-adherence into their models, based on what is observed in practice. For the simulated patients who adhere to the intervention, applying the efficacy estimate directly from the RCT will underestimate the true effect. This is a conservative approach. However, analysts may also want to estimate the effectiveness of an intervention among fully adherent patients through a calibration process, incorporating the adherence observed in the trial, and they should report a sensitivity analysis on different adherence rates.

Different assumptions about adherence can give different results. For example, there are several options when modeling adherence with repetitive screening programs, particularly cancer screening. A 20% non-adherence rate could mean that each time a screening test is recommended a random 20% of the population is non-adherent, or it could mean that 20% of the population never attends the screening program and the remainder of the population is completely adherent, or it could be somewhere between these two extremes. Zauber et al. (2008) incorporated correlation of colorectal cancer screening behavior by assuming that the population was comprised of four risk behavior groups: those who never attend the screening program and those with low, moderate, and high random adherence rates. These concepts can also apply to pharmaceutical therapies, where non-adherence could refer to a population who only take a percentage of the recommended medication, or to a portion of the target population not taking the medication at all.

5.4.5 Analysis of Diagnostic Tests

We include the analysis of diagnostic test strategies as a separate type of extrapolation because studies of diagnostic tests focus primarily on test characteristics and not on patient outcomes. Model projections are necessary to translate the short-term outcomes associated with testing (e.g., true-positive result, false-negative result) to long-term outcomes such as lifetime costs and QALYs. Models are well suited to evaluate the costs, benefits, and harms of test-and-treat strategies and require input data from studies of test accuracy, treatment effectiveness, and disease-specific natural history studies. Aside from cognitive, emotional, and behavioral effects of testing, a test result has little immediate impact on outcomes; rather, benefits and harms accrue based on actions that occur because of the test result (further testing or treatment). The value of testing should be judged based on those downstream outcomes—the expected benefits, harms, and costs of alternative testing strategies (including no testing)—and models are good at piecing together the complete sequences of events. Testing strategies may consist of evaluating alternative positivity criteria for a single test (i.e., evaluation of different operating points on a receiver operating characteristic curve), sequencing multiple tests (e.g., if Test A is positive then do Test B, otherwise treat), or a combination of these. A diagnostic test strategy that accurately detects disease (i.e., true-positive result) and leads to effective treatment can result in overall benefit, although those patients with disease who are not detected (i.e., false-negative result) will not receive benefit but will incur the cost and possible risk of the test itself. Diagnostic tests can also falsely detect disease (i.e., false-positive result) and lead to inappropriate treatment, resulting in some degree of harm. Most of the clinical studies assessing medical tests focus on test performance such as sensitivity and specificity. Information on how test results change diagnostic thinking, treatment decisions, and ultimately person- and population-prognostic outcomes is addressed in other studies, or often not addressed at all. Thus, assessing the value of testing involves combining information from different studies, possibly along with expert opinion on some parameters, and this is typically done through modeling.

When conducting a CEA of alternative test-and-treat strategies, it may be important to consider the immediate consequences of testing in terms of costs; cognitive, behavioral, and emotional outcomes; and health outcomes associated with the test(s). The model structure, however, is ideal for identifying the longer term effects of a positive or negative test result, accounting for the likelihood that a provider will act on the results (further workup or intervention), the likelihood that the patient will follow the provider's recommendations, and the likelihood of occurrence of various costs, benefits, and harms associated with additional workup or interventions.

Analysts should be transparent about assumptions regarding the transferability of estimates of test performance. For example, it is important to be explicit about how estimates transfer across populations at different baseline risks or varying distributions of disease severity. Spectrum bias can occur when the spectrum of disease among the study population (that estimates the sensitivity of the test) is markedly different than the population for which the test will be used in practice (Ransohoff and Feinstein 1978). Another bias when using estimates derived from diagnostic testing studies is verification (or workup) bias (Begg and Greenes 1983). This bias occurs when not everyone with a test result has their true disease status ascertained with a gold standard test *and* the chance of receiving the gold standard test is associated with the test result (e.g., patients with positive test results are more likely to undergo gold standard testing). Mathematical adjustments are available for this type of bias (Begg and Greenes 1983). When modeling combinations of tests, analysts should state their assumptions about whether the tests are conditionally independent of each other (conditional on presence of disease and absence of disease) and should conduct sensitivity analysis on alternative assumptions. Analysts should consider that differences will occur across providers with different experience, which will have implications for tests that involve subjective assessment (e.g., radiological tests). Finally, some test characteristics are reported on a per-lesion basis (e.g., colonoscopy for finding adenomatous polyps or colorectal cancer) or on a per-person basis. The analyst must not use one form to represent the other, and should be clear about the approach taken for translating estimates of one type to the other.

5.4.6 Analysis of Multiple Competing Strategies

Another reason to develop a model when conducting a CEA is that often not all of relevant strategies for a particular problem have been evaluated in a single study and the analyst must rely on data from multiple sources. For example, there are several RCTs that compare annual and biennial colorectal cancer screening with fecal occult blood testing versus no screening. However, a CEA of colorectal cancer screening strategies should include other screening modalities (e.g., screening colonoscopy) and perhaps other screening intervals with a fecal occult blood test. As illustrated above, diagnostic strategies can be complex, with multiple tests and several possible ways to sequence tests with different follow-up decisions. Models are also able to evaluate sequences of pharmaceutical therapies to determine which therapies are best used as first-, second-, or third-line drugs.

Modeling can leverage what we know from studies that provide direct evidence of effectiveness. By clearly and transparently specifying the mechanisms of intervention effects on the natural history of the disease, they can be used to evaluate strategies for which we may not have direct evidence.

5.5 TYPES OF DECISION MODELS

The choice of model type is typically related to the decision problem at hand (Table 5.2). Three factors that a modeler should consider in choosing a modeling framework include (1) how to deal with time, (2) the unit of analysis (individual, cohort, or population), and (3) whether modeled individuals are allowed to interact with each other or other components of the model (**Recommendation 4**). For a question with a relatively short time horizon, such as which alternative strategy to choose for the prevention of postoperative infections with no long-term sequelae, a simple decision tree may suffice. In contrast, questions pertaining to the prevention of infectious (communicable) diseases, such as the benefits of an influenza vaccination program, would require a dynamic (infectious disease) model in order to capture the effects from herd

Table 5.2 Types of decision models

Model type	General description	Type of decision best suited for
Decision tree	Diagrams the risk of events and states of nature over a fixed time horizon	Modeling interventions for which the relevant time horizon is short and fixed
State-transition model, cohort	Simulates a hypothetical cohort of individuals through a set of health states over time	Modeling interventions for diseases or conditions that involve risk over a long time horizon and/or recurrent events
Microsimulation (individual) model	Simulates one individual at a time; tracks the past health states of individual and models risk of future events stochastically	Modeling complex disease processes, when state-transition models require excessively complex number of health states
Dynamic transmission model	System of differential equations that simulates the interactions between individuals and the spread of disease	Modeling interventions for communicable diseases, such as vaccinations, where the nature of disease transmission is important
Dynamic simulation models	Simulates one individual at time with interactions between individuals and within a health care system	Evaluating alternative health care systems (e.g., workflow, staffing, optimal system level resource allocation)

Source: Adapted from Kuntz et al. (2013).

immunity. Similarly, questions pertaining to the evaluation of systems require a model that can account for interactions between individuals and resources in the health care system (e.g., discrete event simulations, agent-based models). If one can assume independence between simulated individuals, the choice of model depends on the level of complexity desired (e.g., cohort models vs individual-level models). For more discussion of the choice of model type, see the conceptual ISPOR-SMDM report (Roberts et al. 2012) and for a more detailed taxonomy of models, see Brennan, Chick, and Davies (2006).

5.5.1 Decision Trees

A decision tree is a model that provides a logical structure for a decision and possible events as they unfold over time. The primary advantage of decision trees over other types of models is that they are generally presented in a logical and easy-to-follow way. Even in cases where the decision tree is quite "bushy," the decision maker can readily view each pathway following a decision option, as well as the pathway probabilities. The primary disadvantage of a decision tree is that it is only applicable to situations in which there are no (or a very limited number of) recurring events and in which the relevant time horizon is relatively short and fixed.

5.5.2 State-Transition Models

State-transition models are commonly used and are appropriate for modeling clinical problems that involve changing health states over time, or when the timing of events is important (Siebert et al. 2012). State-transition models that simultaneously simulate a cohort (also referred to as Markov models) provide a convenient tool for calculating lifetime costs and quality-adjusted life expectancy, the recommended measures in a CEA with a lifetime time horizon. The advantage of using this type of model is that it can capture many of the features present in a clinical process (e.g., risk of disease over time, changing health states over time, episodic events) in a relatively simple and transparent way. The primary disadvantage is the underlying assumption that the probability of moving from one health state to another depends only on the initial state and not on past history—either states visited in the past or time spent in those states. Modelers address this limitation by creating health state descriptions that include past history. For example, health states can be defined according to whether a stroke has occurred, or perhaps even the number or type of stroke. Health states can also be defined to include the number of years spent in a particular state. The difficulty is that the number of states can increase exponentially as the analyst attempts to include all relevant history for a clinical problem, which can result in a very large model that is difficult—sometimes impossible—to manage.

5.5.3 Microsimulation Models

The distinguishing feature of a microsimulation model, or individual-level model, is that it simulates one individual at a time (Siebert et al. 2012). These models can be based on discrete or continuous time. A key feature of a microsimulation model is that it keeps track of each simulated individual's history (by using tracking parameters) so there is no need for a complex set of health states to be defined. Microsimulation models can track multiple comorbidities, whether continuous or not, for each simulated individual and allow comorbidities to interact and affect patient outcomes. They can simulate events one cycle at a time, or they can simulate time to an event by drawing from distributions, thereby modeling in continuous time. The key advantages of microsimulation models are their flexibility for modeling the disease process and interventions and their ability to overcome many of the limitations inherent in state-transition models. The main disadvantage of microsimulation models is that they can consume considerable computer time, as they require sometimes millions of individuals to be simulated in order to obtain a stable estimate of the expected values of costs and effects.

5.5.4 Dynamic Transmission Models

Dynamic transmission models, or infectious disease models, should be used when disease transmission is an important component of the conceptualization of the problem (Pitman et al. 2012). Such models are able to simulate interactions between humans (e.g., direct contact [Ebola], airborne [influenza], or sexually transmitted [HIV] infections) and how these interactions affect the spread of a disease over time. They can also include spatial details pertinent to the spread of communicable disease, such as the location of classrooms in a school affected by an influenza outbreak. Because they include information on how interactions between individuals affect transmission, these models can more accurately quantify the impact of different interventions on health outcomes, such as vaccination and its impact via herd immunity. Brisson and Edmunds (2003) demonstrated the differences between using a Markov model and a dynamic transmission model to characterize varicella vaccination and the ability of the dynamic model to capture the indirect benefits of vaccination. One limitation of these models is that, because of the complexity of programming and the exponential increase in the number of differential equations needed to deal with the added complexity, they may include oversimplifications of complex processes such as screening programs. Examples include dynamic transmission models of human papillomavirus (HPV) and cervical cancer, which have failed to incorporate the detailed screening and triage strategies recommended by policy groups such as the American Society of Colposcopy and Cytopathology (Elbasha, Dasbach, and Insinga 2007).

5.5.5 Dynamic Simulation Models

Dynamic simulation models are used primarily to evaluate systems where there are competing demands for resources; they include system dynamics, discrete event simulation, and agent-based models (Karnon et al. 2012; Marshall et al. 2015). They have been applied to patient scheduling and admission rules, patient routing and flow schemes (Jun, Jacobson, and Swisher 1999), and to resource constraint decisions (e.g., donated livers for liver transplants). An example of the type of applications for which dynamic simulation models are uniquely well designed is the comparison of current laparoscopic surgical practice with a new model system in which patient care is handed off between two anesthesiologists in order to balance patient volume and safety (Stahl et al. 2004). Another example is the evaluation of workflow models of parallel induction of anesthesia in the operating room to optimize facilities and use of resources (Marjamaa et al. 2009).

In summary, there are three major factors that a modeler should consider in choosing a modeling framework: (1) how to deal with time, (2) the unit of analysis (individual, cohort, or population), and (3) whether modeled individuals are allowed to interact with each other or other components of the model. Time can be fixed (as in decision trees or when analysts model immediate consequences with no temporal component), treated as discrete intervals (e.g., discrete time state-transition models), or treated as continuous (e.g., discrete event simulations with or without interactions). The unit of analysis pertains to whether we are interested in cohort-level modeling or individual-level modeling (e.g., microsimulation or discrete event-based), or a population-level analysis. To allow the prognosis of one individual to depend on the state of other individuals requires specific model types (dynamic transmission models); dynamic simulation models go still farther and allow for interactions between individuals, and between individuals and the health care system.

5.6 ELEMENTS OF A MODEL

5.6.1 Structural Assumptions in the Model

The good practice guidelines for decision-analytic modeling proposed by Philips et al. (2004) and Sculpher, Fenwick, and Claxton (2000) used a framework with three themes: structure, data, and consistency. Structural aspects relate to the scope and the mathematical structure of the model. The scope of the CEA problem was covered in section 5.2, above; this section pertains to the mathematical structure of the model (and the assumptions required). Structure includes the conceptualization and classification of disease states, the functional relationship between risk factors and outcomes, and the choice of time horizon, among other modeling elements. Structural modeling assumptions should be made transparent and evaluated in sensitivity analyses (**Recommendation 5**) (see Chapter 11).

Good modeling practice guidelines recommend that models capture the biological/theoretical elements of the disease process (Caro et al. 2012; Philips et al. 2004; Weinstein et al. 2003). In other words, health states should not be defined based on health care utilization alone (e.g., hospitalization) but on characterizations of disease states (e.g. mild, moderate, severe). In this example, the reduction in hospitalizations due to intervention could be derived based on slowing the progression through disease states. Characterizing disease states allows one to capture changes in health-related quality of life in addition to changes in health care utilization. The manner in which the intervention affects the natural history of the disease process (e.g., slows the progression of disease) should be clear.

Model development requires that the analyst make assumptions about the natural history of the disease and how the harms and benefits of the interventions are incorporated into the model. It is important that the analysis adequately describes and justifies each assumption. Structural assumptions can often be incorporated into a model by specifying parameters that are not informed by data but that represent assumptions involving, for example, some form of extrapolation. An example of such a parameter would be the time horizon of an intervention effect. Conducting a sensitivity analysis on these structural parameters would demonstrate the sensitivity of the model results to these structural assumptions.

During model development there are often several ways analysts can structure the decision problem. Sometimes the choice of a certain modeling structure has very good clinical or statistical justification, but at other times there may be several possibilities with no single way being dominant. In these situations, the analyst should plan to conduct structural sensitivity analyses to explore the implications of different structural assumptions. For example, in a model evaluating ovarian cancer screening, Havrilesky et al. (2011) evaluated the impact of modeling ovarian cancer as two phenotypes versus one and found that potential reductions in mortality from a screening program were smaller when two phenotypes were assumed. In a more hypothetical article, Bentley, Weinstein, and Kuntz (2009) evaluated the potential bias associated with different ways of categorizing an inherently continuous variable (e.g., blood pressure) in a state-transition model. Ideally, the modeling team could maintain multiple models with alternative structures that could be used to evaluate these structural assumptions. For example, Jutkowitz et al. (2014) conducted a CEA of different drug therapy options, including sequential strategies, for patients with gout. The authors presented a table of sensitivity analyses conducted on several structural assumptions (reproduced in Table 5.3), for example, that second-line therapy is as effective as first-line therapy, or that patients whose disease was controlled with therapy remained controlled.

5.6.2 Cohort versus Population Simulations

There are alternative ways to define the people for whom costs and benefits accrue; analysts should provide a rationale for their approach (**Recommendation 6**). Models can be used to simulate cohorts (single or multiple) or populations. A cohort simulation is typically conducted with one single-age cohort (or birth cohort). Cohorts can also be characterized by sex, comorbidities, and other relevant factors that are known at the time of the decision. For example, to evaluate the cost-effectiveness of a cancer-screening program starting at age 50 and stopping at age 75, one approach is to simulate a cohort of 50-year-old individuals under various scenarios (e.g., annual screening, no screening) for a lifetime. Another approach to modeling an annual screening program would be to simulate a cohort of persons aged 50 to 75 over their lifetime (i.e., multiple prevalent cohorts), where the age distribution reflects the population under consideration. This approach would project the costs and benefits among all current individuals eligible for the screening program. Dewilde and Anderson (2004) showed that the cost-effectiveness of cervical cancer screening was more unfavorable when multiple prevalent cohorts were simulated simultaneously compared with the single-age cohort of the youngest age.

An alternative way of accumulating the costs and benefits of a program is to consider incident cohorts in addition to the multiple prevalent cohorts. In the screening example, incident cohorts would be the new 50-year-olds becoming eligible for screening each year. In this type of population-based simulation, the entire eligible population would be simulated each year for a specified number of years—that is, the implementation period, which is the time over which the intervention is applied to the simulated population (O'Mahony, Newall, and van Rosmalen 2015). Hoyle and Anderson (2010) showed that the cost-effectiveness of a program changed when incident cohorts were included in the model, and that the number of future incident cohorts modeled (i.e., the length of the planning horizon) influenced the aggregate cost-effectiveness estimate. They also considered the possibility that cost-effectiveness may vary between incident cohorts. For these types of analysis, the analyst must decide on the planning horizon and whether to keep the intervention in place while simulating the remaining cohorts at the end of the planning horizon.

Table 5.3 Cost-effectiveness of gout therapies—structural assumptions*

Strategy	All structural assumptions set to the midpoint of the tested range			Structural assumption of baseline model and testing							
	Lifetime costs, $	QALYs	ICER, $/QALY	Second-line therapy is as effective as first-line therapy: reduce the effect of second-line therapy between 0% and 50% (midpoint, 25%)		Once controlled patients remained controlled: annual probability of becoming uncontrolled† varied between 0.00 and 0.15 (midpoint, 0.075)		Patients discontinued therapy if they remained uncontrolled for 9 mo: probability of becoming uncontrolled on therapy if uncontrolled for 9 mo varied between 0.00 and 1.00 (midpoint, 0.50)		Patients have perfect adherence: annual probability of nonadherence varied between 0.00 and 0.50 (midpoint, 0.25)	
				ICER (low range value, 0%), $/QALY	ICER (high range value, 50%), $/QALY	ICER (low range value, 0.00), $/QALY	ICER (high range value, 0.15), $/QALY	ICER (low range value, 0.00), $/QALY	ICER (high range value, 1.00), $/QALY	ICER (low range value, 0.00), $/QALY	ICER (high range value, 0.50), $/QALY
Allopurinol only (dose escalation)	10,353	12,473	Reference	Reference	Reference	Reference	Reference	Reference	Reference	Reference	Reference
Allopurinol-febuxostat sequential therapy (dose escalation)	11,791	12,493	68,800	58,800	93,300	61,700	75,000	51,100	94,600	91,300	66,600

(continued)

Table 5.3 Continued

Strategy	All structural assumptions set to the midpoint of the tested range			Structural assumption of baseline model and testing							
				Second-line therapy is as effective as first-line therapy: reduce the effect of second-line therapy between 0% and 50% (midpoint, 25%)		Once controlled patients remained controlled: annual probability of becoming uncontrolled† varied between 0.00 and 0.15 (midpoint, 0.075)		Patients discontinued therapy if they remained uncontrolled for 9 mo: probability of becoming uncontrolled on therapy if uncontrolled for 9 mo varied between 0.00 and 1.00 (midpoint, 0.50)		Patients have perfect adherence: annual probability of nonadherence varied between 0.00 and 0.50 (midpoint, 0.25)	
	Lifetime costs, $	QALYs	ICER, $/QALY	ICER (low range value, 0%), $/QALY	ICER (high range value, 50%), $/QALY	ICER (low range value, 0.00), $/QALY	ICER (high range value, 0.15), $/QALY	ICER (low range value, 0.00), $/QALY	ICER (high range value, 1.00), $/QALY	ICER (low range value, 0.00), $/QALY	ICER (high range value, 0.50), $/QALY
Febuxostat-allopurinol sequential therapy (dose escalation)	14,519	12,504	271,900	278,100	261,500	259,400	281,400	289,300	254,600	609,700	188,200

Source: Table 4 in Jutkowitz et al. (2014).

*Results from sensitivity analyses on the key structural assumptions of the model. The first column presents the ICER when all structural assumptions are set to the midpoint of their tested range. Only results from nondominated strategies for all treatment options are shown. Column headers indicate the structural assumption and how it was tested. Strategies are ordered by increasing cost and effectiveness. The ICER represents the additional cost per QALY of the next-most-expensive strategy. If strategies are dominated, they are not used to evaluate an ICER.

† Assumed to remain in uncontrolled-on-therapy state for life.

Abbreviations: ICER = incremental cost-effectiveness ratio; QALY(s) = quality-adjusted life-year(s).

Generally, population-based simulations are appropriate for modeling the prevention of infectious diseases that spread from person to person (i.e., dynamic models). For interventions related to infectious diseases, such as vaccination programs, a population model is typically used in order to capture the person-to-person spread of disease and the indirect effects of prevention (e.g., herd immunity).

The choice between single-age cohort analyses, multiple prevalent cohorts, and population-based analyses may depend on the target audience. Hoyle and Anderson (2010) recommend that CEAs include all current and all future cohorts and report a "combined cohorts ICER." However, Kuntz, Fenwick, and Briggs (2010) questioned whether it is appropriate to aggregate results over multiple cohorts. Similarly, Karnon, Brennan, and Akehurst (2007) noted that Dewilde and Anderson's multi-cohort approach can be used to account for the effect of cohort heterogeneity on aggregate cost-effectiveness but suggested that separate per-cohort analyses be used where interventions can be applied differently to separate cohorts.

O'Mahony et al. (2013) suggest that reporting cost-effectiveness as a single aggregate estimate for all cohorts is inappropriate for several reasons. First, aggregate estimates over many cohorts may hide useful information from decision makers by making implicit the assumption that a common policy decision will apply to all cohorts. Second, the choice of cohorts to include appears logically problematic; aggregate results could differ widely depending on the choice of cohorts to include in the aggregate estimate. Third, aggregate estimates demand that the analyst make significant assumptions about the future (planning horizon), which results in large uncertainty in aggregate estimates. Finally, O'Mahony and colleagues suggest that aggregate modeling prompts broader questions about decision making over multiple periods for health care priority setting, such as falling drug prices over time. They conclude that analysts should estimate the cost-effectiveness of more than just a single incident cohort in cases in which cost-effectiveness is likely to vary between cohorts, with estimates reported on a disaggregate per-cohort basis in addition to the overall estimate for all cohorts. The Second Panel supports the conclusions of O'Mahony et al. but recognizes that there may be reasons for alternative approaches related to the decision-making context (**Recommendation 6**).

5.6.3 Data Sources

The original Panel recommended that a CEA use the best data available (Gold et al. 1996, 308-309), meaning data from the best designed and least biased study or studies. Increasingly, however, best practice is moving beyond this recommendation to the idea that parameters for a CEA should be based on all relevant data, not just the "best" available source or sources (**Recommendation 7**) (see Chapter 9), understanding that this synthesis may require corrections for sources of bias or in recognition of time and resource constraints (see Chapter 6). Methods have moved the farthest in this direction for parameters relating to the effectiveness of interventions, and less for estimates of incidence and prevalence of disease and for costs and utility weights. The guidelines for economic evaluations issued by NICE in 2013 capture current thinking: "Consideration of a comprehensive evidence base is fundamental to the appraisal process. Evidence of various types and from multiple sources may inform the appraisal" (National Institute for Health and Care Excellence [NICE] 2013, 20).

Chapter 9 of this volume details methods for systematically identifying, collecting, and combining evidence on the effectiveness of interventions in order to produce unbiased estimates of effectiveness parameters in the form required by the analysis. Methods typically used for selecting cost data and preference weights are described here.

This chapter's recommendations apply to all evidence used in an analysis. For all the data, whether from a meta-analysis or a single data source, best practice is the same: analysts should select data for an analysis after considering all relevant data sources (within reason—a full systematic review is not always required); the data selected should be appropriate for the interventions and target population; the choice of data sources and the methods used to critically appraise them should be justified; the data, its sources, and its strengths and limitations should be clearly described; and any adjustments to the data, or calculations involving the data, should be described and justified (**Recommendations 7–9**). Notably, the standard hierarchy of evidence quality does not necessarily apply to CEAs, and the process should not be held to the standards used for systematic reviews. The evidence used should be appropriate for the question under consideration. For example, an observational, population-based study, rather than an RCT, generally provides a better estimate for disease incidence. As emphasized elsewhere, transparency is fundamental: the choices made at each step of the CEA should be clearly reported and explained to allow users to evaluate its validity and applicability (**Recommendations 7–9**).

5.6.3.1 Cost Inputs

For trial-based analyses, statistical techniques are available to guide analyses of cost data collected directly within a trial (Glick et al. 2014). For model-based analyses, cost parameters need to be defined and estimated from a variety of data sources (see Chapters 8, and 9). The cost of an intervention may consist of several different parameters (e.g., cost per mg of drug, dispensing fee, office visit). Costs associated with harms should be quantified separately, if possible, to allow for sensitivity analysis. The various disease states of the model should be detailed enough to reflect meaningful differences in state-specific costs (whether pertaining to the disease itself or to the intervention) and the costs assigned to disease states should be net costs. Because many costs are age-dependent (e.g., productivity costs) it is important that age be represented in models (and sex in most cases).

When a CEA is intended to inform a public payer's decisions, the source of costs may be prescribed in the payer's own guidelines for economic evaluations. US analysts often use Medicare costs (more accurately, Medicare payment rates) since they apply to virtually all people age 65 and older, and are sometimes taken to approximate a national payer perspective. In England and Wales NICE requires use of NHS costs (National Institute for Health and Care Excellence [NICE] 2013). In Canada, CADTH does not specify the costs of a particular payer, but it does indicate a preference for microcosting, based on Canadian routine practice (Canadian Agency for Drugs and Technologies in Health [CADTH] 2006).

Deriving the costs for an analysis often requires adjusting and combining data from original sources. For example, the original cost data for tests, outpatient visits, and hospital stays may have been collected in different years and reflect the price levels of those years; they will all need to be adjusted to the price level of a common year for use in the analysis. Alternatively, the costs for a particular age group relevant to the analysis may need to be adjusted upward or downward if costs are only available for the whole population in a particular data source. All such calculations and adjustments should be clearly described and justified.

5.6.3.2 *Preference Weights*

Following the original Panel, the Second Panel also recommends that preference weights for a Reference Case come from a representative sample of the community (see Chapter 7). Both Panels recommend that a preference weights system be preference-based, interval-scaled, and on a scale of 0 (dead) to 1 (perfect health). Any system that meets those requirements is acceptable. When a CEA is conducted for a national payer, the preference weight system may be prescribed by the payer's guidelines. For example, CADTH specifies that analysts should use an appropriate preference-based system that allows the calculation of QALYs and recommends the standard gamble or time trade-off methods when preferences are measured directly (Canadian Agency for Drugs and Technologies in Health [CADTH] 2006). To promote consistency across evaluations conducted for the UK National Health Service, NICE recommends use of the EQ-5D (National Institute for Health and Care Excellence [NICE] 2013), either the three-level (EQ-5D-3L) or the five-level (EQ-5D-5L) version.

Within a single system for eliciting preference weights, the levels of, and variation in, the weights will come from the sample variation, bias, and other characteristics of the sample of people who provided responses to that system. Following the original Panel's recommendation, the preference weights should be elicited from a representative sample of the community. The study selected will, of course, need to include weights for the health states relevant to the CEA. The selection of a particular source will thus be justified in terms of the qualities of the preference elicitation process used, the representativeness of the sample, and the appropriateness of the health states evaluated.

5.6.4 Calibration as Estimation

We define calibration as the process of determining the values of unobserved (possibly unobservable) parameters so that model outputs match ("fit") observed (empirical) data. The observed data, typically as summary measures, are referred to as "calibration targets." Model calibration is an iterative process that continues until consistency is obtained between the model outputs and known data. For example, a model developed to evaluate cancer screening programs that identify precancerous lesions needs to employ calibration methods to estimate the unobserved process of transitioning from no disease to precancerous disease to preclinical cancer. This is because empirical studies that detect precancerous lesions remove them and thus one cannot observe their progression. Using calibration targets of the prevalence of precancerous lesions and the incidence of clinical cancer, one can determine estimates for parameters that describe the underlying disease process through calibration.

There are several possible approaches to calibration, but all should report on the following components (**Recommendation 10**) (Stout et al. 2009):

1. Although data sources are not used directly to inform model parameters, they are used as calibration targets. Thus, **Recommendations 7–9** would apply to calibration targets.
2. Analysts should report the goodness-of-fit metric used to determine the degree of fit of the model output from a particular parameter set with the calibration targets. Goodness-of-fit metrics include likelihood-based measures, distance measures, and visual assessment of fit.
3. The analyst should report the manner in which the search of the parameter space (i.e., all of the possible combinations of the calibrated parameter sets) was carried out. This could be a systematic grid search or a directed search using several computer-based algorithms, such as a simplex algorithm (Kong, McMahon, and Gazelle 2009).
4. The analyst should report the criteria by which the fit was determined to be reasonable.
5. The analyst should indicate the stopping criteria used to determine when the calibration process was complete. Best-fitting parameter sets can be used to conduct probabilistic sensitivity analysis (PSA) on the calibrated parameters (in addition to the other parameters) by randomly selecting a particular parameter set for each PSA simulation with a probability that is equal to the inverse of the goodness-of-fit metric.

In recent systematic reviews of the published literature for evidence- and consensus-based guidance on the conduct and reporting of decision and simulation models (Kuntz et al. 2013; Philips et al. 2004), model calibration methods were identified as areas for future methods research.

5.7 PARAMETER UNCERTAINTY

A critical step in CEA is the analysis and reporting of uncertainty in model parameters that is attributable to the uncertainty about each parameter estimate (including calibration parameters as noted in the previous section). We do not make any specific recommendations in this chapter but refer the reader to Chapter 11 and the ISPOR-SMDM report on model parameter estimation and uncertainty (Briggs et al. 2012).

5.8 MODEL OUTPUT

The analyst should make it clear how the model results are calculated. If an individual-level simulation is performed, the number of iterations per model run should be specified and justified (**Recommendation 11**). If a PSA is performed, the number of simulations per parameter set should be given. In addition, the analyst should note whether expected values are provided as averages over the PSA simulations (as we would recommend) or calculated with mean parameter values.

The variance of an expected value derived by an individual-level simulation decreases as the number of individuals simulated increases. The analysts should perform sufficient analyses to quantify this relationship and then run a sufficiently large number of simulated individuals to ensure that the difference between strategies has a negligible chance of being caused by simulation noise. As stated in the ISPOR-SMDM Task Force report on state-transition models, "To achieve stable results in an individual-based simulation, sufficient individuals must be modeled. Stability of model results is assessed by calculating variance from multiple runs with identical numbers of individuals, which should be much smaller than the smallest difference expected between strategies. Variance reduction techniques (e.g., using common random numbers) can decrease the required numbers" (Siebert et al. 2012, 697).

5.9 VALIDATION

Validation of the decision model should occur throughout the conduct of a CEA (**Recommendation 12**) (Eddy et al. 2012). Face validity requires demonstration that a model is functioning properly technically (internal consistency) and that the model inputs and outputs reflect known evidence (external consistency). It can also refer to the process of obtaining input from disease experts about whether the model captures the most important elements of the disease and interventions. To evaluate internal consistency, modelers need to perform extensive "debugging," in which the decision model is subjected to extreme input conditions to test whether it produces the expected outcomes. In addition, modelers should vary both structural and variable assumptions to ensure that the expected outputs are produced. This process should be done with input from disease and policy experts. Tests for external consistency involve matching the decision model outputs to observed empirical data.

To assess the validity of a cost-effectiveness model, analysts often work with clinical investigators to verify the model's clinical and structural assumptions. In addition, to determine which inputs and parameters exert the most leverage on model outputs, a range of sensitivity analyses should be conducted and results reported. Finally, modelers validate the intermediate and final numerical predictions of their models against existing primary data from clinical trials and large observational studies.

According to the NICE guidelines, "The external validity of the extrapolation should be assessed by considering both clinical and biological plausibility of the inferred outcome as well as its coherence with external data sources such as historical cohort data sets or other relevant clinical trials. Internal validity should be explored and when statistical measures are used to assess the internal validity of alternative models of extrapolation based on their relative fit to the observed trial data, the limitations of these statistical measures should be documented" (National Institute for Health and Care Excellence [NICE] 2013, 51). We agree with this guidance and emphasize the need to fully explore and report the impact of various model assumptions.

The ISPOR-SMDM Task Force recommends that model documentation "should be sufficiently detailed to enable those with the necessary expertise and resources to reproduce the model" (Eddy et al. 2012, 735). We agree with this recommendation, as it provides a level of technical transparency (**Recommendation 13**). In addition, the Cancer Intervention and Surveillance Modeling Network (a National Cancer Institute-funded consortium of cancer modelers) has adopted a comparative modeling approach—also called cross validation—where multiple models are developed independently.

In addition to performing and reporting summary measures required in a CEA, analysts should present the model results in a disaggregated format to make the results more transparent to users (see Chapter 13). For example, a composite measure of QALYs combines life expectancy and health-related quality of life over patients' lifetimes. In order to provide insights into the QALY differences, an analyst should also report unadjusted life expectancy, as well as intermediate outcomes that inform the calculations of quality-adjusted life expectancy. For the latter, these outcomes could be expected to be number of years spent in different health states (with different utility weights and costs assigned), or the number of events that occur in a person's lifetime under different strategies.

5.10 CONCLUSIONS

The use of decision models is standard practice for conducting CEAs, and recommendations for developing such models are included in several country-specific guidelines for conducting CEAs for health technology appraisals. Decision models can range from very simple to complex, and they help structure analysts' thinking and facilitate the communication of assumptions. Decision models provide a structural framework for synthesizing data from disparate sources and allow for extrapolations that are often required to appropriately reflect the decision context. This chapter provides recommendations pertaining to the use of decision models for CEAs, including recommendations related to model structure, data sources, and validity.

5.11 RECOMMENDATIONS

1. We recommend that the analyst perform a broad conceptualization of the decision problem with input from clinical and policy experts. The scope of the cost-effectiveness analysis (CEA) for which the model is being used should be clearly defined (see Chapter 4).
2. The initial conceptualization of the model should be independent of the data identification phase. The model should represent the decision problem and be described in a detailed and transparent manner. The model structure should

accommodate relevant consequences of the alternatives under consideration. The conceptualization process should be iterative with the model development and parameterization phases.

3. Analysts should consider the following factors, ideally in consultation with the decision maker, to inform the use of a decision model: (1) need for extrapolation (e.g., beyond the time horizon of the available data, beyond intermediate study outcomes, to other populations, to other strategies) and/or (2) need to integrate multiple data sources (e.g., evaluate diagnostic tests, multiple strategies, weighing harms with benefits).

4. Use a model that is appropriate for addressing the study questions. Often more than one model type would work. Factors to consider include (1) short-term fixed time horizon or not; (2) the unit of analysis; (3) interactions between simulated individuals or other model components. Use good practices in modeling guidelines (International Society for Pharmacoeconomics and Outcomes Research [ISPOR] and Society for Medical Decision Making [SMDM] Task Force).

5. Full documentation and justification of structural assumptions should be provided. When there are alternative plausible structural assumptions, appropriate uncertainty analyses to examine their effects on model outputs should be undertaken (see Chapter 11).

6. In developing a model, analysts should specify (1) the starting population(s), including all subgroups, and (2) whether they are analyzing a cohort or a population. Analysts should provide their rationale for analyzing a population instead of defined cohorts.

7. Consider all available evidence for informing model parameters and use a summary of that evidence where appropriate. Identify all data sources within reason and justify the choice of evidence used.

8. The methods used to critically appraise sources of data for cost-effectiveness models should be stated.

9. Use appropriate methods to analyze or combine data from different sources.

10. Calibration is an appropriate way to estimate model parameters. When estimating parameters using a calibration approach, the following components should be presented: (1) data sources used for calibration target(s); (2) goodness-of-fit metric used to determine the degree of fit; (3) the manner in which the parameter space was searched; and (4) the criteria used to determine that the fit was reasonable.

11. The analyst should report how the model results are calculated. If an individual-level simulation is performed, specify and justify the number of iterations per model run. If a probabilistic sensitivity analysis (PSA) is performed, specify the number of simulations per parameter set.

12. Validation of the decision model should occur throughout the conduct of a CEA. The analyst should describe and justify how the model was validated. The types of validation to consider are (1) face validity, (2) internal validity (verification), and (3) external validity.

13. Model descriptions should be detailed enough to allow for reproduction. Model results should be presented in a disaggregated format for purposes of model transparency.

5.12 REFERENCES

Australian Government Department of Health. 2013. "Guidelines for preparing submissions to the Pharmaceutical Benefits Advisory Committee. Version 4.4." http://www.pbac.pbs. gov.au/.

Begg, C. B., and R. A. Greenes. 1983. Assessment of diagnostic tests when disease verification is subject to selection bias. *Biometrics* 39 (1):207–215.

Bentley, T. G., M. C. Weinstein, and K. M. Kuntz. 2009. Effects of categorizing continuous variables in decision-analytic models. *Med Decis Making* 29 (5):549–556.

Brennan, A., S. E. Chick, and R. Davies. 2006. A taxonomy of model structures for economic evaluation of health technologies. *Health Econ* 15 (12):1295–1310.

Briggs, A. H., M. C. Weinstein, E. A. Fenwick, J. Karnon, M. J. Sculpher, and A. D. Paltiel. 2012. Model parameter estimation and uncertainty analysis: a report of the ISPOR-SMDM Modeling Good Research Practices Task Force Working Group-6. *Med Decis Making* 32 (5):722–732.

Brisson, M., and W. J. Edmunds. 2003. Economic evaluation of vaccination programs: the impact of herd-immunity. *Med Decis Making* 23 (1):76–82.

Canadian Agency for Drugs and Technologies in Health (CADTH). 2006. *Guidelines for the Economic Evaluation of Health Technologies: Canada.* 3rd ed. Ottawa: CADTH. https:// www.cadth.ca/media/pdf/186_EconomicGuidelines_e.pdf.

Caro, J. J., A. H. Briggs, U. Siebert, and K. M. Kuntz. 2012. Modeling good research practices— overview: a report of the ISPOR-SMDM Modeling Good Research Practices Task Force-1. *Med Decis Making* 32 (5):667–677.

CDC Diabetes Cost-effectiveness Group. 2002. Cost-effectiveness of intensive glycemic control, intensified hypertension control, and serum cholesterol level reduction for type 2 diabetes. *JAMA* 287 (19):2542–2551.

Dewilde, S., and R. Anderson. 2004. The cost-effectiveness of screening programs using single and multiple birth cohort simulations: a comparison using a model of cervical cancer. *Med Decis Making* 24 (5):486–492.

Eddy, D. M., W. Hollingworth, J. J. Caro, J. Tsevat, K. M. McDonald, and J. B. Wong. 2012. Model transparency and validation: a report of the ISPOR-SMDM Modeling Good Research Practices Task Force-7. *Med Decis Making* 32 (5):733–743.

Elbasha, E. H., E. J. Dasbach, and R. P. Insinga. 2007. Model for assessing human papillomavirus vaccination strategies. *Emerg Infect Dis* 13 (1):28–41.

Gandjour, A. 2011. A model to transfer trial-based pharmacoeconomic analyses to clinical practice. *Pharmacoeconomics* 29 (2):97–105.

Gelber, R. D., B. F. Cole, S. Gelber, and A. Goldhirsch. 1995. Comparing treatments using quality-adjusted survival: the Q-Twist method. *Amer Statistician* 49 (2):161–169.

Glick, H. A., J. A. Doshi, S. S. Sonnad, and D. Polsky. 2014. *Economic Evaluation in Clinical Trials.* 2nd ed. Oxford: Oxford University Press.

Gold, M. R., J. E. Siegel, L. B. Russell, and M. C. Weinstein, eds. 1996. *Cost-Effectiveness in Health and Medicine.* New York: Oxford University Press.

Goldman, L., M. C. Weinstein, P. A. Goldman, and L. W. Williams. 1991. Cost-effectiveness of HMG-CoA reductase inhibition for primary and secondary prevention of coronary heart disease. *JAMA* 265 (9):1145–1151.

Guyot, P., N. J. Welton, M. J. Ouwens, and A. E. Ades. 2011. Survival time outcomes in randomized, controlled trials and meta-analyses: the parallel universes of efficacy and cost-effectiveness. *Value Health* 14 (5):640–646.

Havrilesky, L. J., G. D. Sanders, S. Kulasingam, J. P. Chino, A. Berchuck, J. R. Marks, and E. R. Myers. 2011. Development of an ovarian cancer screening decision model that incorporates disease heterogeneity: implications for potential mortality reduction. *Cancer* 117 (3):545–553.

Hlatky, M. A., D. K. Owens, and G. D. Sanders. 2006. Cost-effectiveness as an outcome in randomized clinical trials. *Clin Trials* 3 (6):543–551.

Hoyle, M., and R. Anderson. 2010. Whose costs and benefits? Why economic evaluations should simulate both prevalent and all future incident patient cohorts. *Med Decis Making* 30 (4):426–437.

Hunink, M. G. M., M. C. Weinstein, E. Wittenberg, M. F. Drummond, J. S. Pliskin, J. B. Wong, and P. P. Glasziou. 2014. *Decision Making in Health and Medicine: Integrating Evidence and Values*. 2nd ed. Cambridge: Cambridge University Press.

Johannesson, M., B. Jonsson, J. Kjekshus, A. G. Olsson, T. R. Pedersen, H. Wedel, and the Scandinavian Simvastatin Survival Study Group. 1997. Cost effectiveness of simvastatin treatment to lower cholesterol levels in patients with coronary heart disease. *N Engl J Med* 336 (5):332–336.

Jun, J. B., S. H. Jacobson, and J. R. Swisher. 1999. Application of discrete-event simulation in health care clinics: a survey. *J Oper Res Soc* 50 (2):109–123.

Jutkowitz, E., H. K. Choi, L. T. Pizzi, and K. M. Kuntz. 2014. Cost-effectiveness of allopurinol and febuxostat for the management of gout. *Ann Intern Med* 161 (9):617–626.

Karnon, J., A. Brennan, and R. Akehurst. 2007. A critique and impact analysis of decision modeling assumptions. *Med Decis Making* 27 (4):491–499.

Karnon, J., J. Stahl, A. Brennan, J. J. Caro, J. Mar, and J. Moller. 2012. Modeling using discrete event simulation: a report of the ISPOR-SMDM Modeling Good Research Practices Task Force-4. *Med Decis Making* 32 (5):701–711.

Kong, C. Y., P. M. McMahon, and G. S. Gazelle. 2009. Calibration of disease simulation model using an engineering approach. *Value Health* 12 (4):521–529.

Kuck, K. H., R. Cappato, J. Siebels, and R. Ruppel. 2000. Randomized comparison of antiarrhythmic drug therapy with implantable defibrillators in patients resuscitated from cardiac arrest: the Cardiac Arrest Study Hamburg (CASH). *Circulation* 102 (7):748–754.

Kuntz, K., F. Sainfort, M. Butler, B. Taylor, S. Kulasingam, S. Gregory, E. Mann, J. M. Anderson, and R. L. Kane. 2013. Decision and Simulation Modeling in Systematic Reviews. Methods Research Report. (Prepared by the University of Minnesota Evidence-based Practice Center under Contract No. 290-2007-10064-I.) AHRQ Publication No. 11(13)-EHC037-EF. Rockville, MD: Agency for Healthcare Research and Quality. February 2013. www.effectivehealthcare.ahrq.gov/reports/final.cfm.

Kuntz, K. M., E. Fenwick, and A. Briggs. 2010. Appropriate cohorts for cost-effectiveness analysis: to mix or not to mix? *Med Decis Making* 30 (4):424–425.

Kuntz, K. M., and M. C. Weinstein. 1995. Life expectancy biases in clinical decision modeling. *Med Decis Making* 15 (2):158–169.

Larsen, G., A. Hallstrom, J. McAnulty, S. Pinski, A. Olarte, S. Sullivan, M. Brodsky, J. Powell, C. Marchant, C. Jennings, T. Akiyama, and the AVID Investigators. 2002. Cost-effectiveness of the implantable cardioverter-defibrillator versus antiarrhythmic drugs in survivors of serious ventricular tachyarrhythmias: results of the Antiarrhythmics Versus Implantable Defibrillators (AVID) economic analysis substudy. *Circulation* 105 (17):2049–2057.

Latimer, N. R. 2013. Survival analysis for economic evaluations alongside clinical trials—extrapolation with patient-level data: inconsistencies, limitations, and a practical guide. *Med Decis Making* 33 (6):743–754.

Mandelblatt, J. S., K. A. Cronin, S. Bailey, D. A. Berry, H. J. de Koning, G. Draisma, H. Huang, S. J. Lee, M. Munsell, S. K. Plevritis, P. Ravdin, C. B. Schechter, B. Sigal, M. A. Stoto, N. K. Stout, N. T. van Ravesteyn, J. Venier, M. Zelen, E. J. Feuer, and the Breast Cancer Working Group of the Cancer Intervention and Surveillance Modeling Network (CISNET). 2009. Effects of mammography screening under different screening schedules: model estimates of potential benefits and harms. *Ann Intern Med* 151 (10):738–747.

Marjamaa, R. A., P. M. Torkki, E. J. Hirvensalo, and O. A. Kirvela. 2009. What is the best workflow for an operating room? A simulation study of five scenarios. *Health Care Manag Sci* 12 (2):142–146.

Marshall, D. A., L. Burgos-Liz, M. J. Ijzerman, N. D. Osgood, W. V. Padula, M. K. Higashi, P. K. Wong, K. S. Pasupathy, and W. Crown. 2015. Applying dynamic simulation modeling methods in health care delivery research—the SIMULATE checklist: report of the ISPOR Simulation Modeling Emerging Good Practices Task Force. *Value Health* 18 (1):5–16.

Mushlin, A. I., W. J. Hall, J. Zwanziger, E. Gajary, M. Andrews, R. Marron, K. H. Zou, and A. J. Moss. 1998. The cost-effectiveness of automatic implantable cardiac defibrillators: results from MADIT. Multicenter Automatic Defibrillator Implantation Trial. *Circulation* 97 (21):2129–2135.

National Institute for Health and Care Excellence (NICE). 2013. *Guide to the Methods of Technology Appraisal 2013. NICE article [PMG9]*. London: NICE. http://publications.nice.org.uk/pmg9.

O'Brien, B. J., S. J. Connolly, R. Goeree, G. Blackhouse, A. Willan, R. Yee, R. S. Roberts, and M. Gent. 2001. Cost-effectiveness of the implantable cardioverter-defibrillator: results from the Canadian Implantable Defibrillator Study (CIDS). *Circulation* 103 (10):1416–1421.

O'Brien, B. J., M. F. Drummond, R. J. Labelle, and A. Willan. 1994. In search of power and significance: issues in the design and analysis of stochastic cost-effectiveness studies in health care. *Med Care* 32 (2):150–163.

O'Mahony, J. F., A. T. Newall, and J. van Rosmalen. 2015. Dealing with time in health economic evaluation: methodological issues and recommendations for practice. *Pharmacoeconomics* 33 (12):1255–1268.

O'Mahony, J. F., J. van Rosmalen, A. G. Zauber, and M. van Ballegooijen. 2013. Multicohort models in cost-effectiveness analysis: why aggregating estimates over multiple cohorts can hide useful information. *Med Decis Making* 33 (3):407–414.

Philips, Z., L. Ginnelly, M. Sculpher, K. Claxton, S. Golder, R. Riemsma, N. Woolacoot, and J. Glanville. 2004. Review of guidelines for good practice in decision-analytic modelling in health technology assessment. *Health Technol Assess* 8 (36):iii–iv, ix–xi, 1–158.

Pitman, R., D. Fisman, G. S. Zaric, M. Postma, M. Kretzschmar, J. Edmunds, and M. Brisson. 2012. Dynamic transmission modeling: a report of the ISPOR-SMDM Modeling Good Research Practices Task Force Working Group-5. *Med Decis Making* 32 (5):712–721.

Prosser, L. A., A. A. Stinnett, P. A. Goldman, L. W. Williams, M. G. Hunink, L. Goldman, and M. C. Weinstein. 2000. Cost-effectiveness of cholesterol-lowering therapies according to selected patient characteristics. *Ann Intern Med* 132 (10):769–779.

Raiffa, H. 1968. *Decision Analysis: Introductory Lectures on Choices under Uncertainty.* Reading, MA: Addison-Wesley.

Ransohoff, D. F., and A. R. Feinstein. 1978. Problems of spectrum and bias in evaluating the efficacy of diagnostic tests. *N Engl J Med* 299 (17):926–930.

Revicki, D. A., and L. Frank. 1999. Pharmacoeconomic evaluation in the real world. Effectiveness versus efficacy studies. *Pharmacoeconomics* 15 (5):423–434.

Roberts, M., L. B. Russell, A. D. Paltiel, M. Chambers, P. McEwan, and M. Krahn. 2012. Conceptualizing a model: a report of the ISPOR-SMDM Modeling Good Research Practices Task Force-2. *Med Decis Making* 32 (5):678–689.

Scandinavian Simvastatin Survival Study Group. 1994. Randomised trial of cholesterol lowering in 4444 patients with coronary heart disease: the Scandinavian Simvastatin Survival Study (4S). *Lancet* 344 (8934):1383–1389.

Sculpher, M., E. Fenwick, and K. Claxton. 2000. Assessing quality in decision analytic cost-effectiveness models. A suggested framework and example of application. *Pharmacoeconomics* 17 (5):461–477.

Sculpher, M. J., K. Claxton, M. Drummond, and C. McCabe. 2006. Whither trial-based economic evaluation for health care decision making? *Health Econ* 15 (7):677–687.

Siebert, U., O. Alagoz, A. M. Bayoumi, B. Jahn, D. K. Owens, D. J. Cohen, and K. M. Kuntz. 2012. State-transition modeling: a report of the ISPOR-SMDM Modeling Good Research Practices Task Force-3. *Med Decis Making* 32 (5):690–700.

Singal, A. G., P. D. Higgins, and A. K. Waljee. 2014. A primer on effectiveness and efficacy trials. *Clin Transl Gastroenterol* 5:e45.

Sisk, J. E., W. Whang, J. C. Butler, V. P. Sneller, and C. G. Whitney. 2003. Cost-effectiveness of vaccination against invasive pneumococcal disease among people 50 through 64 years of age: role of comorbid conditions and race. *Ann Intern Med* 138 (12):960–968.

Sox, H. C., M. C. Higgins, and D. K. Owens. 2013. *Medical Decision Making.* 2nd ed. Chichester: John Wiley & Sons Ltd.

Stahl, J. E., D. Rattner, R. Wiklund, J. Lester, M. Beinfeld, and G. S. Gazelle. 2004. Reorganizing the system of care surrounding laparoscopic surgery: a cost-effectiveness analysis using discrete-event simulation. *Med Decis Making* 24 (5):461–471.

Stout, N. K., A. B. Knudsen, C. Y. Kong, P. M. McMahon, and G. S. Gazelle. 2009. Calibration methods used in cancer simulation models and suggested reporting guidelines. *Pharmacoeconomics* 27 (7):533–545.

Weinstein, M. C., B. O'Brien, J. Hornberger, J. Jackson, M. Johannesson, C. McCabe, and B. R. Luce. 2003. Principles of good practice for decision analytic modeling in health-care evaluation: report of the ISPOR Task Force on Good Research Practices—Modeling Studies. *Value Health* 6 (1):9–17.

Willan, A. R., and A. H. Briggs. 2006. *Statistical Analysis of Cost-Effectiveness Data.* Chichester: John Wiley & Sons Ltd.

Zauber, A. G., I. Lansdorp-Vogelaar, A. B. Knudsen, J. Wilschut, M. van Ballegooijen, and K. M. Kuntz. 2008. Evaluating test strategies for colorectal cancer screening: a decision analysis for the U.S. Preventive Services Task Force. *Ann Intern Med* 149 (9):659–669.

6

Identifying and Quantifying
the Consequences of Interventions

Joshua A. Salomon, Thomas A. Trikalinos,
Gillian D. Sanders, and Jeanne S. Mandelblatt

6.1 INTRODUCTION

Chapter 4 focuses on designing a cost-effectiveness analysis (CEA), describing the series of decisions that an analyst must make regarding the overall approach to the study and specific aspects of study design. Chapter 5 focuses on how to then use a decision model as a framework for a CEA. The remaining steps in conducting a CEA are these: (1) to identify and enumerate relevant consequences of the different interventions or strategies being compared; (2) to measure the quantities or frequencies of those consequences; (3) to value them; and (4) to aggregate over them. This chapter begins with the first of these steps, by detailing how analysts should first undertake a systematic identification of the full array of consequences relevant to the decision being evaluated, and it lays the groundwork for the second step, by describing key types of data sources and measurement approaches that can be used to quantify consequences that fall within the defined scope and perspective of the analysis. Toward this latter end, this chapter focuses primarily on data sources and measurement approaches relevant to quantifying health outcomes. Chapters 7 and 8 follow with more details on how specific consequences are measured and valued, with Chapter 7 focusing on valuing health outcomes and Chapter 8 focusing on identifying, quantifying, and valuing resource use and other non-health consequences with the specific objective of expressing the net value of these as costs in a CEA.

This chapter builds on concepts presented in Chapter 5 of the original Panel's book (Mandelblatt, J. S., D. G. Fryback, M. C. Weinstein, L. B. Russell, M. R. Gold, and D. C. Hadorn. 1996. "Assessing the Effectiveness of Health Interventions." In *Cost-Effectiveness in Health and Medicine*, edited by M. R. Gold, J. E. Siegel, L. B. Russell and M. C. Weinstein, 135–175. New York: Oxford University Press).

This chapter takes as its point of departure the chapter titled "Assessing the Effectiveness of Health Interventions" in the original Panel's volume, with the new title and content reflecting a broader scope. Part of the reason for this broadened scope is our emphasis on the applicability of cost-effectiveness methods beyond clinical interventions, and the resulting need to consider a range of consequences beyond the domain of clinical effectiveness. The scope of this chapter is also consistent with our new recommendation for analysts to develop an Impact Inventory as a key step in any CEA; this chapter aims to provide guidance that aids in developing such an inventory.

An important element of a CEA that guides the tasks described in this chapter is the choice of perspective, as discussed in Chapters 3 and 4. The Second Panel reaffirms the recommendation that a Reference Case analysis be included in all CEAs. Departing from the position of the original Panel, we recommend that all studies report on Reference Case analyses from both the healthcare sector perspective and the societal perspective (Chapter 3). As noted in the Reference Case recommendations at the end of Chapter 3, analysts may also wish to conduct and report on additional analyses from other perspectives, where such analyses are indicated by a particular study question or decision problem.

The remainder of this chapter is organized into two main sections. Section 6.2 focuses on the identification of consequences to include in a CEA, providing a typology to aid in conceptualizing the array of different consequences that may be pertinent to comparisons of interventions and strategies in a CEA, and introducing the Impact Inventory as a formal framework for cataloging these consequences. Section 6.3 then turns to the task of quantifying consequences in the Impact Inventory, offering a detailed consideration of measurement approaches and data sources that can inform this quantification, focusing in particular on quantities that pertain to estimation of health outcomes.

6.2 IDENTIFYING CONSEQUENCES FOR A CEA

In seeking to develop guidance for identifying and enumerating consequences in a CEA, we envision two distinct phases of this endeavor, the first distinguished by its broad and inclusive scope and the second by its emphasis on balancing validity and completeness with pragmatic concerns. In the first phase, we recommend that analysts seek to identify *all* consequences of a decision, whether positive or negative, and regardless of whether they occur within or outside of the formal healthcare sector. The second phase of a CEA will typically reflect a narrowing of scope to allow focus on a subset of consequences that will be subject to measurement and valuation in the analysis. In the healthcare sector perspective Reference Case analysis, this narrowing is guided by the exclusion of consequences falling outside the formal healthcare sector, but even in the broader societal perspective some identified consequences may not be explicitly quantified and valued for pragmatic reasons. The recommendations advanced in this chapter include guidance on how the choice of consequences that will be accounted for in the calculation of costs, effectiveness, and cost-effectiveness should be consistent with the choice of perspective, linked to a set of measurement strategies and data sources, and guided by practical considerations.

6.2.1 Identifying All Consequences That Are Relevant to an Analysis

As indicated in Chapters 2–4, a CEA that is intended to inform the broad allocation of health resources needs to take a correspondingly broad view of the potential consequences of the interventions being evaluated. Thus, at the start of the study the analyst should identify all consequences, positive or negative, that could be affected by those interventions (see **Recommendation 1** at the end of this chapter). There are a number of different dimensions along which consequences may be distinguished, and we emphasize three of those dimensions below.

6.2.1.1 *Consequences in Different Sectors of Society*

The first, and perhaps most important, dimension along which consequences may be distinguished relates to the *sector of society* in which the consequences are realized. To correspond to the Reference Case perspectives recommended by the Second Panel, we divide consequences into those that pertain to the formal healthcare sector, costs within the informal healthcare sector (and therefore not part of the Reference Case healthcare sector perspective), and consequences in all other sectors. This division is elaborated below, in Section 6.2.2. We may further distinguish consequences outside the formal healthcare sector according to whether or not these consequences lend themselves naturally to valuation in monetary terms. For example, effects of changes in health on consumption or on the labor market are naturally expressed in monetary units, whereas consequences for education, or for the justice system—while it is conceivable for analysts to monetize—do not necessarily translate as readily into economic metrics.

6.2.1.2 *Consequences in Populations with Different Degrees of Proximity to the Intervention*

The full array of consequences of different interventions includes both those that accrue to members of the target population and those that affect others. A familiar example of this important distinction relates to vaccination against infectious disease, which has health consequences both for the person who receives the vaccine and also for those whom the person might otherwise infect, who are protected by "herd immunity." Other examples include interventions delivered to pregnant women, such as folic acid fortification, that have important consequences for infants. Impacts on individuals who are not direct recipients of an intervention may also derive from social rather than biological links, as in the example of quality-of-life effects in a person who is caring for a spouse with a health condition. To ensure that none of these potential effects are overlooked, it may help to keep three broad groups in mind—the recipients of the intervention; those who are responsible for care of these recipients, including health-care workers, family and other caregivers; and the larger community—and to consider at each stage of identifying consequences whether all significant consequences for each of these groups have been recognized.

6.2.1.3 *Consequences at Different Time Points in Relation to the Intervention*

Many interventions have effects that extend over time, including not just effects that are immediately manifested following the intervention, but those that persist or chains of consequences that emanate from the point of intervention. For example, capturing the consequences of a smoking cessation intervention requires an understanding of the long-term health consequences among smokers and non-smokers, which may be fully realized over a period of decades. Related to the distinction above regarding different degrees of proximity to the intervention, interventions that have external effects related to transmission of infectious disease should also be recognized as having a "long tail" of consequences that can extend far into the future, as effects are realized among multiple generations of potential infections. The guiding principle is to examine a time horizon that is long enough to capture the salient consequences of a given choice. Chapters 4 and 5 in this volume discuss the choice of time horizon as this choice relates to framing of a CEA, and to modeling strategies, respectively.

6.2.2 The Impact Inventory: Cataloging Consequences Across Sectors

We recommend that all Reference Case analyses begin with an Impact Inventory (**Recommendation 2**). The Impact Inventory first lists all consequences of an intervention, within and outside of the formal healthcare sector. Analyses from either the healthcare sector or the societal perspective require the analyst to quantify and value health consequences and resource use that fall within the formal healthcare sector. Analyses from the healthcare sector perspective will integrate this subset of consequences from the Impact Inventory in an incremental cost-effectiveness ratio (ICER). Analyses conducted from a societal perspective require a further step of assessing consequences that fall outside the formal healthcare sector, quantifying and valuing them where possible and exploring how best to summarize them, for example as an additional ICER or in terms of net monetary benefit (NMB) or net health benefit (NHB). When a study features results expressed as ICERs from a healthcare sector perspective, then the Impact Inventory serves the critical function of explicitly identifying additional consequences that are not included in these ICERs because they fall beyond the boundaries of the healthcare sector perspective. This in turn provides an opportunity to consider whether their inclusion would be likely to alter the conclusions from the analysis.

The Impact Inventory provides a framework for organizing, thinking about, and presenting various types of consequences starting from the broad distinction of the sector of society in which the consequences occur. Table 6.1 presents a proposed template for an Impact Inventory. Examples of completed Impact Inventories are provided in the two worked examples presented in Appendix A and Appendix B.

Table 6.1 Impact Inventory template

Sector	Type of impact (list category within each sector with unit of measure if relevant)*	Included in this Reference Case analysis from . . . perspective?		Notes on sources of evidence
		Healthcare sector	Societal	
Formal healthcare sector				
Health	*Health outcomes (effects)*			
	Longevity effects	☐	☐	
	Health-related quality-of-life effects	☐	☐	
	Other health effects (e.g., adverse events and secondary transmissions of infections)	☐	☐	
	Medical costs			
	Paid for by third-party payers	☐	☐	
	Paid for by patients out-of-pocket	☐	☐	
	Future related medical costs (payers and patients)	☐	☐	
	Future unrelated medical costs (payers and patients)	☐	☐	
Informal healthcare sector				
Health	Patient time costs	NA	☐	
	Unpaid caregiver time costs	NA	☐	
	Transportation costs	NA	☐	
Non-healthcare sectors (with examples of possible items)				
Productivity	Labor market earnings lost	NA	☐	
	Cost of unpaid lost productivity due to illness	NA	☐	
	Cost of uncompensated household production	NA	☐	
Consumption	Future consumption unrelated to health	NA	☐	

(continued)

Table 6.1 Continued

Sector	Type of impact (list category within each sector with unit of measure if relevant)*	Included in this Reference Case analysis from . . . perspective?		Notes on sources of evidence
		Healthcare sector	Societal	
Social services	Cost of social services as part of intervention	NA	☐	
Legal/ criminal justice	Number of crimes related to intervention	NA	☐	
	Cost of crimes related to intervention	NA	☐	
Education	Impact of intervention on educational achievement of population	NA	☐	
Housing	Cost of intervention on home improvements (e.g., removing lead paint)	NA	☐	
Environment	Production of toxic waste or pollution by intervention	NA	☐	
Other (specify)	Other impacts	NA	☐	

* Categories listed are intended as examples for analysts.
Abbreviation: NA = not applicable.

The Impact Inventory first divides consequences into those that pertain to the formal healthcare sector, those that pertain to the informal healthcare sector, and those that pertain to all other sectors. Each of these main sections is further divided by major categories of consequences, as discussed below. The rows in the Impact Inventory allow for a listing of specific consequences within each category, and the analyst should provide sufficient detail to distinguish the broad array of consequences that pertain to a particular analysis, especially where the different interventions and strategies under comparison may differ with respect to these consequences. Corresponding to the two recommended Reference Case analyses, the Impact Inventory includes two columns that serve as a checklist that will supply a simple visual summary of the ways the two perspectives differ in terms of the consequences they include. The checklist also enables analysts to identify consequences that in principle belong in one or both of the perspectives, but that are omitted from the analysis for reasons that should be explicitly clarified in the description of the study (as discussed in Section 6.2.3). Finally, we suggest that the Impact Inventory also provides an opportunity to summarize the key types of data that constitute the evidence base for quantifying each type of consequence or other relevant comments. A final column in the template is intended to accommodate notes to this effect.

In the following section, we elaborate on the identification of specific consequences within the formal healthcare sector and within other sectors.

6.2.2.1 *Consequences Within the Formal Healthcare Sector*

Within the formal healthcare sector, CEAs routinely draw a further distinction between health outcomes and the formal healthcare sector resource implications of the actions executed to achieve those health outcomes. As shorthand, we may think of these, respectively, as *effects* and *costs*, the latter reflecting the reality that some expenditure of resources is necessary to provide an intervention and initiate its chain of consequences. Those consequences, in turn, will likely imply further changes in the demand on various resources.

A complete accounting of significant health outcomes (to be quantified and aggregated eventually as quality-adjusted life-years [QALYs] or related measures and explained further in Chapter 7) will depend on the conditions or diseases addressed by the interventions. Analysts should identify all health outcomes that may be affected by the choice of intervention or strategy, including both mortality outcomes and nonfatal outcomes that can be understood in terms of different types of morbidities, levels of function (e.g., disabilities of various kinds), or disease stages. A complete accounting will also include the adverse consequences of an intervention, such as complications from surgery or side effects of a medication. To ensure that the analysis is based on accurate estimates of the net health effects from the interventions, it is as important to account for adverse effects fully and accurately as to account for the interventions' beneficial health effects.

Costs within the formal healthcare sector may be modeled in either of two ways: (1) as total costs for the healthcare sector services required at various points in the intervention (e.g., the cost of screening, follow-up, and hospitalization for surgery, among others), or (2) as counts of resources required at different stages of the intervention (e.g., numbers of tests, doses of medication, days in the hospital), which are then multiplied by the appropriate unit costs to derive total costs. Although it requires more detailed data, the second approach is preferable and was recommended by the original Panel because it allows for flexible analysis of costs, in which the impact of resource use and unit costs on cost-effectiveness can be explored separately. Costs are discussed in much greater detail in Chapter 8.

6.2.2.2 *Consequences Beyond the Healthcare Sector*

The consequences of interventions may be broad, including both positive effects ("benefits") and negative effects (which may have resource implications or at any rate be summarized in terms of "costs") outside the healthcare sector, and this should be reflected in the Impact Inventory.

Through their effects on health, interventions can have consequences for activities such as paid work, education, and crime, which are reflected within various sections of the Impact Inventory. These non-healthcare sector effects should be taken into account, documented, and, if possible, estimated and quantified in terms of the magnitude of their effects. Interventions may also add to or reduce costs outside of the healthcare sector. Some of the additional costs or savings might flow directly from the interventions. An intervention might, for example, require transportation for the patient to and from the care provider or the use of family members' time to care for the patient, or alterations in the construction of the house to accommodate the patient's limitations. These costs fall outside the formal healthcare sector and are often omitted from CEAs, but they involve real resources that could be used for other purposes; the inability to use those resources for those other purposes and the loss of the benefits of those other purposes, represents their opportunity cost when used for the intervention. Other interventions, for example a professional service provided at home, might reduce the need for transportation, or the time required of family members. Again, analysts should consider at the outset of the analysis whether such consequences are likely to be important for the interventions they are evaluating and plan to include them in the analysis as appropriate.

6.2.3 The Rule of Reason

As described above, the Impact Inventory is intended to prompt a broad identification and enumeration of all of the consequences relating to the choice of intervention or strategy, both within the healthcare sector and in other sectors. In most analyses a subset of these consequences will be quantified and valued for inclusion in the analysis. In the next section, we will turn to a consideration of measurement approaches and data sources that can inform this quantification and valuation, focusing in particular on quantities that pertain to estimation of health outcomes.

First, we reiterate a general recommendation articulated by the original Panel with regard to the identification of a subset of consequences, selected from among the full universe of consequences enumerated in the Impact Inventory, that will be included in an analysis. The resulting narrowing of scope of the analysis should (1) reflect the choice of perspective and (2) be subject to the "rule of reason" (**Recommendation 3**). Regarding the implications of choice of perspective, the Second Panel recommends that every CEA include Reference Case analyses that report costs and effects from a healthcare sector perspective and a societal perspective. Regarding the rule of reason, in either the healthcare sector perspective or the societal perspective, consequences that have been identified in the Impact Inventory may not end up being quantified and valued later in the analysis. The rule of reason may be expressed as follows: Consequences that are expected to be trivially small in the context of the analysis, and thus to have little effect on the results, can reasonably be excluded at the analyst's discretion. This exclusion should, however, be explicitly noted and justified.

One purpose of the Impact Inventory is to let readers and users of the analysis know the full range of possible consequences and consider how omitting any of those from the quantification and valuation steps may have altered the conclusions.

6.3 MEASUREMENT APPROACHES AND DATA SOURCES

We turn now to the second major objective of this chapter, which is to begin to consider steps relating to measurement of consequences. Given the choice of consequences to include in an analysis, arrived at through the process described above, consequences can either be measured directly, as in a CEA that is based on a trial, or they must be quantified indirectly based on various inputs that are synthesized using a decision model.

Trial-based CEAs constitute a minority of all CEAs, and thus we offer only the following brief remarks on them here. When both clinical and economic data are available from the same trial, the expected cumulative cost and expected cumulative effectiveness (e.g., expressed as quality-adjusted survival) can be estimated and compared across trial arms (intervention strategies). However, consequences that accrue while a person lives, such as costs, get *censored* when survival times are censored, and this has to be accounted for using appropriate analytic methods (Heitjan, Kim, and Li 2004; Liu 2009; Liu, Huang, and O'Quigley 2008; Tsiatis and Davidian 2004). Otherwise, estimates of the expected cumulative costs and expected survival, and derivative summary measures, such as the ICER or NHB or NMB, may be biased (Bang and Tsiatis 2002). This issue applies equally to CEAs that quantify consequences indirectly using a model, but it is important to mention it specifically in regard to trial-based CEAs, as it may be tempting to equate *direct* measurement of outcomes with *complete* measurement of outcomes.

Most CEAs quantify consequences by combining information from distinct sources, comprising empirical data and expert opinion. For example, consider a CEA that compares screening versus no screening among prospective young competitive athletes to identify those with heart disease (Wheeler et al. 2010). The CEA model returns quality-adjusted life expectancy and expected costs based on incidence of heart disease; incidence of sudden death in those with and without heart disease and in those who engage in competitive athletic activity versus not; effectiveness of treatment for discovered heart disease; sensitivity and specificity of various screening modalities to diagnose underlying heart disease; and costs associated with screening and treatment. The quantification of consequences thus requires estimation of a large number of parameters, some corresponding directly to frequencies or quantities of the consequences and others representing parameters that will influence these quantities' consequences, often in combination with other parameters. In the following sections we propose a broad scheme for organizing the different parameters; describe information sources that are appropriate for various model parameters; consider how the information obtained from empirical data maps to model parameters; and discuss in some detail study designs, estimation, and assessment of the internal and external validity of empirical studies that inform various types of model parameters. We conclude with a discussion of eliciting information from experts.

6.3.1 Empirical Data or Expert Opinion for Informing Model Parameters?

Most model parameters should ideally be estimated from empirical data. Depending on the availability of empirical information, we distinguish three cases. First, empirical data may exist to directly estimate the parameter at hand, e.g., there are study estimates of the sensitivity and specificity of a diagnostic test in a context that is sufficiently similar to the decision context. In the second case, no empirical data exist (or none are practically attainable) to estimate the parameter value directly, but feasible values for the parameter can be inferred by calibrating the model against other data (Rutter, Miglioretti, and Savarino 2009). An example is modeling the natural history of colorectal cancer where there are no directly applicable empirical data on the length of the dwelling time of benign adenomas (the time benign adenomas take to become malignant). Instead, plausible dwelling time values can be discerned by calibrating the models to population-wide longitudinal data on the incidence of colorectal cancer (Kuntz et al. 2011). In the third case, no empirical data exist from which to obtain estimates for the parameters, directly or through calibration-as-estimation, and information must therefore be elicited from experts.

6.3.2 Using Empirical Data to Inform Model Parameters

Consider a model parameter that can be informed by readily available empirical data. Depending on the parameter at hand, the empirical information may come from a completed or de novo analysis of a trial, cohort, registry, or other source. Here we consider how to approach each individual information source; Chapter 9 examines the synthesis of information from multiple sources, including empirical data and expert opinions.

Intuitively, in most cases one cannot simply use estimates from a data analysis directly as model parameters: shortcomings in study design, execution, or analysis can bias results. In addition, study estimates, even if they are free of bias, may not be directly applicable to the decision context. When biases such as measurement error, confounding, and selection bias operate, the estimate differs from the estimand by the net magnitude of all the biases. Furthermore, the contexts of the study and the model often differ, and this can manifest as the non-transferability difference, which expresses potential lack of applicability or generalizability of study results. The direction and magnitude of net bias and non-transferability are unknown, and are typically judged based on an assessment of the internal and external validity of the study. These judgments are subjective and uncertain and can be conveyed by putting prior distributions on the study and context parameters. Subjectivity in the specification of the prior distributions is always present. Making no corrections for bias and non-transferability may be plausible when well-conducted studies exist and are truly applicable to the modeled setting. However, most often, such studies are not available.

Without exception, CEAs require choices about which data to use, how to synthesize data from independent sources, and whether and how to adjust data that are not directly applicable to the decision context of the CEA, or data that come from studies that introduce bias through their design, execution, or analysis. It is not feasible to be purely objective in this process, in that the true applicability and internal validity of each empirical study are unknowable, and each analyst can have a different opinion about how well the study-specific estimates transfer to the parameters in the CEA. Subjectivity, however, is not arbitrariness. The CEA should be planned and executed systematically, subjective choices should be justified or at least motivated and their impact should be explored, and the whole process should be adequately documented. Transparency is attainable.

6.3.3 Study Designs, Study Parameter Estimates, and Assessments of Study Validity

Within the healthcare sector, we suggest that model parameters can be categorized broadly as measures of *occurrence, test performance, effect, preference, and cost and resource use*. This classification scheme is convenient because considerations of study design, parameter estimation, and assessment of study internal and external validity tend to be more similar within these categories than across them. While this chapter focuses in depth on only the first three of these parameters as the categories relating most directly to health outcomes, it is useful to begin with some general remarks that relate to the full array of parameter types. Table 6.2 connects common types of model parameters to study designs that can be used to inform them.

Various schemes exist regarding the hierarchies of sources of evidence according to their susceptibility to bias. The most commonly used hierarchies pertain to sources of evidence about intervention effects. They place randomized controlled trials (RCTs) at the top, followed by cohorts, then case-control studies, case-series, case reports,

Table 6.2 Study designs for informing categories of model parameters

Category	Example	Typical designs	Considerations
Measures of occurrence	Prevalence of condition	Cross-sectional survey	Selection bias; missing data; information bias
	Incidence of condition	Longitudinal (cohort)	Selection bias, attrition bias, measurement bias, transferability
Measures of test performance	Consequences of testing (including sensitivity/ specificity of test)	Cohort, nested case-control, case-control, cross-sectional designs, RCT	Selection bias, information bias, measurement bias, missing data
Measures of effect	Intervention effectiveness	RCT, cohort, self-controlled case-series, case-control	Selection bias; confounding; measurement bias
Measures of preference	Utility weights	Cross-sectional; cohort; case-series	Selection bias; measurement bias; transferability
Cost and resource use measures	Resource use	Cross-sectional survey	Selection bias; measurement bias; transferability
	Unit costs	Survey	Selection bias; measurement bias; transferability

Abbreviation: RCT = randomized controlled trial.

and lastly, expert opinion. The desire for objectivity in technology assessment has popularized the use of such hierarchies in the evidence-based medicine community, often in a stringent and mechanistic fashion (Eddy, Hasselblad, and Shachter 1992; Rothman, Greenland, and Lash 2008; Welton et al. 2012). For example, Cochrane systematic reviews consider only RCTs for intervention effects. Other technology assessments may consider nonrandomized studies as well, but they are often constructed to avoid synthesizing across designs (Institute for Quality and Efficiency in Health Care [IQWiG] 2015; Norris et al. 2011).

The problem is that hierarchies are heuristics and usually preclude meaningful analysis of bias. In principle, all study designs in the "measures of effect" row of Table 6.2, can, if properly analyzed, yield unbiased estimates of intervention effects. In practice, an RCT with large attrition rates can yield more biased estimates than a carefully executed self-controlled case series. A meaningful bias analysis would be a sensitivity analysis that aims to understand the direction and magnitude of bias in a study, along the lines of *quantitative bias analysis* (Greenland 2011; Rosenbaum 2010).

Further, the hierarchies do not capture the applicability (transferability) of study estimates to the decision context of the CEA. For example, in patients with chronic coronary artery disease one can obtain estimates for the relative risk of overall mortality between catheter-based interventions, bypass surgery, and medical treatment from several RCTs (Boden et al. 2007; Hueb et al. 2010) or from analyses of large observational databases (Goodney et al. 2010; Klein et al. 2010) and registries. Well-designed and well-conducted RCTs may be more robust to selection bias and confounding than nonrandomized studies. By contrast, patient enrollment in RCTs is often more restrictive than in observational studies, and it may be less applicable to some target populations: in the chronic coronary artery disease example mentioned above, most trials did not enroll patients with chronic kidney disease or people older than 70 years.

As noted above, a CEA analyst has to account for both bias and non-transferability, and perhaps choose sources that trade one for the other. We recommend that instead of strictly following hierarchies of evidence, a CEA would be better served by a careful examination of each study that might be used to inform a parameter in the analysis. Furthermore, we recommend that estimates of the probabilities or frequencies of health and economic consequences associated with alternative choices be based on the best available evidence, in consideration of the full array of available information from either primary or secondary data sources, including corrections for sources of bias to the extent possible, and in recognition of time and resource constraints (**Recommendation 4**). In the following sections we briefly examine sources of evidence for the first three categories of parameters in Table 6.2. Chapter 7 picks up with discussion of measures of preference, specifically relating to health-related quality of life. Chapter 8 focuses on measures of resource use and costs.

6.3.4 Measures of Occurrence

Commonly used measures of occurrence are incidence time, incidence rate, incidence proportion, and prevalence. These measures are not interchangeable, and care is needed when establishing correspondence between estimates from empirical studies and model parameters. For example, when modeling new cancer cases in a population, one would use estimates of an incidence measure to inform the corresponding model parameter. Conversely, when modeling the uptake of healthcare resources by cancer patients in a population, one would need estimates of the prevalence of cancer (perhaps by stage and age, as applicable). Furthermore, the relationship among the various measures of occurrence is not always straightforward, and in general, one cannot be derived from the other unless additional information is available. Thus direct conversions between different measures of occurrence are rarely practical.

6.3.4.1 *Internal Validity of Studies Estimating Measures of Occurrence*

Selection bias, missing data, and information bias are the most important distortions that threaten the validity of estimates of incidence and prevalence measures. Selection bias operates when study participation is determined by factors that are related to the probability that the event of interest will occur. For example, the observed breast cancer incidence rate in a cohort of self-selected middle-aged women can be a biased estimate of the incidence rate among middle-aged women in the general population if the decision to enroll in the cohort is influenced by whether or not a woman has a blood relative with breast cancer.

Missing data are also an important consideration. When data are *missing completely at random*, sample estimates are unbiased. When data are *missing at random given covariates*, it is possible to obtain unbiased estimates if the censoring mechanism is known and includes measured variables. When data are *missing not at random*, no entirely satisfactory approach exists (Little and Rubin 2002).

Information bias is a distortion secondary to measurement bias, or to shifts in the definition of a condition or event. An example of measurement bias occurs when a proxy measurement or criterion is used instead of a final target measurement to define the presence of a condition. An example of information bias pertains to shifting definitions of conditions. For example, in 2003 the American Diabetes Association lowered the threshold for the diagnosis of impaired fasting glucose tolerance to a blood glucose concentration of 100 mg/dL (Genuth et al. 2003), down from the previous threshold of 110 mg/dL (Gabir et al. 2000). The change in the definition of the condition must be accounted for when assessing empirical data on prevalence or incidence measures of diabetes.

6.3.4.2 *External Validity of Studies Estimating Measures of Occurrence*

The external validity of an empirical study should be evaluated with respect to the target population, which is the population modeled in the CEA. A study has high external validity when estimates from that study are likely to be transferable (applicable) to the target setting. Estimates of prevalence or incidence measures are transferable when the study's catchment population and the target population are similar with respect to all factors that affect the probability that the event of interest occurs. Estimates of the probabilities or frequencies of health and economic consequences associated with alternative choices should be specific to the individuals and groups affected by the intervention. Such estimates may have to be transferred to the target setting from other settings, based on credible understanding of pertinent relationships, and with adequate exploration of the invoked assumptions (**Recommendation 5**).

6.3.5 Measures of Test Performance

Ultimately, the value of any test is measured by whether the information it provides affects decision-relevant outcomes such as mortality, morbidity, and health-related quality of life. Although testing and test results have *direct* cognitive, emotional, social, and behavioral effects (Bossuyt and McCaffery 2009), often the most significant effects of testing are *indirectly exerted* through downstream additional diagnostic workup or treatment (Mushlin 1999).

6.3.5.1 *Direct Consequences of Testing*

The direct consequences of testing can include clinical outcomes; emotional, cognitive, social, and behavioral effects; and costs. The importance of these effects should be examined for the specific test and application at hand, considering relevant evidence (Caulfield et al. 2013); not all tests have important or lasting direct effects.

With respect to direct *clinical outcomes* of testing, some tests can pose direct health risks to patients. A biopsy can cause local hemorrhage, inflammation, or even serious infection; a colonoscopy carries a risk of large intestine perforation; and contrast media used in computed tomography can cause nephropathy or allergic reactions. Direct harms of testing need not be immediate; for example, exposure to ionizing radiation for diagnostic studies might be associated with malignancy in the long term. Some testing procedures can have direct beneficial health effects. In infants with suspected meconium obstruction, a barium enema conducted for diagnostic purposes may relieve the obstruction. In some cases, the diagnostic procedure itself amounts to the indicated treatment. Resection of an intestinal polyp during a diagnostic colonoscopy, for example, can be curative if the polyp is a localized malignant tumor. Similarly, excision of skin lesions or endometrial curettage can be curative procedures if they remove localized lesions with malignant potential, even when performed for diagnostic indications.

The *emotional effects* of testing include changes in anxiety, worry, and depression caused by the prospect of testing, the testing procedure, or the knowledge of testing results. For example, a positive screening test result for cancer can cause often short-lived (Laing et al. 2014; Wade et al. 2013) but sometimes longer-term (Brewer, Salz, and Lillie 2007; Maissi et al. 2005) anxiety or depression. Reciprocally, a negative test result might provide reassurance and thus enhance well-being in some patients but not in others (van Ravesteijn et al. 2012).

The *cognitive effects* of testing include the patients' perceptions and understanding about their health status or their prognosis. Testing for a serious condition, such as testing for BRCA gene mutations in a woman with personal and family history suggestive of familial breast cancer, can cause a woman to ponder her personal risks and preferences for different health states and interventions. In addition, the test result can be important for her children, who may also carry the mutation and be at increased risk themselves. The information conveyed by a test result can be of value to some patients, even if it is not actionable in terms of health. For example, consumers were found to be willing to pay for a hypothetical test for predicting eventual development of Alzheimer's disease, even if the test were not accurate, and often for reasons related to logistics and life planning, such as issuing advanced directives and buying insurance (Neumann et al. 2001). Empirical data from oncology, infectious diseases, obstetrics and gynecology, neurology, endocrinology, and other medical specialties also suggest that patients are willing to pay for test results, not necessarily because they expect improvement in their health outcomes but because they perceive value from knowing the results (Lin et al. 2013).

The *social effects* of testing pertain to the impact of testing and of its results on peoples' social relationships, or on their perceptions about their role in their social environment. A positive HIV test result, for example, especially in the early stages of the HIV epidemic, was a stigmatizing diagnosis for some. The ethical, social, and legal implications of testing can include discrimination in employment, including not hiring someone or not allowing someone to work in a high-risk environment, and difficulty in obtaining insurance (Bank et al. 2004; Godard et al. 2003).

The aforementioned health, emotional, cognitive, and social impact of testing and test results may lead to *behavioral effects* in terms of lifestyle adjustments, such as engaging in exercise, following a healthy diet, or quitting smoking, or in terms of adhering to screening or treatment schedules. For example, screening for colorectal cancer has been shown to increase beneficial health behaviors, such as exercising, that are not highly associated with reduced risk of colorectal cancer per se, compared to not screening (Larsen et al. 2007).

Finally, testing can incur monetary and time costs and other *economic consequences* that that are borne by the patient or the payer. A general discussion of these issues is included in Chapter 8.

6.3.5.2 *Indirect Consequences of Testing*

Most effects of testing are indirect in that they are exerted through downstream decisions about additional testing or interventions. Further, changes in test performance do not necessarily result in changes in health outcomes. From this perspective, measures of test performance such as sensitivity, specificity, positive and negative likelihood ratios, and positive and negative predictive values are surrogates of the downstream desired decision-relevant health outcomes. Typically information on test performance and on the effects of treatments is reported in different studies and has to be pieced together in the CEA model.

6.3.5.3 Measuring the Performance of a Single Test

Test performance is often quantified with measures such as (1) sensitivity and specificity, (2) positive and negative likelihood ratios, and (3) positive and negative predictive values and likelihood ratios. These measures inform on different aspects of test performance, and any of them can be used to estimate model parameters. Other measures of test performance exist (e.g., area under the receiver operating characteristic [ROC] curve, Q^* point, and so on), but their usefulness in parameterizing models is limited. They are reviewed in Rutter and Gatsonis (1995).

6.3.5.4 Measuring the Performance of Tests That Classify Results in More Than Two Categories

The metrics discussed above pertain to classifications in two categories, namely, of people with and without disease. However, in practice, test results can categorize people in more than two categories, which can be ordered or unordered. An example of an ordered categorization is when a continuous measurement is discretized in adjacent categories (e.g., a fasting blood glucose level lower than 100 mg/dL, between 100 and 126 mg/dL, and higher than 126 mg/dL). An example of an unordered categorization is using chest radiography to distinguish between various conditions (round pneumonia, primary nodule, metastasis). In such cases, a straightforward way to describe test results is through a statistical model that predicts the ordered or unordered categorical test result from the test measurements (e.g., actual concentration of blood glucose, or attributes of the chest radiography) combined with other characteristics (such as, age, sex, symptoms, etc., as applicable).

6.3.5.5 Measuring Test Performance in the Absence of an Error-Free Reference Standard for Defining the Disease

When the true disease status is not known, common measures of performance are not easy to estimate. In the classical paradigm for evaluating the performance of an index test, the results of the test are compared with the true status of every tested individual or every tested specimen. Sometimes, this true status is directly observable (e.g., for tests predicting short-term mortality after a procedure). However, in many cases the true status of the tested subject is judged based on another test as a reference method. When the reference test does not mirror the truth adequately, the index test is compared against a faulty standard, and is bound to err. The worse the measurement error in the reference test compared to the unobserved truth, the poorer the estimate of the index test's performance will be. This is otherwise known as "reference standard bias" (Bossuyt 2008; Rutjes et al. 2007; Trikalinos and Balion 2012; Whiting et al. 2004). In the presence of reference standard bias, the naive estimates of test performance that one would obtain by treating the reference standard as error-free can be biased upward or downward.

6.3.5.6 *Measuring the Performance of Combinations of Tests or Repeated Tests*

Cost-effectiveness models often compare strategies that involve combinations of tests. There are at least three common cases. The first case is modeling diagnostic strategies that involve concurrent application of a battery of tests (e.g., using a combination of clinical examination, blood tests, and imaging to diagnose diverticulitis in patients with abdominal pain). The second pertains to modeling conditional sequential tests, where one test is used to triage patients for further diagnostic workup with confirmatory testing (e.g., when evaluating solitary pulmonary nodules, where one may start with an imaging test, and potentially follow up with a biopsy). The third case pertains to repeated applications of the same test, as is the case with longitudinal screening for the diagnosis of chronic disease.

Analysts may have the option to model the testing strategy as a whole, if pertinent empirical data are available. The advantage is that one does not have to deal with the complications of modeling the performance of a test conditional on other tests' results. The disadvantage is that such information is relatively unavailable. More important, perhaps, it is rare that all study participants have been managed with the same diagnostic algorithm. Even in prospective studies of testing, healthcare providers typically have discretion in how to manage their patients, and protocol violations and missing data are common. Furthermore, this approach is not conducive to evaluating alternative testing strategies.

Another approach is to reconstruct the performance of the whole testing strategy based on evidence on the performance of each test. If available, head-to-head data on the comparative performance of two or more tests offer valuable information. Otherwise one would have to make assumptions about how the performance of one test changes conditional on the results of another test.

6.3.5.7 *Study Designs for Estimating Diagnostic Performance*

6.3.5.7.1 Designs for estimating sensitivity, specificity, and likelihood ratios

Conditional measures of test performance, such as the true-positive and false-positive proportions (equivalently, sensitivity and specificity), and positive and negative likelihood ratios can be obtained from cohort, nested case-control, case-control, or even cross-sectional designs. In practice, the populations of those with disease or without disease can be systematically different, and therefore, the estimates of performance measures can also differ (Lijmer et al. 1999).

The testing arm in an RCT that compares testing versus no testing can be used to provide estimates of performance measures, e.g., true-positive and false-positive proportions. In such a case, however, the estimation treats the testing arm as a *cohort* (a group of people defined by an exposure to testing) and does not make use of the control arm.

6.3.5.7.2 Designs for estimating positive and negative predictive values

Metrics that essentially require estimation of the prevalence of the disease, such as the positive and negative predictive values, are estimable from a cohort design or from a cross-sectional design only if the application at hand requires no longitudinal information.

6.3.5.8 *Internal Validity of Studies Estimating Diagnostic Performance*

Selection bias, information and measurement bias, and missing data are the major categories of threats to the internal validity of test performance studies (Whiting et al. 2004; Whiting et al. 2011).

A study should *enroll patients from the target population of people with suspected disease* in an unbiased manner, e.g., as a random sample, or by enrolling all consecutive eligible patients during the study period. Excluding people in whom the diagnosis is very easy (e.g., because they have a pathognomonic symptom or sign) or very difficult changes the composition of the studied population and can result in biased estimates of test performance. Similarly, *exclusion of indeterminate results with the index test* can result in overestimates of test performance (Philbrick et al. 1982). Cohort or cross-sectional study designs sampling from the target population are indicated. Case-control designs can easily result in disease and no-disease groups in which the distributions of test results are more dissimilar that the disease and no-disease groups in the target population, and thus result in inflated estimates of test performance (Lijmer et al. 1999; Whiting et al. 2004).

Biases can also be introduced by problems in the *application and interpretation of the index test.* To minimize measurement bias, index test measurements should be obtained without knowledge of the disease status or the reference standard results. Predefining the threshold for interpreting a test result as positive or negative minimizes the likelihood of bias introduced by data-driven post hoc selection of thresholds (Ewald 2006; Leeflang et al. 2008).

Similarly, biases can be secondary to problems in the *application and interpretation of the reference standard.* For example, reference standard bias refers to cases where the reference test has a non-negligible misclassification rate (Bossuyt 2008; Rutjes et al. 2007; Trikalinos and Balion 2012; Whiting et al. 2004) and can result in upward or downward bias in test performance measures, as described earlier, in Section 6.3.5.5. Interpreting reference test results without knowledge of the index test results can help minimize misclassifications due to measurement bias (Whiting et al. 2004).

The *timing between the measurements with index test and the reference test* matters when these measurements can change over time. On the one hand, if the interval between the index and reference test measurements is substantially long compared to the speed with which measurements change or the disease progresses, then the performance of the index test would be underestimated. On the other hand, if the reference standard is based on follow-up, as is the case with many prognostic tests, a long enough follow-up period should be used to allow reliable identification of people with the disease. Timing may be irrelevant for tests that correspond to characteristics that are constant over time, such as somatic genetic variations.

Finally, it is not uncommon to encounter designs in which a subset of the study population receives the reference standard and the remainder of the group receives a different reference test or none at all. This can happen if the reference standard carries a substantial risk of adverse effects, as happens with an invasive biopsy procedure, or is expensive. *Verification bias* can occur when the probability of receiving the reference standard test depends on the results of the index test. Verification bias can misclassify false-negative test results as true-negative test results, resulting in an overestimation of sensitivity and an underestimation of specificity (Begg and Greenes 1983; de Groot et al. 2011; Panzer, Suchman, and Griner 1987).

6.3.5.9 *External Validity of Studies of Test Performance*

The external validity (generalizability) of estimates from studies of test performance pertains to whether these estimates transfer to a target setting. Thus considerations of external validity are paramount when an analyst examines the applicability of study estimates to the setting specified in the CEA model. The transferability of estimates depends on the definition of the disease, the test threshold, and the distribution of test results in those with and without the disease. It also depends on which test performance measures are examined (Irwig et al. 2002).

Estimates of true-positive and false-positive proportions and other conditional measures are transferable across studies if four assumptions hold. The first assumption is that the *exact definition of the disease is constant*. Many conditions are defined on the basis of criteria that can change over time or across locations, as discussed earlier in Section 6.3.4.2 on the external validity of measures of occurrence. For example, the definition of fasting glucose impairment has changed over time. The second assumption is that *the positivity threshold of the test is constant*. The true-positive and false-positive proportions increase or decrease jointly across thresholds. The *positivity threshold* can be chosen explicitly for quantitative tests and implicitly for qualitative tests (Beam, Layde, and Sullivan 1996) to match the testing setting (screening, diagnosis, prognosis, patient management, treatment planning) and the role of the test in the patient management strategy (sole test, triaging test for subsequent workup, or confirmatory test after a triaging test). The third and fourth assumptions are that the *distributions of test results among people with disease* and *among those without the disease are constant*. These assumptions are not satisfied if the spectrum of disease or non-disease differs between the population in which estimates are obtained and the target population to which estimates should be transferred. For estimates of positive and negative predictive values (or of post-test probabilities of disease) to be transferable, a fifth stronger assumption of *a constant prevalence of disease* is required and is rarely likely to hold, especially across different testing settings (e.g., screening versus diagnosis).

The aforementioned assumptions for the transferability of estimates of diagnostic test performance can be violated in typical applications and should not be invoked uncritically. It is the responsibility of the analyst to judge whether the assumptions are likely to hold. If they are deemed unlikely to hold, then the estimates of test performance are not directly transferable (are biased for the target setting) and must be "corrected" by invoking additional assumptions (e.g., about the direction and magnitude of the bias); or are used as is, with appropriate qualification of the CEA analysis results. At any rate, sensitivity analyses will be required. Chapter 9 provides a general discussion of issues related to nontransferability of estimates.

6.3.6 Measures of Effects of Interventions

Measures of intervention effect are differences in expected outcomes between two interventions, say an intervention and a comparator. Most commonly, effect measures correspond to differences in means of measurements (e.g., in average blood pressure with each intervention); hazard ratios for time-to-event outcomes; incidence rate ratios for count outcomes (e.g., number of heart attacks or strokes per person-year); or risk differences, risk ratios, or odds ratios for categorical outcomes (e.g., proportion of people with complications within 30 days of surgery). Most effect measures of interest in CEAs are causal rather than associational, and depending on the granularity of the modeling, they may be specific to population subgroups.

Two causal effects that are commonly of interest are the intention-to-treat causal effect, and the average effect among the treated. The former measures the impact of the assignment of participants to an intervention, and the latter measures the impact of the intervention. A CEA that explicitly models nonadherence would probably require the causal effect among the treated. By contrast, a coarser model that does not explicitly model nonadherence can be parameterized on the basis of an intention-to-treat effect. While the intention-to-treat effect can be readily estimated in RCTs, irrespective of nonadherence, estimation of the causal effect on the treated can be much more involved, because patients may deviate from their assigned intervention, for reasons related to intervention effectiveness.

The effects of interventions can be different in subgroups defined by age, sex, comorbidities, or disease risk. Obviously, when modeling strategies that pertain to population subgroups, analysts should use estimates of subgroup-specific effects to inform CEA model parameters. However, it may still be desirable to explicitly model subgroups comprising a general population, even if the CEA examines strategies at the level of the general population, and then to integrate over subgroups to obtain summary measures such as the ICER in the general population. This modeling can be important when one considers outcomes that are valued differently across population subgroups, and when the intervention has different effects across subgroups.

Generally speaking, some causal effects can be estimated in a straightforward way in RCTs. Causal inference is possible with nonrandomized designs, but it requires more assumptions and, typically, more complex statistical modeling (Rubin 1974).

6.3.6.1 *Randomized Controlled Trials*

Randomization is an unconfounded intervention assignment mechanism (Rubin 1974). It ensures that, in expectation, the distribution of effect modifiers are the same in all groups, and that differences in the measured outcomes can be causally attributed to the intervention. This is why RCTs are the mainstay of clinical research. The typical RCT has a parallel-arm design, where the enrolled participants are randomly assigned to disjoint groups. In an RCT it is possible to obtain an unbiased estimate of the intention-to-treat effect, which is the causal effect of *the assignment*, by comparing outcome means between arms. However, when data are missing for reasons related to the outcome, when there are protocol deviations in the delivery of the intervention (e.g., contamination or non-adherence) or the ascertainment and measurement of outcomes, or when the interventions are dynamic treatment regimens rather than point exposures, estimation of causal effects can be complex. In such cases, the causal effect among the treated individuals, which is often the needed effect in a CEA model, may have to be estimated based on causally explicit analyses (Toh and Hernan 2008; Tsodikov, Szabo, and Wegelin 2006). Such problems are common in large pragmatic trials that evaluate policy recommendations (e.g., for screening, for lifestyle modifications, or for nutrient intake guidance). In such cases, the RCTs resemble observational studies with baseline randomization, and they should be analyzed as observational studies (Hernán, Hernández-Diaz, and Robins 2013).

6.3.6.2 *Nonrandomized Designs*

Causal effects of interventions can be estimated from nonrandomized designs, but assumptions have to be invoked to make up for the lack of an unconfounded intervention assignment mechanism. Important unmeasured confounders commonly exist when interventions are assigned by physicians to patients, or when study participants self-select what intervention to receive (Miettinen 1983). We rely extensively on nonrandomized designs to estimate causal effects, for many reasons. In principle, all causal questions can be answered with an RCT, but, in practice, RCTs are impractical for getting answers to many questions (e.g., when evaluating screening strategies for breast cancer, there are many plausible strategies and there is need for long follow-up or large sample sizes to attain enough power) or unethical (e.g., to establish whether passive smoking causes cancer). Second, many RCTs enroll highly selected populations and are conducted by specialized personnel in highly controlled conditions, and their findings do not necessarily transfer to other contexts, such as routine care. Thus many interventions that have been found effective in trials and have been recommended in clinical practice guidelines are found to be as effective in clinical practice (Oswald and Bateman 1999; Sonis et al. 1998; Wilson et al. 2000), explaining in part the lack of larger adoption of interventions (Cabana et al. 1999; Ford et al. 1987; Grol et al. 1998; Messerli 2000; Pashos et al. 1994).

To minimize confounding and other biases, a multitude of designs and statistical analyses have been proposed, often quite specific to the problem at hand, but their review is beyond the scope of this book. Many approaches aim to compare like with like, through adjustment, stratification (sub-classification), or matched sampling (Cochran 1968; Gu and Rosenbaum 1993; Rubin 2006). Other approaches aim to estimate a marginal intervention effect (as with marginal structural modeling) (Robins, Hernan, and Brumback 2000), an average treatment effect for a subgroup of participants who may be almost randomly allocated to the interventions of interest (as with instrumental variable analyses) (Baiocchi, Cheng, and Small 2014), or a local intervention effect (as with regression discontinuity designs, when there is precise knowledge of the rules that determine the intervention) (Angrist and Pischke 2008).

6.3.6.3 *Internal Validity of Studies Estimating Measures of Effect*

The major threats to the internal validity of studies of intervention effects are confounding, selection (Hernán, Hernández-Diaz, and Robins 2004), and measurement biases (Hernán and Cole 2009).

6.3.6.3.1 Confounding

Confounding exists when the distribution of effect modifiers is different among individuals who are assigned to different interventions. As mentioned already, randomization is a major defense against confounding. If a quantitative bias analysis (see below) is not possible, to gauge the likelihood of bias, one can consider the balance of participant characteristics at baseline, along with whether the design and execution of the assignment mechanism were adequate.

Some nonrandomized designs or analysis methods address confounding by imitating an RCT, in that they identify subgroups of people in which the allocation is as good as random, provided that underlying assumptions hold. Judging the likelihood that substantial residual confounding exists in an analysis of a nonrandomized design is very challenging. A useful device can be to compare the study at hand with an idealized randomized version of it, and examine key differences (Cochrane Bias Methods Group and Cochrane Non-Randomised Studies Methods Group 2014). Substantial residual confounding is more likely when known confounders are not accounted for, and when key assumptions are unlikely to hold. Identifying the important confounders is context specific, and requires good understanding of the relevant knowledge base (Hernán et al. 2002). Key assumptions for propensity score-based analyses, instrumental variables, regression discontinuity, and marginal structural modeling are discussed in the related literatures and are not expanded here.

6.3.6.3.2 Selection bias

Selection bias operates when those who are selected for analysis are different from those who are eligible. In the presence of selection bias, the association between exposure and outcome among those selected for analysis differs from the association among those eligible. In randomized designs, selection bias typically arises when data are not available on all randomized participants because there is differential loss-to-follow-up (also termed attrition bias), or because of nonresponse, or when there is differential intensity in the diagnostic workup between the compared arms (also termed ascertainment bias). In addition, in nonrandomized designs examples of selection bias include biased sampling of controls in case-control studies, self-selection (volunteer), and or healthy worker biases. All these examples are meaningful to classify as selection biases because they have fundamentally the same structure (Hernán, Hernández-Diaz, and Robins 2004).

6.3.6.3.3 Information/measurement bias and error

Information or measurement bias arises when measurements are made with non-negligible error, even when, on average, the errors cancel out (have zero mean). Measurement error can pertain to the mischaracterization of the received intervention or to the measurement of outcomes and non-outcome variables.

6.3.6.3.4 Assessing the net effect of biases

Judging the likelihood of various types of bias, as well as their overall impact (the magnitude and direction of the net bias), is rather difficult, because most often individual sources of bias have opposing or unclear directions. Ideally, a quantitative bias analysis would be available; alternatively, one has to resort to qualitative bias analysis, which amounts to the analysts' opinions about the presence and relative importance of flaws in the design, execution, and analysis of the study at hand.

Methods for quantitative bias analysis have been in development and application for many decades, and they are reviewed in specialized texts (Lash et al. 2014). Some methods allow correction of measured bias sources, such as measurement error and misclassification or missing data, most of which assume that data are available to allow estimation of parameters in an adjustment method, for example by imputation of the missing correct values (Little and Rubin 2002; Rothman, Greenland, and Lash 2008). Other methods deal with instances where no such measurements exist or are possible, and amount to performing sensitivity analyses based on plausible background information (Eddy, Hasselblad, and Shachter 1992; Flanders and Khoury 1990; Greenland 1996; Rothman, Greenland, and Lash 2008).

Methods for qualitative bias analysis have less rigorous theoretical grounding. The emphasis has been on operationalizing definitions and processes so that they can be applied uniformly. It is unclear whether this standardization is successful, however; examples abound where mechanistic application of qualitative bias analysis were demonstrated to have resulted in superficial treatment of very important topics (see for example an in-depth critique of a qualitative bias analysis of mammography screening trials [Freedman, Petitti, and Robins 2004]). For example, for RCTs, the Cochrane Collaboration instructs its reviewers to evaluate the likelihood of bias domains such as selection, ascertainment, performance, attrition, reporting, or other biases, and then to combine these assessments qualitatively to estimate the likelihood of net bias (Higgins et al. 2011). The assessment of each bias dimension may be aided by the presence of methodological "flags," such as blinding of participants and personnel, and generation and concealment of the randomization sequence. Indicatively, compared to a trial where study personnel and participants are blinded to the allocated treatments, lack of blinding may imply higher risk of ascertainment and performance bias. Assessments of bias depend also on the outcome, e.g., self-reported or subjective outcomes such as pain severity might be more prone to bias than major clinical outcomes, such as death.

To aggregate across the bias dimensions, analysts would consider the likely direction and magnitude of bias per dimension, and then form a judgment about the net magnitude of the bias in the study for the specific outcome. This aggregation is exceedingly difficult to perform consistently in a purely qualitative fashion, and it would be more transparent when done quantitatively (see Manzi et al. [2011] and Turner et al. [2009] for detailed expositions).

6.3.6.4 *External Validity of Studies Estimating Measures of Effect*

Generally speaking, an unbiased effect measure is transferable from the study setting to a target setting if the populations (the distribution of effect modifiers), versions of the intervention, and outcome definitions are the same. Most often there are differences that must be accounted for in some fashion. Identifying conditions for transferring estimates from studies to different settings, as well as performing such extrapolations is an area of ongoing methods research (Bareinboim and Pearl 2013).

6.3.7 Eliciting Experts' Probabilities

As mentioned above, for certain model parameters, there may be limitations in the empirical evidence base that point to the need for expert judgment about uncertain quantities as the best available, or a useful additional, source of information. Expert elicitation (EE) has been defined as "a systematic process of formalizing and quantifying, typically in probabilistic terms, expert judgments about uncertain quantities," and its origins can be traced to the development of decision theory in the 1950s (US Environmental Protection Agency 2009). Expert elicitation may be regarded as a subset of activities within the broader category of expert judgment, with the distinction being that EE focuses on questions of science (i.e., characterizations of the state of knowledge) as opposed to questions of values and preferences (US Environmental Protection Agency 2009).

There are various circumstances in which EE can play an essential role in the measurement of consequences for a CEA. It is often needed to characterize uncertainty where existing data are inadequate and new data collection is not practical or feasible. In such situations, solicitation of parameter estimates from experts who have special knowledge about the values of interest may be appropriate and necessary. Expertise in specific areas may be indicated by relevant publications/grants in a given topic, recommendations/nominations from respected bodies/persons, formal training in areas of interest, or membership or positions held. Such experts, however, should be free of any potential or real conflict of interest, and, in general, solicitation of expert judgment from more than one expert with differing perspectives, backgrounds, and responsibilities is helpful in minimizing biases and increasing the potential validity of the estimate. As in all parameter estimation, the process should be transparent.

A good example of an attempt to develop formal guidance for EE is the White Paper produced by the Expert Elicitation Task Force convened by the US Environmental Protection Agency's Scientific Policy Council (US Environmental Protection Agency 2009). The White Paper offered recommendations around key issues in expert elicitation, including specifying the types of problems that are well suited to this approach; the design and conduct of an EE; selection of experts; presentation and use of results from an EE; and the role of peer review in an EE project.

6.4 CONCLUSIONS

Once an overall approach to the design of a CEA has been established, analysts must identify and enumerate relevant consequences of the different interventions or strategies being compared. Once this has been done, analysts are then faced with the often difficult task of measuring, valuing, and aggregating the benefits and harms. This chapter describes a systematic identification of the full array of consequences, introduces the Impact Inventory, and describes key types of data sources and measurement approaches. In the next two chapters we turn our focus to valuing health outcomes (Chapter 7) and resource use and other non-health consequences (Chapter 8).

6.5 RECOMMENDATIONS

1. A cost-effectiveness analysis (CEA) should identify all *types of consequences* affected by the choice of interventions being compared, relating to health (survival and/or health status), resource use in the healthcare sector, and consequences outside the healthcare sector. Both positive consequences (e.g., health benefits, improvements in non-health outcomes such as education, and reductions in resource use) and negative consequences (e.g., health harms, harms in other sectors, and increases in resource use) should be identified.
2. The comprehensive identification of consequences should be summarized in an Impact Inventory, a required part of the Reference Case. The Impact Inventory should organize consequences based on the sector to which they pertain, and it should indicate, for each of the consequences listed, whether the consequence is included in each of the perspectives used in the analysis.
3. Decisions about which of these consequences to *measure and value* in the analysis should, first, be consistent with the specified perspective of the analysis and, second, strike a reasonable balance between expense and difficulty on the one hand and potential importance in the analysis on the other. Consequences that are deemed likely to be insignificant in the context of the analysis can reasonably be excluded,

and this exclusion should be explicitly noted in the Impact Inventory and justified within the supporting information.

4. Estimates of the probabilities or frequencies of health and economic consequences associated with alternative choices should be based on the best available evidence, in consideration of the full array of available information from either primary or secondary data sources, including corrections for sources of bias to the extent possible, and in recognition of time and resource constraints.

5. Estimates of the probabilities or frequencies of health and economic consequences associated with alternative choices should be specific to the individuals and groups affected by the intervention. Such estimates may have to be transferred to the target setting from other settings, based on credible understanding of pertinent relationships, and with adequate exploration of the invoked assumptions.

6.6 REFERENCES

Angrist, J. D., and J.-S. Pischke. 2008. "Getting a Little Jumpy: Regression Discontinuity Designs." In *Mostly Harmless Econometrics: An Empiricist's Companion*, 251–268. Princenton: Princeton University Press.

Baiocchi, M., J. Cheng, and D. S. Small. 2014. Instrumental variable methods for causal inference. *Stat Med* 33 (13):2297–2340.

Bang, H., and A. A. Tsiatis. 2002. Median regression with censored cost data. *Biometrics* 58 (3):643–649.

Bank, I., M. P. Scavenius, H. R. Buller, and S. Middeldorp. 2004. Social aspects of genetic testing for factor V Leiden mutation in healthy individuals and their importance for daily practice. *Thromb Res* 113 (1):7–12.

Bareinboim, E., and J. Pearl. 2013. A general algorithm for deciding transportability of experimental results. *J Causal Inference* 1 (1):107–134.

Beam, C. A., P. M. Layde, and D. C. Sullivan. 1996. Variability in the interpretation of screening mammograms by US radiologists. Findings from a national sample. *Arch Intern Med* 156 (2):209–213.

Begg, C. B., and R. A. Greenes. 1983. Assessment of diagnostic tests when disease verification is subject to selection bias. *Biometrics* 39 (1):207–215.

Boden, W. E., R. A. O'Rourke, K. K. Teo, P. M. Hartigan, D. J. Maron, W. J. Kostuk, M. Knudtson, M. Dada, P. Casperson, C. L. Harris, B. R. Chaitman, L. Shaw, G. Gosselin, S. Nawaz, L. M. Title, G. Gau, A. S. Blaustein, D. C. Booth, E. R. Bates, J. A. Spertus, D. S. Berman, G. B. Mancini, and W. S. Weintraub. 2007. Optimal medical therapy with or without PCI for stable coronary disease. *N Engl J Med* 356 (15):1503–1516.

Bossuyt, P. M. 2008. Interpreting diagnostic test accuracy studies. *Semin Hematol* 45 (3): 189–195.

Bossuyt, P. M., and K. McCaffery. 2009. Additional patient outcomes and pathways in evaluations of testing. *Med Decis Making* 29 (5):E30–E38.

Brewer, N. T., T. Salz, and S. E. Lillie. 2007. Systematic review: the long-term effects of false-positive mammograms. *Ann Intern Med* 146 (7):502–510.

Cabana, M. D., C. S. Rand, N. R. Powe, A. W. Wu, M. H. Wilson, P. A. Abboud, and H. R. Rubin. 1999. Why don't physicians follow clinical practice guidelines? A framework for improvement. *JAMA* 282 (15):1458–1465.

Caulfield, T., S. Chandrasekharan, Y. Joly, and R. Cook-Deegan. 2013. Harm, hype and evidence: ELSI research and policy guidance. *Genome Med* 5 (3):21.

Cochran, W. G. 1968. The effectiveness of adjustment by subclassification in removing bias in observational studies. *Biometrics* 24 (2):295–313.

Cochrane Bias Methods Group and Cochrane Non-Randomised Studies Methods Group. 2014. "A Cochrane Risk of Bias Assessment Tool: For Non-Randomized Studies of Interventions (ACROBAT-NRSI). Version 1.0.0, 24 September 2014." https://sites.google.com/site/ riskofbiastool/.

de Groot, J. A., P. M. Bossuyt, J. B. Reitsma, A. W. Rutjes, N. Dendukuri, K. J. Janssen, and K. G. Moons. 2011. Verification problems in diagnostic accuracy studies: consequences and solutions. *BMJ* 343:d4770.

Eddy, D. M., V. Hasselblad, and R. Shachter. 1992. *Meta-Analysis by the Confidence Profile Method: The Statistical Synthesis of Evidence*. Boston: Academic Press.

Ewald, B. 2006. Post hoc choice of cut points introduced bias to diagnostic research. *J Clin Epidemiol* 59 (8):798–801.

Flanders, W. D., and M. J. Khoury. 1990. Indirect assessment of confounding: graphic description and limits on effect of adjusting for covariates. *Epidemiology* 1 (3):239–246.

Ford, L. G., C. P. Hunter, P. Diehr, R. W. Frelick, and J. Yates. 1987. Effects of patient management guidelines on physician practice patterns: the Community Hospital Oncology Program experience. *J Clin Oncol* 5 (3):504–511.

Freedman, D. A., D. B. Petitti, and J. M. Robins. 2004. On the efficacy of screening for breast cancer. *Int J Epidemiol* 33 (1):43–55.

Gabir, M. M., R. L. Hanson, D. Dabelea, G. Imperatore, J. Roumain, P. H. Bennett, and W. C. Knowler. 2000. The 1997 American Diabetes Association and 1999 World Health Organization criteria for hyperglycemia in the diagnosis and prediction of diabetes. *Diabetes Care* 23 (8):1108–1112.

Genuth, S., K. G. Alberti, P. Bennett, J. Buse, R. Defronzo, R. Kahn, J. Kitzmiller, W. C. Knowler, H. Lebovitz, A. Lernmark, D. Nathan, J. Palmer, R. Rizza, C. Saudek, J. Shaw, M. Steffes, M. Stern, J. Tuomilehto, P. Zimmet, D., and the Expert Committee on the Diagnosis and Classification of Diabetes Mellitus. 2003. Follow-up report on the diagnosis of diabetes mellitus. *Diabetes Care* 26 (11):3160–3167.

Godard, B., S. Raeburn, M. Pembrey, M. Bobrow, P. Farndon, and S. Ayme. 2003. Genetic information and testing in insurance and employment: technical, social and ethical issues. *Eur J Hum Genet* 11 Suppl 2:S123–S142.

Goodney, P. P., L. Travis, F. L. Lucas, E. S. Fisher, and D. Goodman. 2010. Trends and Regional Variation in Cardiac Revascularization. A Dartmouth Atlas Surgery Report. http://www. dartmouthatlas.org/downloads/reports/Carotid_Revasc_012610.pdf.

Greenland, S. 1996. Basic methods for sensitivity analysis of biases. *Int J Epidemiol* 25 (6):1107–1116.

Greenland, S. 2011. "Bias Analysis." In *International Encyclopedia of Statistical Science*, Vol. 2, edited by M. Lovric, 145–148. New York: Springer Verlag.

Grol, R., J. Dalhuijsen, S. Thomas, C. Veld, G. Rutten, and H. Mokkink. 1998. Attributes of clinical guidelines that influence use of guidelines in general practice: observational study. *BMJ* 317 (7162):858–861.

Gu, X. S., and P. R. Rosenbaum. 1993. Comparison of multivariate matching methods: structures, distances and algorithms. *J Comput Graph Stat* 2:405–420.

Heitjan, D. F., C. Y. Kim, and H. Li. 2004. Bayesian estimation of cost-effectiveness from censored data. *Stat Med* 23 (8):1297–1309.

Hernán, M. A., and S. R. Cole. 2009. Invited Commentary: Causal diagrams and measurement bias. *Am J Epidemiol* 170 (8):959–962; discussion 963–954.

Hernán, M. A., S. Hernández-Diaz, and J. M. Robins. 2004. A structural approach to selection bias. *Epidemiology* 15 (5):615–625.

Hernán, M. A., S. Hernández-Diaz, and J. M. Robins. 2013. Randomized trials analyzed as observational studies. *Ann Intern Med* 159 (8):560–562.

Hernán, M. A., S. Hernández-Diaz, M. M. Werler, and A. A. Mitchell. 2002. Causal knowledge as a prerequisite for confounding evaluation: an application to birth defects epidemiology. *Am J Epidemiol* 155 (2):176–184.

Higgins, J. P., D. G. Altman, P. C. Gøtzsche, P. Jüni, D. Moher, A. D. Oxman, J. Savović, K. F. Schulz, L. Weeks, J. A. Sterne, Cochrane Bias Methods Group, and Cochrane Statistical Methods Group. 2011. The Cochrane Collaboration's tool for assessing risk of bias in randomised trials. *BMJ* 343:d5928.

Hueb, W., N. Lopes, B. J. Gersh, P. R. Soares, E. E. Ribeiro, A. C. Pereira, D. Favarato, A. S. C. Rocha, A. C. Hueb, and J. A. F. Ramires. 2010. Ten-year follow-up survival of the Medicine, Angioplasty, or Surgery Study (MASS II): a randomized controlled clinical trial of 3 therapeutic strategies for multivessel coronary artery disease. *Circulation* 122 (10):949–957.

Institute for Quality and Efficiency in Health Care (IQWiG). 2015. General Methods. Version 4.2 of 22 April 2015. https://www.iqwig.de/download/IQWiG_General_Methods_Version_%204-2.pdf.

Irwig, L., P. Bossuyt, P. Glasziou, C. Gatsonis, and J. Lijmer. 2002. Designing studies to ensure that estimates of test accuracy are transferable. *BMJ* 324 (7338):669–671.

Klein, L. W., F. H. Edwards, E. R. DeLong, L. Ritzenthaler, G. D. Dangas, and W. S. Weintraub. 2010. ASCERT: The American College of Cardiology Foundation–The Society of Thoracic Surgeons Collaboration on the comparative effectiveness of revascularization strategies. *JACC Cardiovasc Interv* 3 (1):124–126.

Kuntz, K. M., I. Lansdorp-Vogelaar, C. M. Rutter, A. B. Knudsen, M. van Ballegooijen, J. E. Savarino, E. J. Feuer, and A. G. Zauber. 2011. A systematic comparison of microsimulation models of colorectal cancer: the role of assumptions about adenoma progression. *Med Decis Making* 31 (4):530–539.

Laing, S. S., A. Bogart, J. Chubak, S. Fuller, and B. B. Green. 2014. Psychological distress after a positive fecal occult blood test result among members of an integrated healthcare delivery system. *Cancer Epidemiol Biomarkers Prev* 23 (1):154–159.

Larsen, I. K., T. Grotmol, K. Almendingen, and G. Hoff. 2007. Impact of colorectal cancer screening on future lifestyle choices: a three-year randomized controlled trial. *Clin Gastroenterol Hepatol* 5 (4):477–483.

Lash, T. L., M. P. Fox, R. F. MacLehose, G. Maldonado, L. C. McCandless, and S. Greenland. 2014. Good practices for quantitative bias analysis. *Int J Epidemiol* 43 (6):1969–1985.

Leeflang, M. M., K. G. Moons, J. B. Reitsma, and A. H. Zwinderman. 2008. Bias in sensitivity and specificity caused by data-driven selection of optimal cutoff values: mechanisms, magnitude, and solutions. *Clin Chem* 54 (4):729–737.

Lijmer, J. G., B. W. Mol, S. Heisterkamp, G. J. Bonsel, M. H. Prins, J. H. van der Meulen, and P. M. Bossuyt. 1999. Empirical evidence of design-related bias in studies of diagnostic tests. *JAMA* 282 (11):1061–1066.

Lin, P. J., M. J. Cangelosi, D. W. Lee, and P. J. Neumann. 2013. Willingness to pay for diagnostic technologies: a review of the contingent valuation literature. *Value Health* 16 (5):797–805.

Little, R. J. A., and D. B. Rubin. 2002. *Statistical Analysis with Missing Data*. 2nd ed. Hoboken, NJ: John Wiley & Sons, Inc.

Liu, L. 2009. Joint modeling longitudinal semi-continuous data and survival, with application to longitudinal medical cost data. *Stat Med* 28 (6):972–986.

Liu, L., X. Huang, and J. O'Quigley. 2008. Analysis of longitudinal data in the presence of informative observational times and a dependent terminal event, with application to medical cost data. *Biometrics* 64 (3):950–958.

Maissi, E., T. M. Marteau, M. Hankins, S. Moss, R. Legood, and A. Gray. 2005. The psychological impact of human papillomavirus testing in women with borderline or mildly dyskaryotic cervical smear test results: 6-month follow-up. *Br J Cancer* 92 (6):990–994.

Manzi, G., D. J. Spiegelhalter, R. M. Turner, J. Flowers, and S. G. Thompson. 2011. Modelling bias in combining small area prevalence estimates from multiple surveys. *J R Stat Soc Ser A Stat Soc* 174 (1):31–50.

Messerli, F. H. 2000. Antihypertensive therapy: beta-blockers and diuretics—why do physicians not always follow guidelines? *Proc (Baylor Univ Med Cent)* 13 (2):128–131.

Miettinen, O. S. 1983. The need for randomization in the study of intended effects. *Stat Med* 2 (2):267–271.

Mushlin, A. I. 1999. Challenges and opportunities in economic evaluations of diagnostic tests and procedures. *Acad Radiol* 6 Suppl 1:S128–S131.

Neumann, P. J., J. K. Hammitt, C. Mueller, H. M. Fillit, J. Hill, N. A. Tetteh, and K. S. Kosik. 2001. Public attitudes about genetic testing for Alzheimer's disease. *Health Aff (Millwood)* 20 (5):252–264.

Norris, S. L., D. Atkins, W. Bruening, S. Fox, E. Johnson, R. Kane, S. C. Morton, M. Oremus, M. Ospina, G. Randhawa, K. Schoelles, P. Shekelle, and M. Viswanathan. 2011. Observational studies in systemic reviews of comparative effectiveness: AHRQ and the Effective Health Care Program. *J Clin Epidemiol* 64 (11):1178–1186.

Oswald, N., and H. Bateman. 1999. Applying research evidence to individuals in primary care: a study using non-rheumatic atrial fibrillation. *Fam Pract* 16 (4):414–419.

Panzer, R. J., A. L. Suchman, and P. F. Griner. 1987. Workup bias in prediction research. *Med Decis Making* 7 (2):115–119.

Pashos, C. L., S. L. Normand, J. B. Garfinkle, J. P. Newhouse, A. M. Epstein, and B. J. McNeil. 1994. Trends in the use of drug therapies in patients with acute myocardial infarction: 1988 to 1992. *J Am Coll Cardiol* 23 (5):1023–1030.

Philbrick, J. T., R. I. Horwitz, A. R. Feinstein, R. A. Langou, and J. P. Chandler. 1982. The limited spectrum of patients studied in exercise test research. Analyzing the tip of the iceberg. *JAMA* 248 (19):2467–2470.

Robins, J. M., M. A. Hernan, and B. Brumback. 2000. Marginal structural models and causal inference in epidemiology. *Epidemiology* 11 (5):550–560.

Rosenbaum, P. R. 2010. *Design of Observational Studies*. New York: Springer. http://www.stewartschultz.com/statistics/books/Design%20of%20observational%20studies.pdf.

Rothman, K. J., S. Greenland, and T. L. Lash. 2008. *Modern Epidemiology*. 3rd ed. Philadelphia: Lippincott Williams & Wilkins.

Rubin, D. B. 1974. Estimating causal effects of treatments in randomized and nonrandomized studies. *J Educ Psychol* 66 (5):688–701.

Rubin, D. B. 2006. *Matched Sampling for Causal Effects*. New York: Cambridge University Press.

Rutjes, A. W., J. B. Reitsma, A. Coomarasamy, K. S. Khan, and P. M. Bossuyt. 2007. Evaluation of diagnostic tests when there is no gold standard. A review of methods. *Health Technol Assess* 11 (50):iii, ix–51.

Rutter, C. M., and C. A. Gatsonis. 1995. Regression methods for meta-analysis of diagnostic test data. *Acad Radiol* 2 Suppl 1:S48–S56; discussion S65-47, S70-41 pas.

Rutter, C. M., D. L. Miglioretti, and J. E. Savarino. 2009. Bayesian calibration of microsimulation models. *J Am Stat Assoc* 104 (488):1338–1350.

Sonis, J., D. Doukas, M. Klinkman, B. Reed, and M. T. Ruffin 4th. 1998. Applicability of clinical trial results to primary care. *JAMA* 280 (20):1746.

Toh, S., and M. A. Hernan. 2008. Causal inference from longitudinal studies with baseline randomization. *Int J Biostat* 4 (1):Article 22.

Trikalinos, T. A., and C. M. Balion. 2012. Chapter 9: options for summarizing medical test performance in the absence of a "gold standard." *J Gen Intern Med* 27 Suppl 1:S67–S75.

Tsiatis, A. A., and M. Davidian. 2004. Joint modeling of longitudinal and time-to-event data: an overview. *Statistica Sinica* 14 (3):809–834.

Tsodikov, A., A. Szabo, and J. Wegelin. 2006. A population model of prostate cancer incidence. *Stat Med* 25 (16):2846–2866.

Turner, R. M., D. J. Spiegelhalter, G. C. S. Smith, and S. G. Thompson. 2009. Bias modelling in evidence synthesis. *J R Stat Soc Ser A Stat Soc* 172 (1):21–47.

US Environmental Protection Agency. 2009. Expert Elicitation Task Force White Paper. January 6, 2009. External Review Draft. http://yosemite.epa.gov/sab/sabproduct.nsf/fedrg-str_activites/F4ACE05D0975F8C68525719200598BC7/$File/Expert_Elicitation_White_Paper-Expert_Elicitation_White_Paper-January_06_2009.pdfJanuary_06_2009.pdf.

van Ravesteijn, H., I. van Dijk, D. Darmon, F. van de Laar, P. Lucassen, T. O. Hartman, C. van Weel, and A. Speckens. 2012. The reassuring value of diagnostic tests: a systematic review. *Patient Educ Couns* 86 (1):3–8.

Wade, J., D. J. Rosario, R. C. Macefield, K. N. Avery, C. E. Salter, M. L. Goodwin, J. M. Blazeby, J. A. Lane, C. Metcalfe, D. E. Neal, F. C. Hamdy, and J. L. Donovan. 2013. Psychological impact of prostate biopsy: physical symptoms, anxiety, and depression. *J Clin Oncol* 31 (33): 4235–4241.

Welton, N. J., A. J. Sutton, N. Cooper, K. R. Abrams, and A. E. Ades. 2012. *Evidence Synthesis for Decision Making in Healthcare.* Chichester: John Wiley & Sons Ltd.

Wheeler, M. T., P. A. Heidenreich, V. F. Froelicher, M. A. Hlatky, and E. A. Ashley. 2010. Cost-effectiveness of preparticipation screening for prevention of sudden cardiac death in young athletes. *Ann Intern Med* 152 (5):276–286.

Whiting, P., A. W. Rutjes, J. B. Reitsma, A. S. Glas, P. M. Bossuyt, and J. Kleijnen. 2004. Sources of variation and bias in studies of diagnostic accuracy: a systematic review. *Ann Intern Med* 140 (3):189–202.

Whiting, P. F., A. W. Rutjes, M. E. Westwood, S. Mallett, J. J. Deeks, J. B. Reitsma, M. M. Leeflang, J. A. Sterne, P. M. Bossuyt, QUADAS-2. Group. 2011. QUADAS-2: a revised tool for the quality assessment of diagnostic accuracy studies. *Ann Intern Med* 155 (8):529–536.

Wilson, S., B. C. Delaney, A. Roalfe, L. Roberts, V. Redman, A. M. Wearn, and F. D. Hobbs. 2000. Randomised controlled trials in primary care: case study. *BMJ* 321 (7252):24–27.

7

Valuing Health Outcomes

David Feeny, Murray Krahn, Lisa A. Prosser,
and Joshua A. Salomon

7.1 INTRODUCTION

As outlined in Chapter 2 and Chapter 6, the measure of health outcomes used in
cost-effectiveness analysis (CEA) is typically the number of quality-adjusted life
years (QALYs) gained. Quality-adjusted life years are calculated by multiplying the
health-related quality of life associated with a health state—often referred to as the
utility or preference score or weight, and measured on the conventional scale in which
dead = 0.00 and perfect health = 1.00—by the duration of that health state. This chapter
focuses on how to determine the utility or preference scores for health states and how
to estimate QALYs.

To explore this topic it is necessary to consider a number of conceptual and practical
issues, beginning with the definition of health-related quality of life. We then examine
preference-based and non-preference-based approaches to measuring health-related
quality of life. We discuss expected utility theory, which provides one foundation for
the preference-based approach needed to estimate QALYs. We describe two main
approaches to assessing preferences for health states: the direct approach, in which
respondents provide a valuation of a health state, and the indirect or multi-attribute
approach, in which respondents complete a questionnaire that is then scored using
pre-existing preference weights, usually derived from members of the community.

The quality and usefulness of QALYs depends on the quality and validity of the
utility scores used to calculate them. Therefore, we discuss the criteria for assessing the
measurement properties of measures of health-related quality of life. A key component of the multi-attribute approach is its scoring system, by which levels on multiple
attributes (domains or dimensions) of health are aggregated into a single score on the

This chapter builds on concepts presented in Chapter 4 of the original Panel's book (Gold,
M. R., D. L. Patrick, G. W. Torrance, D. G. Fryback, D. C. Hadorn, M. S. Kamlet, N. Daniels,
and M. C. Weinstein. 1996. "Identifying and Valuing Outcomes." In *Cost-Effectiveness in Health
and Medicine*, edited by M. R. Gold, J. E. Siegel, L. B. Russell and M. C. Weinstein, 82–134.
New York: Oxford University Press).

one-dimensional 0.00 (= dead) to 1.00 (= perfect health) scale needed for QALYs. We therefore review the major methods for estimating multi-attribute utility functions. Guidance on how to select measures and published scores for use in CEAs is provided. A major decision that needs to be made when conducting a CEA is whether to use utility scores provided by patients or scores provided by the community; we review this topic. Special issues, such as states worse than dead, and special populations, such as children and family members of the ill, are discussed. Finally, our recommendations are presented (Section 7.13). Online appendices presenting important supporting material are available at: http://www.chepa.org/research-papers/valuing-health-outcomes/online-appendices.

7.1.1 Definition of Health-Related Quality of Life

We follow the work of the original Panel (Gold et al. 1996b, 83), which adopted the definition of health-related quality of life provided by Patrick and Erickson (1993): "Health-related quality of life is the value assigned to duration of life as modified by the impairments, functional states, perceptions, and social opportunities that are influenced by disease, injury, treatment, or policy" (Patrick and Erickson 1993, 22). The concept of health-related quality of life incorporates the idea that health is a major determinant of overall well-being while recognizing that factors other than health (e.g., freedom, spirituality) may also affect overall quality of life.

What are the consequences of healthcare and public health interventions? Interventions may affect health status positively or negatively; they may also affect longevity. Therefore, one way of representing the output of the healthcare and public health systems is quality-adjusted survival, that is, how long and how well we live. There are several major approaches (to be discussed below) to quantifying quality-adjusted survival, including QALYs, health-adjusted life expectancy (HALE), and disability-adjusted life years (DALYs). A major advantage of integrative measures such as QALYs is that they provide a common "metric" in which diverse outcomes can all be expressed (e.g., the health losses associated with a certain number of myocardial infarctions can be expressed commensurately with the health losses associated with a certain number of episodes of childhood pneumonia), which assists decision making across different programs.

7.1.2 Preference-Based vs Non-Preference-Based Measures of Health-Related Quality of Life

There are two main approaches to measuring health-related quality of life, which are derived from different academic traditions: the preference-based approach (based on economics and decision science) and the non-preference-based approach (based on a variety of social science and clinical disciplines). Outcomes researchers outside of the discipline of health economics have developed many non-preference-based instruments to measure health. Generic instruments are available to evaluate overall health in adult populations (e.g., the 36-Item Short Form Health Survey [SF-36] [Ware and Sherbourne 1992]). Specific instruments assess health within specific diseases or conditions (e.g., the Western Ontario and McMaster Universities [WOMAC] Osteoarthritis Index [Bellamy 1989]), or targeted symptoms of interest (e.g., the Neck Pain Disability Index [Vernon and Mior 1991]). Similarly, there are both generic and specific preference-based measures. As explained below, a key component of the preference-based approach is that scoring focuses on the value attached to health states.

7.1.3 Interval-Scale Properties

To use utility scores to estimate QALYs, the scores must have interval-scale properties (see **Recommendation 3** in Section 7.13) (Keeney and Raiffa 1993; Torrance 1986)—that is, the difference between 0.4 and 0.6 must be the same as the difference between 0.1 and 0.3. Standard ordinal microeconomic utility theory assumes that people have preferences for outcomes and that those preferences are transitive. Thus if A is strictly preferred to B, and B is strictly preferred to C, then A is preferred to C. Following the seminal work of von Neumann and Morgenstern (Luce and Raiffa 1957; von Neumann and Morgenstern 1944), expected utility theory makes additional assumptions sufficient to generate utility scores with interval-scale properties. Expected utility theory was devised to examine decision making in situations involving risk, that is, situations in which decisions makers do not know with certainty what the outcomes will be. Virtually all decisions in healthcare and public health involve such risk. Von Neumann and Morgenstern expected utility theory is widely regarded as a normative model for decision making under risk (Harsanyi 1955; Keeney 1976).

Keeney and Raiffa (1993) and others extended von Neumann and Morgenstern expected utility theory to accommodate outcomes consisting of more than one attribute. This theory is the foundation for multi-attribute utility measures of health-related quality of life, such as the EuroQol EQ-5D and Health Utilities Index Mark 3 (HUI3), described later in this chapter. Table 7.1 and Online Appendix 7.1 provide brief descriptions of widely used multi-attribute measures.

7.1.4 Preferences for Health States vs Paths

A health state is informally characterized by a recognizable health profile, and more formally by a combination of attributes (domains or dimensions) that are relevant in characterizing health. The EQ-5D-3L, for example, considers health to be characterized by five attributes (mobility, self-care, usual activities, pain/discomfort, and anxiety/depression), each of which has three levels.

For CEA, the concept of health states is highly congruent with certain types of health economic models (state-transition models) that represent the trajectories of individuals or groups by their progress through a set of health conditions. However, health can also be characterized as a series of events, or a path or trajectory through a set of health states. Healthy-year equivalents are an example of the path-state approach (Mehrez and Gafni 1993). For models that represent health outcomes in these ways

Table 7.1 Description of EuroQol 5D-3L (EQ-5D-3L), Health Utilities Index Mark 2 (HUI2) and Mark 3 (HUI3), Quality of Well-Being (QWB), and Short Form 6D (SF-6D) Multi-Attribute Preference-Based measures

Measure	Dimensions of health status (numbers of levels)	Number of unique health states	Scoring function
EQ-5D-3L[a]	Mobility (3); self-care (3); usual activities (3); pain/discomfort (3); anxiety/depression (3)	243 plus unconscious and dead	Ad hoc modified linear additive based on TTO scores from random sample of the population of Great Britain; Ad hoc modified linear additive based on TTO scores from random sample of the population of the United States of America; also similar functions based on TTO scores in many other countries
HUI2	Sensation (4); mobility (5); emotion (5); cognition (4); self-care (4); pain and discomfort (5); fertility (3)	24,000 plus dead	Multiplicative multi-attribute based on SG scores from random sample of parents in general population in Canada
HUI3	Vision (6); hearing (6); speech (5); ambulation (6); dexterity (6); emotion (5); cognition (5); pain and discomfort (5)	972,000 plus dead	Multiplicative multi-attribute based on SG scores from random sample of general population in Canada
QWB	Mobility (3); physical activity (3); social activity (5); symptom/problem complex (27)	1,215 plus dead	Linear additive based on VAS scores from random sample of general population in the United States of America
SF-6D	Physical functioning (6); role limitations (4); social functioning (5); pain (6); mental health (5); vitality (5)	18,000 plus dead	Ad hoc modified linear additive based on SG scores from random sample of general population in the United Kingdom

Source: Adapted from Feeny (2005a, 414).

[a] The EQ-5D-5L has five levels per attribute.

Abbreviations: TTO = time trade-off; SG = standard gamble; VAS = visual analog scale.

(e.g., discrete event simulation, decision trees), it is preferences for paths or events, rather than for states, that may be the focus of measurement.

7.2 QUALITY-ADJUSTED LIFE YEARS (QALYS)

Quality-adjusted life years (**Recommendation 1**) and disability-adjusted life years (DALYs) are health metrics that aggregate two components of health: survival (life expectancy) and a weight reflecting the health-related quality of life of the health outcome, or in the case of DALYs, the severity of a particular disabling health outcome (Gold, Stevenson, and Fryback 2002). Quality-adjusted life years weight survival using measures of preference, and they are usually applied to health states or sequences of health states. In contrast, DALYs weight survival based on disability, and they are usually applied to particular sequelae of a disease or injury.

In the standard approach to QALYs, the quality-adjustment weight for each health state is multiplied by the time spent in that state (which is discounted as discussed in Chapter 10) and then summed to calculate the number of QALYs. An example is displayed in Figure 7.1, in which outcomes are assumed to occur with certainty. Without the health intervention, an individual's health-related quality of life would deteriorate according to the lower curve, and the individual would die at time "Death 1." The area under the curve represents the number of QALYs expected with no intervention. With the health intervention, the individual would deteriorate more slowly, live longer, and

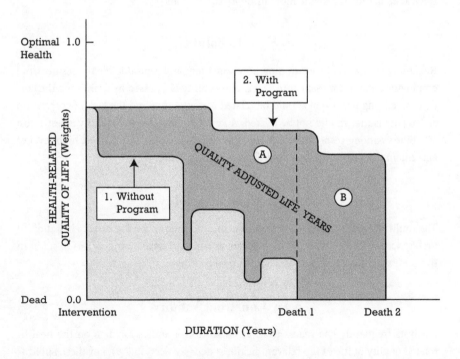

Figure 7.1 Quality-adjusted life years (QALYs) gained from an intervention.
Source: Figure 4.2 in Gold et al. (1996b, 92).

die at time "Death 2." The area between the two curves is the number of QALYs gained by implementing the intervention. The area can be divided into two parts, A and B, as shown in Figure 7.1. Part A represents the number of QALYs gained purely as the result of improvements in health-related quality of life during the time in which the individual would, in any case, have been alive. Part B represents the number of QALYs gained from longer life (i.e., the amount of life extension multiplied by the health-related quality of that life extension). It should be noted that this example is a special case in which there is no decrement in health-related quality of life associated with the process of undergoing treatment. Additional issues associated with the use of QALYs and DALYs are discussed later (see Sections 7.9.4 and 7.9.5), in Online Appendices 7.2–7.4, as well as in Chapter 12 (see also **Recommendation 1**).

7.3 MEASUREMENT PROPERTIES OF PREFERENCE-BASED INSTRUMENTS

As noted above, preference-based measures are needed to estimate QALYs. Therefore the measurement properties of preference-based instruments are an important consideration in CEA. Given the lack of a gold standard measure of health-related quality of life, criterion validity cannot be assessed. As a result, the focus is on reliability, content validity, construct validity, and responsiveness. In the following paragraphs we review these key criteria; elsewhere, Fayers and Machin (2007), Feeny et al. (2013), and Revicki et al. (2000) provide more in-depth discussions.

7.3.1 Reliability

Reliability is assessed by examining how consistent and reproducible the results from employing a certain measure are. Internal reliability is assessed by examining the correlation among items that should be related to each other and the lack of correlation among items that should not be related. A key element of reproducibility is test-retest reliability. Among respondents whose health is stable there should be a high level of agreement between scores at two different points in time.

7.3.2 Content Validity

The multi-attribute measure, or health-state descriptions for the direct elicitation of preference scores, should cover the relevant and important attributes of health status in the context of the intervention(s) and clinical condition(s) being evaluated.

7.3.3 Construct Validity

Analysts frequently use scores from cross-sectional studies for data on the health-related quality of life of the relevant health states (see Section 7.8). For these applications, cross-sectional construct validity—that is, evidence that the measure captures what it is intended to measure—is a key measurement property. In particular, evidence on known-groups construct validity is crucial. Is there evidence that a preference-based measure generates scores that distinguish among levels of severity of a particular condition? Do scores from the measure distinguish between those with the condition who do not have comorbidities and those with the condition who do have comorbidities?

7.3.4 Responsiveness

A key criterion in the context of evaluating the effectiveness of intervention is responsiveness—that is, the ability of the measure to capture within-person change over time when it occurs.

7.4 METHODS FOR MEASURING UTILITIES: OVERVIEW

To illustrate the different ways that health states may be represented for valuation, consider the following description of a health state for a man with prostate cancer following a radical prostatectomy:

> A 68-year-old former teacher was treated 1 year ago for prostate cancer. The surgery was successful but left him with moderate urinary incontinence, such that he occasionally loses control of his bladder. Also, the operation affected his sexual function and is no longer able to have sexual intercourse with his wife. Loss of bladder control has affected his confidence in attending social events. The change in sexual function and the cancer diagnosis have changed his relationship with his wife.

Note that this description includes a diagnosis, symptoms, and function. However, it does not describe the patient's living circumstances, his economic well-being, the type of society he lives in, his spirituality, or his goals and ambitions in life. Thus, we have a description of *health-related* quality of life, but not overall quality of life. To generate a preference score for this patient's state of health for the purpose of conducting a CEA, we have the following options:

i) We could measure his score *directly* by asking him about his preference for his current health using the standard gamble or time-tradeoff methods.
ii) We could generate a description of his health (like the paragraph above) and ask other patients or members of the general population about their preference for this health state using the standard gamble or time-tradeoff. This is also usually considered to be a form of *direct* preference elicitation, even though the respondent is not the patient.
iii) We could ask the patient to complete a health status questionnaire (e.g., EQ-5D or HUI), and use the responses, along with preference weights derived from members of the general population, to generate the score for his health state. That

is, the patient himself would tell us about his health status, but the preference for this health state would come from others. This is *indirect* utility assessment based on the use of a multi-attribute utility measure. Online Appendices 7.1, 7.5, and 7.6 provide additional detail on the development of these scoring systems.

7.5 DIRECT UTILITY MEASUREMENT

Direct methods of measuring utilities have been developed primarily from two theoretical traditions: expected utility theory and psychophysics (judgment of sensation). This chapter focuses primarily on methods based on expected utility theory that provide a foundation for estimating QALYs. Additional details are presented in Online Appendix 7.7.

7.5.1 Expected Utility Approaches

The major approaches based on expected utility theory are choice-based methods such as the standard gamble and time trade-off. The *standard gamble* approach is based on the axioms of expected utility theory and has been widely used to measure health state preferences (Torrance 1986; Weinstein, Torrance, and McGuire 2009). In the standard gamble the respondent is given a choice between (i) a lottery consisting of a preferred health state with probability p (usually perfect health) and a dis-preferred state with probability $1-p$ (usually dead) and (ii) a certain and intermediately ranked state (the state for which the analyst wants a utility score). The probability p is then systematically varied until the respondent is indifferent between the lottery and the sure thing.

The *time trade-off* method presents the respondent with the task of determining what amount of time he or she would be willing to give up to be in a better versus a poorer health state (Torrance, Thomas, and Sackett 1972; Weinstein, Torrance, and McGuire 2009). Here the choice is between two certain states rather than the certain state of the described health state and a lottery between perfect health and dead. The time trade-off method asks respondents to value the alternatives of being in a less desirable health state (A) for a longer period of time, followed by being dead, versus being in a more desirable state (B, usually perfect health) for a shorter period of time, followed by being dead. Different durations for the time spent in state B are offered until the respondent becomes indifferent in choosing between the alternatives. The preference for state A is calculated as life expectancy at the point of indifference in state B divided by the life expectancy in state A. Buckingham and Devlin (2006) provide a rationale in utility theory for the time trade-off method by linking it to the concept of compensating variation; that is, the reduction in the duration of life is compensated for by the improvement in health (going from health state A to B). Online Appendix 7.7 provides additional detail.

7.5.2 Psychophysical Approaches

Direct utility measurement methods derived from the psychophysical tradition include *rating scale* methods and the *paired-comparison* approach (see Online Appendix 7.8).

Rating scale methods, including *category scaling* and *visual analog scales,* require respondents to assign each health state to a number, usually on a scale from 0 (least desirable or dead) to 100 (most desirable or perfect health). Visual aids such as a "Feeling Thermometer," in which the most desirable health state is at the top and the least desirable at the bottom, are used to support this task. Respondents are instructed to place health states along the scale according to their relative desirability, typically with the additional instruction that the spacing between any two points in the scale should be regarded as equivalent. The preference score for each of the states is simply the value associated with its placement on the scale. States worse than dead can be accommodated using these methods.

The paired-comparison approach is a commonly used example from a broader set of ordinal elicitation methods that includes other discrete choice elicitation methods, as well as ranking methods. These methods are further discussed below in Section 7.5.5 and in Online Appendices 7.8 and 7.9.

7.5.3 Direct Elicitation Methods in Practice

Rating scales are believed to produce interval-level values when respondents are instructed to place the health states on the scale such that the intervals between their placements reflect the differences they perceive between the health states. However, concerns regarding scaling characteristics both of category and visual analog scales have been raised. Issues include end-of-scale aversion and context effects (Streiner and Norman 1995; Torrance, Feeny, and Furlong 2001). Rating scale methods typically yield health utility scores that are closer to the middle of the range; they can be lower or higher than scores elicited using standard gamble or time trade-off methods. Nonetheless, rating scales are generally regarded as a useful step early in the elicitation process because they introduce the respondent to the health states to be evaluated and provide information on the ordinal rankings of the health states (Torrance, Feeny, and Furlong 2001). In order to implement the standard gamble and the time trade-off, some information on the ranking of health states is required.

7.5.4 Chronic and Temporary Health States

Conventional standard gamble and time trade-off methods were developed to elicit scores for chronic health states. Using these methods to value temporary health states can be challenging. A number of alternative methods have been tested and applied for the valuation of health states with a duration of less than one year (Wright et al. 2009). These include chained approaches for the standard gamble and time trade-off (Jansen et al. 2000; Locadia et al. 2004; McNamee et al. 2004; Ormel et al. 1994), the waiting trade-off (Swan et al. 2000), the sleep trade-off (Gage, Cardinalli, and Owens 1996; Tosteson and Hammond 2002; Tosteson et al. 2002), and the time trade-off with modifications (Lee et al. 2005; Prosser et al. 2004). Additional detail on these approaches is provided in Online Appendix 7.7.

7.5.5 Choice of Elicitation Methods for Direct Utility Measurement

Different elicitation methods often do not yield the same score when applied to the same specific health states or illnesses (Fryback et al. 1993; Hornberger, Redelmeier, and Petersen 1992; Nease et al. 1995; Nord 1992; Read et al. 1984). Variations in measured scores across methods can occur for reasons that include: the sensitivity (or lack thereof) of a measurement strategy to specific domains of health affected by an illness; cognitive difficulties the measure presents to the population from which elicitations are obtained; the degree to which preferences for health states are affected by risk attitudes implicit in the measurement strategy; the scaling properties particular to the technique used; whether or not scores are elicited in a face-to-face interview; the use of props; the extent of training and experience of the interviewer; the method for ordering the sequence of questions for choice-based techniques (ping-pong; bisection); numeracy of respondents; and time horizon of health states. Because of this heterogeneity, it is important to perform sensitivity analyses to examine the implications of alternative sets of utility scores. The techniques for sensitivity analyses are discussed in Chapter 11.

Until relatively recently, ordinal data collection methods such as ranking tasks were commonly included in health valuation studies, mainly as "warm-up" tasks (Brazier, Roberts, and Deverill 2002; Dolan et al. 1996; Fryback et al. 1993) but not as a basis for deriving cardinal valuations. At the time of the original Panel, there were a few exceptions (Fanshel and Bush 1970; Kind 1982), but since that time, there has been a substantial increase in the number of studies that derive cardinal (interval-scale) values from ordinal information, borrowing techniques that have been widely applied in areas as diverse as consumer marketing (Louviere, Hensher, and Swait 2000), political science (Koop and Poirier 1994), transportation research (Beggs, Cardell, and Hausman 1981), and environmental economics (Adamowicz, Louviere, and Williams 1994). A prominent example of the use of the discrete-choice approach is the program of research to estimate multi-attribute utility functions for the EQ-5D-5L system in various countries (Oppe et al. 2014). In the paired comparisons discrete-choice approach described by Oppe and colleagues, the respondent is asked to choose between two EQ-5D-5L health states, A and B; more specifically the respondent is asked "which is better, state A or state B?" (Oppe et al. 2014, 452). Unlike the process with the standard time trade-off, the respondent is not asked a series of questions to identify a point of indifference. Potential advantages of ordinal data collection approaches include relative ease of comprehension and administration, as well as greater reliability corresponding to reduced measurement error. Particularly in settings or subpopulations in which educational attainment and numeracy are limited, an ordinal measurement strategy may have considerable practical advantages. These issues are further discussed in Online Appendices 7.8 and 7.9.

7.6 INDIRECT OR MULTI-ATTRIBUTE UTILITY MEASUREMENT

7.6.1 Generic Preference-Based Measures

An alternative approach to direct measurement of preferences for health outcomes is the indirect or multi-attribute approach. It is labeled "indirect" because the source of preferences is not the subjects who are experiencing the health state. The label "multi-attribute" refers to the class of generic preference-based measures that include multiple attributes (domains or dimensions) of health status (**Recommendations 4, 5, 6, 7, and 8**). The breadth of coverage of attributes makes these measures useful for making comparisons among groups and health conditions, thus promoting comparability and consistency across studies (**Recommendation 4**).

There are two fundamental components in the multi-attribute approach: (1) a health status classification system and (2) a preference-based scoring system. In this approach, subjects experiencing the health state complete a questionnaire based on the health status classification system of the instrument (self-assessed health status); that health state is then valued with the preference-based scoring system for the instrument, which is typically based on community preferences (community valuation).

Each multi-attribute measure or instrument covers a defined set of attributes. The characteristics of the major multi-attribute measures are described in Table 7.1. As noted in Table 7.1, each measure describes a large number of unique health states (see also Online Appendix 7.1). All of these measures include some combination of function across physical and mental health, but no two measures share identical attributes.

7.6.2 Condition- or Disease-Specific Preference-Based Measures

If the analyst has evidence that generic preference-based measures perform poorly in a particular context, an alternative approach is to create a condition-specific preference-based measure. In some cases investigators create a new condition-specific health status classification system and then estimate a multi-attribute utility function for it; examples include the work of Revicki et al. (1998a) (asthma); Revicki et al. (1998b) (rhinitis); and the Patient-Oriented Prostate Utility Scales (PORPUS) designed for patients with prostate cancer (Krahn et al. 2007). In other cases investigators start with an existing condition-specific health status classification system, and sometimes modify it to facilitate the estimation of a multi-attribute utility function; they then develop a multi-attribute utility function for the condition-specific measure; an example is the work of Brazier et al. (2005) (menopausal health-related quality of life).

If the scores for such measures are anchored on "perfect health" and "dead," then they are, in theory, comparable to scores derived from generic preference-based measures. As with any condition-specific measures, there is the potential to fail to detect adverse effects and to fail to capture the effects of comorbidities. In addition, the scoring function for the condition-specific measure may not reflect potentially important preference interactions between its attributes and comorbidities. Further, the condition is named (identified) in most condition-specific measures (Brazier and Tsuchiya 2010). For instance, an item in the National Eye Institute Visual Functioning Questionnaire-25 is "Do you accomplish less than you would like because of your vision?" When preference scores for condition-specific measures are obtained from members of the general population, the scores may be influenced by the naming of the condition. In some cases, such as cancer, scores when there is a disease label tend to be lower than scores for the same health state description without the disease label (Rowen et al. 2012); in other cases, the disease label may have little or no effect on scores. Further, as Brazier and Tsuchiya (2010) note, condition-specific measures may be subject to focusing effects and may exaggerate the importance of the problems associated with the condition being valued as compared to other conditions. There appears to be a trade-off between the enhanced specificity and potentially greater responsiveness of preference-based condition-specific measures, on the one hand, and decreased comparability with scores from generic preference-based measures on the other.

7.6.3 How to Estimate Scoring Systems for Multi-Attribute Utility Measures

As noted earlier in this chapter, a major method for obtaining utility scores is to have patients in a study complete a questionnaire based on a multi-attribute generic preference-based measure. The completed questionnaire provides information on the health states of respondents. Those health states are then valued with the multi-attribute utility function or the scoring function for that generic measure. Typically, these scoring functions are based on preference data obtained from members of the general population; thus, they represent community preferences.

There is a host of important theoretical and methodological issues involved in estimating multi-attribute utility functions, including the choice of preference elicitation technique, functional form, statistical methods used to estimate the function, and assessment of the validity of the utility scores generated by the function; brief summaries of these characteristics for a number of measures are provided in Table 7.1. Users of these systems need to consider which attributes are included and whether or not the attributes included are appropriate in the context of their application. Users also need to assess the performance of these scoring systems. A key issue in assessing the performance of the estimated multi-attribute utility functions is within-sample and out-of-sample accuracy in predicting directly measured utility scores. Another key issue is the choice of an appropriate functional form for the multi-attribute utility function. These methodological issues are discussed in detail in Online Appendices 7.5 and 7.6.

7.7 THE CONTENT AND MEANING OF UTILITY SCORES

7.7.1 How to Interpret Utility Scores

A key component of attaching meaning to utility scores is the interpretation of differences or changes. In addition to noting that the difference or change is statistically significant, the analyst questions whether its magnitude is clinically important. Relevant concepts include a clinically important difference (Guyatt et al. 2002), a patient-important difference (Guyatt et al. 2004), and a minimal important difference. Schünemann and colleagues define the minimal important difference as "The smallest difference in score in the outcome of interest that informed patients or informed proxies perceive as important, either beneficial or harmful, and that would lead the patient or clinician to consider a change in management" (Schünemann et al. 2005, 82).

For generic multi-attribute preference-based measures, a number of studies using a variety of approaches provide guidance. Although there is heterogeneity in the resulting guidelines, differences or changes in utility scores of 0.03 (3 out of 100) or more for these measures are, in general, regarded as clinically important (Drummond 2001; Feeny et al. 2012; Kaplan 2005; Luo, Johnson, and Coons 2010; Walters and Brazier 2003).

There is less guidance on what constitutes a clinically important difference for directly measured standard gamble, time trade-off, and visual analog scores. For standard gamble and time trade-off scores, on the basis of measurement precision, observed cross-sectional differences in scores, and observed prospective changes in scores, a rule of thumb is that differences or changes of 0.05 (5 out of 100) or more are clinically important (Feeny 2005a, b). For visual analog scale scores, differences or changes of 0.06 to 0.08 (6–8 out of 100) or more are regarded as clinically important (Schünemann et al. 2003).

These criteria are useful for interpreting the differences in change scores in a randomized controlled trial or single study that uses utility scores as an outcome measure. But in many CEAs, it is the expected health-related quality of life of two (or more) interventions that is being compared, drawing on data on utility scores from multiple sources. Further, scores for a number of relevant health states are used to estimate QALYs. There is little guidance in the literature about the magnitude of differences in QALYs that can be regarded as important. In the context of quality-adjusted survival in cancer care, Revicki et al. (2006) suggest that differences of 10% (10 out of 100) or more be regarded as important. Guidance on the interpretation of gains in life expectancy is found in Krahn et al. (1997) and Wright and Weinstein (1998).

7.7.2 Are Productivity Effects Included in Utility Scores?

The original Panel assumed that the effects of morbidity on productivity and leisure were captured by the utility measure (**Recommendation 9**). The Second Panel disagrees and argues that it is unlikely that the effects of morbidity on productivity and leisure are captured by most preference-based measures (see Chapter 8). Of course, to the extent that utility scores do reflect any effects of morbidity on productivity and leisure, the decision by the Second Panel opens up the possibility of double counting—that is, the effects on productivity may be captured in pecuniary terms in the numerator and "counted again" in the estimates of incremental QALYs in the denominator. An important implication of this decision by the Second Panel is that utility scores should ideally be obtained so as to capture the "pure" effects on health on health-related quality of life and not effects on productivity.

7.8 SOURCES OF DATA FOR PREFERENCE SCORES TO ASSIGN VALUE TO HEALTH STATES

Preference scores should ideally be based on data on health status obtained in prospective studies as patients experience the disease or condition, the intervention, and the consequences of that intervention, including adverse events, and gathered with a single validated preference-based instrument. It is, however, very unusual that a single preference set will be available that will be fully adequate for a CEA. In such a case, the analyst should use the best available evidence for scores for the relevant health states. This will often involve the use of prospective and cross-sectional evidence, as well as scores from previously published studies.

What criteria should guide the analyst in selecting utility scores from among those available in the existing literature? Coverage of both treatment effects and the adverse effects of treatment is crucial. Borrowing from clinical epidemiology, the PICO framework is useful: patient, problem, or population (P); intervention (I); comparison (C); and outcomes (O) (Sackett et al. 1997). Do the characteristics of the patients in the potential sources of utility scores match the characteristics of the patients in the CEA? Same disease? Same severity? Given that the extent and severity of comorbidities affects utility scores importantly (Maddigan, Feeny, and Johnson 2005; Pohar and Jones 2009), finding a good match can be challenging. If the potential source of the utility scores was an evaluative study, were the interventions being compared the same as in the CEA? Were outcomes assessed with the same measures used in the CEA?

There is substantial evidence that results based on different generic preference-based measures are often not interchangeable (Feeny et al. 2012; Fryback et al. 2007; Luo et al. 2005; Marra et al. 2005; Peasgood and Brazier 2015). For instance, in one study the mean gain in health-related quality of life associated with elective total hip arthroplasty was 0.10 according to SF-6D, 0.16 according to the standard gamble, 0.22 according to HUI2, and 0.23 according to HUI3 (Feeny, Wu, and Eng 2004). Similarly, there are typically systematic differences in standard gamble, time trade-off, and visual analog scales scores. In general for the same health state, standard gamble scores are higher than time trade-off scores, which are in turn higher than visual analog scale scores. Ideally the analyst would assemble scores all based on the same generic preference-based measure or the same elicitation technique. In practice, the existing body of evidence is often not sufficient to support this strategy. These problems highlight the importance of sensitivity analyses (see Chapter 11). Alternative approaches are discussed in Online Appendices 7.8, 7.10, and 7.11.

7.9 WHOSE PREFERENCES SHOULD BE USED IN CEA?

For the most part, the exposition here focuses on asking respondents to value health states that they themselves are experiencing or could experience. Exposition on asking respondents about health states experienced by others is found in Section 7.9.5 and in Chapter 12. Preferences for health states may be obtained from members of the general population, patients, patient proxies, or health professionals. Some studies have suggested that patients value health states differently than members of the general population. For example, Sackett and Torrance (1978) found that the utility scores that dialysis patients assigned to their own health were much higher than scores assigned by members of the general population (difference in score as much as 0.20). Other studies have found similar results (Boyd et al. 1990; Hurst et al. 1994; Torrance 1986), though differences are not usually large (Gold et al. 1996a). Nonetheless, published studies that have used preference sets from a variety of sources have shown that the source of preferences can qualitatively change the result of model-based evaluations (Cowen et al. 1998; Elkin et al. 2004; Hornberger, Redelmeier, and Petersen 1992). When there are differences, it is often the case that patients assign a higher value to the same health states than do members of the general population.

Whose preferences should be used in broad resource allocation decisions remains controversial. Many health economists, and most published guidelines, advocate the use of social or community preferences (Australian Government Department of Health 2013; Canadian Agency for Drugs and Technologies in Health [CADTH] 2006). Other researchers believe that experience of illness is essential in correctly understanding and valuing health outcomes. The issue of comparisons between direct preference scores provided by patients and scores derived from multi-attribute measures using community preferences is discussed in Online Appendix 7.5.

7.9.1 Source of Preferences and Experience of Illness

The source of preferences must be distinguished from experience of illness. Many members of the general population have experience of illness, either personally or through family members or social connections (Dolan and Kahneman 2008). Patient experiences with respect to illness are also heterogeneous. Few will have experienced all health states relevant to their disease. Patients are more likely to have illness experience relevant to a given health state, but not all patients will have such experience, and not all members of the general population will not. Evaluation of current health status must also be distinguished from evaluation of hypothetical health states. Patients and members of the general population may be asked about either, although patients are usually asked about their current health.

Finally, it is vital to draw a distinction between individual and social valuation of health. An individual may not provide the same valuation for a health state that he or she is experiencing (or will experience) as the value that individual attaches to the same health state that will be experienced by others. How such social judgments can best be arrived at is discussed below and in Chapter 12.

7.9.2 Rationale for Using Community Health Preferences

Cost-effectiveness analyses are used to inform ex-ante resource allocation decisions for a group or population. The main arguments put forth in favor of using community preferences (derived from members of the general population) are the insurance principle, the related concept of the social contract, concern about bias associated with using patient preferences, practical issues, and the comparability across studies.

7.9.2.1 *The Insurance Principle*

The CADTH guideline on economic evaluation states: "It is preferred that analysts measuring preferences directly use a representative sample of the general public, who are suitably informed about the health states being valued. The reasoning is that they are the ultimate payers of the publicly funded health care system and potential patients" (Canadian Agency for Drugs and Technologies in Health [CADTH] 2006, 27). The implicit rationale here is that, as costs are borne by potential beneficiaries of publicly funded healthcare systems prior to the potential for benefit, so health effects should also be considered in an ex-ante way. This is the insurance principle (Dolan and Kahneman 2008; Hadorn and Uebersax 1995).

7.9.2.2 *The Social Contract Principle*

A related argument in favor of using community preferences is that doing so reflects a social contract which states that society should create mechanisms to allocate resources to prevent and reduce illness and improve health and longevity. Because such health systems will benefit virtually all members of society, the preferences of all members of society should be taken into account. A key component of this argument is that it is being a member of the society rather than being a tax payer that justifies the use of community preferences.

7.9.2.3 *Bias*

A concern that has been raised is that patients' valuations of health outcomes may be biased. Rawls's concept of a "veil of ignorance" is often cited in this context. The idea here is that "parties situated behind a veil of ignorance . . . do not know how the various alternatives will affect their particular case, and they are obliged to evaluate principles solely on the basis of general considerations" (Rawls 1972, 136-137). Those who have experienced illness may be inclined to overstate their illness or disability, either because their experience of illness changes their valuation of health status or because of a desire to influence health policy in a manner that will result in personal benefit, for instance by having more healthcare resources allocated to their problem or condition. In practice, this does not seem to happen.

Potential bias unrelated to personal incentives is a more substantive concern. We use "bias" here to characterize the concern that individuals' values may be systematically different from societal values—that is, preferences for the kind of society in which the general population thinks it best to live (Menzel et al. 2002; Ubel, Richardson, and Menzel 2000). Patients experiencing illness, especially chronic illness, often *adapt* to their changed circumstances. Adaptation may involve several elements: (i) denial, or inability to admit how poor one's health actually is; (ii) loss of recognition of full health; (iii) development of greater skill in the abilities that remain; (iv) change in activity to correspond with remaining abilities; (v) adjustment of goals in the light of new circumstances; (vi) altered conceptualization of health; (vii) lowered expectations; and (viii) heightened stoicism (Menzel et al. 2002). Some of these elements of adaptation could theoretically lead to health state valuations that are inappropriate for societal valuation. For example, it may not be appropriate for patients' denial of their actual health status, lowered expectations that come with illness, and stoicism, which may minimize illness severity, to inform social judgments as to the desirability of health outcomes. On the other hand, it is unlikely that individuals without experience of illness would be able to imagine how they could develop their remaining abilities or adjust their activities and life goals in the presence of chronic illness. As Menzel argues, there are aspects of adaptation that weigh both for and against using community preferences. The contrast between the growing role of patient-centered care and the reliance on community preferences in CEA is discussed in Section 7.12 and in Online Appendix 7.12.

7.9.3 Arguments in Favor of Using Patient Preferences

There are several important conceptual arguments against using community preferences. Gandjour (2010) argues that welfare economics as well as several ethical theories support the use of the preferences of those who are directly affected; the implication is that valuations should be based on patient preferences. Gandjour concludes that "a strong argument in favor of using patient preferences . . . is experience with a disease" (Gandjour 2010, E61). Indeed, taking practical considerations into account, there is a strong argument for using patient preferences because, in general, patients are more likely to be well informed about the burden of the disease or condition and the experience of undergoing treatment.

7.9.4 Practical Issues in Favor of Using Community Preferences

Consistent with the insurance and social contract arguments for using community preferences is the practice of eliciting preferences of health states from representative samples of the general population. The preference scores upon which the scoring systems for the major generic preference-based multi-attribute measures are based are drawn from representative samples of community dwelling members of the general population. Note, however, that such samples are not necessarily fully representative of the entire population. Typically those living in long-term care facilities are not sampled. Of course, many of those residents have cognitive or sensory impairments that may affect their ability to participate meaningfully in preference elicitation tasks. Nonetheless, in practice, the scores based on community preferences are likely to be broadly representative.

If one relies instead on patient preferences, the challenges in obtaining a representative sample are more daunting. If, for instance, one has access to a fully comprehensive registry of persons with a disease or health condition, it should be possible to draw a representative sample of the full range of patients. Yet many patients would be unable to provide meaningful preference scores because of disease severity or toxicities associated with treatment or the burdens of comorbidities. Thus the degree of censoring would potentially be substantial.

In conclusion, like the original Panel, the Second Panel favors the use of community preferences for the Reference Case analyses (**Recommendation 4**). Nonetheless we note that there are a number of circumstances (discussed below and in Section 7.13) in which the analyst may also want to use patient preferences.

7.9.5 Are All QALYs Equal?

In the standard approach to estimating QALYs, an intervention that generates marginal gains for many people may be approximately equal to an intervention that generates substantial gains for a small number of people, yet society may favor the latter. Similarly, some investigators have argued that treating those who initially experience highly impaired health is more valuable than treating those with good baseline health (see Chapter 12 and Online Appendix 7.2). A number of authors have suggested that some sort of equity weights should be included in the estimation of QALYs to reflect these concerns (Nord 2015). Empirical applications of this approach have been introduced in several countries, including Norway (Norheim et al. 2014) and the Netherlands (van de Wetering et al. 2013). One inference from these and similar efforts is that the general population does care about equity issues. In contrast, many of these studies have relied on somewhat ad hoc empirical approaches and many have not specified an explicit social welfare function or underlying ethical principle to guide the adjustments for equity and other concerns.

Alternative approaches to addressing these equity issues include multi-criteria decision making and multi-criteria decision analysis (see Chapter 1). An example of the former is the health technology assessment framework developed for the Ontario Health Technology Advisory Committee (OHTAC) (Johnson et al. 2009). The framework recommendation is that OHTAC consider evidence on four criteria when making recommendations about new healthcare technologies: (1) overall clinical benefit; (2) consistency with societal and ethical values; (3) value for money; and (4) feasibility of adoption into the health system. Thus the incremental cost per QALY gained, related to criterion 3, is only one component in the decision-making process. Further, in this way ethical issues can be taken into account without the complications involved in modifying the estimation of QALYs.

There are also several potential important practical problems with regard to use of QALYs. First, QALYs may not accurately reflect the burden of short-lived but intense experiences. The path-state approach discussed in Section 7.1.4 is one approach to this problem. Second, as Fryback and Lawrence (1997) note, in general, life years saved due to an intervention are often not experienced by people in perfect health (**Recommendations 2 and 7**). Fryback and Lawrence argue that the unit of analysis should be the person, not the disease or health condition. Thus even if the intervention prevents disease "x," the person may still have other health problems and comorbidities and thus not be experiencing perfect health.

A related issue is maximal endurable time (Stalmeier and Verheijen 2013; Sutherland et al. 1982; Weyler and Gandjour 2011). The score for a health state that includes some dysfunction may increase with duration over some range but then decrease once the maximal endurable time has been reached. In such a situation the analyst who has a score for the health state for a particular duration may be at risk of distorting the analysis when using that score to compute QALYs over a different duration. Again the path-state approach is useful in this context.

Finally, the Second Panel recommends that when an intervention increases longevity, all subsequent healthcare costs should be included in the estimate of costs (see Chapter 8). Concomitantly, the effects of those interventions on health should also be included in the estimate of the QALYs gained. To the extent that utility scores for the long-term health outcomes are obtained from natural history cohort studies, obtaining scores for the health outcomes should not be overly challenging.

7.10 SPECIAL ISSUES AND POPULATIONS

7.10.1 States Worse Than Being Dead

Recall that the conventional scale required for estimating QALYs is one in which the score 0.00 is assigned to the health state "dead," and 1.00 is assigned to "perfect health." Some health states, however, may be regarded as worse than being dead. This issue has been noted since some of the earliest preference measurement studies, for example, the early work on the Health Utilities Index Mark 1 (Torrance 1982; Torrance, Boyle, and Horwood 1982). While the issue is not confined to the time trade-off technique, we will introduce the problem of valuing states worse than dead using the time trade-off as a concrete example.

One of the most widely used protocols for eliciting time trade-off responses was introduced in the landmark Measurement and Valuation of Health (MVH) study in the United Kingdom (Centre for Health Economics 1994). In the MVH protocol, valuation of a health state using the time trade-off begins with a question to determine whether the state is regarded as better than dead (BTD) or worse than dead (WTD).

For a BTD state, respondents are then asked a series of questions to determine how many years of life lived in perfect health, followed by immediate death, would be equivalent to 10 years of life lived in the health state being valued, followed by immediate death. For a WTD state, respondents are asked questions to determine how many years spent in the health state being valued, followed by a period of perfect health, summing to 10 years, would be equivalent to immediate death. Under the assumptions of expected utility theory, with additional assumptions described by Pliskin, Shepard, and Weinstein (1980), responses to these time trade-off questions can be used to locate an individual's valuation for a particular health state on an interval scale. In theory, values from the time trade-off for BTD states are located within the interval 0 to 1, whereas WTD valuations fall in the interval $-\infty$ to 0. In practice, the lowest possible valuation using the MVH protocol is –39 (due to reporting of responses in ¼-year increments).

Using –39 or some similar value would have a large impact on the mean and would distort the results of a study that includes WTD states, challenging face validity (Dolan et al. 1996). To deal with this problem, a number of researchers have proposed various transformations of the WTD responses (see, e.g., Dolan et al. [1996]; Shaw, Johnson, and Coons [2005]; and Lamers [2007]). These transformations are pragmatic approaches for developing an estimator based on the mean of a set of individual responses, which respects the orderings in these responses (more favorable responses imply higher valuations), while also generating plausible results. Raw scores are transformed onto the –1.00 to 0.00 interval. However, these approaches have been criticized for lacking a strong theoretical basis (Craig and Busschbach 2009; Lamers 2007; Robinson and Spencer 2006). Where alternative transformations of WTD responses have been compared, the choice of transformation has sometimes been found to affect the results substantially (Bansback et al. 2012). It should be noted that the positive linear transformation used by Shaw, Johnson, and Coons (2005) for EQ-5D-3L and Feeny et al. (2002) for HUI3 is consistent with von Neumann-Morgenstern expected utility theory. Additional discussion is presented in Online Appendix 7.7.

7.10.2 Special Populations: General

Certain populations may have characteristics that would make available generic utility instruments less applicable. One category of special population includes those for whom the relevant domains of health may be different from those included in generic utility instruments, such as populations of cognitively impaired patients, psychiatrically ill patients, or family members of ill patients. Existing generic instruments may include one mental health domain, such as anxiety/depression or emotion, but would not likely capture the full range of loss in health associated with other mental health conditions (schizophrenia, bipolar disorder). Another example is a condition associated with rash and itchiness, which may not be adequately addressed with a generic instrument such as the EQ-5D. A second category includes populations, such as children, for whom the most important domains of health may be different, and the preference weights for existing domains may also be different (Petrou and Kupek 2009;

Prosser, Grosse, and Wittenberg 2012; Ungar 2010). For special populations, the use of a generic instrument should be carefully considered, and alternatives (e.g., direct elicitation) should be examined. For many of these populations, a proxy population may be required for eliciting patient ratings.

7.10.3 Children

For children, existing generic preference-based instruments have scoring systems with varying degrees of applicability. The HUI2 scoring system is based on standard-gamble elicitation questions asking the adult respondents to envision themselves as a 10-year-old child who will live in that health state until age 70 (Torrance et al. 1996). This represents an appropriate choice for school-aged children or older but may not apply to younger children. The HUI3 scoring system is based on preference scores collected from members of the community 16 years of age or older (Feeny et al. 2002). Most EQ-5D-3L scoring systems are also based on weights for adult health states. These instruments may be used for adolescents, but they have not been validated for valuing the health of very young children. The EQ5D-Y, a youth version of the EQ-5D, includes the same attributes and levels as the adult version, but with level descriptions appropriate for school-age children; however, at present, an associated preference-based scoring system is not available. The Child Health Utility 9D (CHU-9D) has been developed for children ages 7 to 17 years, but the scoring function is derived from elicitations framed for adult respondents (Stevens 2009). Weights may differ for infants and adolescents. The lack of generic utility instruments for children is due, at least in part, to the methodological difficulties in eliciting weights for childhood health states, which have been noted in the literature (Petrou and Gray 2005; Prosser, Hammitt, and Keren 2007). Additional discussion can be found in Online Appendix 7.7.

7.10.4 Capturing Spillover Effects on Family Members/Caregivers

Existing valuation methods may also fall short for family members/caregivers of chronically ill patients, for whom "spillover effects" are important. The effects of a family member's illness on a caregiver's quality of life have been well documented (Basu and Meltzer 2005; Brouwer 2006). Some of this burden can be attributed to effects on the physical health of the caregiver, but there is increasing evidence that the spillover effects extend beyond the physical domain and that spillover loss of quality of life on family members is not correlated with the level of caregiving (Bobinac et al. 2011; Prosser et al. 2015). To date, few studies have attempted to isolate and measure spillover effects using a health utility measure. While the spillover effects on family members' health-related quality of life can be important and measurable, there is no clear standard for their measurement. Available approaches include both direct and indirect methods (Brouwer et al. 2006; Tilford and Payakachat 2015; Wittenberg and Prosser 2013). Some include domains that are beyond those typically considered as part of the health-related quality of life construct but that have been consistently identified with the caregiver experience (Brouwer et al. 2006), such as fulfillment and relational problems. For this reason, these measures may not be appropriate for the estimation of QALYs in a CEA (Al-Janabi, Flynn, and Coast 2011; Tilford and Payakachat 2015). If spillover effects on family/caregivers are likely to represent an important category of health outcomes associated with an intervention that averted or reduced the severity of an illness of a family member, an attempt should be made to value these effects and incorporate them into the CEA. Further, these spillover effects should be included in Reference Case analyses for both the healthcare sector and societal perspectives.

7.11 TOWARD CONSISTENCY ACROSS STUDIES: CATALOGS OF WEIGHTS

A consistent set of community weights for health conditions and health states used across studies intended to inform resource allocation could improve the comparability of CEAs. Since the publication of Gold et al. (1996b), there have been a number of developments, including the creation of the Tufts Medical Center Cost-Effectiveness Analysis Registry (Center for the Evaluation of Value and Risk in Health n.d.) and publication of a number of papers based on that database (Bell et al. 2001; Brauer et al. 2006; Neumann et al. 2005; Neumann et al. 2015). There have also been a number of other studies that report utility scores based on various instruments for a large number of health conditions (Franks, Hanmer, and Fryback 2006; Hanmer et al. 2016; Hanmer, Hays, and Fryback 2007; Hanmer et al. 2006; Mittmann et al. 2001; Mittmann et al. 1999; Nyman et al. 2007; Petrou and Kupek 2009; Sullivan and Ghushchyan 2006; Sullivan, Lawrence, and Ghushchyan 2005).

The CEA Registry lists some 16,000 utility weights from 4,300 cost-utility studies through 2013, and updates are ongoing. Analyses have shown that published cost-utility analyses have relied on a mix of direct elicitation, generic preference-based instruments, and clinical judgment. One study found, for example, that through 2001, 36% of cost-utility analyses used direct elicitation methods (standard gamble, time trade-off, or rating scale), 23% used generic preference-based measures (EQ-5D, HUI, etc.), and 25% estimated weights based on clinical judgment (Brauer et al. 2006). Increasingly, studies have cited other published utility scores (Brauer et al. 2006). Brauer and colleagues also found that despite the large number of utility scores included, many clinical areas were still poorly represented in the utility catalog—for example, some high morbidity conditions such as musculoskeletal diseases have few utility estimates available.

As noted above in Section 7.8, utility scores from the major generic preference-based measures are, in general, not interchangeable. Furthermore, as noted above, standard gamble and time trade-off scores typically differ, sometimes substantially. An implication may be that it would be constructive to create separate catalogs of scores for each major generic preference-based measure, as well as for standard gamble and time trade-off scores. Systematically using scores from a particular instrument or elicitation method in a CEA would enhance consistency and comparability. Nonetheless, it should be noted that several studies have found that adjusting life years for their quality often has relatively little impact on results of CEAs (Chapman et al. 2004; Greenberg and Neumann 2011).

7.12 PREFERENCES FOR USE IN THE REFERENCE CASE

We recommend that in the Reference Case analyses from both the healthcare sector and societal perspectives, community preferences derived using an instrument that is fit for purpose, be used. By "fit for purpose," we mean an instrument whose measurement properties (reliability, content validity, construct validity, and responsiveness) are adequate to measure the differences and changes in health across the programs, drugs, or devices under consideration. More fundamentally, the criterion for judging adequacy would be empirical evidence from previous studies in the same clinical context supporting the validity and responsiveness of the instrument(s) chosen. Further, the scores from the instrument should exhibit interval-scale properties. Given that a major motivation for the Reference Case is to enhance comparability across studies, we recommend that, in general, generic preference-based measured be used. Although scores from these measures sometimes differ from one another, these measures enhance comparability because as generic measures they all cover a comprehensive range of physical and mental health items, and they all employ the conventional dead = 0.00 to perfect health = 1.00 scale.

This recommendation is based both on theoretical and practical grounds. We continue to endorse the view that "the best articulation of society's preferences for particular health states would be gathered from a representative sample of fully informed members of the community" (Gold et al. 1996a, 99). This recommendation is also based on a desire to maintain and enhance the consistency and comparability of economic evaluations. A consistent approach to health valuation improves the credibility and interpretability of CEA studies as a guide to social decision making.

Like the original Panel we have chosen not to endorse a particular generic preference-based measure. Evidence reviewed in this chapter and in Online Appendices 7.1, 7.5, and 7.6 indicates that each of the major generic preference-based measures has its advantages and disadvantages and may be quite suitable in one context but perform poorly in another. Relying exclusively on one particular measure in contexts in which that measure lacks validity and responsiveness poses a serious risk of missing or understating the effects of intervention. Thus, while relying on one particular measure seemingly serves comparability, clearly an important criterion, it may also attenuate validity. These issues are further discussed by Fryback (2010), Feeny (2013a), and Feeny (2013b).

In general, we have retained most of the recommendations made by the original Panel. Nonetheless, on the basis of methodological developments and empirical experience that has emerged since the publication of Gold et al. (1996b), we have changed or qualified a number of recommendations. More specifically, as discussed in Section 7.7.2 and in Chapter 8, we do not think that productivity effects of changes in morbidity are captured in the estimated QALYs; they should therefore be captured in pecuniary terms and included in the numerator. Further, we recommend that in situations in which analysts have evidence that relying on generic preference-based measures is less than ideal, or that the direct elicitation of scores for relevant health states from the general population is less than ideal, the analyst should incorporate alternative approaches such as the use of patient-derived preferences. Situations in which this may arise include (but are not limited to) cases in which generic preference-based measures are known to lack responsiveness and/or construct validity; cases in which there are important spillovers from the intervention, such as effects on caregivers and other members of the patient's family; and cases in which it is difficult for those who have not experienced or observed the health states associated with the condition and/or its treatment to understand them sufficiently well to provide meaningful scores for those health states. We therefore also recommend that community-derived preference weights be supplemented by preference scores elicited from patients when there are important concerns about the extent to which instruments based on community preferences can represent an informed social judgment about the desirability of a particular condition or outcome.

The focus on community preferences for CEA contrasts substantially with practice in the outcome measurement and recent trends toward patient-centered care. In the fields of health-related quality of life and patient-reported outcomes, it is taken as given that patients are the experts in reporting on the effects of disease and treatment. Furthermore, in healthcare there is an increased role for patient-centered care and patient decision making. In addition, many health technology assessment agencies now include formal patient engagement programs. These important issues are discussed further in Online Appendix 7.12.

7.13 RECOMMENDATIONS

1. For Reference Case analyses from both the healthcare sector and societal perspectives, the health consequences of changes in morbidity and mortality should be aggregated into a single measure using quality-adjusted life years (QALYs).
2. In general, because people whose lives have been saved or extended by an intervention will not be in perfect health, a saved life year will count as less than 1 full QALY.
3. To satisfy the QALY concept, the quality weights must be preference-based, interval-scaled, and measured or transformed onto an interval scale where the reference point "dead" has a score of 0.0 and the reference point "perfect health" has a score of 1.0.
4. Community preferences for health states are the most appropriate ones for use in the Reference Case analyses. In general, we recommend the use of generic preference-based measures such as the EuroQol 5D (EQ-5D), Health Utilities Index (HUI), Short Form 6D (SF-6D), and Quality of Well-Being (QWB). But we have also noted that there are situations in which using patient preferences would be preferable.

5. When community preferences are used and the program (treatment or prevention) is related to an illness or condition, a sensitivity analysis that furnishes information on preferences of persons with the condition will provide important ancillary information. Such sensitivity analyses may be based on the direct elicitation of preference scores from people with the condition and/or the development of alternative scoring functions based on preference scores from those with the condition.

6. If distinct subgroup preferences are identified that will markedly affect a cost-effectiveness ratio, the Reference Case analyses should provide this information and include separate sensitivity analyses that reflect this difference.

7. The health-related quality of life of those whose lives have been saved or extended by a health intervention may be influenced by characteristics such as the age, sex, race, or socioeconomic status of the population involved. See, for instance, Bentley et al. (2011), Pereira et al. (2011), Robert et al. (2009), and Sellers et al. (2013). This may affect the Reference Case analyses in ways that are ethically problematic. In these instances, we recommend that sensitivity analysis be conducted to indicate explicitly how the analysis is affected by these characteristics.

8. A cost-effective analysis (CEA) should be based on a health-state classification system that reflects attributes (domains or dimensions) that are important for the particular problem under consideration. If the CEA is intended for use in a Reference Case analysis from either the healthcare sector or societal perspective, the preference measure used should be a generic one or one capable of being compared to a generic system. More fundamentally, a key criterion is empirical evidence on the validity and responsiveness of the instrument in that context.

9. In general, the effects of morbidity on productivity and leisure are probably not adequately reflected in the estimated QALYs and should therefore be estimated in pecuniary terms and included in the numerator in a CEA. This recommendation introduces some risk of double counting. Appropriate sensitivity analyses may be informative. (See Section 7.7.2 and Chapter 8.)

7.14 REFERENCES

Adamowicz, W., J. Louviere, and M. Williams. 1994. Combining revealed and stated preference methods for valuing environmental amenities. *J Environ Econ Manage* 26 (3):271–292.

Al-Janabi, H., T. N. Flynn, and J. Coast. 2011. QALYs and carers. *Pharmacoeconomics* 29 (12):1015–1023.

Australian Government Department of Health. 2013. "Guidelines for preparing submissions to the Pharmaceutical Benefits Advisory Committee. Version 4.4." http://www.pbac.pbs.gov.au/.

Bansback, N., A. Tsuchiya, J. Brazier, and A. Anis. 2012. Canadian valuation of EQ-5D health states: preliminary value set and considerations for future valuation studies. *PLoS ONE [Electronic Resource]* 7 (2):e31115.

Basu, A., and D. Meltzer. 2005. Implications of spillover effects within the family for medical cost-effectiveness analysis. *J Health Econ* 24 (4):751–773.

Beggs, S., S. Cardell, and J. Hausman. 1981. Assessing the potential demand for electric cars. *J Econometrics* 17 (1):1–19.

Bell, C. M., R. H. Chapman, P. W. Stone, E. A. Sandberg, and P. J. Neumann. 2001. An off-the-shelf help list: a comprehensive catalog of preference scores from published cost-utility analyses. *Med Decis Making* 21 (4):288–294.

Bellamy, N. 1989. Pain assessment in osteoarthritis: experience with the WOMAC osteoarthritis index. *Semin Arthritis Rheum* 18 (4 Suppl 2):14–17.

Bentley, T. G., M. Palta, A. J. Paulsen, D. Cherepanov, N. C. Dunham, D. Feeny, R. M. Kaplan, and D. G. Fryback. 2011. Race and gender associations between obesity and nine health-related quality-of-life measures. *Qual Life Res* 20 (5):665–674.

Bobinac, A., N. J. van Exel, F. F. Rutten, and W. B. Brouwer. 2011. Health effects in significant others: separating family and care-giving effects. *Med Decis Making* 31 (2):292–298.

Boyd, N. F., H. J. Sutherland, K. Z. Heasman, D. L. Tritchler, and B. J. Cummings. 1990. Whose utilities for decision analysis? *Med Decis Making* 10 (1):58–67.

Brauer, C. A., A. B. Rosen, D. Greenberg, and P. J. Neumann. 2006. Trends in the measurement of health utilities in published cost-utility analyses. *Value Health* 9 (4):213–218.

Brazier, J., J. Roberts, and M. Deverill. 2002. The estimation of a preference-based measure of health from the SF-36. *J Health Econ* 21 (2):271–292.

Brazier, J., and A. Tsuchiya. 2010. Preference-based condition-specific measures of health: what happens to cross programme comparability? *Health Econ* 19 (2):125–129.

Brazier, J. E., J. Roberts, M. Platts, and Y. F. Zoellner. 2005. Estimating a preference-based index for a menopause specific health quality of life questionnaire. *Health Qual Life Outcomes* 3:13.

Brouwer, W. B. 2006. Too important to ignore: informal caregivers and other significant others. *Pharmacoeconomics* 24 (1):39–41.

Brouwer, W. B., N. J. van Exel, B. van Gorp, and W. K. Redekop. 2006. The CarerQol instrument: a new instrument to measure care-related quality of life of informal caregivers for use in economic evaluations. *Qual Life Res* 15 (6):1005–1021.

Buckingham, K., and N. Devlin. 2006. A theoretical framework for TTO valuations of health. *Health Econ* 15 (10):1149–1154.

Canadian Agency for Drugs and Technologies in Health (CADTH). 2006. *Guidelines for the Economic Evaluation of Health Technologies: Canada.* 3rd ed. Ottawa: CADTH. https://www.cadth.ca/media/pdf/186_EconomicGuidelines_e.pdf.

Center for the Evaluation of Value and Risk in Health. n.d. The Cost-Effectiveness Analysis Registry [Internet]. Institute for Clinical Research and Health Policy Studies, Tufts Medical Center, Boston. Available from: www.cearegistry.org.

Centre for Health Economics. 1994. Time Trade-Off User Manual: Props and Self-Completion Methods. York, UK: Centre for Health Economics, University of York. http://www.york.ac.uk/che/pdf/op20.pdf.

Chapman, R. H., M. Berger, M. C. Weinstein, J. C. Weeks, S. Goldie, and P. J. Neumann. 2004. When does quality-adjusting life-years matter in cost-effectiveness analysis? *Health Econ* 13 (5):429–436.

Cowen, M. E., B. J. Miles, D. F. Cahill, R. B. Giesler, J. R. Beck, and M. W. Kattan. 1998. The danger of applying group-level utilities in decision analyses of the treatment of localized prostate cancer in individual patients. *Med Decis Making* 18 (4):376–380.

Craig, B. M., and J. J. Busschbach. 2009. The episodic random utility model unifies time trade-off and discrete choice approaches in health state valuation. *Popul Health Metr* 7:3.

Dolan, P., C. Gudex, P. Kind, and A. Williams. 1996. The time trade-off method: results from a general population study. *Health Econ* 5 (2):141–154.

Dolan, P., and D. Kahneman. 2008. Interpretations of utility and their implications for the valuation of health. *Econ J* 118 (525):215–234.

Drummond, M. 2001. Introducing economic and quality of life measurements into clinical studies. *Ann Med* 33 (5):344–349.

Elkin, E. B., M. E. Cowen, D. Cahill, M. Steffel, and M. W. Kattan. 2004. Preference assessment method affects decision-analytic recommendations: a prostate cancer treatment example. *Med Decis Making* 24 (5):504–510.

Fanshel, S., and J. W. Bush. 1970. A health-status index and its application to health-services outcomes. *Oper Res* 18 (6):1021–1066.

Fayers, P. M., and D. Machin. 2007. *Quality of Life: The Assessment, Analysis and Interpretation of Patient-Reported Outcomes.* 2nd ed. Chichester: John Wiley & Sons Ltd.

Feeny, D. 2005a. "Preference-Based Measures: Utility and Quality-Adjusted Life Years." In *Assessing Quality of Life in Clinical Trials*, 2nd ed, edited by P. Fayers and R. Hays, 405–429. Oxford: Oxford University Press.

Feeny, D. 2005b. "The Roles for Preference-Based Measures in Support of Cancer Research and Policy." In *Outcomes Assessment in Cancer: Measures, Methods, and Applications*, edited by J. Lipscomb, C. C. Gotay and C. Snyder, 69–92. New York: Cambridge University Press.

Feeny, D. 2013a. Health-related quality-of-life data should be regarded as a vital sign. *J Clin Epidemiol* 66 (7):706–709.

Feeny, D. 2013b. Standardization and regulatory guidelines may inhibit science and reduce the usefulness of analyses based on the application of preference-based measures for policy decisions. *Med Decis Making* 33 (3):316–319.

Feeny, D., W. Furlong, G. W. Torrance, C. H. Goldsmith, Z. Zhu, S. DePauw, M. Denton, and M. Boyle. 2002. Multiattribute and single-attribute utility functions for the Health Utilities Index Mark 3 system. *Med Care* 40 (2):113–128.

Feeny, D., K. Spritzer, R. D. Hays, H. Liu, T. G. Ganiats, R. M. Kaplan, M. Palta, and D. G. Fryback. 2012. Agreement about identifying patients who change over time: cautionary results in cataract and heart failure patients. *Med Decis Making* 32 (2):273–286.

Feeny, D., L. Wu, and K. Eng. 2004. Comparing short form 6D, standard gamble, and Health Utilities Index Mark 2 and Mark 3 utility scores: results from total hip arthroplasty patients. *Qual Life Res* 13 (10):1659–1670.

Feeny, D. H., E. Eckstrom, E. P. Whitlock, and L. A. Perdue. 2013. A Primer for Systematic Reviewers on the Measurement of Functional Status and Health-Related Quality of Life in Older Adults. (Prepared by the Kaiser Permanente Research Affiliates Evidence-based Practice Center under Contract No. 290-2007-10057-I.) AHRQ Publication No. 13-EHC128-EF. Rockville, MD: Agency for Healthcare Research and Quality. September 2013. www.effectivehealthcare.ahrq.gov/reports/final.cfm.

Franks, P., J. Hanmer, and D. G. Fryback. 2006. Relative disutilities of 47 risk factors and conditions assessed with seven preference-based health status measures in a national U.S. sample: toward consistency in cost-effectiveness analyses. *Med Care* 44 (5):478–485.

Fryback, D. G. 2010. "Measuring health-related quality of life." Paper prepared for the Workshop on Advancing Social Science Theory: The Importance of Common Metrics, National Academies, Washington, DC, February 25-26.

Fryback, D. G., E. J. Dasbach, R. Klein, B. E. Klein, N. Dorn, K. Peterson, and P. A. Martin. 1993. The Beaver Dam Health Outcomes Study: initial catalog of health-state quality factors. *Med Decis Making* 13 (2):89–102.

Fryback, D. G., N. C. Dunham, M. Palta, J. Hanmer, J. Buechner, D. Cherepanov, S. A. Herrington, R. D. Hays, R. M. Kaplan, T. G. Ganiats, D. Feeny, and P. Kind. 2007. US norms for six generic health-related quality-of-life indexes from the National Health Measurement Study. *Med Care* 45 (12):1162–1170.

Fryback, D. G., and W. F. Lawrence, Jr. 1997. Dollars may not buy as many QALYs as we think: a problem with defining quality-of-life adjustments. *Med Decis Making* 17 (3):276–284.

Gage, B. F., A. B. Cardinalli, and D. K. Owens. 1996. The effect of stroke and stroke prophylaxis with aspirin or warfarin on quality of life. *Arch Intern Med* 156 (16):1829–1836.

Gandjour, A. 2010. Theoretical foundation of patient v. population preferences in calculating QALYs. *Med Decis Making* 30 (4):E57–E63.

Gold, M. R., D. L. Patrick, G. W. Torrance, D. G. Fryback, D. C. Hadorn, M. S. Kamlet, N. Daniels, and M. C. Weinstein. 1996a. "Identifying and Valuing Outcomes." In *Cost-Effectiveness in Health and Medicine*, edited by M. R. Gold, J. E. Siegel, L. B. Russell and M. C. Weinstein, 82–134. New York: Oxford University Press.

Gold, M. R., J. E. Siegel, L. B. Russell, and M. C. Weinstein, eds. 1996b. *Cost-Effectiveness in Health and Medicine*. New York: Oxford University Press.

Gold, M. R., D. Stevenson, and D. G. Fryback. 2002. HALYs and QALYs and DALYs, oh my: similarities and differences in summary measures of population health. *Annu Rev Public Health* 23:115–134.

Greenberg, D., and P. J. Neumann. 2011. Does adjusting for health-related quality of life matter in economic evaluations of cancer-related interventions? *Expert Rev Pharmacoecon Outcomes Res* 11 (1):113–119.

Guyatt, G., V. Montori, P. J. Devereaux, H. Schünemann, and M. Bhandari. 2004. Patients at the center: in our practice, and in our use of language. *ACP J Club* 140 (1):A11–A12.

Guyatt, G. H., D. Osoba, A. W. Wu, K. W. Wyrwich, G. R. Norman, and the Clinical Significance Consensus Meeting Group. 2002. Methods to explain the clinical significance of health status measures. *Mayo Clin Proc* 77 (4):371–383.

Hadorn, D. C., and J. Uebersax. 1995. Large-scale health outcomes evaluation: how should quality of life be measured? Part I—Calibration of a brief questionnaire and a search for preference subgroups. *J Clin Epidemiol* 48 (5):607–618.

Hanmer, J., D. Cherepanov, M. Palta, R. M. Kaplan, D. Feeny, and D. G. Fryback. 2016. Health condition impacts in a nationally representative cross-sectional survey vary substantially by preference-based health index. *Med Decis Making* 36 (2):264–274.

Hanmer, J., R. D. Hays, and D. G. Fryback. 2007. Mode of administration is important in US national estimates of health-related quality of life. *Med Care* 45 (12):1171–1179.

Hanmer, J., W. F. Lawrence, J. P. Anderson, R. M. Kaplan, and D. G. Fryback. 2006. Report of nationally representative values for the noninstitutionalized US adult population for 7 health-related quality-of-life scores. *Med Decis Making* 26 (4):391–400.

Harsanyi, J. C. 1955. Cardinal welfare, individualistic ethics, and interpersonal comparisons of utility. *J Polit Economy* 63 (4):309–321.

Hornberger, J. C., D. A. Redelmeier, and J. Petersen. 1992. Variability among methods to assess patients' well-being and consequent effect on a cost-effectiveness analysis. *J Clin Epidemiol* 45 (5):505–512.

Hurst, N. P., P. Jobanputra, M. Hunter, M. Lambert, A. Lochhead, and H. Brown. 1994. Validity of Euroqol—a generic health status instrument—in patients with rheumatoid arthritis. Economic and Health Outcomes Research Group. *Br J Rheumatol* 33 (7):655–662.

Jansen, S. J., A. M. Stiggelbout, P. P. Wakker, M. A. Nooij, E. M. Noordijk, and J. Kievit. 2000. Unstable preferences: a shift in valuation or an effect of the elicitation procedure? *Med Decis Making* 20 (1):62–71.

Johnson, A. P., N. J. Sikich, G. Evans, W. Evans, M. Giacomini, M. Glendining, M. Krahn, L. Levin, P. Oh, and C. Perera. 2009. Health technology assessment: a comprehensive framework for evidence-based recommendations in Ontario. *Int J Technol Assess Health Care* 25 (2):141–150.

Kaplan, R. M. 2005. The minimally clinically important difference in generic utility-based measures. *COPD* 2 (1):91–97.

Keeney, R. L. 1976. A group preference axiomatization with cardinal utility. *Manage Sci* 23 (2):140–145.

Keeney, R. L., and H. Raiffa. 1993. *Decisions with Multiple Objectives: Preferences and Value Tradeoffs*. New York: Cambridge University Press.

Kind, P. 1982. A comparison of two models for scaling health indicators. *Int J Epidemiol* 11 (3):271–275.

Koop, G., and D. J. Poirier. 1994. Rank-ordered logit models: an empirical analysis of Ontario voter preferences. *J Appl Econometrics* 9 (4):369–388.

Krahn, M., K. E. Bremner, G. Tomlinson, P. Ritvo, J. Irvine, and G. Naglie. 2007. Responsiveness of disease-specific and generic utility instruments in prostate cancer patients. *Qual Life Res* 16 (3):509–522.

Krahn, M. D., G. Naglie, D. Naimark, D. A. Redelmeier, and A. S. Detsky. 1997. Primer on medical decision analysis: Part 4—Analyzing the model and interpreting the results. *Med Decis Making* 17 (2):142–151.

Lamers, L. M. 2007. The transformation of utilities for health states worse than death: consequences for the estimation of EQ-5D value sets. *Med Care* 45 (3):238–244.

Lee, G. M., J. A. Salomon, C. W. LeBaron, and T. A. Lieu. 2005. Health-state valuations for pertussis: methods for valuing short-term health states. *Health Qual Life Outcomes* 3:17.

Locadia, M., P. F. Stalmeier, F. J. Oort, M. H. Prins, M. A. Sprangers, and P. M. Bossuyt. 2004. A comparison of 3 valuation methods for temporary health states in patients treated with oral anticoagulants. *Med Decis Making* 24 (6):625–633.

Louviere, J. J., D. A. Hensher, and J. D. Swait. 2000. *Stated Choice Methods: Analysis and Application*. New York: Cambridge University Press.

Luce, R. D., and H. Raiffa. 1957. *Games and Decisions: Introduction and Critical Survey*. New York: John Wiley & Sons, Inc.

Luo, N., J. Johnson, and S. J. Coons. 2010. Using instrument-defined health state transitions to estimate minimally important differences for four preference-based health-related quality of life instruments. *Med Care* 48 (4):365–371.

Luo, N., J. A. Johnson, J. W. Shaw, D. Feeny, and S. J. Coons. 2005. Self-reported health status of the general adult U.S. population as assessed by the EQ-5D and Health Utilities Index. *Med Care* 43 (11):1078–1086.

Maddigan, S. L., D. H. Feeny, and J. A. Johnson. 2005. Health-related quality of life deficits associated with diabetes and comorbidities in a Canadian National Population Health Survey. *Qual Life Res* 14 (5):1311–1320.

Marra, C. A., A. A. Rashidi, D. Guh, J. A. Kopec, M. Abrahamowicz, J. M. Esdaile, J. E. Brazier, P. R. Fortin, and A. H. Anis. 2005. Are indirect utility measures reliable and responsive in rheumatoid arthritis patients? *Qual Life Res* 14 (5):1333–1344.

McNamee, P., S. Glendinning, J. Shenfine, N. Steen, S. M. Griffin, and J. Bond. 2004. Chained time trade-off and standard gamble methods. Applications in oesophageal cancer. *Eur J Health Econ* 5 (1):81–86.

Mehrez, A., and A. Gafni. 1993. Healthy-years equivalents versus quality-adjusted life years: in pursuit of progress. *Med Decis Making* 13 (4):287–292.

Menzel, P., P. Dolan, J. Richardson, and J. A. Olsen. 2002. The role of adaptation to disability and disease in health state valuation: a preliminary normative analysis. *Soc Sci Med* 55 (12):2149–2158.

Mittmann, N., D. Chan, K. Trakas, and N. Risebrough. 2001. Health utility attributes for chronic conditions. *Dis Manag Health Out* 9 (1):11–21.

Mittmann, N., K. Trakas, N. Risebrough, and B. A. Liu. 1999. Utility scores for chronic conditions in a community-dwelling population. *Pharmacoeconomics* 15 (4):369–376.

Nease, R. F., Jr., T. Kneeland, G. T. O'Connor, W. Sumner, C. Lumpkins, L. Shaw, D. Pryor, and H. C. Sox. 1995. Variation in patient utilities for outcomes of the management of chronic stable angina. Implications for clinical practice guidelines. Ischemic Heart Disease Patient Outcomes Research Team. [Erratum appears in *JAMA* 1995;274 (8):612]. *JAMA* 273 (15):1185–1190.

Neumann, P. J., D. Greenberg, N. V. Olchanski, P. W. Stone, and A. B. Rosen. 2005. Growth and quality of the cost-utility literature, 1976-2001. *Value Health* 8 (1):3–9.

Neumann, P. J., T. Thorat, J. Shi, C. J. Saret, and J. T. Cohen. 2015. The changing face of the cost-utility literature, 1990-2012. *Value Health* 18 (2):271–277.

Nord, E. 1992. An alternative to QALYs: the saved young life equivalent (SAVE). *BMJ* 305 (6858):875–877.

Nord, E. 2015. Cost-value analysis of health interventions: introduction and update on methods and preference data. *Pharmacoeconomics* 33 (2):89–95.

Norheim, O. F., B. Allgott, B. Aschim, R. Førde, G. K. Gjul, T. Gundersen, M. Kakad, A. Kjellevold, S. Kvinnsland, H. O. Melberg, A. Moen, O. Maeland, J. A. Olsen, and S. Sjoli. 2014. Åpent og rettferdig—prioriteringer i helsetjenesten [Open and fair—priority setting in the health service]. Official Norwegian Reports 2014: 12. Oslo: Departementenes sikkerhets- og serviceorganisasjon.

Nyman, J. A., N. A. Barleen, B. E. Dowd, D. W. Russell, S. J. Coons, and P. W. Sullivan. 2007. Quality-of-life weights for the US population: self-reported health status and priority health conditions, by demographic characteristics. *Med Care* 45 (7):618–628.

Oppe, M., N. J. Devlin, B. van Hout, P. F. Krabbe, and F. de Charro. 2014. A program of methodological research to arrive at the new international EQ-5D-5L valuation protocol. *Value Health* 17 (4):445–453.

Ormel, J., M. VonKorff, T. B. Ustun, S. Pini, A. Korten, and T. Oldehinkel. 1994. Common mental disorders and disability across cultures. Results from the WHO Collaborative Study on Psychological Problems in General Health Care. *JAMA* 272 (22):1741–1748.

Patrick, D. L., and P. Erickson. 1993. *Health Status and Health Policy: Quality of Life in Health Care Evaluation and Resource Allocation*. New York: Oxford University Press.

Peasgood, T., and J. Brazier. 2015. Is meta-analysis for utility values appropriate given the potential impact different elicitation methods have on values? *Pharmacoeconomics* 33 (11):1101–1105.

Pereira, C. C., M. Palta, J. Mullahy, and D. G. Fryback. 2011. Race and preference-based health-related quality of life measures in the United States. *Qual Life Res* 20 (6):969–978.

Petrou, S., and R. Gray. 2005. Methodological challenges posed by economic evaluations of early childhood intervention programmes. *Appl Health Econ Health Policy* 4 (3):175–181.

Petrou, S., and E. Kupek. 2009. Estimating preference-based Health Utilities Index Mark 3 utility scores for childhood conditions in England and Scotland. *Med Decis Making* 29 (3):291–303.

Pliskin, J. S., D. S. Shepard, and M. C. Weinstein. 1980. Utility functions for life years and health status. *Oper Res* 28:206–224.

Pohar, S. L., and C. A. Jones. 2009. The burden of Parkinson disease (PD) and concomitant comorbidities. *Arch Gerontol Geriatr* 49 (2):317–321.

Prosser, L. A., S. D. Grosse, and E. Wittenberg. 2012. Health utility elicitation: is there still a role for direct methods? *Pharmacoeconomics* 30 (2):83–86.

Prosser, L. A., J. K. Hammitt, and R. Keren. 2007. Measuring health preferences for use in cost-utility and cost-benefit analyses of interventions in children: theoretical and methodological considerations. *Pharmacoeconomics* 25 (9):713–726.

Prosser, L. A., K. Lamarand, A. Gebremariam, and E. Wittenberg. 2015. Measuring family HRQoL spillover effects using direct health utility assessment. *Med Decis Making* 35 (1):81–93.

Prosser, L. A., G. T. Ray, M. O'Brien, K. Kleinman, J. Santoli, and T. A. Lieu. 2004. Preferences and willingness to pay for health states prevented by pneumococcal conjugate vaccine. *Pediatrics* 113 (2):283–290.

Rawls, J. 1972. *A Theory of Justice*. Oxford: Clarendon Press.

Read, J. L., R. J. Quinn, D. M. Berwick, H. V. Fineberg, and M. C. Weinstein. 1984. Preferences for health outcomes. Comparison of assessment methods. *Med Decis Making* 4 (3):315–329.

Revicki, D. A., D. Feeny, T. L. Hunt, and B. F. Cole. 2006. Analyzing oncology clinical trial data using the Q-TWiST method: clinical importance and sources for health state preference data. *Qual Life Res* 15 (3):411–423.

Revicki, D. A., N. K. Leidy, F. Brennan-Diemer, S. Sorensen, and A. Togias. 1998a. Integrating patient preferences into health outcomes assessment: the multiattribute Asthma Symptom Utility Index. *Chest* 114 (4):998–1007.

Revicki, D. A., N. K. Leidy, F. Brennan-Diemer, C. Thompson, and A. Togias. 1998b. Development and preliminary validation of the multiattribute Rhinitis Symptom Utility Index. *Qual Life Res* 7 (8):693–702.

Revicki, D. A., D. Osoba, D. Fairclough, I. Barofsky, R. Berzon, N. K. Leidy, and M. Rothman. 2000. Recommendations on health-related quality of life research to support labeling and promotional claims in the United States. *Qual Life Res* 9 (8):887–900.

Robert, S. A., D. Cherepanov, M. Palta, N. C. Dunham, D. Feeny, and D. G. Fryback. 2009. Socioeconomic status and age variations in health-related quality of life: results from the National Health Measurement Study. *J Gerontol B Psychol Sci Soc Sci* 64 (3):378–389.

Robinson, A., and A. Spencer. 2006. Exploring challenges to TTO utilities: valuing states worse than dead. *Health Econ* 15 (4):393–402.

Rowen, D., J. Brazier, A. Tsuchiya, T. Young, and R. Ibbotson. 2012. It's all in the name, or is it? The impact of labeling on health state values. *Med Decis Making* 32 (1):31–40.

Sackett, D. L., W. S. Richardson, W. C. Rosenberg, and R. B. Haynes. 1997. *Evidence-Based Medicine: How to Practice and Teach EBM*. New York: Churchill Livingstone.

Sackett, D. L., and G. W. Torrance. 1978. The utility of different health states as perceived by the general public. *J Chronic Dis* 31 (11):697–704.

Schünemann, H. J., L. Griffith, R. Jaeschke, R. Goldstein, D. Stubbing, and G. H. Guyatt. 2003. Evaluation of the minimal important difference for the feeling thermometer and the St. George's Respiratory Questionnaire in patients with chronic airflow obstruction. *J Clin Epidemiol* 56 (12):1170–1176.

Schünemann, H. J., M. Puhan, R. Goldstein, R. Jaeschke, and G. H. Guyatt. 2005. Measurement properties and interpretability of the chronic respiratory disease questionnaire (CRQ). *COPD* 2 (1):81–89.

Sellers, S., D. Cherepanav, J. Hanmer, D. G. Fryback, and M. Palta. 2013. Interpersonal discrimination and health-related quality of life among black and white men and women in the United States. *Qual Life Res* 22 (6):1307–1312.

Shaw, J. W., J. A. Johnson, and S. J. Coons. 2005. US valuation of the EQ-5D health states: development and testing of the D1 valuation model. *Med Care* 43 (3):203–220.

Stalmeier, P. F., and A. L. Verheijen. 2013. Maximal endurable time states and the standard gamble: more preference reversals. *Eur J Health Econ* 14 (6):971–977.

Stevens, K. 2009. Developing a descriptive system for a new preference-based measure of health-related quality of life for children. *Qual Life Res* 18 (8):1105–1113.

Streiner, D. L., and G. R. Norman. 1995. *Health Measurement Scales: A Practical Guide to their Development and Use.* 2nd ed. Oxford: Oxford University Press.

Sullivan, P. W., and V. Ghushchyan. 2006. Preference-Based EQ-5D index scores for chronic conditions in the United States. *Med Decis Making* 26 (4):410–420.

Sullivan, P. W., W. F. Lawrence, and V. Ghushchyan. 2005. A national catalog of preference-based scores for chronic conditions in the United States. *Med Care* 43 (7):736–749.

Sutherland, H. J., H. Llewellyn-Thomas, N. F. Boyd, and J. E. Till. 1982. Attitudes toward quality of survival. The concept of "maximal endurable time." *Med Decis Making* 2 (3):299–309.

Swan, J. S., D. G. Fryback, W. F. Lawrence, F. Sainfort, M. E. Hagenauer, and D. M. Heisey. 2000. A time-tradeoff method for cost-effectiveness models applied to radiology. *Med Decis Making* 20 (1):79–88.

Tilford, J. M., and N. Payakachat. 2015. Progress in measuring family spillover effects for economic evaluations. *Expert Rev Pharmacoecon Outcomes Res* 15 (2):195–198.

Torrance, G. W. 1982. "Multiattribute Utility Theory as a Method of Measuring Social Preferences for Health States in Long-Term Care." In *Values and Long-Term Care*, edited by R. L. Kane and R. A. Kane, 127–156. Lexington, MA: Lexington Books.

Torrance, G. W. 1986. Measurement of health state utilities for economic appraisal. *J Health Econ* 5 (1):1–30.

Torrance, G. W., M. H. Boyle, and S. P. Horwood. 1982. Application of multi-attribute utility theory to measure social preferences for health states. *Oper Res* 30 (6):1043–1069.

Torrance, G. W., D. Feeny, and W. Furlong. 2001. Visual analog scales: do they have a role in the measurement of preferences for health states? *Med Decis Making* 21 (4):329–334.

Torrance, G. W., D. H. Feeny, W. J. Furlong, R. D. Barr, Y. Zhang, and Q. Wang. 1996. Multiattribute utility function for a comprehensive health status classification system. Health Utilities Index Mark 2. *Med Care* 34 (7):702–722.

Torrance, G. W., W. H. Thomas, and D. L. Sackett. 1972. A utility maximization model for evaluation of health care programs. *Health Serv Res* 7 (2):118–133.

Tosteson, A. N., and C. S. Hammond. 2002. Quality-of-life assessment in osteoporosis: health-status and preference-based measures. *Pharmacoeconomics* 20 (5):289–303.

Tosteson, A. N., T. S. Kneeland, R. F. Nease, and W. Sumner. 2002. Automated current health time-trade-off assessments in women's health. *Value Health* 5 (2):98–105.

Ubel, P. A., J. Richardson, and P. Menzel. 2000. Societal value, the person trade-off, and the dilemma of whose values to measure for cost-effectiveness analysis. *Health Econ* 9 (2):127–136.

Ungar, W. J., ed. 2010. *Economic Evaluation in Child Health.* Oxford: Oxford University Press.

van de Wetering, E. J., E. A. Stolk, N. J. van Exel, and W. B. Brouwer. 2013. Balancing equity and efficiency in the Dutch basic benefits package using the principle of proportional shortfall. *Eur J Health Econ* 14 (1):107–115.

Vernon, H., and S. Mior. 1991. The Neck Disability Index: a study of reliability and validity. *J Manipulative Physiol Ther* 14 (7):409–415.

von Neumann, J., and O. Morgenstern. 1944. *Theory of Games and Economic Behavior*. Princeton: Princeton University Press.

Walters, S. J., and J. E. Brazier. 2003. What is the relationship between the minimally important difference and health state utility values? The case of the SF-6D. *Health Qual Life Outcomes* 1 (1):4.

Ware, J. E., Jr., and C. D. Sherbourne. 1992. The MOS 36-item short-form health survey (SF-36). I. Conceptual framework and item selection. *Med Care* 30 (6):473–483.

Weinstein, M. C., G. Torrance, and A. McGuire. 2009. QALYs: the basics. [Erratum appears in *Value Health* 2010;13 (8):1065]. *Value Health* 12 Suppl 1:S5–S9.

Weyler, E. J., and A. Gandjour. 2011. Empirical validation of patient versus population preferences in calculating QALYs. *Health Serv Res* 46 (5):1562–1574.

Wittenberg, E., and L. A. Prosser. 2013. Disutility of illness for caregivers and families: a systematic review of the literature. *Pharmacoeconomics* 31 (6):489–500.

Wright, D. R., E. Wittenberg, J. S. Swan, R. A. Miksad, and L. A. Prosser. 2009. Methods for measuring temporary health states for cost-utility analyses. *Pharmacoeconomics* 27 (9):713–723.

Wright, J. C., and M. C. Weinstein. 1998. Gains in life expectancy from medical interventions—standardizing data on outcomes. *N Engl J Med* 339 (6):380–386.

8

Estimating Costs and Valuations
of Non-Health Benefits
in Cost-Effectiveness Analysis

Anirban Basu

8.1 INTRODUCTION

This chapter examines the process of identifying, quantifying, and valuing the resource costs associated with healthcare interventions that arise due to the use and consequences of those interventions. A primary objective of cost-effectiveness analysis (CEA) is to incorporate a consideration of resource consumption into decisions about healthcare. An explicit examination of resources allows an assessment of costs relative to the health benefits of an intervention.

Costs associated with a healthcare or public health intervention have two components: (1) resources used during the process of production, delivery, and consumption of the intervention and (2) the resources used or saved as a consequence of the use of healthcare or public health interventions. Some of these consequences may fall outside the healthcare sector. We categorize the types of resources that most interventions affect and describe generally how they are included in a CEA. We then describe the process of developing cost estimates by identifying, quantifying, and then valuing the resources associated with an intervention. It is the cumulative result of this process, rather than any single element of it, that comprises cost. Although we focus much of this chapter on the construction of measures of costs from the components of resource units and their values, sometimes called *micro-costing*, we also comment on more aggregative *gross-costing* approaches that may be a useful alternative for some analyses.

As detailed in Chapter 3, the Second Panel recommends that all studies report a Reference Case analysis based on a healthcare sector perspective and a Reference Case

This chapter builds on concepts presented in Chapter 6 of the original Panel's book (Luce, B. R., W. G. Manning, J. E. Siegel, and J. Lipscomb. 1996. "Estimating Costs in Cost-Effectiveness Analysis." In *Cost-Effectiveness in Health and Medicine*, edited by M. R. Gold, J. E. Siegel, L. B. Russell and M. C. Weinstein, 176–213. New York: Oxford University Press). This new chapter is dedicated to the memory of Willard G. Manning (1946–2014).

analysis based on a societal perspective. To make this evaluation more explicit and transparent to users of an analysis, the Second Panel also recommends inclusion of an Impact Inventory (see Chapters 4, 6, and 13) in the Reference Case analyses. The main purpose of the Impact Inventory is to describe impacts both inside and outside the formal healthcare sector. The Impact Inventory lists the broad health and non-health impacts of an intervention.

Analysts may wish to present results from other perspectives in addition to the Reference Case perspectives, if these other perspectives are of interest to specific decision makers. Therefore, we discuss costing of all potential categories of resource use, some or all of which might be relevant under alternative perspectives.

8.1.1 A Graphic Illustration of Costs and Effects in CEA

The introduction and use of a healthcare or public health intervention has potentially far-reaching economic implications, whether that intervention is a behavioral or health educational intervention, a new drug, a screening test, a treatment device, or a procedure. In CEA, the relative value of an intervention in comparison to its alternative is expressed as an incremental cost-effectiveness ratio (ICER), which is the ratio of the incremental costs between the intervention and the alternative over incremental benefits. As already mentioned, the costs associated with an intervention are driven by resources used during the production, delivery, and consumption of the intervention, and the resources used or saved as a consequence of this consumption. We recommend that both of these cost categories be included in the numerator of the ICER. The specific components of the costs of using an intervention and those of the costs of consequences from the intervention that should be included in an analysis would depend on the perspective of the analysis. For example, the resources would include the "time" inputs from the individual receiving the intervention when a societal perspective is taken but not when a healthcare sector perspective is taken. All resource use that is both germane to the analysis and non-trivial in magnitude should be included in the Reference Case analyses from both the healthcare sector and societal perspectives (see **Recommendation 2** in Section 8.6). Valuation of these resources generally follows the principle of opportunity costs, which represent the long-term marginal or incremental value forgone due to the use of these resources (**Recommendation 3**). Unlike the original Panel on Cost-Effectiveness in Health and Medicine (Gold et al. 1996), the Second Panel argues that the production values (morbidity and mortality costs, both in the formal and informal markets) of the changes in health status associated with the intervention are not well captured by measures such as quality-adjusted life years (QALYs). The Second Panel will therefore suggest that explicit monetary valuation of morbidity and mortality costs should be included in the numerator of the ICER.

Very much like the life-years metric, quality-adjusted life years are meant to reflect a measure of health. Valuation of health under welfarist and extra-welfarist perspectives are discussed in Chapters 2 and 7.

Figure 8.1, a modified version of the original Panel's Figure 6.1, illustrates the entire chain of effects with elements that flow one to another, beginning with the intervention

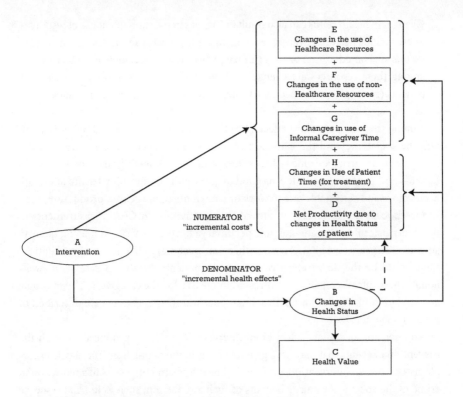

Figure 8.1 Economic consequences of health interventions: the incremental cost-effectiveness ratio (ICER) from a societal perspective.
Source: Adapted from Figure 6.1 in Gold et al. (1996).

(oval A), for example, a screening procedure. The intervention itself requires healthcare resources such as a lab test and pathologist's time (rectangle E), and may require other types of resources, such as transportation or friction costs (rectangle F) or an informal (unpaid) caregiver's assistance (rectangle G). Usually, the intervention will require "time" inputs from the individual receiving the intervention (rectangle H). Note that in Figure 8.1 we present all possible categories of resource uses that reflect an ICER from a societal perspective. The Reference Case healthcare sector perspective should consider specific components of these resource uses as described below.

The purpose of the intervention is to improve health or to delay declines in health. These gains can be measured either as reductions in an undesired health state, such as morbidity and mortality, or as increases in a desired state, such as improved life expectancy and health-related quality of life (oval B). Changes in health have potential pecuniary (economic) and non-pecuniary effects. Among the potential pecuniary effects are these:

1. Changes in health status that affect the amount of productive activity that an individual engages in, in the formal and informal labor markets and within the household; this is referred to as a change in productivity (rectangle D).

2. Changes in health status can also result in changes in the subsequent use of resources. These include healthcare resources (rectangle E), as well as resources that may fall in sectors such as education or the criminal justice system (rectangle F). Also included among these resources are changes in time that caregivers devote to assisting ill patients (rectangle G). All pecuniary effects are measured in terms of dollars.

Among the non-pecuniary effects, health in and of itself is valued by individuals and the society beyond the valuation of its pecuniary effects. For example, health can have both intrinsic value—that is, the pleasure of knowing that one is in good health—and instrumental value, as good health can help one enjoy leisure and work hours more and can enable one to work or contribute to household production, even if one chooses not to engage in any of those activities. In CEA, measurements of these intrinsic and instrumental non-pecuniary effects are carried out using quality-adjusted life years (QALYs). Among other non-pecuniary effects of an intervention, there could be the direct effect of changes in patients' health on caregivers' well-being. These effects can also be expressed in QALYs for the caregivers. The rationale and valuation principles for QALYs of patients and their caregivers are described in detail in Chapter 7.

Another non-pecuniary effect of an intervention could be produced through the prevention of events that may have general effects in the population. The classic example arises when an intervention, say a mental health treatment, results in a reduction of crime in the society. Pecuniary benefits of such a reduction, such as judicial resource cost savings and property damage cost savings, are accounted for on the pecuniary side. But the well-being of individuals who are the likely victims of crime would certainly be improved with the reduction of crime. Similarly, the whole community may benefit from an environment with lower crime. These type of non-pecuniary benefits are typically not measured through QALYs. There are examples in the literature on cost-benefit analysis of valuing these benefits through willingness-to-pay approaches. We discuss how to account for these benefits in CEA, given the limitations on methods that exist today.

It should be noted here that QALYs can sometimes be interpreted as the utility function of health but not necessarily overall welfare, as they do not include the utility from consumption. However, maximization of QALYs is viewed to be equivalent to maximization of overall welfare under the assumptions that overall utility is multiplicative between utility of consumption and QALYs, and that the utility of consumption is constant over time (Bleichrodt and Quiggin 1999). Further discussion of this measure can be found in Chapter 3. Moreover, the temporal change in the utility of consumption can be accommodated in CEA from a societal perspective through the discounting factor (see Chapter 10).

An ideal CEA begins by identifying all of the consequences of adopting one intervention versus another, including use of resources (medical services use, public health program costs, non-healthcare sector costs, informal caregiving, and patient time costs—rectangles D–H in Figure 8.1) and the effects of the intervention on health status (oval B). The amount or magnitude of each change is quantified. Finally, these changes are valued: changes in resource use are converted into a summary cost using dollar values for each input. The incremental difference in input costs and the costs of consequences forms the basis for the cost element in the CEA. The changes in health status and life expectancy are converted into QALYs or another summary health effect measure.

The distinction between components to be included in the numerator versus the denominator is relevant only for constructing an ICER. Because the ICER is expressed as a cost per QALY, it is recommended that only the quantification of health as measured by QALYs enter the denominator of the ICER, while all other aspects of costs and effects of an intervention enter the numerator (**Recommendation 1**). Note that both the numerator and the denominator represent changes in their respective quantities to reflect incremental effects between two interventions (i.e., an intervention and its comparator). When QALYs are valued using specific societal- or healthcare sector-specific willingness-to-pay thresholds (or, alternatively, the net costs in the numerator are converted to QALYs using the inverse of the threshold), alternative measures of net value can be expressed as net health benefit (NHB) or net monetary benefit (NMB) metrics, which are formed by linear combination of the effects on costs and effectiveness scales (Stinnett and Mullahy 1998). More discussions on this valuing of QALYs can be found in Chapter 2.

The remainder of this chapter is organized into three broad sections. In the first (Section 8.2), we lay out the types of cost categories that should be considered in a CEA. We revisit some of the theoretical issues related to the inclusion of these categories in CEA (see Chapter 2) and discuss some of the debates surrounding various categories. In the second section (Section 8.3), we illustrate the categories that enter the two Reference Case perspectives. Finally, in Section 8.4, we discuss the valuation of resources in these categories.

8.2 CONCEPTUAL COST CATEGORIES

8.2.1 Types of Resource Costs

For the purpose of CEA in health and medicine, resources can be broadly categorized into those that fall within the formal healthcare sector and those that fall outside of it. The latter includes the informal healthcare sector. With this categorization, the concepts of "direct" and "indirect" costs, as defined by the original Panel and reflecting the literature at the time they wrote, become obsolete. Different components of costs and effects could be deemed to be "direct" depending on the perspective of the analyses. For example, from a societal perspective all components that affect public welfare are assumed to be direct, although these effects can fall in a variety of sectors. The valuation of these resources should not include the value of health in and of itself, because health is captured by valuation of the QALY measure. Instead, a more intuitive grouping of resource use may be expressed as the consumption costs of an intervention and the costs (or savings) of consequences due to the intervention, either of which can fall in multiple sectors of the economy. For example, a public health program that introduces a physical check-up and exercise program for middle school children should consider both the costs of medical staff (healthcare sector) and the costs of school staff and facility use (education sector) as consumption costs of the intervention.

In the next section we consider the types of resources within each sector that can contribute to either the consumption or the consequence of an intervention.

8.2.2 Costs Within the Formal Healthcare Sector

There are two types of costs within the healthcare sector, those that arise from the use or consumption of the intervention and those that arise as a consequence of this consumption. Either of these types of costs may include all or some of the costs of drugs, devices, physician and allied healthcare time/services, inpatient care, outpatient visits, and special/assistive devices (rectangle E in Figure 8.1). Depending on the specific healthcare system under consideration (e.g., US versus UK), costs of long-term care and home care may also be included. For example, the healthcare costs of mammography screening include the costs associated with the screening itself, such as those of the mammogram procedure and physician time. In addition, they include the costs of further tests to follow up both false-positive and true-positive results and the downstream costs (or savings) associated with cases of breast cancer, such as hospitalization and treatment costs.

These healthcare costs should be counted in Reference Case analyses conducted from both the healthcare sector and societal perspectives. However, some of the costs of an intervention may fall outside the formal healthcare sector—for example, time costs for patients and their caregivers, transportation costs, and other sector costs. We recommend that these costs not be included in the healthcare sector perspective Reference Case analysis but should be accounted for in the societal perspective Reference Case analysis (see Chapter 4). In certain instances, a specific healthcare sector or organization may bear some of these intervention costs that fall outside the formal healthcare sector. In those instances, an additional analysis from the perspective of the relevant decision maker should be conducted. For example, the US Department of Veteran's Affairs (VA) pays for transportation costs for patients residing in rural settings, who have to travel to seek care in VA hospitals in urban areas. An analysis from the VA perspective should account for these costs as part of the numerator in the ICER, but they should not be included in the Reference Case healthcare perspective.

The healthcare consequences of an intervention would also include the components of resource uses listed above. All resources within the formal healthcare sector that lead to total healthcare costs should be accounted for over the lifetime of the patients under each intervention (**Recommendation 6**). Two debates arise in this context: (1) Whether "unrelated" costs during the time when subjects are alive under either intervention should be accounted for and (2) whether related or unrelated or both, healthcare costs should be accounted for during the additional life-years produced by an intervention over the alternative.

In the literature, healthcare consequences are often divided into "related" versus "unrelated" healthcare costs. Related healthcare costs are usually defined as expenditures that are incurred as a result of the conditions for which intervention is delivered. For example, treatment of acute sinusitis is likely to affect only the medical costs of treating acute sinusitis but not other healthcare-related costs. All other costs are defined as "unrelated."

The two issues related to the inclusion of related and unrelated costs are highlighted in a stylized example in Figure 8.2, which illustrates the cumulative trajectory of total healthcare costs for a subject over time under two alternative treatments. Under treatment 1, the patent incurs a steeper rate of accumulation of total costs and dies at the end of year 8. Under treatment 2, the accumulation rate of total costs is slower, and the patient lives until the end of year 10. Therefore, the first issue concerns whether unrelated costs should be accounted for while measuring cost difference in the first 8 years (i.e., the portion marked "Area A" in Figure 8.2). The second issue concerns how cost differences between two treatments should be accounted for during years 9 and 10, when the patient is alive only under treatment 2 (i.e., the portion marked "Area B" in Figure 8.2).

The original Panel did not directly deal with the first issue. This was because if some of the healthcare costs are truly unrelated to the condition, their population distributions should be the same in either intervention during the period when patients are expected to be alive. Consequently, when related costs are identified, the incremental healthcare cost parameter is identical irrespective of whether only related or total costs are considered, as unrelated costs should cancel out with the difference. While related costs can be identified relatively easily for some conditions (e.g., asthma or

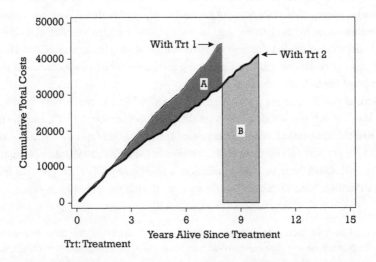

Figure 8.2 Stylized example showing differences in cumulative costs for a patient under two alternative treatments.

acute sinusitis), they are more difficult to identify for others (e.g., diabetes), especially when the condition is behavioral in nature (e.g., smoking habits). Consequently, in some cases researchers are forced to consider all healthcare costs (Weaver et al. 2009), while in others they opt to consider only related costs (Hoogendoorn et al. 2013). The primary reason for excluding unrelated costs, where related costs are readily identified, is a statistical one, because most cost estimations are based on (finite) sample distribution of costs and not their population distribution. Even though the population distribution of "truly" unrelated costs should be identical under two alternatives, the (finite) sample distributions may deviate, thereby adding noise to the estimation of incremental total costs. Therefore, it makes sense to focus exclusively on related costs for the estimation of incremental healthcare costs in cases where survivals under alternative interventions are the same and the analyst can effectively identify related cost components.

The second issue—whether related or unrelated or both types of healthcare costs should be accounted for during the additional life years produced by an intervention over the alternative—was discussed briefly by the original Panel. These costs are part of the *mortality costs* or *future costs*, as described below, but they include only healthcare costs. Suppose, for example, that we contemplate instituting a suicide prevention program in a high school. Imagine that the program is highly effective and reduces teenage suicide by 50%. Students who would otherwise have died now lead lives of normal length and have medical care utilization comparable to that of the average person their age. Should the future costs of healthcare that these students consume be counted as costs of the intervention? Weinstein and Stason (1977) and Drummond et al. (2015) have argued that they should be counted, whereas Russell (1986) has argued that they should not. The former view argues that the future added costs represent an opportunity cost for the healthcare sector, that is, that the additional expenditure could have been spent toward other people's healthcare needs. The latter view argues that, from a societal perspective, if we account for healthcare expenditures, why not account for expenditures on food, clothing, and so on during the added years of life? The original Panel recommended that related costs should always be accounted for. However, they did not reach consensus on including unrelated future healthcare costs in CEA because of the lack of theoretical reasoning.*

Several works since the publication of the original Panel's report have shed light on this topic, which is discussed in greater detail below (Section 8.2.4.1), and the much-debated theoretical reasoning points toward the inclusion of all costs incurred during the added years of life (Feenstra et al. 2008; Garber and Phelps 1997; Lee 2008; Meltzer 1997, 2006, 2008; Nyman 2004). Weinstein and Manning (1997) argue that it is not only difficult to identify related healthcare costs during the added years of life, but also

---

* The original Panel discussed the argument of Garber and Phelps (1997) that the inclusion or exclusion of any component of future costs would not change the relative rankings of treatments, in terms of ICERs, as long as all analyses follow the approach of including or excluding future costs in a consistent manner. They pointed out that this result holds true only if the "unrelated" components of costs from "related" disease are also excluded, which would be difficult, if not impossible, to accomplish.

that, even if those costs can be identified, both related and unrelated costs should be attributed to the intervention producing extension of life. Theoretical underpinnings about future costs, as discussed below (Section 8.2.4.2), support this assertion. This is especially true from a budgetary perspective within a healthcare sector, as extension of lives due to one intervention is bound to use additional resources that could otherwise have been spent on other interventions and/or other patients. Therefore, all healthcare costs, related and unrelated, irrespective of whether related costs can be identified, should be considered during the estimation of incremental future costs when survivals under alternative interventions are not the same.

In summary, we recommend that all healthcare costs, related and unrelated, should be considered either when survival under alternative interventions is not the same or when cost components cannot be readily identified as related to the target condition (**Recommendation 7**).

8.2.3 Costs Outside the Healthcare Sector

Costs discussed under this heading should be counted in Reference Case analyses conducted from the societal perspective but not the healthcare sector perspective.

8.2.3.1 *Productivity Costs*

Productivity costs reflect the production value of time in society. This is reflected as a cost because poor health can force one's time to be unproductive. Conversely, interventions that improve health can produce benefits by enabling time to be productive. Productive activities include those conducted in the household, the informal labor market, and the labor market. Valuation of these effects is discussed below (Section 8.4.2.1). Here we consider whether productivity costs should be measured explicitly and incorporated with other resource costs in the numerator of the ICER, or whether these costs are already captured in the health state valuation measures (QALYs) in the denominator of the ICER, as was suggested by the original Panel, so that any additional inclusion of these costs would lead to "double counting" (Brouwer, Koopmanschap, and Rutten 1997; Weinstein et al. 1997).

There are both theoretical and empirical reasons to believe that productivity benefits or costs should not be included in QALYs. The theoretical reason stems from the fact that if QALYs do capture productivity, there is no reason why those QALYs should be valued against a threshold that is the shadow price of a healthcare budget (see Chapter 2), which is allocated to maximize health and not productivity. The empirical reasons can be summed with two distinct questions: (1) Do QALY measurements capture *any* effects of an intervention on the productivity of patients? (2) Are QALYs reliable measures for capturing *all* of the productivity effects of an intervention? The second question becomes irrelevant if the answer to the first question is negative.

Research since the original Panel's recommendations has shown that QALYs typically do not reliably capture measures of productivity. In most cases, productivity effects are simply not considered by the respondents to preference elicitation questions. QALYs measured with generic health state valuation indices such as the Health Utilities Index (HUI) and EuroQol EQ-5D have been shown not to vary with changes in productivity (Krol, Brouwer, and Sendi 2006). In fact, respondents are explicitly asked to ignore income effects during the elicitation of HUI (Sculpher and O'Brien 2000).

In a randomized experiment, Meltzer, Weckerle, and Chang (1999) found that "spontaneous inclusion" by respondents of income when the time trade-off question is silent on the issue is relatively uncommon; this contrasts with the original Panel's suggestion. The authors concluded that "economic costs of illness are unlikely to be reflected in QOL [quality-of-life] questions, so these need to be counted separately." Similarly, in a survey of health professionals, Sendi and Brouwer (2005) found that the effects of ill health on income were not routinely incorporated in the valuation of health states. A 2010 review of seven empirical surveys (Tilling et al. 2010) shows that the proportion of respondents who spontaneously assumed income reduction without being instructed to do so varied widely, thereby raising doubt as to the reliability of the QALY measure in capturing productivity effects.

This evidence suggests that QALYs are not reliable measures for capturing productivity effects; therefore, these effects should be explicitly measured and included in the numerator of the ICER. Consequently, we have moved rectangle D in Figure 8.1, which captures the morbidity and mortality cost components, from the denominator (so the original Panel) to the numerator of the ICER. Although current evidence suggests that doing so does not imply double counting productivity effects when eliciting utility weights (Meltzer, Weckerle, and Chang 1999; Sendi and Brouwer 2005; Shiroiwa et al. 2013; Tilling et al. 2010), one can be more confident about avoiding double counting "by instructing individuals to provide QALY weights based on the assumption that their financial circumstances would not vary with health states" (Meltzer and Johannesson 1999). However, more research is needed to identify methods that would minimize double counting.

A comparison of productivity costs over the life span of patients under alternative interventions would tend to capture both morbidity and mortality costs. However, mortality costs that are incurred as a result of differential survival of patients under alternative interventions must net consumption costs from the measurements of productivity gains. We discuss these issues in greater detail under "Future Costs" below (see Section 8.2.4.1). Moreover, such calculations should also include friction costs associated with these productivity changes, especially when interventions lead to large-scale changes in productivity. This topic is discussed in greater detail under "Friction Costs" below (see Section 8.2.4.2).

8.2.3.2 Time Costs

There are two forms of time costs that are not captured in productivity costs. These reflect real changes to the use of resources by patients and society; therefore, they should be considered in CEAs from some perspectives. The first is the time a patient spends to access care and participate in or undergo an intervention (rectangle H, Figure 8.1). This use of time is, in effect, a part of the intervention, but its costs are rarely borne by the healthcare sector. Relevant time costs include travel and waiting time, as well as the time spent actually receiving treatment. The second form of time costs involves the time spent by informal (unpaid) caregivers in caring for patients, both during the treatment period and also in the future (rectangle G, Figure 8.1).

Because the healthcare sector perspective does not include these costs, CEAs conducted from this perspective have an inherent bias against interventions that rely on time inputs that are purchased and paid for by the healthcare sector and in favor of those that rely on unpaid patient time or informal support (Russell 2009). In many cases, these time costs represent significant investments in the care of patients (Yabroff and Kim 2009). The societal perspective provides an important complementary perspective when such time costs are significant.

Patients' time cost in the numerator is only the opportunity cost of time in treatment, and it does not include any adjustment for the unpleasantness of the intervention. To the extent that an intervention is unusually unpleasant or painful, an adjustment in the denominator QALY is necessary, while the time component remains in the numerator. For example, if prevention of heart disease involved a regimen of daily swimming, the monetary value of the time spent would be included in the numerator, and any appreciable increase (or decrease) in health-related quality of life from enjoyment (or dislike) of the swimming would be assessed in the QALY.

Although the costs of time in treatment are real costs of an intervention, they may be omitted from an analysis if (and only if) they are small or the alternatives being analyzed involve very similar time costs. In this respect, costs of time receiving an intervention are like other costs. If they are trivially small or do not differ across regimens, their inclusion will have little effect on the final results of an analysis, and they may therefore be omitted at the analyst's discretion (following the "rule of reason"). Analysts should take note, however, that if costs have been excluded from an analysis because they are similar across regimens, total program costs of the intervention would need to be re-evaluated if the program is assessed in relation to a different comparator.

8.2.3.3 *Other Sector Costs*

Many health interventions—especially public health interventions that aim to promote health—incur consequences that fall outside the healthcare sector. Some of these effects occur because of changes in individual behaviors. Examples are plentiful in the literature, for example, with alcohol abuse treatments (see, e.g., Zarkin et al. [2010] and the illustrative study presented in Appendix A), substance abuse treatments (Ettner et al. 2006; Humphreys, Wagner, and Gage 2011), mental health prevention programs (Drost et al. 2013), and public health programs (Basu et al. 2012). In other cases, costs or savings in non-healthcare sectors accrue as part of the intervention itself, such as when lead pipes used for delivery of water are replaced in an effort to mediate exposure to lead. In the United States, some of these costs and effects fall on local, county, or other public health system budgets, which are typically not considered to be part of the healthcare sector. For example, substance abuse treatments can have direct effects on the use of respite and homeless shelters, whose costs are borne by counties. An important sector outside of healthcare to consider is the criminal justice system, as many health and public health interventions produce consequences that reduce involvement of their beneficiaries with that system. In addition, certain interventions may affect other sectors, such as the education system (e.g., AHDH monitoring and treatment in school-aged children). As with any other cost component, exclusion of impacts to a particular sector in a CEA should be based on the analyst's discretion ("rule of reason") as long as the analyst can effectively defend such a choice. Impacts that will have little effect on the final results of an analysis may be omitted.

When non-healthcare sector impacts are substantial, they should be explicitly documented in the Impact Inventory and included in the Reference Case analysis from a societal perspective, even though they are not included in the Reference Case analysis from a healthcare sector perspective. In these instances, CEA analysis from additional perspectives, such as a public health perspective or the perspective of a local jurisdiction, may become relevant.

8.2.4 Other Cost Categories

8.2.4.1 Future Costs

As noted earlier, another area in economic evaluations in healthcare where there has been debate since the original Panel's recommendations is the issue of whether costs incurred during added years of life ("future costs") due to an intervention or policy should be attributed to that intervention or policy. These costs include not only healthcare costs (which should be included, as explained in Section 8.2.2) but also productivity and consumption consequences. Taking a pure healthcare sector perspective mitigates this argument, but it cannot be neglected from a societal perspective. For example, such arguments have been used in economic evaluations of mass screening programs where future costs were included (Mushlin and Fintor 1992).

Recent works on this topic have dealt with this problem formally, based on welfare economic theory (Feenstra et al. 2008; Garber and Phelps 1997; Lee 2008; Meltzer 1997, 2006, 2008; Nyman 2004). This literature provides a useful reminder of the complexity of thinking about the issue of future costs in economic evaluations in health and medicine. It has shown convincingly that careful analysis done using a consistent theoretical perspective continues to support the inclusion of future costs in CEA. This argument can be supported with analyses with varying degrees of complexity ranging from a simple perspective of an N person economy, in which only a smaller number of persons live to a second period (Meltzer 2006, 2008), to a more complex model based on consumptions conditional on survival over a lifetime (Feenstra et al. 2008; Meltzer 1997).

Much of the debate on future costs has focused on identifying the appropriate methodology from a societal perspective, where the main issue is whether future productivity and earnings should be accounted for. The original Panel considered these to be "mortality costs" and recommended against including them in the ICER because it was thought that they were included implicitly in the QALY estimates. However, as discussed above (Section 8.2.3.1), it is unlikely that QALY estimates capture these consequences. Hence, net future resources used during added years of life under one intervention versus another should be explicitly considered.

Nyman (2004) argues that consumption costs and earnings during the added years of life should not be accounted for because QALYs do not capture utility of consumption. However, under the assumption laid out by Bleichrodt and Quiggin (1999), under which QALY maximization is equivalent to welfare maximization, failure to capture the utility of consumption is inconsequential (see Chapter 2). Nevertheless, developing new measures of well-being that can potentially capture the effects of an intervention on health and consumption and the interactions between them could be of great value (Nyman 2011).

Net resource use can be captured by the following equation:

$$[(Healthcare\ Costs + Non\text{-}Healthcare\ Consumption\ Costs) - Productivity]$$

Productivity benefits (expressed in dollars) and healthcare costs during the added years of life are automatically accounted for when these items are cumulated over the life years of each subject under alternative arms of the intervention. An important part of accounting for net future costs is to also account for the non-healthcare consumption costs during the added years of life (**Recommendation 10**). When a healthcare sector perspective is taken, future costs should include only the total healthcare sector costs incurred during added years of life from one intervention versus another (**Recommendation 6**). Table 8.1 summarizes the different cost components included in the two Reference Case perspectives.

Interestingly, the direction in which inclusion of future costs affects an ICER depends on the ratio between the incremental life year gains over the incremental QALY gains from alternative interventions (Meltzer 1997). To see this, let us write total incremental costs as: $\Delta C_{Total} = \Delta C_{Present} + \Delta C_{Future}$, where $\Delta C_{Present}$ are the incremental costs that do not account for the costs accruing during the added year of life. Under the approximation (Meltzer 1997) that the mortality changes resulting from an intervention are concentrated at the time of the intervention and that annual future costs are roughly constant (= C), then $\Delta C_{Future} = C \cdot \Delta LEs$, where ΔLEs represents incremental life expectancy. The ICER including future costs can be expressed as:

$$\frac{\Delta C_{Total}}{\Delta QALYs} = \frac{\Delta C_{Present} + C \cdot \Delta LEs}{\Delta QALYs} = \frac{\Delta C_{Present}}{\Delta QALYs} + C \cdot \frac{\Delta LEs}{\Delta QALYs}$$

Therefore, the bias due to the omission of future costs can go in either direction depending on the sign of C and the ratio of $\Delta LE / \Delta QALYs$. Naturally, when $\Delta LEs = 0$, there is no bias. If C is positive (which may be the case if consumption expenditures surpass production), then for an intervention that increases life expectancy along with QALYs, omitting the future costs would yield a lower ICER for the intervention, thereby favoring those interventions that extend life over interventions that improve its quality.

Indeed, the inclusion of future costs (health care and non-healthcare) is now standard in many governmental agencies. For example, Swedish guidelines now recommend the routine inclusion of future costs in medical CEAs (Rappange et al. 2008), and the National Institute of Health and Care Excellence (NICE) in the United Kingdom includes such costs in its health technology appraisals. For example, a recent appraisal of trabectedin for the treatment of relapsed ovarian cancer included not only costs relating to treatment but also all other costs related to the management of stable disease, progressive disease, and adverse events in the economic model during the lifetime of the patients (National Institute for Health and Care Excellence [NICE] 2011). Because use of trabectedin was found to increase life expectancy, this amounted to inclusion of future healthcare costs in the analysis, although NICE considers only "related" future healthcare costs. For example, in the trabectedin case, all healthcare costs related to ovarian cancer incurred during the additional years of life were included. As Sculpher points out, there is "no logical basis to ignore unrelated 'downstream' costs and include unrelated 'downstream' benefits" (Sculpher 2013, 4). Because increased life expectancy (or decreased mortality) is always considered to be a benefit of a health intervention or policy, it is logical to attribute all healthcare expenditures incurred during these additional life years to that intervention or policy. From the healthcare sector perspective, these are the sum of the opportunity costs of this specific intervention that could have otherwise been spent on treating other patients (Weinstein and Manning 1997).

Another example of the inclusion of future costs is the detailed return-on-investment portfolio generated for the State of Washington on all preventive and intervention programs and policies within the state (Lee et al. 2012). The analyses followed a life-cycle approach, where all future costs were included in the analyses.

A recent survey of representatives from health technology assessment (HTA) bodies worldwide revealed that at least half of those bodies take a societal perspective in assessing cost-effectiveness, with a much higher percentage among HTA bodies in Europe (Stephens, Handke, and Doshi 2012). Therefore, these discussions are likely to have a meaningful impact on these decision-making bodies.

Many previous recommendations in this field (World Health Organization 2003), including those of the original Panel, asserted that as long as analysts are consistent with the inclusion or exclusion of future costs in their analyses, the results will be comparable. While that is true, cost-effectiveness as a tool for decision making should not only strive to make analyses comparable but also to make them useful in informing the optimal allocation of resources in a society. Inclusion and exclusion of future costs and effects can change the relative rankings of interventions. Moreover, failure to reflect these resources ignores real opportunity costs and benefits for the future generations in a society.

There are many distributional consequences of including future costs in CEAs as well (see Chapter 12). While these are important to most decision makers, it may be more convenient to deal with these distributional issues outside of the CEA. As we mention throughout this report, CEA presents only one set of inputs to the wider decision making process. These inputs would consist not only of the ICER but also the Impact Inventory showing the distribution of costs and effects falling to different sectors of the economy (Chapter 13). A separate estimate for the net future costs may also be presented for these considerations.

8.2.4.2 *Friction Costs*

Friction costs associated with, but distinct from, productivity gains and losses associated with illness or lost life should be counted when relevant. Friction costs are non-healthcare costs—transaction costs—associated with the replacement of a worker. For example, if substitute labor is never quite as productive as the labor it replaces, and the difference in productivity is not fully captured by wage rates, then the discrepancy is a friction cost. Similarly, if there are training costs for new or temporary employees, friction costs accrue to the employer, and these are real societal costs (DeLeire and Manning 2004). Similarly, costs associated with the facilitation of transfer payments in the society should be counted when relevant.

8.2.4.3 *Transfer Costs*

Income transfers involving the redistribution of money are not real costs to society and should not be included in the societal perspective Reference Case ICER. The exchange of money per se does not necessarily indicate that resources have been consumed. Programs that provide welfare or disability payments transfer money from one group of people to another (e.g., from the working population to people with disabilities), but those income transfers do not change the aggregate value of the resources available to society. We encourage analysts to track and report transfers when they are significant, because redistributional effects of interventions are often of concern to the audience of a CEA (see Chapter 12). When describing transfer costs, it is important to emphasize that they should not be added to the real societal resource costs in the analysis (**Recommendation 11**).

When analyses are conducted from a viewpoint other than the societal, transfer costs may represent lost or gained access to resources from the perspective of the analysis. In this case, the transfer costs should be included in the ICER. For example, Javitt, Canner, and Sommer (1989) incorporate avoided disability payments for blindness in an analysis on preventive ophthalmology conducted from a governmental perspective.

While transfers themselves are not costs to society, the process of transferring money may involve real resource costs. For example, determining eligibility for transfer programs and monitoring continuing eligibility requires administrative expenses, and the participant incurs application and compliance costs. Raising the money for transfer payments (i.e., with taxes) often requires real administrative costs. Another cost results when the payment of a tax or receipt of a subsidy changes the work choices of those involved.

Strictly speaking, these costs should be included, although the transfer payment itself is not. Often, however, the costs associated with transfer payments will not be important enough to merit inclusion. Analysts can assess whether, for example, real welfare losses from inappropriate financial incentives or the administrative cost of operating a transfer program will affect the results of an analysis, and proceed with an analysis of these effects if they are significant. See Starrett (1988) for approximations to the welfare cost of using taxation as a source of funding in the context of cost–benefit analysis; similar qualitative conclusions also apply to CEA.

8.2.4.4 Fixed Costs

Certain resource uses may not change despite increasing (scaling up) the number of intervention units served, especially in the short term. Such resources are known as "fixed costs." A classic example is the use of a magnetic resonance imaging (MRI) in screening. When an MRI machine is purchased, a fixed cost is incurred; the number of MRI readings with that machine will not change that cost. However, over the long term, investment in a second machine may be required. Therefore, even though the upfront costs of the MRI machine are fixed in the short term, these costs would change with the growth in demand for MRI services. In well-functioning markets, the price of MRI service should have internalized the upfront cost of investing in the MRI machine. Therefore, separate consideration of the cost of buying the MRI machine is not necessary when evaluating the cost-effectiveness of screening via MRI versus some other modality.

Another area where consideration of fixed costs becomes important is the research and development (R&D) costs and other first-copy costs associated with a new drug. The short-term marginal costs of production and distribution of a drug are often significantly lower than the market price, especially during the period of patent protection, and the handling of these costs can affect the outcome of an analysis. However, when dynamic efficiency, in terms of investments in R&D and production, is considered from a societal perspective, the short-term marginal cost of production alone would be an insufficient measure of drug costs. Instead, the long-term or social marginal costs of production for the drug, including the R&D investments required to produce the drug, should be considered (**Recommendation 8**). The social marginal costs will be higher than the short-term marginal costs. However, they are typically lower than the market price, especially during the patent period. The difference between the market price and the social marginal costs reflects the mark-up that contributes toward the social producer surplus. Because the producer surplus should be included as value generated from the societal perspective, this marked-up market price should not be used to represent the opportunity costs of a drug from a societal perspective (Cutler and Ericson 2010; Garrison et al. 2010). Rather, the social marginal costs should be used. However, obtaining estimates for the social marginal costs of production is often difficult if not impossible. Over the long term, because the class of drugs must break even—that is, have revenues large enough to cover R&D, production, and distribution costs—prevailing transaction prices with a social insurer will usually act as a serviceable way to reflect the production costs of the drugs from a societal perspective. More research is needed to ascertain whether an additional deflator of these transaction prices is needed to better approximate the social marginal costs. We discuss some of the alternatives that could be used now in Section 8.4.1.1.

For perspectives other than societal, the price paid by the decision maker for the good or service is the relevant one, inclusive of whatever return on investment in R&D or rent to the patent holder or copyright holder has been incorporated into the price. If, for example, a patient or insurance carrier pays a price for Provenge—a drug used in the treatment of metastatic prostate cancer—that reflects patent restrictions, then the relevant price for a CEA is the one paid. Similarly, if a health plan obtains large bulk discounts or uses generics in its formulary, then those discounted transaction prices are the relevant ones for the CEA. Analysts are encouraged to conduct a formal sensitivity analysis to check robustness of the CEA results to variations in base prices used.

8.3. DECIDING ON WHICH CATEGORIES TO ACCOUNT FOR IN REFERENCE CASE ANALYSES

Table 8.1 lists the different cost components to be included in the calculation of the ICER from the two Reference Case perspectives. Note that the healthcare sector perspective includes only healthcare costs that are related to the supply side of healthcare.

Table 8.1 Cost components included in the two Reference Case perspectives

Cost component	Reference Case perspective	
	Healthcare	Societal
Formal healthcare sector:*		
Paid for by third-party payers	✓	✓
Paid for by patients out-of-pocket	✓	✓
Informal healthcare sector:		
Patient time	–	✓
Unpaid caregiver time	–	✓
Transportation costs	–	✓
Non-healthcare sectors:		
Productivity	–	✓
Consumption	–	✓
Social services	–	✓
Legal or criminal justice	–	✓
Education	–	✓
Housing	–	✓
Environment	–	✓
Other (e.g., friction costs)	–	✓

*Includes current and future costs, related and unrelated to the condition under consideration.

8.4 METHODS FOR VALUING RESOURCES IN MONETARY TERMS FOR SPECIFIC CATEGORIES

Estimation of the total costs of an intervention follows one common approach: Identify the resources consumed and produced as a consequence of an intervention, measure those resource uses, and value them using unit cost estimates (**Recommendation 4**). From a societal perspective, these unit costs reflect the opportunity costs of the resources, which is the long-term marginal value forgone as a result of the use of these resources. It is possible that relevant unit costs from a private payer perspective deviate from the opportunity costs of resources in the society. When exact unit cost estimates are not available, a probabilistic approach is warranted, where the variance in unit costs is acknowledged through distribution functions. More discussion of the specification of variance function and the probability distribution function is provided in Chapter 11.

The discreteness with which resource types are defined and their unit costs are assigned determines the nature of costing approaches. On one end of the spectrum, there are approaches that call for the direct enumeration and costing out of every input consumed and produced as a consequence of the treatment of a particular patient. On the other end of the spectrum are such gross approaches as estimating the cost of an event—for example, a hospitalization for a heart attack—by assigning a national average figure such as the Medicare-derived (diagnosis related group [DRG]) reimbursement rate, or estimating the total costs of an episode of care following the intervention using econometric methods to longitudinal claims data set. We refer to the former approach as *micro*-costing and the more aggregative method as *gross-costing*. In most CEAs, a hybrid approach is adopted, where inputs consumed in treatment are estimated with micro-costing approaches, and the consequences of the treatment are measured with gross-costing approaches.

It is important to note that neither approach can claim to be accurate or precise in all situations. The appropriate use of an approach would depend on the specific types of resources to be measured and valued.

It is particularly important to use micro-costing when the cost of an input is integral to the analysis. For example, in examining different protocols for autologous bone marrow transplant, use of a previously collected cost-per-case measure would obscure cost differences related to the protocols under consideration. Alternatively, if it were thought that differences in resources consumed per service or unit of output are small but volume is large, then it would be appropriate to account painstakingly for the small differences. Micro-costing is also clearly indicated when the gross measure (such as a DRG or an average payment for a service) corresponds poorly to resource cost (Shrestha, Sansom, and Farnham 2012). For example, a relatively intensive cholesterol counseling program within a physician's office would require additional resources but might not affect a gross measure such as reimbursement rates for the office visit.

For many analyses, gross-costing estimates are adequate, and because they do not require the intensive research that may be needed to generate micro-cost estimates, they are generally much easier and less expensive to obtain. Gross-cost estimates are acceptable when using a more exact micro-cost estimate cost would not have an important effect on the analysis. In essence, a gross-costing approach follows a micro-costing principle but is applied to less discretely categorized resources. For example, cost estimates might be obtained for hospital stays or doctor visits rather than for the procedures and professional time expended during these encounters. The advantages of gross-costing are its simplicity, practicality, and, if data are obtained broadly, robustness to geographic, institutional, and other sources of variation. Its disadvantage is that relatively little attention is given to examination of the interventions involved in treating illnesses, the site of healthcare delivery, or other details that contribute to cost.

8.4.1 Costs Within the Healthcare Sector

8.4.1.1 Micro-Costing

The most highly specific micro-costing approach, which is frequently associated with primary data collection within randomized controlled trials (RCTs) or observational research studies, involves the prospective collection of data on the exact number and type of each healthcare resource consumed by the patient. These designs track resource consumption and intervention effects as they occur (Ruger et al. 2008). Unit cost multipliers are applied to the quantity of each type of service consumed, and the results are summed to obtain total cost, either for the entire inpatient stay or for that subset of inpatient services germane to the analysis at hand. Several methods exist for carrying out micro-costing studies (Frick 2009), and more research is needed to understand if one or more methods are more appropriate in specific settings. Indeed, development of a checklist to conduct, report, and appraise micro-costing studies is underway (Ruger and Reiff 2015).

Micro-costing studies generally do not continue long enough to capture the full economic (and health) consequences of an intervention. Models are therefore required to estimate the likelihood of utilization and health consequences occurring in the future (i.e., after the study period ends). These consequences are often captured by assessing the likelihood that a patient will remain in a specific health state over time and then assigning an average estimate of healthcare costs for that health state. Such average costs are typically estimated from data on medical care utilization, which may be collected manually or electronically from encounter or billing systems. In addition, however, some categories of relevant resource use are not routinely captured by bills. Out-of-plan utilization and out-of-pocket expenditures generally require separate data collection efforts, such as diaries or interviews, because neither nonmedical resource consumption nor time consumed in treatment is routinely tracked by any administrative systems.

Market prices for healthcare resources reflect the appropriate unit costs for those resources when the relevant markets are competitive. For example, the wages of a registered nurse or the charge for an office visit generally provide an adequate measure of the value of the resources consumed. In other cases, market prices may not reflect the true opportunity cost to society of the resources used to produce the good or service (**Recommendation 5**). This is so because the resources include a component of profit in excess of an actuarially fair rate of return on investment and allowance for risk, as is typically the case when there is any form of market distortion or imperfection of market power. An example of this in the US market is that the list price that hospitals charge for a service, such as a coronary artery bypass graft or a neonatal intensive care unit day, will exceed the opportunity cost to society of the resources used. In order to obtain an estimate of opportunity costs of the resources, a cost-to-charge ratio can be used to deflate the charges. The Medicare Cost Reports provide easily accessible data that can be used to calculate cost-to-charge ratios. The analyst must consider the specific needs of the analysis when applying this remedy. An average correction for the difference between costs and charges for the hospital as a whole may not provide the right correction for a particular service provided by that hospital. Cost-to-charge ratios for the specific service should be obtained when necessary. Additional discussions on unit costs in the United States and other countries can be found in Glick et al. (2007).

For pharmaceuticals, finding average transaction prices is not straightforward, at least not in the United States. It is now widely accepted that the average wholesale prices (AWPs) are no longer a reliable estimate of the transaction prices (Academy of Managed Care Pharmacy 2009). In fact, many vendors have stopped publishing AWPs. There are, however, nine different possible alternative benchmarks identified (Curtiss, Lettrich, and Fairman 2010), highlighting the complexity of the transactions for pharmaceutical payments in the United States. While there is no consensus on what is the most accurate measure of transaction prices for pharmaceuticals, we recommend using the Federal Supply Schedule (FSS), a publicly available source of information of the cost paid for drugs by many federal agencies in the United States (**Recommendation 9**). Determining the extent to which this reflects the true social marginal costs of a drug remains an area for future work. While these prices may be used for both the healthcare sector and the societal perspective Reference Case analyses, other payer perspectives must use the pharmaceutical prices transacted for. In such analyses, pharmaceutical prices need not remain constant over time. Anticipating price changes that may occur with the loss of patent in the future should be accounted for in the analysis.

8.4.1.2 *Gross-Costing*

When payer reimbursement and out-of-pocket expenditures are directly observed, such as in electronic claims data, a gross-costing approach to valuing resources used during an episode of care or a specified time period in a health state avoids the problem of finding market price for each individual component of service use and its adjustment. A large literature exists on the econometric modeling of individual-level expenditure data, which are well known for their idiosyncrasies. Many excellent reviews of this literature are available (Jones 2000, 2011). Four distinct messages are apparent in this literature:

1. The assumption that observations of costs are identically distributed is wrong. Cost data are inherently heteroskedastic and skewed, and statistical analyses that do not account for these features could lead to misleading results.
2. Avoid transformation models, where a dependent variable is transformed by the natural logarithm or a power transformation to eliminate the skewness in the error or to make the model linear in parameters. It has been well established that a very difficult and unreliable retransformation process is often required to obtain effects on raw scale expenditure from these models (Manning 1998; Manning and Mullahy 2001).
3. Perform extensive goodness-of-fit tests to assess the appropriateness of any model specification (Basu, Arondekar, and Rathouz 2006).
4. Explicitly deal with censoring in longitudinal cost data, even if censoring is random in nature like the type of censoring that arises from administrative censoring (Bang and Tsiatis 2000; Basu and Manning 2010; Lin 2000, 2003; Lin et al. 1997; O'Hagan and Stevens 2004; Raikou and McGuire 2004).

In addition, directly estimating incremental costs of an intervention on the basis of retrospective data is subject to selection biases that arise because alternative interventions are not randomly assigned to individuals, but rather are chosen by the patient or the patient's provider. To the extent that these decisions are driven by factors that affect expenditures, a naïve comparison of intervention-specific mean expenditures would produce a biased estimate of the incremental treatment effect. Careful attention should be paid to dealing with these factors appropriately, some of which may be observed in the data at hand, while others remain omitted (Polsky and Basu 2012).

8.4.2 Costs Outside the Healthcare Sector

8.4.2.1 Productivity Costs and Future Healthcare-Unrelated Costs

Productivity costs represent the production value of time spent on formal labor markets, informal labor markets, and in household production (**Recommendation 14**). In the formal market, earnings lost because of patients' health status can be measured by means of a human capital approach, accounting for expected earnings in each time period in the patients' lifetime. Because an individual would be employed in the market only if the marginal product of labor is at least as large as the wages plus fringe benefits offered, the marginal value of a unit of time in the formal labor market is given by the wages plus fringe benefits. Annual expected earnings can be imputed based on the product of the following two parameters: (1) the health-status-specific likelihood of a person's participating in the labor market and (2) the mean annual salary plus fringe benefits in that market. In 2014, on average, fringe benefits in the United States accounted for 31.6% of the total compensation (i.e., fringe rate ~ 46%; Bureau of Labor Statistics [2015]).

The human capital approach typically assumes that time lost by an individual in the labor market is not compensated for by an otherwise unproductive person. Although it is often believed that this assumption holds only for developed countries, where unemployment rates are low (Koopmanschap et al. 1995), it may also hold for many developing countries with high unemployment rates, where people outside the labor force are productive in the informal market and the household sectors. In contrast, the friction costs approach to valuing productivity in the formal market assumes that the productivity costs consist only of the uncompensated part of lost productive time (Koopmanschap et al. 1995). From an employer perspective, this may make sense if the employer can restrict productivity losses associated with the health of their employees by substituting for missed labor through internal reserves within the firm, and by hiring externally, without incurring additional costs. However, such functioning of a firm does not often align with the neoclassical economic theory of firms or with empirical observations (Johannesson and Karlsson 1997). Naturally, estimates of productivity costs obtained with a friction cost approach usually yield smaller estimates than estimates obtained with a human capital approach (Jacob-Tacken et al. 2005; van Asselt et al. 2008). However, from a societal perspective, a friction cost approach implies that the person who is compensating for the time of the sick individual was otherwise completely unproductive in the society, not only in terms of labor market production, but also in terms of informal market and household productions. Because of the severity of this assumption, we recommend using the human capital approach for analyses conducted from the societal perspective.

A more nuanced micro-costing approach to productivity losses would also measure the extent of absenteeism (an employee's intentional or habitual absence from work) and presenteeism (attending work while sick) even though the individual has not formally left the labor market. Standardized questionnaires are available to measure absenteeism and presenteeism (Kessler et al. 2003). Nonproductive time due to these two channels should also be costed on the basis of wages plus fringe benefits.

There are many distributional questions surrounding this approach. Should we allow these parameters to vary by age and sex? Should the mean annual salary be health status-specific? Traditional cost–benefit analysis typically would use targeted estimates of these two parameters, based on age, sex, health status, and other characteristics of patients, to reflect the true resource use in the society. However, decision making with such estimates runs into the challenge of comparing the social value of interventions for children, who do not work, versus the elderly, who are likely to be retired, versus those who are primary participants in the labor market. Moreover, a population whose members are less likely to hold a high-paying job, on average, such as people with severe mental illnesses, would be disadvantaged if their disease-specific salaries were used for evaluation purposes. At the same time, ignoring the productivity costs would bias evaluation in favor of those interventions that have only life expectancy gains. For example, the value of a new drug for people with schizophrenia that improves cognition, which in turn leads to better functional outcomes, including labor market participation, would be seriously underestimated if these productivity benefits were not considered. While the appropriate weighting for productivity gains would depend on the institution and the social context, it must be noted that a consistent process should be developed within that institution in order to evaluate all interventions in a consistent fashion. Moreover, one must be aware that whatever the final process, it has implications for the distributional consequences of resources. Hence, we do not prescribe any one method to weigh these productivity gains (**Recommendation 16**). Often a sensitivity analysis using different weighting schemes may be useful. In the worked example on alcohol abuse treatment in Appendix A, we use age-specific labor force participation and common wage and fringe benefit rates to value time across all individuals. Sensitivity analysis revealed that the results were robust to other weighting schemes. Table 8.2 provides estimates for 2014 average earnings (which can be converted to wage rates) by age in the United States. Population surveys, such as the Current Population Surveys in the United States, can also be used to estimate the rates of labor market participation.

The above method to measure and value productivity gains is obviously geared toward those who participate in formal labor markets. Naturally, with this approach there is a distributional bias with respect to age (especially after retirement age, e.g., 65 years; this issue is discussed further in Chapter 12). However, a growing body of work has shown how elderly individuals are contributing in informal labor markets by volunteering time for various activities (e.g., baby-sitting), counseling, and mentoring younger people (Hank and Stuck 2008; Mutchler, Burr, and Caro 2003). For example, consider an emeritus professor who is no longer paid by the university, but who works substantial hours mentoring students and junior faculty. In fact,

Table 8.2 Average annual consumption costs by age (2014 US dollars)

Age group	Average annual expenditures per person					
	Total expenditures		Healthcare expenditures		Non-healthcare expenditures	
	Mean	SE	Mean	SE	Mean	SE
All ages	$20,440	$329	$1,452	$34	$18,988	$330
Age < 25	$15,187	$688	$472	$53	$14,715	$691
25 ≤ age ≤ 34	$17,174	$574	$782	$48	$16,392	$576
35 ≤ age ≤ 44	$17,289	$516	$938	$73	$16,352	$521
45 ≤ age ≤ 54	$22,416	$680	$1,408	$70	$21,009	$683
55 ≤ age ≤ 64	$26,615	$702	$2,085	$86	$24,530	$707
65 ≤ age ≤ 74	$24,609	$897	$2,731	$79	$21,878	$901
75 ≤ age	$21,489	$908	$3,069	$104	$18,420	$914

Note: The original table provided annual expenditures per consumer units. To estimate annual expenditures per person, we divided the annual expenditures by the average number of people in the consumer unit that was provided in the same table.

Source: Bureau of Labor Statistics. Consumer Expenditure Survey. Washington DC: US Department of Labor Statistics, 2014. http://www.bls.gov/cex/2013/combined/age.pdf.

some evidence suggests that individuals are likely to *reduce* their leisure hours after retirement (Nimrod, Janke, and Kleiber 2008). A treatment that alleviates negative health states and enables an elderly person to participate in informal labor production should be rewarded. With the growing number of retirees in the United States and other industrialized nations, failure to incorporate these benefits could unintentionally carry resources away from this population. More research is needed to appropriately characterize the time spent by retirees in doing informal productive work. These times can then be valued using the same principle employed in valuing formal productive time.

Using the same principle, time contributed by formal (paid) and informal (unpaid) caregivers in caring for patients should be valued in the same way as productivity costs (**Recommendation 15**). However, hourly rates for both should be based on the marginal pre-tax wage rate plus fringe benefits observed in the formal caregiver's market. Informal caregivers may derive additional value through caregiving, which should be captured through their QALYs.

Another channel of productivity costs occurs through the production of household activities that include time spent caring for and helping children and adults in the household. Household production can be defined to include activities such as housework; food preparation, cooking and clean-up; household management; shopping; obtaining services; and travel related to household activity (Grosse, Krueger, and Mvundura 2009). Because the health of an individual may affect that individual's capability to contribute toward these activities, the value of replacing those lost contributions should be included as productivity costs. Grosse, Krueger, and Mvundura (2009) present detailed estimates of age- and sex-specific estimates of these household productivity times in the United States. These times can be valued with the same principle employed in valuing formal productive time. However, learning how alternative interventions may affect household productivity times would require more research and more a detailed micro-costing approach for measuring the impact on specific dimensions of household productivity.

Finally, as discussed above, mortality costs that are incurred due to the differential survival of patients under alternative medical interventions must net consumptions costs from the measurements of productivity gains. Because healthcare consumption is already accounted for under healthcare costs, one must estimate an average annual non-healthcare-related consumption for the patients (**Recommendation 17**). Table 8.3 illustrates estimates for the average healthcare-related and non-healthcare-related consumption costs from the Consumer Expenditure Surveys in the United States. Again, as in the discussions around valuing productivity costs, one can use an age-specific estimate of consumption (to reflect the fact that the elderly may have lower consumption on average than younger people) or use a generic overall estimate of consumption costs. The degree of targeting (e.g., by age, sex, other factors) should be consistent between earnings and consumption, and the choice of the appropriate valuation methods and level of targeting will depend on the decision maker or the institution to which such analyses are catering (**Recommendation 18**). Consumption costs can be ignored if the survival curves under alternative interventions are similar.

Table 8.3 Average annual earnings by age (2014 US dollars)

Age group	Average annual earnings per person	
	Mean	SE
All ages	$44,245	$316
Age < 25	$20,398	$462
25 ≤ age ≤ 34	$39,907	$537
35 ≤ age ≤ 44	$51,366	$733
45 ≤ age ≤ 54	$52,749	$721
55 ≤ age ≤ 64	$53,329	$825
65 ≤ age ≤ 74	$41,317	$1,568
75 ≤ age	$37,300	$3,432

Source: Author's calculations using the Current Population Survey 2014 July data set. http://thedataweb.rm.census.gov/ftp/cps_ftp.html#cpsbasic.

8.4.2.2 *Time Costs*

Time spent seeking and receiving healthcare is usually thought to come from one's leisure time. Under the traditional economics of labor markets, one chooses to participate in leisure by not engaging in productive activities. Therefore, the marginal value of a unit of time of leisure should be at least as large as the amount the individual could have earned by working. We recommend using the post-tax wage rate plus fringe benefits to estimate the value of time as a tractable means for obtaining estimates for the societal perspective Reference Case analysis (**Recommendation 12**). In 2014, the effective individual income tax rate in the United States was estimated to be 9.2% (Tax Policy Center 2013). Post-tax wage rate plus fringe benefits applies to time spent by patients in seeking care but not by caregivers in providing care to patients. This is because the latter is considered to be a productive activity by the caregiver and should be valued as described above (Section 8.4.2.1). In addition, as discussed in Section 8.4.2.1, whether such wage rates should be age-specific, disease-specific, or a unitary number that applies to all would depend on the decision-making context and institutional preferences. It is recommended that sensitivity analyses should be carried out with alternative forms of valuation of time.

The use of wages to value time assumes that the person obtains no direct satisfaction from the provision of the time. The time consumed is lost leisure or lost work, but it is of no intrinsic value. However, if one dislikes waiting in a doctor's office, and these time costs represent a substantial amount of costs in the analyses, then attention should be paid to measuring these preferential aspects through health-related quality-of-life measures (**Recommendation 13**).

For adults unable to work and for children in general, there are no wage data. We encourage research into how to better value the time for these two groups. In the meantime, we make the following suggestions. For teenagers, one could use the solution used for homemakers and informal caregivers, namely, basing the wage rate on teenagers in the labor force and adjusting as necessary for the selection bias of using observed market wages for teenagers not in the labor force. For younger children and adults unable to work, there is no easy alternative. Another possible alternative for all of these groups is to use questionnaires to elicit willingness-to-pay for the time costs, which could be done on standard populations in much the same way that weights can be derived for health states. Given the potential importance of the costs of time in treatment for these three groups, we encourage research into methods and estimates of the opportunity cost of time.

8.4.2.3 *Other Sector Costs*

The impact of healthcare and public health interventions on resource use in sectors outside of healthcare should be valued by the respective market prices for those resources in those sectors. For example, when alcohol abuse treatments reduce crime, the costs savings associated with this reduction can be measured by the gross costs of an arrest (or micro-costing each of the specific inputs that goes into arresting, e.g., police time, monitoring costs, etc.), the gross costs involved with the justice system (or micro-costing the time of judges, lawyers, and clerks, among others), and the gross costs of incarceration if a person is convicted. In addition, one must account for the gross costs of physical damages caused by the crime (e.g., tangible damages to health and property). These costs can be obtained by recording prevailing prices of these resources. Similarly, costs falling to the education sector, where an intervention may, for example, need additional nurses in schools, must be accounted for by the cost of employing an additional nurse for specific periods of time.

Interventions that have substantial effects on the levels of education and training for individuals must account for labor market returns to these increased human capital investments over the long term. The importance of human capital has long been recognized in labor economics (Becker 1975). Individuals with more education have better performance in terms of labor market outcomes (Card 1999). Empirically, such labor market returns have been consistently demonstrated in a long and extensive literature in labor economics (Carneiro, Heckman, and Vytlacil 2011; Sianesi and Van Reenen 2002). Even if the wage rate in the labor market is assumed to be constant for everyone, following the discussions above, human capital returns may become manifest in terms of increased probability of participation in labor markets (Card 1999, 2001; Heckman, Lochner, and Todd 2006). In fact, recent empirical analysis has also found causal effects of education on general health and well-being (Cutler and Lleras-Muney 2010). Establishing methods to incorporate the long-term health effects of education in CEAs needs further work.

As with time costs, the valuation of the use of these resources assumes there is no additional satisfaction or dissatisfaction associated with them. For example, prevention of crime by a public health intervention would not only reduce the costs related to the crime rate but would likely also have an intangible benefit to the society as a whole. That is, potential victims of crimes would place an incremental value on a society where there is less crime. Such intangible benefits or costs are difficult to monetize. One possibility is to elicit willingness-to-pay for these benefits from citizens at large, as is typically done in cost–benefit analysis. There may be other ways to value these intangible effects by developing measures, such as measuring QALYs for each sector and then valuing them based on the marginal threshold for the respective sectors. However, more work is needed to quantify these intangible benefits and costs. In the absence of methods to value these benefits in QALY terms, we recommend that they be explicitly included in the Impact Inventory created for a CEA. In addition, for a Reference Case analysis from a societal perspective, intrinsic non-healthcare benefits, such as the psychological benefits of lower crime, should be valued in monetary terms and be included in the numerator of the ICER. However, the methods of valuation would depend on the jurisdiction of the analysis. In the United States, willingness-to-pay would be an acceptable method. Sensitivity analysis should be conducted by presenting the societal ICER with and without these benefits (**Recommendation 19**).

8.5 OTHER ISSUES

8.5.1 Price Inflation

When the data on prices used in a CEA come from different time periods, or when the study is projecting costs for different time periods, market prices can vary because of general inflation or because some particular resource is becoming more or less scarce. The usual approach for handling price changes is to bring past prices into current terms, so that they reflect the opportunity cost of the resources in common dollar terms; one can directly add 2005 dollars, but it is not meaningful to add 1999 dollars and 2009 dollars because their real purchasing power was different (**Recommendation 20**).

Analysts should select an appropriate index for use in adjusting the prices of various resources. The most commonly used measure to adjust for inflation is the Consumer Price Index (CPI). If the price being brought up to date is a wage or some other measure that rises at the rate of general price inflation, then the CPI provides a serviceable way to correct for inflation. However, if the good or input has a different rate of price change than the economy as a whole, a more specific measure should be used. Unfortunately, there is no gold standard for adjusting for inflation in medical expenditures. The CPI accounts only for out-of-pocket expenditure and therefore may not be appropriate for inflating total medical care expenditures, but it may be appropriate for certain medical care components. Unfortunately, the medical care component of the CPI, which was constructed to account for the differential price change in the medical sector, is fraught with measurement errors (Newhouse 2001). Recent work (Grosse and Zuvekas 2015) has highlighted that the GDP deflator or the personal consumption expenditure (PCE) price index can be used when the analysis is meant to reflect total purchasing power. However, this is rarely the goal of a CEA. Instead, it is proposed that disease-specific costs could be inflated using the Personal Health Care (PHC) Expenditure deflator developed by the Centers for Medicare and Medicaid Services (CMS) (Grosse and Zuvekas 2015) and also supported by the Agency for Healthcare Research and Quality (AHRQ). However, these indices are only available with a lag-time of two years. Therefore, we recommend the use of the PHC deflator up to the most recent year available, and then apply the PCE to update to the current year (Agency for Healthcare Research and Quality 2015). Adjustments using PCE and PHC estimates appear to produce very close results (Grosse and Zuvekas 2015). Where appropriate, costs used in a CEA should reflect the costs in the jurisdiction where the intervention is or will be implemented (**Recommendation 21**).

8.5.2 Returns to Scale

Most analysis of costs in CEA is thought of in terms of the assumptions of constant returns to scale. This is especially true when estimates of resource use are obtained from small studies, such as small RCTs. When the marginal costs of resources are likely to change with the scale of the intervention, then it is necessary to estimate a cost function and derive the marginal cost that is reflective of the scope of the intervention. Many healthcare interventions will exhibit no important economies or diseconomies of scale or scope. When that is the case, average costs and marginal costs will be equal, and the correction may be based on average costs; estimates of incremental or marginal costs thus need not be developed.

8.5.3 Discounting

Costs should be discounted at the same rate as health effects (**Recommendation 22**). More discussion on this topic can be found in Chapters 2 and 10. Sensitivity to alternative discount rates should be studied.

8.6 RECOMMENDATIONS

1. In cost-effectiveness analysis (CEA), all resource use should be valued in monetary terms and be included in the numerator of an incremental cost-effectiveness ratio (ICER). The denominator of an ICER should reflect only health as expressed in quality-adjusted life years (QALYs).
2. All resource use that is both germane to the analysis and non-trivial in magnitude should be included in the Reference Case analyses from both the healthcare sector perspective and the societal perspective. Resource use should be reflected regardless of whether a monetary transaction takes place.
3. From a long-term perspective, costs in CEA should reflect the opportunity costs of the resources used, which represent the marginal or incremental costs of resources, rather than average costs. Therefore, attention should be paid to instances in which

constant return-to-scale for resources used may not apply when implementing an intervention in a population.

4. In principle, the full three-step approach to determining costs, entailing the identification, measurement (quantification), and valuation of resource use, is preferred. The choice between mirco-costing and gross-costing approaches should reflect the importance of precise cost estimates, feasibility, and cost.

5. To the extent that prices reflect opportunity costs, they are an appropriate basis for valuing changes in resources. If prices do not adequately reflect opportunity costs because of market distortions, they should be adjusted; when substantial bias is present and adjustment is not feasible, another proxy for opportunity cost should be used. Sometimes the opportunity costs of a resource may be different for the healthcare sector perspective than for the societal perspective.

6. All healthcare resources consumed over the lifetime of the patients as part of, or as a result of, an intervention should be valued in monetary terms and included in the numerator of an ICER.

7. All healthcare costs, related or unrelated, should be considered either when survivals under alternative interventions are not the same or when cost components cannot be readily identified as related to the target condition.

8. Fixed costs for research and development of a healthcare intervention should always be taken into account, unless these fixed costs are similar across all the comparator interventions.

9. In the United States, the Federal Supply Schedule (FSS) for drug prices should be used to reflect the social marginal costs of drugs for Reference Case analyses from both the healthcare sector perspective and the societal perspective. In CEAs conducted from other perspectives, costs should reflect the transaction prices from the perspective of the analysis.

10. In addition to **Recommendation 6**, for a Reference Case analysis from a societal perspective, all non-healthcare resources consumed over the lifetime of the patients as part of, or as a result of, an intervention should be valued in monetary terms and included in the numerator of an ICER.

11. For a Reference Case analysis from a societal perspective, non-healthcare resources include patients' time costs, caregivers' time costs, productivity benefits, consumption costs, friction/administrative costs, and relevant costs from all other sectors of the economy outside of healthcare. Costs that are transferred from one section of the population to another should not be included.

12. For a Reference Case analysis from a societal perspective, patients' time costs reflect the time spent receiving an intervention. This time resource is assumed to displace leisure time of the patients and is therefore valued at the marginal post-tax wage rate plus fringe benefits. Under compelling evidence that such time spent replaces labor time and not leisure time, it should be valued as productive time as explained in **Recommendation 14**.

13. For a Reference Case analysis from a societal perspective, if the time spent receiving an intervention has a significant positive or negative impact on health-related

quality of life, this impact should be incorporated into the denominator of an ICER, leaving the time component in the numerator.

14. For a Reference Case analysis from a societal perspective, three types of productive time for patients should be considered: (a) time spent in formal labor markets; (b) time spent in informal labor markets; and (c) time spent in household production. Where sufficient data exist, all three types of productive time should be valued with the marginal pre-tax wage rate plus fringe benefits.

15. For a Reference Case analysis from a societal perspective, both formal (paid) and informal (unpaid) caregivers' time should be viewed as productive time and valued with marginal pre-tax wage rate plus fringe benefits in the formal caregiver market.

16. The degree to which marginal wage rates, tax rates, and fringe benefit rates should be stratified based on age, sex, and/or disease conditions depends on the needs of the decision makers that the analysis aims to inform. If stratified estimates are used, the distributional consequences of such an approach should be discussed.

17. For a Reference Case analysis from a societal perspective, consumption costs should reflect the non-healthcare consumptions. Consumption costs should be considered only where there is differential survival across comparator interventions.

18. As with wage rates, stratification of consumption costs should meet the needs of decision makers. Distributional consequences arising as a result of stratification should be discussed.

19. For a Reference Case analysis from a societal perspective, intrinsic non-healthcare benefits, such as the psychological benefits of a lower crime rate, should be valued in monetary terms and included in the numerator of an ICER. The methods of valuation would depend on the jurisdiction of the analysis. In the United States, willingness-to-pay to value these outcomes would be an acceptable method. Sensitivity analysis should be conducted by presenting the societal ICER with and without these benefits.

20. Cost-effectiveness analyses should be conducted in constant dollars that remove general price inflation. If the prices in question change at a rate different from general price levels, that variation should be reflected in the adjustments used. For example, in the United States, the personal consumption expenditure (PCE) price index and the Personal Health Care (PHC) Expenditure deflator should be used to adjust for inflation in healthcare expenditures. For non-healthcare sector expenditures, the regular Consumer Price Index (CPI) should be used.

21. The costs used in a CEA should reflect the costs in the jurisdiction where the intervention is or will be implemented.

22. Costs should be discounted at the same rate as health effects.

8.7 REFERENCES

Academy of Managed Care Pharmacy. 2009. AMCP Guide to Pharmaceutical Payment Methods, 2009 Update (Version 2.0). *J Manag Care Pharm* 15 (6 Suppl A):S3-S57, quiz S58-S61.

Agency for Healthcare Research and Quality. 2015. "Medical Expenditure Panel Survey (MEPS). Using Appropriate Price Indices for Analyses of Health Care Expenditures or Income Across Multiple Years." Last Modified April 3, 2015. Accessed March 4, 2016. http://meps.ahrq.gov/about_meps/Price_Index.shtml.

Bang, H., and A. Tsiatis. 2000. Estimating medical costs with censored data. *Biometrika* 87 (2): 329-343.

Basu, A., B. V. Arondekar, and P. J. Rathouz. 2006. Scale of interest versus scale of estimation: comparing alternative estimators for the incremental costs of a comorbidity. *Health Econ* 15 (10):1091-1107.

Basu, A., R. Kee, D. Buchanan, and L. S. Sadowski. 2012. Comparative cost analysis of housing and case management program for chronically ill homeless adults compared to usual care. *Health Serv Res* 47 (1 Pt 2):523-543.

Basu, A., and W. G. Manning. 2010. Estimating lifetime or episode-of-illness costs under censoring. [Erratum appears in *Health Econ* 2011;20 (1):125-126]. *Health Econ* 19 (9): 1010-1028.

Becker, G. S. 1975. *Human Capital: A Theoretical and Empirical Analysis, with Special Reference to Education.* 2nd ed. New York: Columbia University Press.

Bleichrodt, H., and J. Quiggin. 1999. Life-cycle preferences over consumption and health: when is cost-effectiveness analysis equivalent to cost-benefit analysis? *J Health Econ* 18 (6):681-708.

Brouwer, W. B., M. A. Koopmanschap, and F. F. Rutten. 1997. Productivity costs measurement through quality of life? A response to the recommendation of the Washington Panel. *Health Econ* 6 (3):253-259.

Bureau of Labor Statistics. 2015. *Employer Costs for Employee Compensation Historical Listing: March 2004-March 2015.* Washington, DC: Bureau of Labor Statistics. National Compensation Survey. www.bls.gov/ncs/ect/sp/ececqrtn.pdf.

Card, D. 1999. "The Causal Effect of Education on Earnings." In *Handbook of Labor Economics,* Vol. 3A, edited by O. Ashenfelter and D. Card, 1801-1863. Amsterdam: Elsevier Science B.V.

Card, D. 2001. Estimating the return to schooling: progress on some persistent econometric problems. *Econometrica* 69 (5):1127-1160.

Carneiro, P., J. J. Heckman, and E. J. Vytlacil. 2011. Estimating marginal returns to education. *Am Econ Rev* 101 (6):2754-2781.

Curtiss, F. R., P. Lettrich, and K. A. Fairman. 2010. What is the price benchmark to replace average wholesale price (AWP)? *J Manag Care Pharm* 16 (7):492-501.

Cutler, D. M., and K. M. Ericson. 2010. Cost-effectiveness analysis in markets with high fixed costs. *Pharmacoeconomics* 28 (10):867-875.

Cutler, D. M., and A. Lleras-Muney. 2010. Understanding differences in health behaviors by education. *J Health Econ* 29 (1):1-28.

DeLeire, T., and W. Manning. 2004. Labor market costs of illness: prevalence matters. *Health Econ* 13 (3):239-250.

Drost, R.M., A.T. Paulus, D. Ruwaard, and S.M. Evers. 2013. Inter-sectoral costs and benefits of mental health prevention: towards a new classification scheme. *J Ment Health Policy Econ* 16 (4):179-186.

Drummond, M. F., M. J. Sculpher, K. Claxton, G. W. Torrance, and G. L. Stoddart. 2015. *Methods for the Economic Evaluation of Health Care Programmes*. 4th ed. Oxford: Oxford University Press.

Ettner, S. L., D. Huang, E. Evans, D. R. Ash, M. Hardy, M. Jourabchi, and Y. I. Hser. 2006. Benefit-cost in the California treatment outcome project: does substance abuse treatment "pay for itself?" [Erratum appears in *Health Serv Res* 2006;41 (2):613]. *Health Serv Res* 41 (1): 192–213.

Feenstra, T. L., P. H. van Baal, A. Gandjour, and W. B. Brouwer. 2008. Future costs in economic evaluation. A comment on Lee. *J Health Econ* 27 (6):1645–1649; discussion 1650–1641.

Frick, K. D. 2009. Microcosting quantity data collection methods. *Med Care* 47 (7 Suppl 1): S76–S81.

Garber, A. M., and C. E. Phelps. 1997. Economic foundations of cost-effectiveness analysis. *J Health Econ* 16 (1):1–31.

Garrison, L. P., Jr., E. C. Mansley, T. A. Abbott, 3rd, B. W. Bresnahan, J. W. Hay, and J. Smeeding. 2010. Good research practices for measuring drug costs in cost-effectiveness analyses: a societal perspective: the ISPOR Drug Cost Task Force report—Part II. *Value Health* 13 (1):8–13.

Glick, H. A., J. A. Doshi, S. S. Sonnad, and D. Polsky. 2007. *Economic Evaluation in Clinical Trials*. Oxford: Oxford University Press.

Gold, M. R., J. E. Siegel, L. B. Russell, and M. C. Weinstein, eds. 1996. *Cost-Effectiveness in Health and Medicine*. New York: Oxford University Press.

Grosse, S. D., K. V. Krueger, and M. Mvundura. 2009. Economic productivity by age and sex: 2007 estimates for the United States. *Med Care* 47 (7 Suppl 1):S94–S103.

Grosse, S. D., and S. H. Zuvekas. 2015. The price is right: on adjusting health expenditures for inflation. Centers for Disease Control and Prevention Mimeo 2015 [unpublished].

Hank, K., and S. Stuck. 2008. Volunteer work, informal help, and care among the 50+ in Europe: further evidence for "linked" productive activities at older ages. *Soc Sci Res* 37 (4): 1280–1291.

Heckman, J. J., L. J. Lochner, and P. E. Todd. 2006. "Earnings Functions, Rates of Return and Treatment Effects: The Mincer Equation and Beyond." In *Handbook of the Economics of Education*, Vol. 1, edited by E. Hanushek and F. Welch, 307–458. Amsterdam: Elsevier B.V.

Hoogendoorn, M., M. J. Al, K. M. Beeh, D. Bowles, J. M. Graf von der Schulenburg, J. Lungershausen, B. U. Monz, H. Schmidt, C. Vogelmeier, and M. P. Rutten-van Molken. 2013. Cost-effectiveness of tiotropium versus salmeterol: the POET-COPD trial. *Eur Respir J* 41 (3):556–564.

Humphreys, K., T. H. Wagner, and M. Gage. 2011. If substance use disorder treatment more than offsets its costs, why don't more medical centers want to provide it? A budget impact analysis in the Veterans Health Administration. *J Subst Abuse Treat* 41 (3):243–251.

Jacob-Tacken, K. H., M. A. Koopmanschap, W. J. Meerding, and J. L. Severens. 2005. Correcting for compensating mechanisms related to productivity costs in economic evaluations of health care programmes. *Health Econ* 14 (5):435–443.

Javitt, J. C., J. K. Canner, and A. Sommer. 1989. Cost effectiveness of current approaches to the control of retinopathy in type I diabetics. *Ophthalmology* 96 (2):255–264.

Johannesson, M., and G. Karlsson. 1997. The friction cost method: a comment. *J Health Econ* 16 (2):249–255; discussion 257–249.

Jones, A. M. 2000. "Health Econometrics." In *Handbook of Health Economics*, Vol. 1, edited by A. J. Culyer and J. P. Newhouse, 265–344. Amsterdam and New York: Elsevier.

Jones, A. M. 2011. "Models for Health Care." In *The Oxford Handbook or Economic Forecasting*, edited by M. P. Clements and D. F. Hendry. New York: Oxford University Press.

Kessler, R. C., C. Barber, A. Beck, P. Berglund, P. D. Cleary, D. McKenas, N. Pronk, G. Simon, P. Stang, T. B. Ustun, and P. Wang. 2003. The World Health Organization Health and Work Performance Questionnaire (HPQ). *J Occup Environ Med* 45 (2):156–174.

Koopmanschap, M. A., F. F. Rutten, B. M. van Ineveld, and L. van Roijen. 1995. The friction cost method for measuring indirect costs of disease. *J Health Econ* 14 (2):171–189.

Krol, M., W. Brouwer, and P. Sendi. 2006. Productivity costs in health-state valuations: does explicit instruction matter? *Pharmacoeconomics* 24 (4):401–414.

Lee, R. H. 2008. Thinking rigorously about future costs in cost effectiveness analysis. *J Health Econ* 27 (6):1650–1651.

Lee, S., S. Aos, E. Drake, A. Pennucci, M. Miller, and L. Anderson. 2012. *Return on Investment: Evidence-Based Options to Improve Statewide Outcomes. April 2012 Update (Publication No. 12-04-1201)*. Olympia: Washington State Institute for Public Policy. http://www.wsipp.wa.gov/pub.asp?docid=12-04-1201.

Lin, D. Y. 2000. Linear regression analysis of censored medical costs. *Biostatistics* 1 (1):35–47.

Lin, D. Y. 2003. Regression analysis of incomplete medical cost data. *Stat Med* 22 (7):1181–1200.

Lin, D. Y., E. J. Feuer, R. Etzioni, and Y. Wax. 1997. Estimating medical costs from incomplete follow-up data. *Biometrics* 53 (2):419–434.

Manning, W. G. 1998. The logged dependent variable, heteroscedasticity, and the retransformation problem. *J Health Econ* 17 (3):283–295.

Manning, W. G., and J. Mullahy. 2001. Estimating log models: to transform or not to transform? *J Health Econ* 20 (4):461–494.

Meltzer, D. 1997. Accounting for future costs in medical cost-effectiveness analysis. *J Health Econ* 16 (1):33–64.

Meltzer, D. 2006. "Future Costs in Medical Cost-Effectiveness Analysis." In *The Elgar Companion to Health Economics*, edited by A. M. Jones, 447–454. Cheltenham, UK: Edward Elgar Publishing Limited.

Meltzer, D. 2008. Response to "Future costs and the future of cost-effectiveness analysis." *J Health Econ* 27 (4):822–825.

Meltzer, D., and M. Johannesson. 1999. Inconsistencies in the "societal perspective" on costs of the Panel on Cost-Effectiveness in Health and Medicine. *Med Decis Making* 19 (4):371–377.

Meltzer, D. O., C. E. Weckerle, and L. M. Chang. 1999. Do people consider financial effects in answering quality of life questions? *Med Decis Making* 19 (3):517.

Mushlin, A. I., and L. Fintor. 1992. Is screening for breast cancer cost-effective? *Cancer* 69 (7 Suppl):1957–1962.

Mutchler, J. E., J. A. Burr, and F. G. Caro. 2003. From paid worker to volunteer: leaving the paid workforce and volunteering in later life. *Soc Forces* 81 (4):1267–1293.

National Institute for Health and Care Excellence (NICE). 2011. *Trabectedine for the Treatment of Relapsed Ovarian Cancer. April 2011. NICE technology appraisal guidance [TA222]*. London: NICE. http://www.nice.org.uk/guidance/ta222.

Newhouse, J. P. 2001. Medical Care Price Indices: Problems and Opportunities/The Chung-Hua Lectures. National Bureau of Economic Research Working Paper Series No. 8168. March 2001. DOI: 10.3386/w8168. http://www.nber.org/papers/w8168.

Nimrod, G., M. C. Janke, and D. A. Kleiber. 2008. Expanding, reducing, concentrating and diffusing: activity patterns of recent retirees in the United States. *Leisure Sciences* 31 (1):37–52.

Nyman, J. A. 2004. Should the consumption of survivors be included as a cost in cost-utility analysis? *Health Econ* 13 (5):417–427.

Nyman, J. A. 2011. Measurement of QALYS and the welfare implications of survivor consumption and leisure forgone. *Health Econ* 20 (1):56–67.

O'Hagan, A., and J. W. Stevens. 2004. On estimators of medical costs with censored data. *J Health Econ* 23 (3):615–625.

Polsky, D., and A. Basu. 2012. "Selection Bias in Observational Data." In *The Elgar Companion to Health Economics*, 2nd ed, edited by A. M. Jones, 490–501. Cheltenham, UK; and Northampton, MA: Edward Elgar Publishing, Inc.

Raikou, M., and A. McGuire. 2004. Estimating medical care costs under conditions of censoring. *J Health Econ* 23 (3):443–470.

Rappange, D. R., P. H. van Baal, N. J. van Exel, T. L. Feenstra, F. F. Rutten, and W. B. Brouwer. 2008. Unrelated medical costs in life-years gained: should they be included in economic evaluations of healthcare interventions? *Pharmacoeconomics* 26 (10):815–830.

Ruger, J. P., and M. Reiff. 2015. Protocol for Development of a Checklist for the Conduct, Reporting and Appraisal of Micro-costing Studies in Health Care. Working paper [unpublished].

Ruger, J. P., M. C. Weinstein, S. K. Hammond, M. H. Kearney, and K. M. Emmons. 2008. Cost-effectiveness of motivational interviewing for smoking cessation and relapse prevention among low-income pregnant women: a randomized controlled trial. *Value Health* 11 (2):191–198.

Russell, L. B. 1986. *Is Prevention Better Than Cure?* Washington, DC: The Brookings Institution.

Russell, L. B. 2009. Completing costs: patients' time. *Med Care* 47 (7 Suppl 1):S89–S93.

Sculpher, M. 2013. "Can a life-extending drug be cost-ineffective even if offered for free? The curious economics of costs in added years of life." ISPOR Issues Panel, New Orleans, May 2013. http://www.ispor.org/meetings/neworleans0513/releasedpresentations/IP2_Mark_Sculpher.pdf.

Sculpher, M. J., and B. J. O'Brien. 2000. Income effects of reduced health and health effects of reduced income: implications for health-state valuation. *Med Decis Making* 20 (2):207–215.

Sendi, P., and W. B. Brouwer. 2005. Is silence golden? A test of the incorporation of the effects of ill-health on income and leisure in health state valuations. *Health Econ* 14 (6):643–647.

Shiroiwa, T., T. Fukuda, S. Ikeda, and K. Shimozuma. 2013. QALY and productivity loss: empirical evidence for "double counting." *Value Health* 16 (4):581–587.

Shrestha, R. K., S. L. Sansom, and P. G. Farnham. 2012. Comparison of methods for estimating the cost of human immunodeficiency virus-testing interventions. *J Public Health Manag Pract* 18 (3):259–267.

Sianesi, B., and J. Van Reenen. 2002. The returns to education: a review of the empirical macroeconomic literature. IFS Working Papers W02/05. Institute for Fiscal Studies: London, UK. http://www.ifs.org.uk/publications/2016. DOI: 10.1920/wp.ifs.2002.0205.

Starrett, D. A. 1988. *Foundations of Public Economics*. New York: Cambridge University Press.

Stephens, J. M., B. Handke, and J. A. Doshi. 2012. International survey of methods used in health technology assessment (HTA): does practice meet the principles proposed for good research? *Comp Eff Res* 2:29–44.

Stinnett, A. A., and J. Mullahy. 1998. Net health benefits: a new framework for the analysis of uncertainty in cost-effectiveness analysis. *Med Decis Making* 18 (2 Suppl):S68–S80.

Tax Policy Center. 2013. "Table T13-0174: Average Effective Federal Tax Rates by Filing Status; by Expanded Cash Income Percentile, 2014. Preliminary Results, July 25, 2013." http://www.taxpolicycenter.org/numbers/displayatab.cfm?DocID=3933.

Tilling, C., M. Krol, A. Tsuchiya, J. Brazier, and W. Brouwer. 2010. In or out? Income losses in health state valuations: a review. *Value Health* 13 (2):298–305.

van Asselt, A. D., C. D. Dirksen, A. Arntz, and J. L. Severens. 2008. Difficulties in calculating productivity costs: work disability associated with borderline personality disorder. *Value Health* 11 (4):637–644.

Weaver, M. R., C. J. Conover, R. J. Proescholdbell, P. S. Arno, A. Ang, K. K. Uldall, and S. L. Ettner. 2009. Cost-effectiveness analysis of integrated care for people with HIV, chronic mental illness and substance abuse disorders. *J Ment Health Policy Econ* 12 (1):33–46.

Weinstein, M. C., and W. G. Manning, Jr. 1997. Theoretical issues in cost-effectiveness analysis. *J Health Econ* 16 (1):121–128.

Weinstein, M. C., J. E. Siegel, A. M. Garber, J. Lipscomb, B. R. Luce, W. G. Manning, Jr., and G. W. Torrance. 1997. Productivity costs, time costs and health-related quality of life: a response to the Erasmus Group. *Health Econ* 6 (5):505–510.

Weinstein, M. C., and W. B. Stason. 1977. Foundations of cost-effectiveness analysis for health and medical practices. *N Engl J Med* 296 (13):716–721.

World Health Organization. 2003. Making Choices in Health: WHO Guide to Cost-Effectiveness Analysis. Geneva, Switzerland: WHO. www.who.int/choice/publications/p_2003_generalised_cea.pdf.

Yabroff, K. R., and Y. Kim. 2009. Time costs associated with informal caregiving for cancer survivors. *Cancer* 115 (18 Suppl):4362–4373.

Zarkin, G. A., J. W. Bray, A. Aldridge, M. Mills, R. A. Cisler, D. Couper, J. R. McKay, and S. O'Malley. 2010. The effect of alcohol treatment on social costs of alcohol dependence: results from the COMBINE study. *Med Care* 48 (5):396–401.

9

Evidence Synthesis for Informing Cost-Effectiveness Analysis

Thomas A. Trikalinos, Louise B. Russell,
and Gillian D. Sanders

9.1 INTRODUCTION

Chapter 4 described the elements that organize a cost-effectiveness analysis (CEA): the objective of the analysis, the interventions to be analyzed and compared, the target population, the time horizon, and so forth. That framework begins to establish the data needed for the analysis. Chapter 6 then laid out the kinds of health and non-health outcomes and costs that might be considered as the framework is developed into a detailed analytical plan, and discussed the types of data that can be used for each category. This chapter continues with evidence synthesis for informing CEAs. Throughout, we refer to CEAs that use simulation modeling to quantify, value, and aggregate consequences using data from different sources because these are more common than CEAs based on a single source. However, the concepts discussed here apply more generally to all CEAs.

In the process of developing a CEA model, after choices about model structure have been made, the analysts will be called upon to interpret, adjust, and synthesize empirical data from various sources to justify the model structure and to estimate model parameters. By maximizing the use of available data, it is possible to minimize bias and increases the likelihood of arriving at a high-quality decision.

All approaches to evidence synthesis involve pre-analytical, analytical, and post-analytical phases. In the pre-analytical phase one defines a question and identifies pertinent data from distinct sources. In the analytical phase (synthesis proper), one *posits and learns* relationships across data from distinct sources. In the post-analytical phase one *conjectures* on the implications of the learned relationships for the question at hand.

Informing CEAs using the totality of relevant information increases the likelihood of high-quality decisions. Thus, ideally, CEAs should be rigorous and systematic in identifying, assessing, synthesizing, and interpreting evidence (National Institute for Health and Care Excellence [NICE] 2013), but in, practice, they often are not. In this chapter, we discuss evidence synthesis approaches that have matured and evolved within the evidence-based medicine (EBM) movement and beyond. We propose a systematic process for evidence synthesis in the context of a CEA, which builds on current guidance for systematic reviews and meta-analyses but then departs from it, because evidence synthesis to inform CEAs has specific goals and needs, as explained below.

9.2 HOW DOES EVIDENCE SYNTHESIS INFORM CEA MODEL PARAMETERS?

We subscribe to the maxim that informing CEA models using the totality of relevant information increases the likelihood of making high-quality decisions. What we know in health and medicine we know from empirical data, and thus modeling of health and healthcare should be grounded in empirical data.

Here we introduce the concept of an *evidence synthesis model* for use in CEA. An evidence synthesis model is analogous to a regression model that describes the distribution of data points that, most commonly, are summary statistics from individual studies but that can also include individual participant data (Riley et al. 2008) and even experts' input, appropriately elicited (Garthwaite, Kadane, and O'Hagan 2005; O'Hagan et al. 2006). We present evidence synthesis (meta-analytical) models through a regression framework in Section 9.5. The evidence synthesis model is *learned* from the data, that is, its parameters are estimated by fitting the model to the available data points.

Even more generally, the evidence synthesis model can be rolled into the CEA model, so that estimation of CEA model parameters and calculation of aggregate measures such as the incremental cost-effectiveness ratio (ICER) happen simultaneously. In that case the evidence synthesis model and the CEA model are one and the same, and calibration of CEA model parameters to external data is a form of evidence synthesis, as it amounts to estimation of CEA/evidence synthesis model parameters. For examples, see Eddy (1989); Eddy, Hasselblad, and Shachter (1992); Cooper et al. (2004); and Sutton et al. (2008).

Figure 9.1 outlines our conceptualization of the role of evidence synthesis in the context of a CEA. In brief, informing the value of a parameter in the CEA model amounts to (1) learning an evidence synthesis model that describes the relationship between study characteristics and study estimates that are free of bias and (2) using the evidence synthesis model to predict the value of the parameter of interest in the context of the CEA model.

9.2.1 Accounting for Bias in Study Estimates

The conceptual outline in Figure 9.1 requires that the analysts make judgments about the magnitude and direction of bias in each study, and that they adjust (correct) study estimates for the quantified bias. Every CEA or decision model includes implicit or explicit accounting for bias in study estimates. The most common way to account for

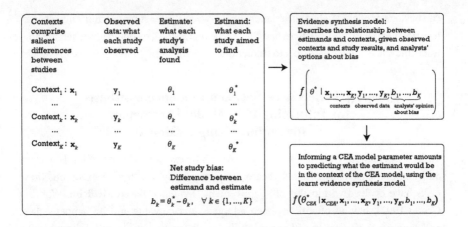

Figure 9.1 Conceptual representation of the role of evidence synthesis in cost-effectiveness analyses (CEAs). Informing model parameters from data implies learning an evidence model that describes how the observed study results relate to salient characteristics of the study's context. The K information sources (studies) are identified in the pre-analytical phase of the evidence synthesis, when judgments about the bias in each study are also made. Learning the evidence synthesis model, and making predictions about the quantity of interest in the context of the CEA, are part of the analytical phase. Incorporating the quantities of interest θ^*_{CEA} in the CEA model, and doing sensitivity and stability analyses, are part of the post-analytical phase of evidence synthesis.

bias is to limit the evidence base to studies that are deemed to be at low risk of bias and to make no further explicit adjustments. In the framework of Figure 9.1, this is equivalent to quantifying the bias in each study as having a magnitude of zero and a variance of zero. An alternative way to think about it is that, by excluding studies that are deemed to be at high risk of bias, analysts assume that the corresponding bias terms have infinite variance, which essentially cancels those studies' contribution in the likelihood function of the evidence synthesis model.

Alternatively, analysts may opt to include in the evidence base studies deemed to have different risks of bias, quantify the magnitude and variance of bias in each study, and incorporate these quantifications in the likelihood of the evidence synthesis model (Turner et al. 2009). While we prefer that all adjustments for bias are made formally in the evidence synthesis model, we are comfortable with implicit adjustments (e.g., by limiting the evidence synthesis only to studies at low risk of bias), as long as all decisions are transparent and explicit in the exposition of the CEA model.

9.2.2 Accounting for Non-Transferability from the Study Context to the CEA Context

By nature, the parameter value that will be used in the CEA model is conditional on the context of the CEA model, but study estimates do not necessarily transfer across contexts. The differences in the context between the studies and the CEA model should always be accounted for. Analogously to the aforementioned adjustments for bias, this can be done explicitly (when the relationship between study estimands and study characteristics is explicitly modeled, perhaps in a meta-regression), or implicitly, when the analysts limit the evidence base only to studies that have the same context as the CEA model.

9.2.3 Differences Between Evidence Synthesis for Informing CEA Model Parameters vs for Summarizing Evidence

Tasks for evidence synthesis to inform CEAs can be executed at varying levels of rigor and comprehensiveness. In healthcare applications, approaches to executing these tasks have evolved within the EBM movement (Evidence-Based Medicine Working Group 1992), having oftentimes been adopted on face-value and by happenstance, and sometimes rigorously and purposefully (Djulbegovic, Guyatt, and Ashcroft 2009; Trikalinos et al. 2013).

Our outlook on evidence synthesis for modeling is congruent with EBM's tenet to minimize bias through systematic, comprehensive, and transparent approaches, but it differs from traditional conceptualizations of systematic reviews in several important ways. These differences imply deviations from standard guidance on how to perform standalone systematic reviews and meta-analyses, which are explained in the following paragraphs (Sections 9.2.3.1 through 9.2.3.6).

9.2.3.1 *Differences in the Acceptable Degree of Comprehensiveness in Evidence Synthesis*

Authors of traditional systematic reviews generally focus on carefully defined questions of clinical efficacy and go to great lengths to identify and include eligible studies, aiming to minimize bias and increase statistical precision in estimating summary effects (Centre for Reviews and Dissemination 2009; Chandler et al. 2013; Chang et al. 2012; Eden et al. 2011; Slutsky et al. 2010). Thus, they run sensitive searches, often in multiple databases, to identify published (and often unpublished) studies. However, in the context of a CEA, analysts may have to conduct evidence syntheses for several parameters, and it may not be practical to be as comprehensive in identifying evidence. Section 9.4.2.1 expands on this difference and proposes workable solutions.

9.2.3.2 *Differences in the Goal of Evidence Synthesis: Description vs Prediction*

The primary goal of standalone systematic reviews is to describe diversity in the characteristics of eligible studies, summarize study findings and limitations, and describe the statistical heterogeneity in study results. Standalone systematic reviews do not always include a quantitative synthesis (meta-analysis). Further, even when a meta-analysis is conducted, the evidence synthesis makes only qualitative statements about biases and non-transferability (applicability) of the findings of individual studies.

By contrast, an evidence synthesis coupled with a CEA is intended to provide a prediction of the parameter of interest in the CEA model context, and it must adjust explicitly for study biases and characteristics of the context. A detailed discussion is provided in Sections 9.5 and 9.7.

9.2.3.3 Differences Regarding Synthesizing Data Across Different Study Designs

Another more specific difference arises for intervention effects. To minimize bias, standalone systematic reviews avoid combining estimates of intervention effects across different study designs (Higgins and Green 2011). The rationale is that, compared to randomized designs, nonrandomized studies are more susceptible to confounding bias. In evidence synthesis for CEAs, the use of models allows the analyst to adopt a more inclusive attitude toward evidence, and to combine information across different study designs with approaches that either model bias (Eddy, Hasselblad, and Shachter 1990; Kaizar 2006, 2015) or correct for bias (Greenland 2005; Lash et al. 2014). We discuss these considerations in Section 9.4.2.

9.2.3.4 Differences Regarding the Need to Grade the "Strength of the Evidence"

Current standards for (standalone) systematic reviews encourage grading the "strength of evidence," usually summarized into categories such as "high," "moderate," or "low" (Agency for Healthcare Research and Quality 2014; Chandler et al. 2013; Eden et al. 2011). These strength of evidence assessments are a qualitative aggregation of judgments about the likelihood that the results of the evidence synthesis are unbiased, applicable (transferable) to the setting of interest, and clinically important. Within a decision analytic framework of CEA, while we encourage an analytical description and critique of the studies in the evidence base (Chapter 6), we discourage traditional strength of evidence gradings because these gradings are explicitly done through the evidence synthesis model and the CEA model.

9.2.3.5 Differences in the Statistical Modeling for Evidence Synthesis

Standalone systematic reviews tend to use relatively simple analysis models when meta-analyses are undertaken. By contrast, evidence synthesis modeling in the context of a CEA model may have to account for complexities that mandate use of advanced modeling, as discussed in Section 9.5. In evidence synthesis for CEA models, the CEA model itself can be seen as the evidence synthesis/analytic machinery (Cooper et al. 2004; Eddy 1989; Eddy, Hasselblad, and Shachter 1992; Sutton et al. 2008).

9.2.3.6 *Differences in the Relative Emphasis Placed on Objectivity vs Transparency*

In standalone systematic reviews, objectivity and transparency are emphasized equally. We argue that for evidence syntheses that aim to inform CEA models, transparency is more attainable than objectivity. With no exception, analysts performing CEAs will have to make choices about which data sources to use, how to synthesize data from various sources, and whether and how to adjust data that are not directly applicable to the decision context of the CEA, or that come from studies with problems in their design, conduct, or analysis. It is not possible to be purely objective in this process. Subjectivity, however, is not arbitrariness. The CEA should be planned and executed systematically, subjective choices should be justified or at least motivated, their impact should be explored, and the whole process should be adequately documented. Transparency is an attainable goal.

9.2.4 Development of Guidance for Evidence Synthesis for Informing CEAs

We repurpose the extensive existing guidance for systematic reviews in healthcare to account for the differences outlined above.

Numerous standards and good practice recommendations exist for evidence synthesis in healthcare and beyond. Examples include the Institute of Medicine's (IOM's) 21 standards and 82 elements of performance for publicly funded systematic reviews (Eden et al. 2011), as well as guidance from programs and initiatives that perform systematic reviews worldwide, such as the Cochrane Collaboration (Chandler et al. 2013), the Agency for Healthcare Research and Quality (AHRQ) Effective Health Care Program (Agency for Healthcare Research and Quality 2014; Chang et al. 2012; Chou et al. 2010; Helfand and Balshem 2010; Owens et al. 2010; Slutsky et al. 2010; Whitlock et al. 2010), and the Centre for Reviews and Dissemination (Centre for Reviews and Dissemination 2009). The Patient-Centered Outcomes Research Institute (PCORI) fully adopts the IOM and AHRQ recommendations (PCORI [Patient-Centered Outcomes Research Institute] Methodology Committee 2013).

We build upon this foundation with recommendations specific to systematic reviews that aim to inform CEAs. Not all of the proposed recommendations are of equal importance, validity, and feasibility. Authors of CEAs are expected to use systematic evidence synthesis approaches (National Institute for Health and Care Excellence [NICE] 2013), but generally they do not. In the remainder of this chapter (Sections 9.3 through 9.10), we describe the process of evidence synthesis for CEA, which differs from standard systematic review practice, as discussed in Section 9.2.3. Our recommendations for good practices are listed at the end of the chapter (Section 9.11). Most correspond to important deviations from the standard guidance. Thus, our overarching recommendation is that analysts should follow established guidance on systematic reviews and meta-analyses, modified as indicated in **Recommendation 1**.

9.3 OVERVIEW OF EVIDENCE SYNTHESIS

The process of evidence synthesis for informing CEA model inputs can be described in three phases. The *pre-analytical phase* includes the tasks of assembling the evidence synthesis team, defining the target question, identifying evidence, and extracting information. This phase is very similar to the pre-analytical phases of standalone systematic reviews and meta-analyses.

In the *analytical phase* the analysts obtain estimates for the target CEA model parameters. The relevant tasks are these: conducting a quantitative synthesis of information; assessing risk of bias and accounting for potential bias; and assessing the transferability of study estimates to the CEA setting and accounting for potential non-transferability.

In the *post-analytical phase* the modelers will use the (adjusted) estimates in the model and report the process and miscellanea, including sensitivity analyses. The post-analytical phase is therefore part of the modeling exercise. Not all evidence syntheses conducted to inform CEAs will be published as standalone systematic reviews. If such a publication is desirable, then the systematic review should follow existing guidance for reporting systematic reviews and meta-analyses (e.g., the Preferred Reporting Items for Systematic Reviews and Meta-Analyses [PRISMA] by Moher et al. 2009, for systematic reviews of interventions). In practice, a standalone systematic review would probably focus on describing the existing studies and describing and explaining between-study diversity. Most often it would synthesize studies and qualify their findings for bias or non-transferability without attempting to correct for the latter, although exceptional examples exist (Manzi et al. 2011).

The aforementioned tasks can be performed at varying levels of rigor. In the next section we introduce the concept of the importance of CEA model parameters; for parameters that are *not important*, it may be justifiable to do non-comprehensive searches, and to forgo corrections for bias or non-transferability. For parameters that are *important*, however, it is difficult to justify anything short of a comprehensive approach.

9.4 PRE-ANALYTICAL CONSIDERATIONS

The prevailing guidance on the pre-analytical phase of systematic reviews, summarized in Table 9.1, generally applies to the evidence syntheses that aim to inform CEAs.

9.4.1 Evidence Synthesis Team and Goals

9.4.1.1 The Evidence Synthesis Team

9.4.1.1.1 Expertise

The evidence synthesis, model development, and analysis teams may overlap fully, in part, or not at all. From the evidence synthesis perspective, the team should include or have access to researchers with good knowledge of, and preferably experience and expertise in, literature identification, study design, statistics, and meta-analysis.

Table 9.1 Pre-analytical phase: salient points from the Institute of Medicine Guidance (Eden et al. 2011) and our discussion

IOM #	IOM recommendation	Practical advice for a CEA
Initiating a systematic review: the review team		
2.1	Establish a team with appropriate expertise and experience to conduct the systematic review	Seek advice from clinical experts, librarians, and others as necessary to supplement the expertise on the CEA team
2.2	Manage bias and conflict of interest (COI) of the team conducting the systematic review	Ask members of the research team, and those consulted by the team, to disclose potential biases. Include a statement listing any potential biases in the report of the analysis.
2.3	Ensure user and stakeholder input as the review is designed and conducted	
2.4	Manage bias and COI for individuals providing input into the systematic review	
Initiating a systematic review: the review protocol		
2.5	Formulate the topic for the systematic review	Prepare a written protocol stating the parameters(s) addressed, eligibility criteria for studies, databases to search, and procedures for searching them; include the data extraction form.
2.6	Develop a systematic review protocol	
2.7	Submit the protocol for peer review	
2.8	Make the final protocol publicly available, and add any amendments to the protocol in a timely fashion	Make the written protocol available to reviewers and editors.
Finding and assessing individual studies		
3.1	Conduct a comprehensive systematic search for evidence	Conduct a comprehensive systematic search for evidence following the written protocol.
3.2	Take action to address potentially biased reporting of research results	
3.3	Screen and select studies	Screen and select studies according to the written protocol.
3.4	Document the search	Document databases searched and terms used in the report. Prepare a PRISMA flow chart.
3.5	Manage data collection	Complete the data extraction form for each study. **Best**: two reviewers independently extract data for each study and compare forms. **Acceptable**: second reviewer checks a sample of studies.
3.6	Critically appraise each study	The data extraction form should include details on study design, population, and other features that reflect study quality.

Abbreviations: IOM = Institute of Medicine; CEA = cost-effectiveness analysis; PRISMA = Preferred Reporting Items for Systematic Reviews and Meta-Analyses.

Analysts conducting CEAs often have developed experience in, for example, literature searches or meta-analysis; alternatively, consultations with experts—for example, librarians or statisticians, respectively—can suffice.

If different teams are responsible for evidence synthesis and model development, special emphasis should be given to coordinating these elements, because the focus of the evidence synthesis will be determined by choices made during model development (**Recommendation 2**). At the same time, evidence synthesis findings can influence structural and other modeling choices. For example, if no data exist on the modification of the treatment effect by a clinical subgroup, then the analysts may opt not to model the subgroup, effectively marginalizing (integrating over) the subgroup-defining variables. If data exist, the modeling decisions (Graham et al. 2011) may be different. Reciprocally, if there is evidence of differential treatment effects across subgroups, modeling the subgroup effects opens up the possibility of performing subgroup-specific analyses. Thus, ideally, model development and evidence synthesis are concurrent and highly interlinked processes.

This interlinkage is automatically achieved when the same analysts develop the CEA model and perform the evidence synthesis. Otherwise, a substantive and integral coordination must be ensured. Coordination can be facilitated if members of the evidence synthesis and CEA modeling teams are familiar with both tasks; if the teams overlap partially; and if projects are managed in such a way that related tasks are advanced in parallel, with adequate communication between teams.

9.4.1.1.2 Disclosure and management of potential conflicts of interest

As discussed in Chapter 13, all members of the CEA team, including those doing the evidence synthesis, must disclose potential financial and non-financial conflicts of interest (Eden et al. 2011; Graham et al. 2011). Disclosures should be given by everyone whose input can affect the conclusions of the CEA. The goal is to manage important conflicts of interest, and this does not necessarily require excluding from the project those who disclose conflicts. It is not uncommon for the most sought-out consultants to have conflicts, and excluding them might result in loss of valuable input. Conflicts can be managed by including experts with competing interests or by ensuring that determination of the final decisions (and the responsibility for them) lies with unconflicted team members.

9.4.1.2 *Prioritizing Which Parameters to Assess with Evidence Synthesis (Formulating the Evidence Synthesis Questions)*

Because of resource constraints, analysts will have to decide which parameters are important enough to prioritize for evidence synthesis, and how comprehensive to be about each step of the evidence synthesis process. The set of important parameters may be revised as the team learns more about the literature and the topic, and as the model's structure and parameterization matures. No hard-and-fast rules exist for prioritizing parameters for evidence synthesis. Analysts should make decisions on a case-by-case basis, guided by the following principles (**Recommendation 3**): Important parameters are those that are (1) influential on model results or (2) critical to the (perceived) validity of the model.

9.4.1.2.1 Parameters that are influential in a quantitative sense

Experienced analysts often have intuition about which parameters will greatly influence model results. We define as influential parameters that, when varied, change the model output substantially or fast (Box 9.1). Especially for simpler models, analysts can accurately predict which parameters will be influential, and thus prioritize them for evidence synthesis with some confidence. For more complex models, however, a formal quantitative sensitivity analysis may be required. This implies that a (preliminary) version of the model is available, and that model development and evidence synthesis proceed in parallel and iteratively. The structure of the preliminary model should be as close to that of the final model as is feasible, and its (preliminary) parameter inputs should have values that are accurate to the best of the analysts' knowledge. The preliminary model can then be run to determine the influential parameters and guide their selection for evidence synthesis. As the model is being revised (in terms of structure, or as better estimates for some parameters become available), the ranking of parameters in terms of influence can change.

9.4.1.2.2 Parameters that are critical to the validity or perceived validity of the model

Some parameters may be perceived as critical for the validity of the model, irrespective of whether they are influential on results in one or more of the ways defined in Box 9.1. For example, many treatments for cancer have a small effect on life expectancy, which may correspond to an even smaller effect on quality-adjusted survival. Even if the treatment effect is not an influential variable in the analysis, it may still be desirable to obtain good estimates about the treatment effect in a CEA. Candidate parameters that may be deemed important in a contextual sense are those that correspond directly to the question examined by the CEA, such as treatment effects, test performance measures, and patient preferences. Engaging stakeholders during the framing of the CEA can help identify such parameters, and thus guide the evidence synthesis. The obvious exception is when the CEA is meant as a sensitivity analysis that aims to document that even implausible values of the parameters of interest would be unlikely to result in a decision change.

9.4.1.3 Selecting Empirical Data

Analysts should include in the evidence base studies that meet protocol-defined eligibility criteria (see Section 9.4.1.5). Briefly, these criteria define characteristics of the context in which the study was done, the study sample, the measurements, and aspects of the design. For example, for studies assessing measures of effect, the eligibility

Box 9.1 Influential Parameters Can Be Defined in Various Ways

More accurately, the degree of "influence" of parameters can be defined in various ways (Rabitz 1984).

- Global influence refers to how much the output of the model varies when the parameter *is changed over a predefined sensitivity analysis interval.*
- Local influence refers to how fast the output varies for *infinitesimal perturbations of the parameter at a given parameter value.* For deterministic parameters, local influence relates to a partial derivative (or differential) of the output with respect to the parameter at hand. For stochastic parameters, it relates to the corresponding functional derivative (or functional differential) (Rabitz 1984).

A parameter can be influential globally, locally, or both.

The precise definition of the influence of a parameter on model output is related to sensitivity analysis concepts, and requires (at least a preliminary version of) the model to be available.

The value of information analyses discussed in Chapter 11—specifically, the expected value of perfect parameter information (EVPPI)—can identify parameters that have a bearing on the *uncertainty around the expected cost and effectiveness* in a CEA. It is likely—but not necessary—that parameters that have high Expected Value of Partial Perfect Information (EVPPI) will also have large local or global influence. The concepts behind the above definitions of the influence of parameters and of value of information analyses are distinct.

criteria define the population, compared interventions or exposure levels, and outcomes (Counsell 1997).

Selecting data sources for model parameters should be guided by epidemiological and statistical principles. Chapter 6 discusses which study designs can be used to obtain estimates for measures of exposure, effect, test performance, preference weights, and costs.

We maintain an inclusive outlook toward evidence from different sources, and we even consider synthesizing information obtained from different study designs if it represents the best pertinent evidence.

9.4.1.4 *Using Existing Research Syntheses vs Producing De Novo Ones*

Substantial economy of resources can be achieved by using existing systematic reviews or meta-analyses. Key considerations when examining whether and how to use existing systematic reviews or meta-analyses pertain to whether the systematic review/meta-analysis can provide the needed parameter estimates, and whether it is current and was well-conducted. By considering these issues, CEA analysts can select which systematic review/meta-analysis to utilize (if more than one exist), and how to utilize it.

9.4.1.4.1 Assessing whether an existing systematic review/meta-analysis can provide the needed parameter estimates

It is possible that an existing systematic review/meta-analysis provides an estimate of the parameter of interest. If the review is deemed current and well-conducted, the appropriate meta-analytic result can be used directly. For example, suppose that the CEA model parameter that we wish to inform is the average treatment effect of bypass surgery versus optimal medical treatment in older women with diabetes who have received the intended treatment (the average treatment effect on the treated). However, more often than not, the summary result from a systematic review/meta-analysis does not correspond directly to the parameter estimate.

The most common reason for a lack of correspondence is that the systematic review result pertains to a different population, intervention, or outcome. In the example presented here, the systematic review may only summarize intention-to-treat results irrespective of patient age, sex, or diabetic status, but the CEA model may require the average effect on treated older women with diabetes. We refer to this concept as the non-transferability (non-generalizability) of the estimate of the systematic review. Chapter 6 expands on assessments of the transferability of study estimates for various types of parameters.

Another reason for a lack of correspondence is that all studies in the systematic review may have overt problems and high likelihood of bias. Most systematic reviews do not aim to correct estimates for bias, but estimates of model parameters should be free of bias, necessitating some correction.

The last reason for a lack of correspondence pertains to the statistic that must be obtained to inform the CEA model parameter. As we discuss in Section 9.5, we require a prediction of the value of the parameter in the context of the CEA model based on the evidence synthesis model and the results of the synthesized studies. Typically, systematic reviews and meta-analyses do not report such statistics, and they may have to be re-analyzed to obtain those data.

However, even when a result from an existing systematic review or meta-analysis cannot be used directly, substantial economy of resources can still be achieved by re-using parts of an existing systematic review.

9.4.1.4.2 Assessing whether a systematic review/meta-analysis is current and well-conducted

Judging whether a systematic review is current is straightforward by examining whether the search period is recent enough for the topic at hand.

Judging whether a systematic review is well-conducted is more complicated. While fatal flaws (e.g., a naïve search that returns implausibly few papers) can be identified easily, it is not easy to distinguish well-done from not-so-well-done systematic reviews. Using source as a proxy for rigor (NICE, AHRQ) offers at best modest assurance. Tools such as the Assessment of Multiple Systematic Reviews (AMSTAR) aim to assess the likelihood that a systematic review will generate unbiased results

(Shea et al. 2007). AMSTAR focuses on items related to how the systematic review was planned (presence of a protocol); how data were identified (comprehensiveness of literature search, double and independent study identification and data extraction); ways data were assessed (assessment of risk of bias, assessment of likelihood of publication bias); approaches to data synthesis (appropriateness of synthesis methods), and means of reporting (availability of included and excluded reference citations). Because they rely on the published systematic review report, AMSTAR and similar tools (Kung et al. 2010) assess both the comprehensiveness of a systematic review and the reporting (writing) skills of its authors. Such tools can perhaps be of use in identifying overt problems in systematic reviews.

9.4.1.4.3 Re-using parts of existing systematic reviews

The analysts may opt to use study-level data reported in the systematic review to conduct the analyses they need (e.g., subgroup analyses or adjustments for bias or non-transferability). An out-of-date systematic review can be updated efficiently, using the original search strategy and focusing only on the data of interest. Alternatively, the systematic review can be used as a compendium of relevant studies, which can be retrieved in full text and assessed and analyzed in detail.

9.4.1.4.4 What to do when multiple systematic reviews exist

When many systematic reviews exist, it may be more time consuming to sort out the differences between them than to perform a focused analysis de novo. Provided that existing systematic reviews agree in their conclusions, one approach is to select a recent review that most closely corresponds to the parameter of interest, and proceed from there as described above. If the reviews disagree, it is likely that they differ in the questions they address, and these differences should be understood to select the review that most closely corresponds to the CEA parameter of interest.

9.4.1.5 *The Evidence Synthesis Protocol*

An a priori developed protocol is important because it involves planning the evidence synthesis, which can help anticipate potential problems; promote transparency; and discourage haphazard selection of studies and extraction of data. To this end, authors of systematic reviews are encouraged to register their protocols online prospectively. The Preferred Standards for Reporting of Systematic Reviews and Meta-analysis Protocols (PRISMA-P) group has developed standards for evidence synthesis protocols (Shamseer et al. 2015).

We adopt existing guidance for systematic reviews (Agency for Healthcare Research and Quality 2014; Centre for Reviews and Dissemination 2009; Chandler et al. 2013; Eden et al. 2011; Shamseer et al. 2015; Slutsky et al. 2010) and suggest that a protocol for evidence synthesis in a CEA should (1) state and explain which parameter estimates will be obtained with evidence synthesis, along with the rationale for the selection; (2) list and justify eligibility criteria for studies (e.g., patient population, interventions evaluated, health outcomes measured); (3) specify study identification tasks (e.g., which database, draft search strategy, and process for citation screening); (4) describe the data extraction procedures to be followed; (5) list data extraction items; (6) describe the approach for the analytic phase of the evidence synthesis; and (7) describe whether and how the evidence synthesis will deal with suspected biases in the individual study results and in the meta-analysis results, and with meta-analysis estimates that are not directly transferable to the CEA model setting.

The protocol is a record of the decisions made by the research team at the outset of the review. As the review unfolds it may be necessary to revisit one or more of those decisions. For example, studies may report outcomes in unanticipated ways. Important changes should be recorded in the protocol. At the end of the review the protocol provides a complete record of the initial decisions and changes in those decisions. For most CEAs, we believe that the protocol for the evidence synthesis need not be a stand-alone document that is accessible to non-experts. A relatively short exposition with crisp and precise descriptions can be entirely satisfactory. The evidence synthesis protocol is a component of (or addendum to) the protocol of the CEA itself. Chapter 13 provides details about the protocol of the CEA.

9.4.2 Identifying and Extracting Information

9.4.2.1 Identifying Relevant Evidence

Standards for systematic reviews emphasize the importance of being comprehensive in the searching stage. For example, IOM and Cochrane's Methodological Expectations of Cochrane Intervention Reviews (MECIR) standards suggest that searches should be as extensive as possible and that, depending on the subject, it may also be appropriate to search national, regional, or subject databases; trial registries like ClinicalTrials.gov and the World Health Organization's (WHO's) International Clinical Trials Registry Platform; and databases of theses, reports, and conference abstracts (Chandler et al. 2013). See Chapter 3 of Eden et al. (2011, 81–154) for more information.

The degree of rigor in this step is a matter of pecuniary calculation: for most CEA models, it is unrealistic to demand exhaustive searches for all model parameters that are informed by empirical data. A workable compromise may be to expend more effort in identifying evidence for important parameters (those that are most influential or critical for the perceived validity of the model) and accept a less comprehensive treatise of other parameters.

We first review the aims and attributes of a comprehensive search, and we then propose principles for operationalizing less comprehensive, but "good-enough" searches.

9.4.2.1.1 What constitutes a comprehensive search?

A comprehensive study identification process has three aims. The first is to *maximize the information included in the evidence synthesis* by identifying as many relevant studies as possible. The second is to *minimize selection bias in the identified evidence base* by searching across multiple sources. Selection bias in the evidence base can occur if a study's findings determine the probability that a study is published (publication bias) (Rothstein, Sutton, and Borenstein 2005), included in a specific database (database bias) (Egger and Smith 1998), or reported in English or another language (language bias) (Juni et al. 2002), among other things. A third aim is to *enhance the face validity of the evidence synthesis.*

The terms used in the search will usually specify the health condition or population of interest, the interventions being evaluated, and eligible study designs. As an example, to identify randomized controlled trials (RCTs) of interventions, standard guidance suggests at minimum expert electronic searches of PubMed/MEDLINE, Embase, and the Cochrane Central Register of Controlled Trials (a database that also includes studies identified by hand-searching a large number of journals), as well as searches of the "grey" literature (Chandler et al. 2013; Eden et al. 2011). The latter can include, for example, unpublished studies, dissertations, dossiers prepared for federal agencies. Specialized databases also exist and should be considered where appropriate. For example, the Cumulative Index to Nursing and Allied Health Literature (CINAHL) indexes study reports on nursing. Behavioral and psychological interventions are often indexed in the Psychological Information Database (PyscINFO), and the Education Resources Information Center (ERIC) database indexes educational interventions.

Expert searches require knowledge of the available databases, their indexing schemes, and the syntax for querying them, and they can take time to finalize. Expert searches typically return anywhere from a thousand citations to tens of thousands of citations (e.g., 1,000 to over 20,000, depending on the topic), of which only a few hundred (e.g., between 2% and 20%) may be reviewed in full text, and only a few dozen may be finally eligible.

9.4.2.1.2 Practical approaches for a "good-enough" search

Instead of designing de novo searches, CEA analysts can start from the literature identified in existing systematic reviews that address the same question or a broader question.

Alternatively, and for common diseases and interventions, it may suffice to examine studies published in English and indexed in a major database, such as PubMed. Empirically, most studies identified by systematic reviews that report searching multiple databases are included in PubMed, and including versus excluding additional studies has little impact on the statistical precision of meta-analysis estimates (Halladay et al. 2015). In terms of selection bias in study inclusion, empirical evidence suggests that within-database variance is typically larger than between-database variance in study findings for common topics (Halladay et al. 2015; Sampson et al. 2003). Similarly, empirical data from meta-analyses that include reports published in multiple languages suggest that within-language variation is generally larger than between-language variation (Juni et al. 2002).

Analysts conducting a CEA should think critically about the appropriateness of the above operationalizations. For example, it has been claimed that Chinese studies of acupuncture report systematically different results than studies conducted in Western countries (Vickers et al. 1998). Thus a CEA of an acupuncture intervention may want to consider studies published in multiple databases in the local Chinese and other Asian literatures or in languages other than English (Cogo et al. 2011).

9.4.2.1.3 Screening citations for eligibility

To minimize the likelihood of mistakes in identifying the eligible citations among the citations returned by the searches, it is good practice to (1) ensure that all members of the team follow the screening criteria in the same way (e.g., by piloting the screening phase and discussing potential disagreements); (2) be systematic in managing the logistics of the screening (tracking work progress and recording screening decisions for all citations); and (3) employ quality control, for example, through (multiple) double screening in full or in part, applying computer algorithms to detect potentially missed studies (Wallace et al. 2013; Wallace et al. 2010), and so on. After articles have been identified as eligible for the systematic review, they will be downloaded in full for further screening and data extraction. At this point it is a good idea to peruse the reference lists in the eligible articles to identify additional studies.

9.4.2.2 *Extracting Information from Identified Sources*

Data should be extracted in extraction forms, to ensure that all needed information is recorded in the same way for all articles and by all extractors, and to help minimized recording of needless information. The data extraction form is typically developed as part of the protocol, and it undergoes revisions during the data extraction process. Electronic (paperless) data extraction is possible in several software systems and may have advantages in terms of ease of use, ability to extract data from different locations, and data management; it may also facilitate eventual updates (Ip et al. 2012).

Items to be extracted should be clearly defined. Elements to be extracted generally include information about the populations, exposures, and outcomes of interest; numerical data needed for meta-analysis; and information that may be useful for quantitative bias analysis, such as the number of dropouts per arm, or the number of people crossing between arms, or internally conflicting and inconsistent data. The extracted data will be used for quantitative analyses and to support assessments of, and perhaps adjustments for, bias and non-transferability of estimates.

9.4.2.2.1 Practical approaches to data extraction

Data extraction is generally laborious, but it can be done efficiently when it is very targeted, as is expected for evidence syntheses conducted to inform CEA models. Because errors in data extraction are common (Gotzsche et al. 2007), it is important to employ quality control measures. These may involve doing the data extraction in duplicate and fully independently—a preferred option (Buscemi et al. 2006)—or using less resource intensive options such as double checking the extraction of some papers or only part of the extracted data in all papers, or prioritizing checking according to the experience of the extractor. There is no substitute for attention to detail and care—for example, empirical data suggest that the more experienced extractors are not necessarily more accurate (Horton et al. 2010).

If double extraction is used, then the extraction forms should be compared and differences should be identified and resolved. In case of a difference, at least one of the extractions will be wrong or incomplete.

9.5 ANALYTICAL CONSIDERATIONS

The first step in creating a CEA is to provide an analytic description of the included studies, which involves assessing studies' internal validity (to gauge the likelihood of bias and inform any bias adjustments) and external validity (to gauge the likelihood that results transfer to the context of the CEA). Items to consider when assessing the internal and external validity of individual studies are discussed in Chapter 6. The next step is evidence synthesis proper, which aims to predict the estimate of the parameter of interest in the CEA context given the available study results, and based on an evidence synthesis model that postulates relationships between the study results.

9.5.1 Analytical Description and Critique of the Evidence Base

In developing a CEA, analysts should provide an analytical description and a critique of the evidence base (**Recommendation 4**). The analytical description should communicate to users of the CEA the salient attributes of the setting in which studies were conducted, their design, and potential limitations. It probably suffices to provide concise descriptions in the form of a table that summarizes the included populations; tests, interventions, or exposures (if and as applicable); study design and size; and outcome definitions or measurement methods used in each study.

Apart from a study-specific description, it is important to convey to users of the CEA the analysts' judgments about the magnitude of biases in the included studies and in the evidence base as a whole, and about how transferable the results of individual studies would be to the context of the CEA model (see Section 9.7).

Unless the systematic review is slated for a standalone publication, it is likely that the table constructed for analytic description will be a supplementary document, and the extent of detail in the exposition should be commensurate with the rule of reason.

9.5.2 Qualitative Synthesis

Qualitative synthesis refers to describing patterns in study results overall (e.g., whether all or most studies have effects in one direction or another) or in relation to study characteristics. Qualitative pattern finding often amounts to "vote counting" or similar informal heuristics and cannot replace formal statistical analysis (meta-analyses and meta-regressions) (Bushman 1994). Most commonly, qualitative synthesis guides quantitative explorations or contextualizes and interprets the findings of quantitative analyses. The role of qualitative synthesis in the context of a CEA is limited, in that a quantitative estimate for parameters is always required. For example, using the range of observed estimates as the range for a sensitivity analysis could be considered a qualitative synthesis task.

9.5.3 Regression as a General Framework for Evidence Synthesis

When we think of meta-analysis, we typically think of taking an average over findings from different sources. However, it is preferable to adopt a more general view of evidence synthesis as a model of data points. In this case, the data points happen to be study results rather than individual patient measurements.

We first recast evidence synthesis in a regression framework and discuss why this is advantageous. We then proceed to discuss the subtle yet important point of exactly what estimate from the regression model corresponds to the target CEA model parameter that the evidence synthesis informs. For simplicity, we assume that no measurement, confounding, or selection bias exists, and that we do not have to make any further extrapolations to transfer estimates to the CEA model setting. We expand on these complications in following sections.

9.5.3.1 *Modeling Study Results as a Study-Level Regression*

The advantage of recasting evidence synthesis in a regression framework is that we can use well-developed theory for estimation, inference, and prediction to enable learning across studies.

9.5.3.1.1 Modeling study results without considering study-level predictors

Assume that we have K studies (indexed by $k = 1,...,K$), each reporting a quantity of interest, such as a mean y. To start, think of y as a scalar (a single number), such as the mean of a measurement (e.g., the mean fasting glucose level) or the expectation of an effect measure (e.g., the mean difference in fasting glucose levels between two groups). In the k-th study, y_k is the sample estimate of the unobserved population parameter θ_k, and σ_k is the standard error of the mean.

An evidence synthesis model consists of an *observational part*, which connects the observed data in each study to the study-specific population parameters

$$y_k \sim N(\theta_k, \sigma_k^2) \tag{1}$$

and a *structural part*, which explains the relationship between the study-specific parameters. The structural part is the mathematical specification of the analysts' beliefs about the way in which results of similar studies are similar. The simplest structure is the common-effect (also known as equal- or fixed-effect) model, in which all studies have the same population effect

$$\theta_k = \Theta, \text{ for all } k. \tag{2}$$

Marginally, equations (1) and (2) can be combined in the intercept-only regression

$$y_k = \Theta + \varepsilon_k, \varepsilon_k \sim N(0, \sigma_k^2) \tag{3}$$

in which the residuals $\varepsilon_k = (y_k - \Theta)$ have different variances, each equal to the corresponding study's sampling variance σ_k^2. Figure 9.2 illustrates the common-effect regression model in equation (3).

The assumption in equation (2) that all studies have the same population effect is often implausible, because studies are conducted in different contexts and can estimate different population effects. An alternative is to assume that population effects in the K studies are distinct but follow a distribution. It is common to assume that the θ_k are exchangeable through a normal distribution

$$\theta_k \sim N(\Theta, \tau^2) \tag{4}$$

with mean Θ and between-study variance (heterogeneity) τ^2. Different specifications of the random-effects distribution in equation (4) (e.g., a mixture of normal

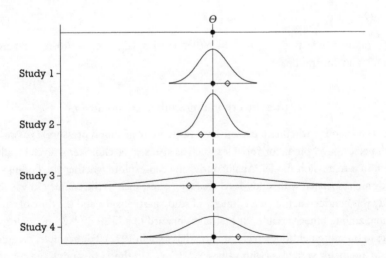

Figure 9.2 Schematic representation of the common-effect model in equation (3). Schematic representation of the model in common-effect meta-analysis. Shown are four studies, represented by four normal distributions. The common-effect model assumes that the true (unobserved) effect θ_k in all four studies (circles) is the same and equal to a common effect Θ. The observed effect y_k in each study (diamond) deviates from the common effect because of sampling variance.

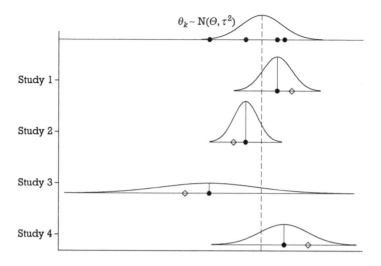

$\theta_k \sim N(\Theta, \tau^2)$

Study 1

Study 2

Study 3

Study 4

Figure 9.3 Schematic representation of the random-effects model in equation (5). The layout is similar to that in Figure 9.2. The random-effects model assumes that the study-specific true effects θ_k (circles) can differ between studies, but are exchangeable through a normal distribution with mean Θ and between-study variance τ^2. The observed effect in each study (diamond) deviates from its own underlying true effect (circle) and from Θ.

distributions instead of a single normal distribution) allow for greater flexibility in evidence synthesis (Karabatsos, Talbott, and Walker 2015). Marginally, combining equations (1) and (4), we obtain the random-intercept regression

$$y_k = \Theta + \zeta_k + \varepsilon_k \tag{5}$$

with random effects $\zeta_k = (\Theta - \theta_k) \sim N(0, \tau^2)$ and $\varepsilon_k \mid \zeta_1, \ldots, \zeta_K \sim N(0, \sigma_k^2)$. Figure 9.3 provides an illustration.

9.5.3.1.2 Incorporating study-level predictors

One can examine whether a person-level response (e.g., blood pressure) is associated with person-level predictor variables, such as age, sex, or cholesterol level, by adding them in a regression model. Analogously, one can explore whether the findings of a study are associated with study-level characteristics, such as the country in which the study was conducted, the race/ethnicity of study participants, and the dose of a medication, among other variables. It is straightforward to add study-level predictor variables to the aforementioned regression models (Rubin 1992). For example, accounting for M predictor variables (with values $x_{k1}, \ldots, x_{kM}$ in the k-th study), the common-effect model in equation (3) becomes the heteroskedastic regression

$$y_k = \underbrace{\Theta_0 + \beta_1 x_{k1} + \cdots + \beta_M x_{kM}}_{\text{mean response conditional on } x\text{'s}} + \varepsilon_k \tag{6}$$

where Θ_0 is the mean effect conditional on all x's being zero, β_1 is the difference in the conditional mean effect for one unit difference in the first variable, and so on for all M variables. Analogously, the random-effects model in equation (5) becomes

$$y_k = \underbrace{\Theta_0 + \beta_1 x_{k1} + \cdots + \beta_M x_{kM}}_{\text{mean response conditional on } x\text{'s}} + \zeta_k + \varepsilon_k \tag{7}$$

which is a random-intercept fixed-slope heteroskedastic regression. Variations of equation (7) to include random slopes are possible and are discussed elsewhere (Amatya et al. 2015; Normand 1999; van Houwelingen, Arends, and Stijnen 2002).

9.5.3.1.3 Which Model to Choose for Evidence Synthesis?

In general, we favor random-effects models over common-effect models for synthesis. More often than not, studies are so diverse in terms of enrolled populations, definitions and measurement of outcomes, and other aspects of study design that the common-effect assumption is implausible.

We do not favor relying on goodness-of-fit or heterogeneity testing to choose between the common-effect model in equation (3) and the random-effects model in equation (5), in part because these tests are generally underpowered for the number of studies typically included in a meta-analysis (Hardy and Thompson 1998), and in part because, between the two choices, random-effects models seem to be more plausible. More generally, however, when choosing between alternative random-effects models (i.e., models that specify alternative distributions for the random effects across studies) or between models that differ in the study-level predictors they use, some consideration of model fit is unavoidable (Panagiotou and Trikalinos 2015).

9.5.3.1.4 Evidence synthesis for two or more parameters

When more than one parameter should be informed by evidence synthesis, a separate evidence synthesis model per parameter can be used. However, if two (or more) parameters are related, it may be important to analyze them jointly to ensure that their estimates are consistent with one another, using multivariate methods. An example where joint analysis may be needed is when a subset of parameters is constrained. For example, in a discrete time Markov model, for each health state, the transition probabilities are constrained to sum to one (are mutually exclusive and exhaustive) and should be analyzed jointly in a way that respects this constraint. Separate evidence syntheses (one per transition probability) do not guarantee that the constraint will be satisfied and can result in inconsistencies (model bugs). Other examples refer to parameters that are stochastically dependent because they are estimates in the same patients. Section 9.5.5 provides details on multivariate meta-analysis.

9.5.3.2 *Informing Model Parameters from Data Is a Prediction Task.*

When obtaining values for a parameter of the CEA model, we predict the value of a study-level response in the context of the CEA θ_{CEA}, based on the observed study results and an evidence synthesis model (which posits how the observed study results relate to one another). Thus θ_{CEA} is a different quantity from the mean Θ in the evidence synthesis model.

For example, consider an evidence synthesis with the random-effects model in equation (5) (where there are no study-level predictors). The prediction of the effect in the context of the CEA is:

$$\theta_{CEA} \sim N(\Theta, \tau^2) \tag{8}$$

The point estimate of θ_{CEA} is Θ, but its variance is larger than the variance of Θ, because it also incorporates between-study heterogeneity.

If, instead, one were to use an evidence synthesis model that describes the expected effect based on M salient characteristics of the context in which each study was performed, one would fit the model in equation (7), and obtain the prediction

$$\theta_{CEA} \sim N(\Theta_0 + \beta_1 x_{CEA,1} + \cdots + \beta_M x_{CEA,M}, \tau^2). \tag{9}$$

9.5.3.2.1 Fitting evidence synthesis models and obtaining predictions

One can fit all models described in the above equations and use them to obtain predictions of parameters in the CEA context with freely available software, as described in Section 9.10. We thus recommend that quantitative evidence syntheses should use methods that (1) model statistical variability of data, (2) allow for between-study heterogeneity, and (3) yield consistent estimates for all model parameters informed by the synthesis (**Recommendation 5**).

9.5.4 Quantitative Synthesis for Specific Types of Parameters

In general, the evidence synthesis models outlined in Section 9.5.3 can be used for any evidence synthesis. However they rely on normal approximations to the within-study likelihood, as per equation (1), which are not satisfactory in all situations. In the following sections we describe our preferred evidence synthesis models for synthesizing common types of parameters.

9.5.4.1 *Meta-Analysis for Measures of Occurrence*

As discussed in Chapter 6, common measures of occurrence can be proportions (e.g., prevalence, incidence proportion), rates of events over an exposure period (e.g., incidence rate), and measures of time-to-event (incidence times).

9.5.4.1.1 Proportions and rates

Based on theory and simulation studies, we prefer to conduct evidence synthesis for proportions or rates using generalized linear mixed models (GLMMs) namely, random-effects logistic or Poisson regressions, respectively (Hamza, van Houwelingen, and Stijnen 2008; Trikalinos, Trow, and Schmid 2013).

9.5.4.1.2 Incidence times

In practice, synthesizing information on the average time to the incidence of an event (e.g., average time to death) requires access to person-level data, and for this reason, it is not routine practice. Methods have been proposed to synthesize survival curves, but they typically require information about censoring and about the functional form of the survival curve that is not reported in the individual studies (Arends, Hunink, and Stijnen 2008). Thus, to use them, analysts typically have to make assumptions that are difficult to verify.

9.5.4.2 *Synthesis of Intervention Effects*

The effects of interventions are measured as differences in expected outcomes between groups of people who receive different interventions. Depending on the analyzed outcome, intervention effects may correspond to differences in mean measurements for continuous outcomes (e.g., in average systolic blood pressure); hazard ratios for time-to-event outcomes; incidence rate ratios for count outcomes (e.g., number of heart attacks or strokes per person-year); or risk differences, risk ratios, or odds ratios for categorical outcomes (e.g., proportion of people with complications within 30 days of surgery).

In the simplest case, a CEA compares strategies involving only two versions of an intervention (e.g., revascularization using stents versus bypass surgery to treat patients with stable ischemic heart disease) (Zhang et al. 2015). In this case, the meta-analysis amounts to averaging intervention effects across studies. A simple approach is a two-step procedure where one first estimates a study-specific effect and subsequently averages the study-specific estimates, as described in the general approach to meta-analysis described in Section 9.5.3. A somewhat more involved approach is to perform the analysis in a single step, using a two-level hierarchical model, where the first level models data within studies, and the second level models between-study variance.

In most cases, however, a CEA examines strategies that involve more than two interventions. As an example, for three interventions, say A, B and C, one can define three pairwise effect measures (A versus B, A versus C, and B versus C), of which two are needed to parameterize a CEA model: either A versus B and A versus C; or A versus B and B versus C; or A versus C and B versus C. These three options are mathematically equivalent, and choosing between them has no bearing on the estimation of the ICER in the CEA model (apart from considerations of numerical stability).

More generally, among T interventions, one can define $T(T-1)/2$ pairwise intervention effects, and there are $T^{(T-2)}$ mathematically equivalent ways to select the $T-1$

effects needed to parameterize a CEA model. This requires that estimates of any set of $T-1$ effects from a meta-analysis should be internally consistent, that is, that CEA models parameterized with them would find exactly the same results. To ensure this result, it is necessary to analyze all available information simultaneously, using network meta-analysis (Higgins and Whitehead 1996; Lu and Ades 2004; Lumley 2002). Network meta-analysis can use information from studies comparing any subset of the T interventions, respecting the stratification of data by study and allowing for between-study heterogeneity in the treatment effects.

Network meta-analysis can be used to obtain estimates for treatment effects that have not been compared head-to-head in a study by comparing them to a common reference. For example, it can estimate the effect of A versus B as the difference of the effect of A versus C minus that of B versus C. Indirect comparisons are valid if there are no differences in the distribution of effect modifiers across the populations enrolled in the meta-analyzed studies, and if all studies use equivalent versions of the interventions (Salanti 2012). If these assumptions are violated, it does not make sense to analyze the studies jointly and to then use them for decision making. In practice it is difficult to examine whether these assumptions hold. It is possible to test for inconsistency in the results of studies in a network, which would indicate that one or both of the above-mentioned assumptions is violated, but inconsistency tests are generally underpowered (Dias et al. 2013b).

9.5.4.3 *Synthesis of Data on Test Performance*

As mentioned in Chapter 6, the summary measures of test performance that are most likely to be transferable across settings are the true-positive proportion (sensitivity) and the false-positive proportion (equal to the complement of specificity). The assessment of diagnostic performance is a bivariate problem, because it involves two outcomes from each study. Within each study the true-positive and false-positive proportions are independent, because they are estimated in disjoint samples (in people with disease and those without disease, respectively). Across studies, however, the true-positive and false-positive proportions involve correlation, because of the threshold effect.

Two summaries of data on test performance are commonly used. Sometimes a helpful way to summarize medical test studies is to provide a "summary point," that is, a summary true-positive proportion and a summary false-positive proportion (or equivalently, sensitivity and specificity). Other times, when the sensitivity or specificity estimates vary widely or when the test threshold varies, it is more helpful to synthesize data using a "summary line" that describes how the average sensitivity changes with the average specificity. Deciding whether a "summary point" or a "summary line" is more helpful as a synthesis is largely subjective (Trikalinos et al. 2012).

9.5.4.3.1 Summarizing test performance with a "summary point"

It may be helpful to use a summary point estimate of test performance that does not vary widely across studies. A summary point is most easily interpretable when all studies have the same explicit test positivity threshold. However, an explicit common threshold is neither sufficient nor necessary for opting to synthesize data with a summary point; a summary point can be helpful whenever test performance estimates do not vary widely across studies.

A frequently used approach uses a bivariate generalized linear mix to model test results in people with and without disease (Macaskill 2004; Reitsma et al. 2005). Detailed descriptions of the model and its variations, their estimation, and their behavior in real applications are found in the literature (Dahabreh et al. 2013; Dahabreh et al. 2012).

9.5.4.3.2 Summarizing test performance with a "summary line"

When the sensitivity and specificity of various studies vary over a large range, it may be more helpful to describe how the average true-positive proportion and the average false-positive proportion relate by means of a summary line. This common situation can be secondary to explicit or implicit variation in the threshold for a positive test result, heterogeneity in populations, reference standards, or the index tests, study design, chance, or bias.

The typical model for summarizing data using a summary line is the hierarchical summary receiver operating characteristic (HSROC) model (Rutter and Gatsonis 1995).

In the absence of covariates, the HSROC model and the aforementioned bivariate model (for obtaining a summary point) are fundamentally connected: one is a reparameterization of the other (Harbord et al. 2007).

9.5.4.3.3 Some advanced topics on evidence synthesis for test performance measures that will be important in CEAs

In practice, evaluation of test performance may involve complicated assessments. In several cases it is not practical or possible to ascertain the presence or absence of the disease (condition) of interest, because the reference test has a non-negligible misspecification rate. In that case, additional information on the performance of the reference test is needed to estimate the performance of the index test. An explanation of the problem and an outline of solutions are provided elsewhere (Trikalinos and Balion 2012). In analogy to network meta-analysis of interventions, which analyzes evidence on the comparison between three or more interventions, methods have been developed for analyzing the comparative performance of multiple index tests (Trikalinos et al. 2014). Several methods have also been proposed for meta-analyzing studies that report diagnostic performance measures at multiple positivity thresholds (Dukic and Gatsonis 2003), extending the meta-analysis methods mentioned above, which employ information from one threshold per study.

9.5.4.4 Synthesis of Data on Costs or Utilization Rates

The original Panel recommended micro-costing, which builds costs from estimates of resources used and unit costs for those resources. Micro-costing often takes resource estimates from clinical guidelines for appropriate care (e.g., which tests are recommended, at what intervals, followed by what treatment if a risk factor or disease is detected). Resource estimates can also come from a single provider, creating obvious problems for generalizing the results of the analysis. We may need to think differently about meta-analyzing the kinds of data used for micro-costing and the kinds used for more aggregate costing of entire disease events.

9.5.4.4.1 Synthesis of data on costs

As discussed already, it may be that unit costs (when micro-costing) are deemed to be parameters for which the notion of an empirical evidence base is irrelevant. This can be true if the CEA takes the perspective of a specific decision maker for whom unit costs are fixed quantities. Examples are NICE, which requires National Health Service (NHS) costs (National Institute for Health and Care Excellence [NICE] 2013) and the Canadian Agency for Drugs and Technologies in Health (CADTH), which uses the costs of the provincial health plan (Canadian Agency for Drugs and Technologies in Health [CADTH] 2006). US analysts often use Medicare payment rates because they apply to virtually all people over the age of 65 and are the closest to a national payer perspective in the United States.

However, for CEAs that model total costs (e.g., when micro-costing is not practical), it is conceivable that an associated evidence base for data on total costs exists, from which it is meaningful to learn. The sources of data need not be published studies—they can be total costs obtained from various states, hospitals, or other levels of aggregation, or total costs over periods of time (deflated), as long as it is deemed that one can learn across them.

Total costs are often modeled with heavy-tailed positive value distributions (e.g., a gamma distribution, or a log-normal, is a popular choice), to allow for large values in a small percentage of the population.

9.5.4.4.2 Synthesis of data on resource use

Resource use is usually quantified using a measure of occurrence, which corresponds to a proportion or a rate measure. Thus, meta-analysis of resource use measures can be done as described in Section 9.5.4.1.1.

9.5.4.5 *Synthesis of Data on Preference Weights or Utilities*

In some cases it can be argued that model parameters related to preference weights or utilities should be elicited directly from the decision maker.

Perhaps more commonly, however, it can be argued that existing studies can be used to inform such parameters. The prevalent current practice is to use a single data source. For preference weights, this means two things: a single preference weight system (which may be prescribed by the sponsor—e.g., the NHS requires the EQ-5D-5L) and a single sample of people's responses to questions based on that system. However, because preference weights for the Reference Case analyses should come from a representative sample of the community (see Chapter 7), it may be possible to synthesize evidence from several studies if more than one exist. Examples of meta-analyses of preference weights have been published (Wyld et al. 2012).

9.5.4.5.1 Considerations for synthesis of preference weights

When selecting the analytic approach for the meta-analysis of preference weights, the following are among the issues to consider: (1) the dimensions of instruments such as the EQ-5D are correlated, and it may be advantageous to synthesize them jointly, with multivariate models, rather than with separate analyses (Section 9.5.5); (2) the error associated with translating measurements between various instruments, or when translating from an instrument (e.g., EQ-5D) to utility weights should be modeled; (3) some preference weights are strictly ordinal, that is, one cannot be smaller than another. Ideally the meta-analysis approach should account for that.

9.5.5 Multivariate Meta-Analysis

In most CEAs it will be desirable to obtain estimates for several outcomes. For example, a CEA comparing revascularization with stents versus bypass surgery in patients with acute coronary artery syndromes may require effect measures for several outcomes, including nonfatal heart attacks, nonfatal strokes, and deaths from heart disease or from other causes. These outcomes are stochastically dependent because they are mutually exclusive (e.g., the more people die of heart disease, the fewer are at risk to die of other causes) (Schmid, Trikalinos, and Olkin 2014; Trikalinos and Olkin 2008). Another example pertains to measurements of preference weights: the dimensions of EQ-5D are correlated because they are measured in the same patients. Because these are multivariate problems, they are naturally meta-analyzed with multivariate methods. Multivariate meta-analysis can synthesize information from stochastically dependent outcomes by using information on the correlations between them (Gleser and Olkin 2009). For parameterizing CEA models, the main advantage of multivariate meta-analysis is that analyzing all information jointly yields estimates that are consistent across outcomes (Welton et al. 2012). In addition, it is often the case that not all outcomes are reported in all studies, in which case multivariate meta-analysis can be used to "borrow information" from the more completely reported outcome to increase the precision in the meta-analysis of the less completely reported outcome (Kirkham, Riley, and Williamson 2012; Riley et al. 2007), as long as non-reported outcomes are missing at random in a given study.

Multivariate meta-analysis requires that information on correlations between the effect measures of different outcomes is available or can be estimated, which is not always true.

9.6 ACCOUNTING FOR BIAS IN EVIDENCE SYNTHESIS MODELS

Whenever external information is used to inform the parameters of a CEA model, bias in the information sources should be accounted for (Figure 9.1). Parameters in a CEA model are bias-free. But what do we mean by bias, and how are bias adjustments made?

9.6.1 Biases in Evidence Synthesis

Figure 9.1 defined study net bias as the expected difference between what a study estimated and what that study aimed to find. At the study level, the main categories of bias are confounding, selection, and information (measurement) bias. Depending on the type of parameter being examined and the study design, one may describe specific mechanisms of bias. For example, in studies measuring the effects of interventions, verification bias is a type of measurement bias, and population stratification is a type of confounding bias in population-based genetic association studies. Analysts can gauge the likelihood of bias by considering issues related to the internal validity of studies, as described in Chapter 6. At the same time, bias can operate at the level of the evidence base if the studies included are selected based on their results, as is the case with publication bias and selective reporting bias.

9.6.1.1 *Analysis of Bias in Each Study*

The magnitude of bias in any given study is unknowable. However, CEA analysts must make judgments about the likelihood that any given study is biased, and about how large the net bias might be. These judgments are by nature subjective, and they come about in two ways, namely qualitative and quantitative bias analysis.

Bias analysis typically starts by decomposing net or total bias in several dimensions, to facilitate descriptions and organize the exposition of arguments. The overall goal is to characterize the magnitude, direction, and uncertainty of bias in each dimension for each study outcome, and then somehow aggregate along these dimensions to obtain an estimate of the net bias (Lash et al. 2014). Bias analysis may help temper overconfidence in research results and their interpretation (Savitz 2003).

9.6.1.1.1 Qualitative bias analysis per study

Schemes for qualitative bias analysis exist primarily for RCTs and effect measures, but also for other designs and measures (e.g., diagnostic cohorts for test performance data). Chapter 6 discusses items to consider when assessing the internal validity of various designs for a range of common measures used in parameterizing CEA models.

As an example, for RCTs, the Cochrane Collaboration advises systematic review authors to evaluate the likelihood of bias domains such as selection, ascertainment, performance, attrition, reporting, or other biases, and then to combine these assessments qualitatively to estimate the likelihood of net bias (Higgins et al. 2011; Higgins and Green 2011). The assessment of each bias dimension may be aided by the presence of methodological "flags," such as blinding of participants and personnel, and generation and concealment of the randomization sequence (in large-scale empirical analyses such flags were not associated with differences in study effects for most types of outcomes [Savovic et al. 2012]). For example, compared to a trial where study personnel and participants are blinded to the allocated treatments, lack of blinding may imply higher risk of ascertainment and performance bias. Assessments of bias also depend on the outcome; for example, self-reported or subjective outcomes such as pain severity might be more prone to bias than major clinical outcomes such as death.

To aggregate across the bias dimensions, analysts consider the likely direction and magnitude of bias per dimension, and then they make judgments about the net magnitude of the bias in the study for the specific outcome. This aggregation is exceedingly difficult to perform consistently in a purely qualitative fashion. It may be somewhat easier when all biases are judged to have the same direction rather than opposing directions. Arguably, this aggregation can be made more transparent when bias in each dimension is elicited from the analysts in the form of a probability density and then quantitatively combined, typically assuming additivity over the examined dimensions of bias (as discussed in the next paragraph). Detailed expositions are available in the literature (Manzi et al. 2011; Turner et al. 2009).

9.6.1.1.2 Quantitative bias analysis per study

Methods for quantitative bias analysis have been in development and application for many decades, and are reviewed in specialized texts (Lash, Fox, and Fink 2009; Lash et al. 2014). Some methods allow correction of measured bias sources, such as measurement error and misclassification or missing data, most of which assume that data are available to allow estimation of parameters in an adjustment method, for example, by imputation of the missing correct values (Lash, Fox, and Fink 2009; Little and Rubin 2002; Rothman, Greenland, and Lash 2008). Other methods deal with instances where no such measurements exist or are possible, and amount to performing sensitivity analyses based on plausible background information (Eddy, Hasselblad, and Shachter 1992; Flanders and Khoury 1990; Greenland 1996; Rothman, Greenland, and Lash 2008).

9.6.1.2 *Biases That Pertain to the Whole Evidence Base*

Several forms of information bias operate at the level of the evidence base, including publication bias, time lag bias, selective outcome reporting bias, selective analysis bias, and fraud—all undermining the validity of evidence synthesis. Publication bias encompasses selectivity in the preparation, submission, and publication of research findings based on the nature and direction of the results (Dickersin and Goodman 2005; Hopewell et al. 2009; Rosenthal 1979). Time lag bias, related to publication bias, includes delayed publication of statistically insignificant ("negative") studies and rapid publication of statistically significant ("positive") findings (Ioannidis 1998; Ioannidis and Trikalinos 2005). Selective outcome reporting bias includes reporting of only a subset of available and original study outcomes based on the magnitude of the treatment effect or its statistical significance (Chan and Altman 2005; Chan et al. 2004; Hutton and Williamson 2000). Selective analysis bias includes use of analysis methods that yield the most favorable outcomes instead of the most appropriate methods (e.g., presenting the multivariable model that yields the most statistically significant results, or choosing effect measures or specifying predictors so that results are statistically significant). The extent to which research fraud permeates the literature is unknown, although there are indications that fraud is not exceedingly rare (Fanelli 2009). Many FDA compliance and research misconduct violations are never corrected, noted, or retracted from publications (Seife 2015). Even when identified, fraudulent publications survive in the literature for several years (Trikalinos, Evangelou, and Ioannidis 2008).

Systematic reviewers have pursued two broad types of methods for dealing with information bias. The first involves detecting (and correcting results for) information bias using only the identified studies—for example, using funnel-plot based methods (Duval and Tweedie 2000; Egger et al. 1997; Harbord, Egger, and Sterne 2006; Rucker, Carpenter, and Schwarzer 2011) or various selection models (Copas and Shi 2000; Copas and Shi 2001; Hedges and Vevea 1996). With these methods one tries to infer what was not included in a meta-analysis based on what was included; this requires many assumptions about how studies are generated and exactly how information bias "censors" studies. Methodological guidance discourages relying exclusively on such analyses to judge the likelihood of information bias (Higgins et al. 2011). We favor analysis of information bias in a sensitivity analysis framework (Copas and Shi 2000; Copas and Shi 2001).

The second method involves obtaining information on the number and results of unidentified studies by examining trial registries, surveying researchers, and perusing conference proceedings and other sources. Arguably the best way to obtain empirical data on the prevalence and impact of information bias (and perhaps to mitigate its impact) is through prospective clinical trial registries (e.g., ClinicalTrials.gov) and registry networks (e.g., International Clinical Trials Registry Platform, ICTRP) that also include submission of full study protocols and summarized results. Regulations established in 1997, and expanded under the US Food and Drug Administration Amendments Act of 2007 (Pub. L. No. 110-85, 121 Stat. 823) and International Committee of Medical Journal Editors (ICMJE) guidance (De Angelis et al. 2004), have motivated industry sponsors and academic researchers to register their studies prospectively. Empirical analyses of prospective registry data give information on the time between study completion and publication, the number of unpublished studies, the fidelity of studies to registered protocols, and the congruence of study results between result registries and publications (Chan et al. 2004; Roest et al. 2015; Vedula et al. 2009; Vedula, Li, and Dickersin 2013). However, apart from documenting the presence of unidentified studies, searches of the grey literature do not necessarily provide means of correcting the ill effects of bias (unless reliable reports of results of "censored" studies are identified to include in the evidence synthesis).

9.6.2 Accounting for Bias in Evidence Synthesis

For a quantitative accounting of bias one can include in the evidence synthesis models described in Section 9.5.3, the density of bias (obtained through eliciting experts' probabilities, as in Turner et al. [2009] and Manzi et al. [2011], or quantitative bias analysis, as in Lash, Fox, and Fink [2009]). A complete framework for the treatment of bias in evidence synthesis was proposed by Eddy and colleagues in their framework for meta-analysis with the confidence-profile method (Eddy 1989; Eddy, Hasselblad, and Shachter 1990, 1992).

Most commonly, however, bias is dealt with indirectly, by restricting the analysis to information sources that are deemed to be at low risk of bias (and thus in no need of explicit adjustment). No matter what course the CEA analysts adopt, they should be explicit about whether and how bias in each study and across studies was handled. The goal of the evidence synthesis should be to produce bias-corrected estimates (**Recommendation 6**).

9.7 ACCOUNTING FOR NON-TRANSFERABILITY OF ESTIMATES

Figure 9.1 clarifies that the goal of the evidence synthesis is to predict what the estimate of the parameter would be in the context of the CEA model, given the information in the available studies.

It is likely that a single study exists that is conducted in *exactly* the same setting as the setting of the CEA model. For example, CEA analyses that are based on a data set from a single trial are by construction conducted in the same context as the trial itself, and no adjustment is required for transferability between contexts. In that case, it may be desirable to borrow some information from other studies while using primarily the index study estimate to inform the model parameter. In a Bayesian framework, this is achieved by obtaining the posterior (shrunken) estimate of the index study result, given the evidence synthesis model and the other studies in the evidence base.

If such an index study does not exist, then the best prediction for the parameter in the context of the CEA model is obtained as indicated in Sections 9.5.3.1.2 and 9.5.3.2, using equations such as equation (9) if study-level predictors were used in the evidence synthesis model, or equation (7) if no study-level predictors were used.

In either case, the evidence synthesis must be explicit about whether and how estimates were adjusted for transferability. The goal of the synthesis should be to produce estimates applicable to the modeled setting (**Recommendation 7**).

9.8 META-ANALYSIS OF INDIVIDUAL PARTICIPANT DATA

Meta-analysis of individual patient data can be used to address questions that are not answerable with meta-analyses of aggregate data. A typical example is the synthesis of information on the modification of the intervention effect by patient-level factors, which involves estimation of interactions between the intervention and effect modifiers. In practice, studies do not report sufficient statistics to allow such analyses. Instead, the analyses must be carried out de novo from individual participant data. The advantages of using individual participant data are that one can standardize definitions of outcomes and exposures, explore a wider range of statistical analyses (e.g., analyze time-to-event data, or different explanatory variables), allow analyses that explore the impact of or account for missing data (e.g., sensitivity analyses for the impact of missingness, and missing value imputation), and allow estimation of effect measures in a target population subgroup, defined by covariates (Debray et al. 2015). Meta-analysis of individual participant data can also incorporate information from studies for which only aggregate data exist (Debray et al. 2015). The main disadvantages are logistical; it takes substantial effort and resources to perform such analyses, and they are typically done for questions about which there is substantial controversy, and which have a high opportunity cost (high value of information).

9.9 SENSITIVITY AND ROBUSTNESS ANALYSES

Evidence synthesis and model development should proceed in parallel, and they are, to some extent, iterative. To prioritize parameters for a systematic evidence synthesis, it may be necessary that model structure and parameterization are at a mature stage. At the same time, information obtained during an evidence synthesis may motivate changes to the model structure and parameterization (e.g., recognizing important effect modifiers that may have to be accounted for in modeling, or realizing that important outcomes have been omitted). Thus, during evidence synthesis analysts can identify sources of structural uncertainty that should be examined in a robustness analysis, as described in Chapter 5.

Further, analysts make many operational judgments during all phases of evidence synthesis. For example, to select evidence applicable to patients with diabetes, an operational criterion may have been used that at least 80% of a study's population should have diabetes. Sensitivity of the synthesis results to this arbitrary cutoff should be examined, especially if large studies are excluded only because they barely miss the cutoff. Similarly, a range of analytical and post-analytical choices in evidence synthesis may have to be examined in sensitivity analyses to allow better understanding of their impact on the CEA model results. In general, we recommend that analysts enumerate scenarios for sensitivity analyses for (1) structure and (2) parameter values based on the findings of the qualitative synthesis and assumptions made when accounting for/dealing with biases and transferability of estimates in the quantitative synthesis (**Recommendation 8**). Most sensitivity analyses can be done without running the whole CEA model if results do not change materially. If estimates change substantially, it may be important to examine how the variables analyzed affect the findings of the CEA model.

9.10 SOFTWARE

All meta-analysis models can be recast in a regression/generalized linear (mixed) modeling framework (Dias et al. 2013a; Normand 1999; Panagiotou and Trikalinos

2015) and can, with some care, be specified in general statistical packages such as R/ S-plus, Stata, and SAS. The same meta-analysis models (with additional specification of prior distributions for parameters) can be estimated in the Bayesian framework numerically, with Markov Chain Monte Carlo (MCMC) numerical integration. Estimates based on MCMC samplers can be coded explicitly in statistical or general programming languages. Alternatively, they are made accessible in software such as WinBUGS/BUGS (Lunn et al. 2000) and JAGS (Plummer 2003) and more recently in specialized packages in software, such as SAS and Stata.

Alternatively, it may be more convenient to use dedicated meta-analysis packages that facilitate data entry, back-calculation of sufficient statistics from each study, and sensitivity analysis, and thereby make specification of complex models easy. These may be libraries such as *metafor* in R (Viechtbauer 2010) and macros such as *metan* in Stata (Harris et al. 2008) or specialized meta-analysis software including, but not limited to, OpenMeta-Analyst (an open-source R-based graphical user interface program) (Wallace et al. 2012), MIX (a Microsoft Excel-based software) (Bax et al. 2006), and Comprehensive Meta-Analysis (a proprietary software) (Borenstein, Rothstein, and Cohen 2005). As of this writing, only OpenMeta-Analyst can fit models using the preferred exact likelihood approaches discussed here. A review of meta-analysis software solutions is provided in Wallace et al. (2009).

9.11 RECOMMENDATIONS

1. Follow established guidance on systematic reviews and meta-analyses, modified as per **Recommendations 2** through **8**, below.
2. The cost-effectiveness analysis (CEA) team and the evidence synthesis team (if separate) should coordinate to refine the scope and goals of the evidence synthesis.
3. Identify the important model parameters. Important parameters are those that are (i) influential on model results or (ii) critical to the (perceived) validity of the model. Estimates of important parameters should be informed by an evidence synthesis.
4. Provide an analytical description and a critique of the evidence base.
5. Quantitative evidence syntheses should use methods that (i) model statistical variability of data, (ii) allow for between-study heterogeneity, and (iii) yield consistent estimates for all model parameters informed by the synthesis.
6. The evidence synthesis should be explicit about whether and how bias in each study and across studies was handled. The goal of the synthesis should be to produce bias-corrected estimates.
7. The evidence synthesis must be explicit about whether and how estimates were adjusted for transferability. The goal of the synthesis should be to produce estimates applicable to the modeled setting.
8. Enumerate scenarios for sensitivity analyses for (i) structure and (ii) parameter values based on the findings of the qualitative synthesis and assumptions made when accounting for/dealing with biases and transferability of estimates in the quantitative synthesis.

9.12 REFERENCES

Agency for Healthcare Research and Quality. 2014. Methods Guide for Effectiveness and Comparative Effectiveness Reviews. AHRQ Publication No. 10(14)-EHC063-EF. Rockville, MD: Agency for Healthcare Research and Quality. January 2014. Chapters available at: www.effectivehealthcare.ahrq.gov.

Amatya, A., D. K. Bhaumik, S. L. Normand, J. Greenhouse, E. Kaizar, B. Neelon, and R. D. Gibbons. 2015. Likelihood-based random-effect meta-analysis of binary events. *J Biopharm Stat* 25 (5):984–1004.

Arends, L. R., M. G. Hunink, and T. Stijnen. 2008. Meta-analysis of summary survival curve data. *Stat Med* 27 (22):4381–4396.

Bax, L., L. M. Yu, N. Ikeda, H. Tsuruta, and K. G. Moons. 2006. Development and validation of MIX: comprehensive free software for meta-analysis of causal research data. *BMC Med Res Methodol* 6:50.

Borenstein, M., D. Rothstein, and J. Cohen. 2005. Comprehensive meta-analysis: a computer program for research synthesis [computer program]. Englewood, NJ: Biostat.

Buscemi, N., L. Hartling, B. Vandermeer, L. Tjosvold, and T. P. Klassen. 2006. Single data extraction generated more errors than double data extraction in systematic reviews. *J Clin Epidemiol* 59 (7):697–703.

Bushman, B. J. 1994. "Vote-Counting Procedures in Meta-Analysis." In *The Handbook of Research Synthesis*, edited by H. Cooper and L. V. Hedges, 193–213. New York: Russell Sage Foundation.

Canadian Agency for Drugs and Technologies in Health (CADTH). 2006. *Guidelines for the Economic Evaluation of Health Technologies: Canada*. 3rd ed. Ottawa: CADTH. https://www.cadth.ca/media/pdf/186_EconomicGuidelines_e.pdf.

Centre for Reviews and Dissemination. 2009. *Systematic Reviews: CRD's Guidance for Undertaking Reviews in Health Care*. York, UK: Centre for Reviews and Dissemination, University of York.

Chan, A. W., and D. G. Altman. 2005. Identifying outcome reporting bias in randomised trials on PubMed: review of publications and survey of authors. *BMJ* 330 (7494):753.

Chan, A. W., A. Hrobjartsson, M. T. Haahr, P. C. Gotzsche, and D. G. Altman. 2004. Empirical evidence for selective reporting of outcomes in randomized trials: comparison of protocols to published articles. *JAMA* 291 (20):2457–2465.

Chandler, J., R. Churchill, J. Higgins, T. Lasserson, and D. Tovey. 2013. Methodological Expectations of Cochrane Intervention Reviews (MECIR): Methodological Standards for the Conduct of New Cochrane Intervention Reviews. Version 2.3, 02 December 2013. http://editorial-unit.cochrane.org/mecir.

Chang, S. M., D. B. Matchar, G. W. Smetana, and C. A. Umscheid (editors). 2012. Methods Guide for Medical Test Reviews. AHRQ Publication No. 12-EC017. Rockville, MD: Agency for Healthcare Research and Quality; June 2012. http://www.ncbi.nlm.nih.gov/books/NBK98241/. Also published as a special supplement to the *Journal of General Internal Medicine*, July 2012.

Chou, R., N. Aronson, D. Atkins, A. S. Ismaila, P. Santaguida, D. H. Smith, E. Whitlock, T. J. Wilt, and D. Moher. 2010. AHRQ series paper 4: assessing harms when comparing medical interventions: AHRQ and the effective health-care program. *J Clin Epidemiol* 63 (5):502–512.

Cogo, E., M. Sampson, I. Ajiferuke, E. Manheimer, K. Campbell, R. Daniel, and D. Moher. 2011. Searching for controlled trials of complementary and alternative medicine: a comparison of 15 databases. *Evid Based Complement Alternat Med* 2011:858246.

Cooper, N. J., A. J. Sutton, K. R. Abrams, D. Turner, and A. Wailoo. 2004. Comprehensive decision analytical modelling in economic evaluation: a Bayesian approach. *Health Econ* 13 (3):203–226.

Copas, J., and J. Q. Shi. 2000. Meta-analysis, funnel plots and sensitivity analysis. *Biostatistics* 1 (3):247–262.

Copas, J. B., and J. Q. Shi. 2001. A sensitivity analysis for publication bias in systematic reviews. *Stat Methods Med Res* 10 (4):251–265.

Counsell, C. 1997. Formulating questions and locating primary studies for inclusion in systematic reviews. *Ann Intern Med* 127 (5):380–387.

Dahabreh, I. J., M. Chung, G. D. Kitsios, T. Terasawa, G. Raman, A. Tatsioni, A. Tobar, J. Lau, T. A. Trikalinos, and C. H. Schmid. 2013. Survey of the methods and reporting practices in published meta-analyses of test performance: 1987 to 2009. *Res Synth Methods* 4 (3):242–255.

Dahabreh, I. J., T. A. Trikalinos, J. Lau, and C. Schmid. 2012. An Empirical Assessment of Bivariate Methods for Meta-Analysis of Test Accuracy. Methods Research Report. (Prepared by Tufts Evidence-based Practice Center under Contract No. 290-2007-10055-I.) AHRQ Publication No 12(13)-EHC136-EF. Rockville, MD: Agency for Healthcare Research and Quality. November 2012. www.effectivehealthcare.ahrq.gov/reports/final/cfm.

De Angelis, C., J. M. Drazen, F. A. Frizelle, C. Haug, J. Hoey, R. Horton, S. Kotzin, C. Laine, A. Marusic, A. J. Overbeke, T. V. Schroeder, H. C. Sox, M. B. Van Der Weyden, and International Committee of Medical Journal Editors. 2004. Clinical trial registration: a statement from the International Committee of Medical Journal Editors. *N Engl J Med* 351 (12):1250–1251 [Editorial].

Debray, T. P., K. G. Moons, G. van Valkenhoef, O. Efthimiou, N. Hummel, R. H. Groenwold, and J. B. Reitsma. 2015. Get real in individual participant data (IPD) meta-analysis: a review of the methodology. *Res Synth Methods* 6 (4):293–309.

Dias, S., A. J. Sutton, A. E. Ades, and N. J. Welton. 2013a. Evidence synthesis for decision making 2: a generalized linear modeling framework for pairwise and network meta-analysis of randomized controlled trials. *Med Decis Making* 33 (5):607–617.

Dias, S., N. J. Welton, A. J. Sutton, D. M. Caldwell, G. Lu, and A. E. Ades. 2013b. Evidence synthesis for decision making 4: inconsistency in networks of evidence based on randomized controlled trials. *Med Decis Making* 33 (5):641–656.

Dickersin, K., and S. Goodman. 2005. The long and creative arm of the drug industry. *Lancet* 365 (9460):656.

Djulbegovic, B., G. H. Guyatt, and R. E. Ashcroft. 2009. Epistemologic inquiries in evidence-based medicine. *Cancer Control* 16 (2):158–168.

Dukic, V., and C. Gatsonis. 2003. Meta-analysis of diagnostic test accuracy assessment studies with varying number of thresholds. *Biometrics* 59 (4):936–946.

Duval, S., and R. Tweedie. 2000. Trim and fill: a simple funnel-plot-based method of testing and adjusting for publication bias in meta-analysis. *Biometrics* 56 (2):455–463.

Eddy, D. M. 1989. The confidence profile method: a Bayesian method for assessing health technologies. *Oper Res* 37 (2):210–228.

Eddy, D. M., V. Hasselblad, and R. Shachter. 1990. An introduction to a Bayesian method for meta-analysis: the confidence profile method. *Med Decis Making* 10 (1):15–23.

Eddy, D. M., V. Hasselblad, and R. Shachter. 1992. *Meta-Analysis by the Confidence Profile Method: The Statistical Synthesis of Evidence*. Boston: Academic Press.

Eden, J., L. Levit, A. Berg, and S. Morton, eds. 2011. *Finding What Works in Health Care: Standards for Systematic Reviews*. Washington, DC: The National Academies Press.

Egger, M., G. Davey Smith, M. Schneider, and C. Minder. 1997. Bias in meta-analysis detected by a simple, graphical test. *BMJ* 315 (7109):629–634.

Egger, M., and G. D. Smith. 1998. Bias in location and selection of studies. *BMJ* 316 (7124):61–66.

Evidence-Based Medicine Working Group. 1992. Evidence-based medicine. A new approach to teaching the practice of medicine. *JAMA* 268 (17):2420–2425.

Fanelli, D. 2009. How many scientists fabricate and falsify research? A systematic review and meta-analysis of survey data. *PLoS One* 4 (5):e5738.

Flanders, W. D., and M. J. Khoury. 1990. Indirect assessment of confounding: graphic description and limits on effect of adjusting for covariates. *Epidemiology* 1 (3):239–246.

Garthwaite, P. H., J. B. Kadane, and A. O'Hagan. 2005. Statistical methods for eliciting probability distributions. *J Amer Statistical Assoc* 100 (470):680–701.

Gleser, L. J., and I. Olkin. 2009. "Stochastically Dependent Effect Sizes." In *The Handbook of Research Synthesis and Meta-Analysis*, 2nd ed, edited by H. Cooper, L. V. Hedges and J. C. Valentine, 357–376. New York: Russell Sage Foundation.

Gotzsche, P. C., A. Hrobjartsson, K. Maric, and B. Tendal. 2007. Data extraction errors in meta-analyses that use standardized mean differences. [Erratum appears in *JAMA* 2007 298 (19):2261–2263]. *JAMA* 298 (4):430–437.

Graham, R., M. Mancher, D. M. Wolman, S. Greenfield, and E. Steinberg, eds. 2011. *Clinical Practice Guidelines We Can Trust*. Washington, DC: The National Academies Press.

Greenland, S. 1996. Basic methods for sensitivity analysis of biases. *Int J Epidemiol* 25 (6):1107–1116.

Greenland, S. 2005. Multiple-bias modelling for analysis of observational data. *J R Stat Soc Ser A Stat Soc* 168 (2):267–306.

Halladay, C. W., T. A. Trikalinos, I. T. Schmid, C. H. Schmid, and I. J. Dahabreh. 2015. Using data sources beyond PubMed has a modest impact on the results of systematic reviews of therapeutic interventions. *J Clin Epidemiol* 68 (9):1076–1084.

Hamza, T. H., H. C. van Houwelingen, and T. Stijnen. 2008. The binomial distribution of meta-analysis was preferred to model within-study variability. *J Clin Epidemiol* 61 (1):41–51.

Harbord, R. M., J. J. Deeks, M. Egger, P. Whiting, and J. A. Sterne. 2007. A unification of models for meta-analysis of diagnostic accuracy studies. [Erratum appears in *Biostatistics* 2008;9 (4):779]. *Biostatistics* 8 (2):239–251.

Harbord, R. M., M. Egger, and J. A. Sterne. 2006. A modified test for small-study effects in meta-analyses of controlled trials with binary endpoints. *Stat Med* 25 (20):3443–3457.

Hardy, R. J., and S. G. Thompson. 1998. Detecting and describing heterogeneity in meta-analysis. *Stat Med* 17 (8):841–856.

Harris, R., M. Bradburn, J. Deeks, R. Harbord, D. Altman, and J. Sterne. 2008. Metan: fixed- and random-effects meta-analysis. *Stata J* 8 (1):3–28.

Hedges, L. V., and J. L. Vevea. 1996. Estimating effect size under publication bias: small sample properties and robustness of a random effects selection model. *J Educ Behav Stat* 21 (4):299–332.

Helfand, M., and H. Balshem. 2010. AHRQ series paper 2: principles for developing guidance: AHRQ and the effective health-care program. *J Clin Epidemiol* 63 (5):484–490.

Higgins, J. P., D. G. Altman, P. C. Gøtzsche, P. Jüni, D. Moher, A. D. Oxman, J. Savović, K. F. Schulz, L. Weeks, J. A. Sterne, Cochrane Bias Methods Group, and Cochrane Statistical Methods Group. 2011. The Cochrane Collaboration's tool for assessing risk of bias in randomised trials. *BMJ* 343:d5928.

Higgins, J. P., and A. Whitehead. 1996. Borrowing strength from external trials in a meta-analysis. *Stat Med* 15 (24):2733–2749.

Higgins, J. P. T., and S. Green, eds. 2011. *Cochrane Handbook for Systematic Reviews of Interventions*: Version 5.1.0 [updated March 2011]. The Cochrane Collaboration. Available from: www.cochrane-handbook.org.

Hopewell, S., K. Loudon, M. J. Clarke, A. D. Oxman, and K. Dickersin. 2009. Publication bias in clinical trials due to statistical significance or direction of trial results. *Cochrane Database of Systematic Reviews* (1):MR000006.

Horton, J., B. Vandermeer, L. Hartling, L. Tjosvold, T. P. Klassen, and N. Buscemi. 2010. Systematic review data extraction: cross-sectional study showed that experience did not increase accuracy. *J Clin Epidemiol* 63 (3):289–298.

Hutton, J. L., and P. R. Williamson. 2000. Bias in meta-analysis due to outcome variable selection within studies. *J R Stat Soc Ser C Appl Stat* 49 (3):359–370.

Ioannidis, J. P. 1998. Effect of the statistical significance of results on the time to completion and publication of randomized efficacy trials. *JAMA* 279 (4):281–286.

Ioannidis, J. P., and T. A. Trikalinos. 2005. Early extreme contradictory estimates may appear in published research: the Proteus phenomenon in molecular genetics research and randomized trials. *J Clin Epidemiol* 58 (6):543–549.

Ip, S., N. Hadar, S. Keefe, C. Parkin, R. Iovin, E. M. Balk, and J. Lau. 2012. A Web-based archive of systematic review data. *Syst Rev* 1:15.

Juni, P., F. Holenstein, J. Sterne, C. Bartlett, and M. Egger. 2002. Direction and impact of language bias in meta-analyses of controlled trials: empirical study. *Int J Epidemiol* 31 (1):115–123.

Kaizar, E. E. 2006. "Combining Information from Diverse Sources." Ph.D. Dissertation, Carnegie Mellon University.

Kaizar, E. E. 2015. Incorporating both randomized and observational data into a single analysis. *Annu Rev Stat Appl* 2 (1):49–72.

Karabatsos, G., E. Talbott, and S. G. Walker. 2015. A Bayesian nonparametric meta-analysis model. *Res Syn Meth* 6 (1):28–44.

Kirkham, J. J., R. D. Riley, and P. R. Williamson. 2012. A multivariate meta-analysis approach for reducing the impact of outcome reporting bias in systematic reviews. *Stat Med* 31 (20):2179–2195.

Kung, J., F. Chiappelli, O. O. Cajulis, R. Avezova, G. Kossan, L. Chew, and C. A. Maida. 2010. From systematic reviews to clinical recommendations for evidence-based health care: validation of revised assessment of multiple systematic reviews (R-AMSTAR) for grading of clinical relevance. *Open Dent J* 4:84–91.

Lash, T. L., M. P. Fox, and A. K. Fink. 2009. *Applying Quantitative Bias Analysis to Epidemiologic Data*. New York: Springer Science + Business Media.

Lash, T. L., M. P. Fox, R. F. MacLehose, G. Maldonado, L. C. McCandless, and S. Greenland. 2014. Good practices for quantitative bias analysis. *Int J Epidemiol* 43 (6):1969–1985.

Little, R. J. A., and D. B. Rubin. 2002. *Statistical Analysis with Missing Data*. 2nd ed. Hoboken, NJ: John Wiley & Sons, Inc.

Lu, G., and A. E. Ades. 2004. Combination of direct and indirect evidence in mixed treatment comparisons. *Stat Med* 23 (20):3105–3124.

Lumley, T. 2002. Network meta-analysis for indirect treatment comparisons. *Stat Med* 21 (16):2313–2324.

Lunn, D. J., A. Thomas, N. Best, and D. Spiegelhalter. 2000. WinBUGS—a Bayesian modelling framework: concepts, structure, and extensibility. *Stat Comput* 10:325–337.

Macaskill, P. 2004. Empirical Bayes estimates generated in a hierarchical summary ROC analysis agreed closely with those of a full Bayesian analysis. *J Clin Epidemiol* 57 (9):925–932.

Manzi, G., D. J. Spiegelhalter, R. M. Turner, J. Flowers, and S. G. Thompson. 2011. Modelling bias in combining small area prevalence estimates from multiple surveys. *J R Stat Soc Ser A Stat Soc* 174 (1):31–50.

Moher, D., A. Liberati, J. Tetzlaff, D. G. Altman, and P. Group. 2009. Preferred reporting items for systematic reviews and meta-analyses: the PRISMA statement. *BMJ* 339:b2535.

National Institute for Health and Care Excellence (NICE). 2013. *Guide to the Methods of Technology Appraisal 2013. NICE article [PMG9]*. London: NICE. http://publications.nice.org.uk/pmg9.

Normand, S. L. 1999. Meta-analysis: formulating, evaluating, combining, and reporting. *Stat Med* 18 (3):321–359.

O'Hagan, A., C. E. Buck, A. Daneshkhah, J. R. Eiser, P. H. Garthwaite, D. J. Jenkinson, J. E. Oakley, and T. Rakow. 2006. *Uncertain Judgements: Eliciting Experts' Probabilities*. Chichester: John Wiley & Sons Ltd.

Owens, D. K., K. N. Lohr, D. Atkins, J. R. Treadwell, J. T. Reston, E. B. Bass, S. Chang, and M. Helfand. 2010. AHRQ series paper 5: grading the strength of a body of evidence when comparing medical interventions—Agency for Healthcare Research and Quality and the effective health-care program. *J Clin Epidemiol* 63 (5):513–523.

Panagiotou, O. A., and T. A. Trikalinos. 2015. Commentary: On effect measures, heterogeneity, and the laws of nature. *Epidemiology* 26 (5):710–713.

PCORI (Patient-Centered Outcomes Research Institute) Methodology Committee. 2013. The PCORI Methodology Report. http://www.pcori.org/research-results/research-methodology/pcori-methodology-report.

Plummer, M. 2003. "JAGS: A Program for Analysis of Bayesian Graphical Models Using Gibbs Sampling." 3rd International Workshop on Distributed Statistical Computing (DSC 2003), March 20-22; Vienna, Austria. http://www.ci.tuwien.ac.at/Conferences/DSC-2003/.

Rabitz, H. 1984. "Sensitivity Methods for Mathematical Modeling." In *Sensitivity of Functionals with Applications to Engineering Sciences: Proceedings of a Special Session of the American Mathematical Society Spring Meeting held in New York City, May 1983*, edited by V. Komkov, 77–92. New York: Springer Verlag.

Reitsma, J. B., A. S. Glas, A. W. Rutjes, R. J. Scholten, P. M. Bossuyt, and A. H. Zwinderman. 2005. Bivariate analysis of sensitivity and specificity produces informative summary measures in diagnostic reviews. *J Clin Epidemiol* 58 (10):982–990.

Riley, R. D., K. R. Abrams, P. C. Lambert, A. J. Sutton, and J. R. Thompson. 2007. An evaluation of bivariate random-effects meta-analysis for the joint synthesis of two correlated outcomes. [Erratum appears in *Stat Med* 2011;30 (4):400]. *Stat Med* 26 (1):78–97.

Riley, R. D., P. C. Lambert, J. A. Staessen, J. Wang, F. Gueyffier, L. Thijs, and F. Boutitie. 2008. Meta-analysis of continuous outcomes combining individual patient data and aggregate data. *Stat Med* 27 (11):1870–1893.

Roest, A. M., P. de Jonge, C. D. Williams, Y. A. de Vries, R. A. Schoevers, and E. H. Turner. 2015. Reporting bias in clinical trials investigating the efficacy of second-generation antidepressants in the treatment of anxiety disorders: a report of 2 meta-analyses. *JAMA Psychiatry* 72 (5):500–510.

Rosenthal, R. 1979. The file drawer problem and tolerance for null results. *Psychol Bull* 86 (3):638–641.

Rothman, K. J., S. Greenland, and T. L. Lash. 2008. *Modern Epidemiology*. 3rd ed. Philadelphia: Lippincott Williams & Wilkins.

Rothstein, H. R., A. J. Sutton, and M. Borenstein, eds. 2005. *Publication Bias in Meta-Analysis: Prevention, Assessment and Adjustments.* Chichester: John Wiley & Sons Ltd.

Rubin, D. B. 1992. Meta-analysis: literature synthesis or effect-size surface estimation? *J Educ Behav Stat* 17 (4):363–374.

Rucker, G., J. R. Carpenter, and G. Schwarzer. 2011. Detecting and adjusting for small-study effects in meta-analysis. *Biometrical Journal* 53 (2):351–368.

Rutter, C. M., and C. A. Gatsonis. 1995. Regression methods for meta-analysis of diagnostic test data. *Acad Radiol* 2 Suppl 1:S48–S56; discussion S65-47, S70-41 pas.

Salanti, G. 2012. Indirect and mixed-treatment comparison, network, or multiple-treatments meta-analysis: many names, many benefits, many concerns for the next generation evidence synthesis tool. *Res Synth Methods* 3 (2):80–97.

Sampson, M., N. J. Barrowman, D. Moher, T. P. Klassen, B. Pham, R. Platt, P. D. St John, R. Viola, and P. Raina. 2003. Should meta-analysts search Embase in addition to Medline? *J Clin Epidemiol* 56 (10):943–955.

Savitz, D. A. 2003. *Interpreting Epidemiologic Evidence: Strategies for Study Design and Analysis.* New York: Oxford University Press.

Savovic, J., H. E. Jones, D. G. Altman, R. J. Harris, P. Juni, J. Pildal, B. Als-Nielsen, E. M. Balk, C. Gluud, L. L. Gluud, J. P. Ioannidis, K. F. Schulz, R. Beynon, N. J. Welton, L. Wood, D. Moher, J. J. Deeks, and J. A. Sterne. 2012. Influence of reported study design characteristics on intervention effect estimates from randomized, controlled trials. *Ann Intern Med* 157 (6):429–438.

Schmid, C. H., T. A. Trikalinos, and I. Olkin. 2014. Bayesian network meta-analysis for unordered categorical outcomes with incomplete data. *Res Synth Methods* 5 (2):162–185.

Seife, C. 2015. Research misconduct identified by the US Food and Drug Administration: out of sight, out of mind, out of the peer-reviewed literature. *JAMA Intern Med* 175 (4):567–577.

Shamseer, L., D. Moher, M. Clarke, D. Ghersi, A. Liberati, M. Petticrew, P. Shekelle, L. A. Stewart, and the Prisma-P Group. 2015. Preferred reporting items for systematic review and meta-analysis protocols (PRISMA-P) 2015: elaboration and explanation. *BMJ* 349:g7647.

Shea, B. J., J. M. Grimshaw, G. A. Wells, M. Boers, N. Andersson, C. Hamel, A. C. Porter, P. Tugwell, D. Moher, and L. M. Bouter. 2007. Development of AMSTAR: a measurement tool to assess the methodological quality of systematic reviews. *BMC Med Res Methodol* 7:10.

Slutsky, J., D. Atkins, S. Chang, and B. A. Sharp. 2010. AHRQ series paper 1: comparing medical interventions: AHRQ and the effective health-care program. *J Clin Epidemiol* 63 (5):481–483.

Sutton, A. J., N. J. Cooper, S. Goodacre, and M. Stevenson. 2008. Integration of meta-analysis and economic decision modeling for evaluating diagnostic tests. *Med Decis Making* 28 (5):650–667.

Trikalinos, N. A., E. Evangelou, and J. P. Ioannidis. 2008. Falsified papers in high-impact journals were slow to retract and indistinguishable from nonfraudulent papers. *J Clin Epidemiol* 61 (5):464–470.

Trikalinos, T. A., and C. M. Balion. 2012. Chapter 9: options for summarizing medical test performance in the absence of a "gold standard." *J Gen Intern Med* 27 Suppl 1:S67–S75.

Trikalinos, T. A., C. M. Balion, C. I. Coleman, L. Griffith, P. L. Santaguida, B. Vandermeer, and R. Fu. 2012. Chapter 8: meta-analysis of test performance when there is a "gold standard." *J Gen Intern Med* 27 Suppl 1:S56–S66.

Trikalinos, T. A., I. J. Dahabreh, B. C. Wallace, C. H. Schmid, and J. Lau. 2013. Towards a Framework for Communicating Confidence in Methodological Recommendations for Systematic Reviews and Meta-Analyses. Methods Research Report. (Prepared by Tufts Evidence-based Practice Center under Contract No. 290-2007-10055-I.) AHRQ Publication No. 13-EHC119-EF. Rockville, MD: Agency for Healthcare Research and Quality; September 2013. www.effectivehealthcare.ahrq.gov/reports/final.cfm.

Trikalinos, T. A., D. C. Hoaglin, K. M. Small, N. Terrin, and C. H. Schmid. 2014. Methods for the joint meta-analysis of multiple tests. Res Syn Meth 5 (4):294–312.

Trikalinos, T. A., and I. Olkin. 2008. A method for the meta-analysis of mutually exclusive binary outcomes. Stat Med 27 (21):4279–4300.

Trikalinos, T. A., P. Trow, and C. H. Schmid. 2013. Simulation-Based Comparison of Methods for Meta-Analysis of Proportions and Rates. Methods Research Report. (Prepared by the Tufts Medical Center Evidence-based Practice Center under Contract No. 290-2007-10055-I.) AHRQ Publication No. 13(14)-EHC084-EF. Rockville, MD: Agency for Healthcare Research and Quality; November 2013. www.effectivehealthcare.ahrq.gov/reports/final.cfm.

Turner, R. M., D. J. Spiegelhalter, G. C. S. Smith, and S. G. Thompson. 2009. Bias modelling in evidence synthesis. J R Stat Soc Ser A Stat Soc 172 (1):21–47.

van Houwelingen, H. C., L. R. Arends, and T. Stijnen. 2002. Advanced methods in meta-analysis: multivariate approach and meta-regression. Stat Med 21 (4):589–624.

Vedula, S. S., L. Bero, R. W. Scherer, and K. Dickersin. 2009. Outcome reporting in industry-sponsored trials of gabapentin for off-label use. N Engl J Med 361 (20):1963–1971.

Vedula, S. S., T. Li, and K. Dickersin. 2013. Differences in reporting of analyses in internal company documents versus published trial reports: comparisons in industry-sponsored trials in off-label uses of gabapentin. PLoS Med 10 (1):e1001378.

Vickers, A., N. Goyal, R. Harland, and R. Rees. 1998. Do certain countries produce only positive results? A systematic review of controlled trials. Control Clin Trials 19 (2):159–166.

Viechtbauer, W. 2010. Conducting meta-analyses in R with the metafor package. J Stat Softw 36 (3):1–48.

Wallace, B. C., I. J. Dahabreh, C. H. Schmid, J. Lau, and T. A. Trikalinos. 2013. Modernizing the systematic review process to inform comparative effectiveness: tools and methods. J Comp Eff Res 2 (3):273–282.

Wallace, B. C., I. J. Dahabreh, T. A. Trikalinos, J. Lau, P. Trow, and C. H. Schmid. 2012. Closing the gap between methodologists and end-users: R as a computational back-end. J Stat Softw 49 (5):1–15.

Wallace, B. C., C. H. Schmid, J. Lau, and T. A. Trikalinos. 2009. Meta-Analyst: software for meta-analysis of binary, continuous and diagnostic data. BMC Med Res Methodol 9:80.

Wallace, B. C., T. A. Trikalinos, J. Lau, C. Brodley, and C. H. Schmid. 2010. Semi-automated screening of biomedical citations for systematic reviews. BMC Bioinformatics 11:55.

Welton, N. J., A. J. Sutton, N. Cooper, K. R. Abrams, and A. E. Ades. 2012. Evidence Synthesis for Decision Making in Healthcare. Chichester: John Wiley & Sons Ltd.

Whitlock, E. P., S. A. Lopez, S. Chang, M. Helfand, M. Eder, and N. Floyd. 2010. AHRQ series paper 3: identifying, selecting, and refining topics for comparative effectiveness systematic reviews: AHRQ and the effective health-care program. J Clin Epidemiol 63 (5):491–501.

Wyld, M., R. L. Morton, A. Hayen, K. Howard, and A. C. Webster. 2012. A systematic review and meta-analysis of utility-based quality of life in chronic kidney disease treatments. PLoS Med 9 (9):e1001307.

Zhang, Z., P. Kolm, M. V. Grau-Sepulveda, A. Ponirakis, S. M. O'Brien, L. W. Klein, R. E. Shaw, C. McKay, D. M. Shahian, F. L. Grover, J. E. Mayer, K. N. Garratt, M. Hlatky, F. H. Edwards, and W. S. Weintraub. 2015. Cost-effectiveness of revascularization strategies: the ASCERT study. J Am Coll Cardiol 65 (1):1–11.

10

Discounting in Cost-Effectiveness Analysis

Anirban Basu and Theodore G. Ganiats

10.1 INTRODUCTION

There is broad agreement that in cost-effectiveness analysis (CEA), as in any other economic evaluation, future costs and health effects should be discounted and their present values calculated to form a cost-effectiveness ratio (see **Recommendation 1**, Section 10.6). Only then will the interventions' cost-effectiveness ratios be appropriately adjusted for the differential timing of costs and health effects so that the decision maker can compare each ratio from the same temporal baseline.

Economic theory implies that in a perfectly competitive, risk-free, tax-free world in which all commodities (including something called "health") are "perfectly divisible"—so that individual decision makers could precisely adapt their consumption of goods and services over time—the returns to savings (i.e., the consumption rate of return) equals the return on private sector investments. In this situation, there would be only *one* interest rate, which could be used as the appropriate discount rate. This would also coincide with the observed market interest rate.

In the social decision-making context, as opposed to individual decision making, explicit development of the investment processes and the objective functions determining consumption values can be used to define an optimal social discount rate (Claxton et al. 2011; Claxton et al. 2006; Gravelle and Smith 2001; Ramsey 1928). This chapter presents a general outline of this theory of social discounting.

Key recommendations on discounting from the original Panel included the use of a 3% discount rate and discounting of costs and health effects at the same rate. The Second Panel maintains these recommendations, but the reasons for using the same rate for costs and health effects are different than those laid out by the original

This chapter builds on concepts presented in Chapter 7 of the original Panel's book (Lipscomb, J., M. C. Weinstein, and G. W. Torrance. 1996. "Time Preference." In *Cost-Effectiveness in Health and Medicine*, edited by M. R. Gold, J. E. Siegel, L. B. Russell, and M. C. Weinstein, 214–246. New York: Oxford University Press).

Panel. The original Panel argued that differential discounting was logically inconsistent. Those arguments were based on principles such as Keeler and Cretin's paradox (Keeler and Cretin 1983), Weinstein and Stason's chain of logic argument (Weinstein and Stason 1977), and Viscusi's equivalence argument (Viscusi 1995). Although each of these arguments points out a real logical inconsistency with differential discounting, none of them addresses the underlying problems of decision making and resource allocation over time that may drive to differential discounting (Nord 2011; Paulden 2014). In this chapter, we review some recently discussed principles for discounting from a resource allocation point of view, and we summarize some key current debates before presenting the Second Panel's recommendations.

10.2 OVERVIEW OF DISCOUNTING

The most common computational process for discounting is based on an exponential model. A description of this model can start with the concept of interest on an investment. One can calculate the future value of an investment using the compound interest rate formula

$$FV = PV\,(1+r)^t, \tag{1}$$

where FV is future value, PV is present value, r is the interest rate, and t is time. Instead of determining the future value of a present outcome, as in equation (1), discounting calculates the present value of a future outcome. The formula for the calculation is simply a rearrangement of the interest rate formula to

$$PV = FV\,/(1+r)^{t-1}, \tag{2}$$

where FV, PV, and t are the same (adjusted to $t-1$ to account for not discounting the first year), and r is the discount rate.

Virtually all CEAs in health expand equation (2) and use some variant of the following "discrete-time" model. Let $O_j(t)$ be an outcome (cost or health effect) in time period t for individuals who receive intervention j, and let $O_b(t)$ be the outcome expected for the group with the comparator (baseline) intervention. If the interventions were initiated at period 1 and continued through period T, then the present value of the outcome (from the vantage point of the start of period 1) can be calculated from equation (2) as

$$\Delta O = \sum_1^T [O_j(t) - O_b(t)]/(1+i)^{t-1} \tag{3}$$

where i is the discount rate selected to convert future consequences to their present value. Typically, the calculations are performed twice, once for the economic outcomes (costs) and once for the non-economic outcomes (e.g., quality-adjusted life years [QALYs]), and these two results are used to calculate the cost-effectiveness ratio for the intervention relative to the comparator.

Table 10.1 Example of incremental costs and health effects over 3 years

Year	Incremental cost	Incremental QALYs gained
1	$10,000	2
2	$12,000	4
3	$8,000	3

Abbreviation: QALY = quality-adjusted life year.

To illustrate, suppose a 3-year intervention has been proposed with the anticipated streams of costs and health effects relative to the status quo listed in Table 10.1.

Given a 5% discount rate, the present value of costs (*C*) and of health effects (*E*) over the 3 years may be expressed, respectively, as

$$\Delta C = \$10,000 + \$12,000 / (1 + 0.05)^1 + \$8,000 / (1 + 0.05)^2 = \$28,685$$

and

$$\Delta E = 2 + 4 / (1 + 0.05)^1 + 3 / (1 + 0.05)^2 = 8.53 \text{ QALYs},$$

so the cost-effectiveness ratio is $\Delta C / \Delta E = \$3,363 / \text{QALY}$.

For the above discounting calculations, we adopt the convention of assuming that outcomes occur in the middle of each time interval (year), and that discounting does not occur in the first year. One could just as easily assume that these outcomes accrue at the end of each interval, or at the beginning, and many CEAs do one or the other.

This exponential model has been the standard approach in both CEA and cost–benefit analysis since Samuelson proposed the discounted utility model in 1937 (Frederick, Loewenstein, and O'Donoghue 2002; Samuelson 1937). Key to exponential discounting is the constant rate, so that in any two time periods of equal length, the proportional decrease in value will be the same. For example, if the value decreases 5% during the second year, then it will also decrease by 5% in the twentieth year. Naturally, just as the absolute increase in value grows with a constant compound interest rate (as the principal grows), the absolute decrease in value slows with a constant discount rate (as the value shrinks). For example, using equation (2), we can see that the present value of $1,000 in the second year, discounted at 5%, is $952, a decrement of $48 from the first year. But the present value of $1,000 in the twentieth year, discounted at 5%, is $395, a decrement of only $20 from the value in the nineteenth year.

Central to the process is the selection of a discount rate for outcomes that is appropriate for the analytic perspective. Thus, if the decision maker is indifferent to incurring $100 of cost this year versus $110 of cost next year, this implies (solving for *r* in equation [2]) an annual discount rate of 10%.

While the mechanistic application of discounting is straightforward, the appropriate discount rates for costs and health effects have been the subjects of debate. The assumption that economic and noneconomic outcomes have equal discount rates and alternatives to the assumption of an exponential model for the discount rate are discussed later in Sections 10.4.2 and 10.5 in this chapter.

10.3 A GENERAL FRAMEWORK FOR DISCOUNTING IN CEA

The general rationale for discounting is that social decision makers want to maximize an objective function (e.g., utility or health) while making a fair assessment about the value of this objective function that is derived today rather than tomorrow. However, the valuation of this objective function changes over time. For example, in order to make the utility derived from a marginal consumption dollar in the present equivalent to that derived from the marginal consumption dollar in the future, where consumption is more plentiful, the consumption in the future would have to be discounted. We present two decision-making scenarios that are relevant for the two Reference Case analyses recommended in this book: (1) for the societal perspective analysis, a welfarist scenario where the consumption value of health is maximized given an omnibus budget and (2) for the healthcare sector perspective analysis, an extra-welfarist scenario where only health is maximized given a fixed healthcare budget.

10.3.1 A Welfarist, Omnibus Budget Scenario

We start with a welfarist perspective where a social welfare function is defined by the aggregation of utilities over consumption (C) and health (H), and the society faces an omnibus budget constraint. Under this circumstance, one can achieve the desired objective by maximizing the consumption value of health derived from the social welfare function (Claxton et al. 2011; Gravelle et al. 2007). Let the consumption value of health for time period 1 be $V_1 \cdot H_1$. Here V represents the consumption value of health in any given period and reflects the amount of consumption that is equivalent to one unit of health in any given period.*

Consider two periods where the present consumption value of health gained and forgone in each of the two periods is determined by accepting a technology with total costs S, which includes both healthcare costs (E) and non-healthcare costs (F) that fall on consumption (Table 10.2).

In Table 10.2, λ represents the *inverse of the marginal utility of income or consumption* for the respective periods. The pure social rate of time preference (describing impatience) for consumption is denoted by ρ_C. Some investigators have argued that, for a social decision maker, this should be zero, since it would be unethical to

---

* Based on the discussions in Chapter 2, if one represents utility to be multiplicative between health and consumption, i.e., if $U(C,H) = V(C) * H$, then at the optimal levels of consumption and health, C^* and H^*, the consumption value of health is given by $\partial V(C^*) \cdot H^* / \partial H^* = V(C^*)$.

Table 10.2 Health and cost effects in terms of current consumption

Time period	1	2
Present value of utilities gained	$V_1 \cdot \Delta H_1$	$\dfrac{V_2 \cdot \Delta H_2}{(1+\rho_C)}$
Present consumption value forgone	$\dfrac{\Delta S_1}{\lambda_1}$	$\dfrac{\Delta S_2}{\lambda_2(1+\rho_C)}$

value the utility of future consumption lower than the utility of current consumption purely as a result of impatience (Solow 1974). However, others have pointed out that a zero rate of pure time preference implies a savings rate excessively higher than what is typically observed in real-world savings behavior, leading to paradoxical results (Arrow 1995).

In this context, the decision to adopt the technology would be based on whether

$$V_1 \cdot \Delta H_1 + \frac{V_2 \cdot \Delta H_2}{(1+\rho_C)} \geq \frac{\Delta S_1}{\lambda_1} + \frac{\Delta S_2}{\lambda_2(1+\rho_C)}$$

Therefore, when employing a decision-making criterion in period 1 based on net present valuation, the utilitarian value of the costs in the second period $\left(\text{i.e., } \dfrac{\Delta S_2}{\lambda_2(1+\rho_C)} \right)$ must account for the growth in the marginal utility of income. Moreover, the consumption value of health may also be changing from period 1 to period 2 because of the change in consumption between the periods. This growth, under an assumption of constant consumption elasticity of marginal utility,* would be represented by the negative of the rate of growth in the marginal utility of consumption. This is because as consumption grows, the marginal utility of consumption decreases, and therefore, at the margin, one would need more units of consumption to value the same unit of health. Hence,

$$V_2 = V_1(1-g_C), \text{ and}$$

$$\lambda_2 = \lambda_1(1+g_C),$$

---

* Because $\lambda = 1/(\partial V(C^*) \cdot H * /\partial C)$, i.e., the inverse of the marginal utility of income, it will grow at the inverse of the same rate as the marginal utility of consumption, $\partial V(C^*)/\partial C$, keeping H constant. Then, under the assumption of constant consumption elasticity of marginal utility, $\left(\dfrac{\partial V(C^*_1)}{\partial C} \right) / \left(\dfrac{\partial V(C^*_2)}{\partial C} \right) = \left(\dfrac{V(C^*_1)}{V(C^*_2)} \right)$, $V(C^*)$ would grow at the same rate as $\dfrac{\partial V(C^*)}{\partial C}$. Therefore, λ and $V(C^*)$ will grow at the same rate but in opposite directions.

where g_c is the growth in the marginal utility of consumption. Thus the decision to adopt a technology would be written as:

$$V_1 \cdot \Delta H_1 + \frac{V_1(1-g_c) \cdot \Delta H_2}{(1+\rho_c)} \geq \frac{\Delta S_1}{\lambda_1} + \frac{\Delta S_2}{\lambda_1(1+g_c)(1+\rho_c)}$$

Because g_c and ρ_c are small, the above expression can be approximated as:

$$V_1 \cdot \Delta H_1 + \frac{V_1 \cdot \Delta H_2}{(1+\rho_c+g_c)} \geq \frac{\Delta S_1}{\lambda_1} + \frac{\Delta S_2}{\lambda_1(1+\rho_c+g_c)}$$

Therefore, the social discount rate in this scenario can be denoted as $r = \rho_c + g_c$.

Ramsey (1928) showed that this social discount rate can be expressed as $r = \rho_c + \theta \cdot g$, where

- ρ_C is the social decision maker's pure time preference;
- θ is the consumption elasticity of marginal utility, that is, how fast the utility from marginal consumption decreases with consumption; and
- g is the growth rate of consumption (or how fast consumption is increasing).

This represents conceptualizing an optimal discount rate for CEA from a societal perspective and implies that the same discount rate should be used for both costs and the consumption value of health. In what follows, we consider the case where an explicit budget constraint has been specified for healthcare so that all costs relating to the purchase of healthcare fall on this budget, and there are no effects on consumption. Moreover, the objective function to maximize may follow an extra-welfarist approach to maximize just health and not its consumption value.

10.3.2 An Extra-Welfarist, Fixed Healthcare Budget Scenario

Under an extra-welfarist view, an explicit social goal may be to maximize health, not its consumption value, given an exogenous budget for healthcare (Claxton et al. 2011). Under these circumstances, the two-period outcomes for a technology can be represented as shown in Table 10.3.

Table 10.3 Health and cost effects in terms of current health

Time period	1	2
Present value of health gained	ΔH_1	$\dfrac{\Delta H_2}{(1+\rho_H)}$
Present consumption value forgone	$\dfrac{\Delta E_1}{k_1}$	$\dfrac{\Delta E_2}{k_2(1+\rho_H)}$

Note that here ρ_H represents the social time preference for health, which may be different from the social time preference for consumption. Here, k_t represents the health forgone due to marginal dollars spent on healthcare, that is, the cost-effectiveness threshold at time t. Hence, a decision based on the net present value of health would be to accept the technology if

$$\Delta H_1 + \frac{\Delta H_2}{\left(1+\rho_H\right)} \geq \frac{\Delta E_1}{k_1} + \frac{\Delta E_2}{k_1\left(1+\rho_H+g_k\right)}$$

10.4 SUMMARIZING THE THEORETICAL IMPLICATIONS FOR DISCOUNTING

The general framework for discounting laid out in the previous section implies that the appropriate discount rates for costs and health effects would depend on the fixed nature of the healthcare budget, the social objective of maximizing welfare versus health, changes in the consumption value of health and in the cost-effectiveness threshold, and the social time preference (which may be different for health versus consumption). The implied discount rates are summarized in Table 10.4.

10.4.1 Implications for Discount Rate from the Societal Perspective

For CEA from a societal perspective, represented by our welfarist scenario with an omnibus budget, the same discount rate should be used for both costs and the consumption value of health. Moreover, that discount rate is given by the Ramsey (1928) equation: $r = \rho_C + \theta \cdot g$.

The societal pure time preference for consumption (ρ_C) rate has been estimated to be between 1% and 2%, averaging to about 1.5% (Evans and Sezer 2002, 2004).

Table 10.4 Appropriate discount rate for costs and health effects from alternate scenarios

Scenario	Discount rate for health	Discount rate for costs
Welfarist, omnibus budget	$\rho_C + \theta \cdot g$	$\rho_C + \theta \cdot g$
Extra-welfarist, fixed healthcare budget	ρ_H	$\rho_H + g_k$

Notation:
ρ_C: social rate of time preference for consumption
ρ_H: social rate of time preference for health
θ: consumption elasticity of marginal utility of consumption
g: growth rate of consumption
g_k: growth rate of the cost-effectiveness threshold

Blundell, Browning, and Meghir (1994), using a lifetime consumption model, estimated the elasticity of the marginal utility of consumption (θ) to be between 1.2% and 1.4%. The growth rate of consumption (g) varies across countries. Latest estimates of the growth rate in consumption expenditure for the United States and the United Kingdom are around 1.7% and 1.1%, respectively (World Bank 2014). A typical estimate of a social discount rate is then given by (1.5 + 1.3*1.4) or about 3.0% to 3.5%. For example, in 2004, following this Ramsey (1928) formula, the UK National Institute for Health and Care Excellence (NICE) required that CEAs discount both costs and health effects at the 3.5% social discount rate (National Institute for Health and Care Excellence [NICE] 2004), even though NICE evaluations did not follow a societal perspective. The 2013 NICE recommendation continues to be 3.5% (National Institute for Health and Care Excellence [NICE] 2013). Similarly, the Australian Pharmaceutical Benefits Advisory Committee recommends a discount rate of 5% to be applied to both costs and health effects (Australian Government Department of Health 2013).

10.4.2 Implications for Discount Rate from a Healthcare Sector Perspective

Typically, a healthcare sector perspective represents having a fixed healthcare budget with the aim of maximizing health by itself. In this situation, the discount rate for costs is theoretically different than the discount rate for health if the cost-effectiveness threshold (k) changes over time. To determine whether the discount rate for costs would be greater or lower than that of health, one must determine the directionality (sign) of this change. Theoretically, the sign for this growth rate remains ambiguous. On the one hand, if the healthcare budget grows while holding technology constant, the cost-effectiveness threshold may increase. On the other hand, when health improves considerably over time, healthcare budgets may fall, and so would the cost-effectiveness threshold. There is no conclusive empirical evidence from the economic literature to suggest that the marginal productivity of healthcare dollars, as reflected in the cost-effectiveness threshold, is changing in one direction or the other over time, and this factor remains an area for future research. In any case, it is unlikely that the cost-effectiveness thresholds would change dramatically over short periods of time. Therefore, it is prudent to assume that $g_k = 0$, although more research is needed to better understand the directionality and the rate of change of the threshold.

When g_k is assumed to be zero, a common discount rate may be applied to both costs and health effects from the healthcare perspective. When just health is being maximized, this common discount rate is given as the social time preference for health, ρ_H. Paulden and Claxton (2012) further show that the social rate of time preference for health is revealed by the allocation of healthcare budgets over time. In fact, they show that the rate of time preference for health can be expressed as the real rate of return on investment (ρ_S) minus the growth rate of the cost-effectiveness threshold, that is, $\rho_H = \rho_S - g_k$. With g_k assumed to be zero, $\rho_H = \rho_S$.

Estimates for real rates of return vary by country. In the United States, the real rate of return for governmental bonds ranges from 2% to 4% (Thornburg Investment Management 2014), while the overall real rate of return for governmental tax revenue could be even higher (Burgess and Zerbe 2013).

10.4.3 Recommendations for Reference Case Analyses

Considerable uncertainty exists around each of the parameters that together comprise the appropriate discount rates from the societal and the healthcare sector perspectives. Because the goal of the Reference Cases is to promote comparability across studies, we recommend that a 3% interest rate be used for both costs and health effects in both the societal and the healthcare sector perspective analyses (**Recommendations 2 and 3.1**). This preserves the recommendation made by the original Panel. It is always advisable to perform sensitivity analysis around any baseline discount rates used, especially when costs and health effects are incurred at different times for different interventions. In practice, sensitivity analyses are performed by varying the rates (**Recommendation 3.2**) from the lower bound of 2%–3% to an upper bound of 8%–9%. This has been the standard of CEA practice within most industrialized countries and their assessment bodies (Gravelle and Smith 2001), including NICE in the United Kingdom and the Office of Management and Budget in the United States, although the NICE 2013 recommendations are for a sensitivity analysis at 3.5% for both costs and health effects (National Institute for Health and Care Excellence [NICE] 2013).

10.5 ALTERNATIVE DISCOUNTING METHODS

As already described above, discounting usually uses an exponential model. Over the last 30 years empirical research on time preference has demonstrated several inadequacies of the discounted utility model originally proposed by Samuelson (1937) as a descriptive model for human behavior (Frederick, Loewenstein, and O'Donoghue 2002). For example, many people would choose $100 today over $110 tomorrow. However, even though the delay is the same (1 day), those same people would choose the $110 in 31 days over $100 in 30 days, contrary to what would be predicted by the discounted utility model. These demonstrated inadequacies of the standard discounted utility model have led to a variety of alternative discounting methodologies. Doyle (2013) surveyed 20 such models. Here we describe two popular models.

10.5.1 Hyperbolic Discounting

Whereas the discount rate is stable over time in the exponential model, hyperbolic discounting changes the discount rate over time in a specific way. Ainslie (1992) showed that the discount functions in human behavior are often hyperbolic. Specifically, a discount rate that is higher in the near term and lower in the more distant future better represents people's preferences when they make decisions than does a constant discount rate (Ben-Zion, Rapoport, and Yagil 1989; Chapman and Elstein 1995; Redelmeier and Heller 1993; Thaler 1981). For example, in Thaler (1981), the discount rate for $15 now vs money 1 month, 1 year, and 10 years in the future was 345%, 120%, and 19%, respectively. To what extent such individual preferences translate to social discount rates remains to be studied.

10.5.2 Declining Discount Rate

Another approach to a non-stochastic discount rate is to determine *a priori* a declining discount rate (DDR). The primary reasons for using a DDR are (1) as healthcare budgets continue to grow in real terms, the productivity of health investments may decline, thereby relaxing the constraint of investment and (2) future discount rates are inherently uncertain, and to reflect this uncertainty one must use certainty equivalents of discount rates that naturally decline over time (Arrow et al. 2013). Sensitivity analyses are performed using alternative DDR schedules. While the United Kingdom uses DDR for cost–benefit analysis when the time horizon is greater than 30 years (HM Treasury 2003), it is not accepted by NICE for CEA (National Institute for Health and Care Excellence [NICE] 2013).

10.5.3 Conclusions: Discount Rate Method

Of the three methods discussed here, exponential discounting is the most commonly used in CEA. Hyperbolic discounting has the advantage of being descriptive (i.e., consistent with human behavior), but it is not yet a standard. While, as noted, DDRs are accepted under some jurisdictions, they are used primarily in the context of CBA with a long (at least 30-year) time horizon. To date, there is insufficient evidence to change from the current standard of the exponential method.

10.6 RECOMMENDATIONS

1. In cost-effectiveness analyses (CEAs) from both the societal and the healthcare sector perspectives, the costs and health effects of all interventions should be expressed in terms of their present value to society, as a prerequisite for generating cost-effectiveness ratios.

2. In the Reference Case analyses from both the societal and healthcare sector perspectives, costs and health effects should be discounted at the same rate.

3.1. The discount rate should be subject to review, and possible revision, over time in light of significant changes in the underlying economic data. However, to retain comparability with existing analyses, we recommend that 3% continue to be used in base-case analyses from both Reference Case perspectives for at least the next 10 years.

3.2. Sensitivity analyses should be conducted on the discount rate used in a CEA.

10.7 REFERENCES

Ainslie, G. 1992. *Picoeconomics: The Strategic Interaction of Successive Motivational States within the Person.* Cambridge: Cambridge University Press.

Arrow, K. 1995. "Intergenerational Equity and the Rate of Discount in Long-Term Social Investment." Eleventh World Congress of the International Economic Association (IEA), Tunis, Tunisia, December 1995. Stanford Economics Department Faculty Papers Archive, Paper 97-005. http://www-siepr.stanford.edu/workp/swp97005.pdf.

Arrow, K., M. Cropper, C. Gollier, B. Groom, G. Heal, R. Newell, W. Nordhaus, R. Pindyck, W. Pizer, P. Portney, T. Sterner, R. S. Tol, and M. Weitzman. 2013. Environmental economics. Determining benefits and costs for future generations. *Science* 341 (6144):349–350.

Australian Government Department of Health. 2013. "Guidelines for preparing submissions to the Pharmaceutical Benefits Advisory Committee. Version 4.4." http://www.pbac.pbs.gov.au/.

Ben-Zion, U., A. Rapoport, and J. Yagil. 1989. Discount rates inferred from decisions: an experimental study. *Manage Sci* 35 (3):270–284.

Blundell, R., M. Browning, and C. Meghir. 1994. Consumer demand and the life-cycle allocation of household expenditures. *Rev Econ Stud* 61:57–80.

Burgess, D. F., and R. O. Zerbe. 2013. The most appropriate discount rate. *Journal of Benefit-Cost Analysis* 4 (3):392–400.

Chapman, G. B., and A. S. Elstein. 1995. Valuing the future: temporal discounting of health and money. *Med Decis Making* 15 (4):373–386.

Claxton, K., M. Paulden, H. Gravelle, W. Brouwer, and A. J. Culyer. 2011. Discounting and decision making in the economic evaluation of health-care technologies. *Health Econ* 20 (1):2–15.

Claxton, K., M. Sculpher, A. Culyer, C. McCabe, A. Briggs, R. Akehurst, M. Buxton, and J. Brazier. 2006. Discounting and cost-effectiveness in NICE—stepping back to sort out a confusion. *Health Econ* 15 (1):1–4.

Doyle, J. R. 2013. Survey of time preference, delay discounting models. *Judgm Decis Mak* 8 (2):116–135.

Evans, D., and H. Sezer. 2002. A time preference measure of the social discount rate for the UK. *Appl Econ Letters* 34:1925–1934.

Evans, D., and H. Sezer. 2004. Social discount rates for six major countries. *Appl Econ Letters* 11:557–560.

Frederick, S., G. Loewenstein, and T. O'Donoghue. 2002. Time discounting and time preference: a critical review. *J Econ Lit* 40 (2):351–401.

Gravelle, H., W. Brouwer, L. Niessen, M. Postma, and F. Rutten. 2007. Discounting in economic evaluations: stepping forward towards optimal decision rules. *Health Econ* 16 (3):307–317.

Gravelle, H., and D. Smith. 2001. Discounting for health effects in cost-benefit and cost-effectiveness analysis. *Health Econ* 10 (7):587–599.

HM Treasury. 2003. The Green Book: Appraisal and Evaluation in Central Government. London: The Stationery Office (TSO). https://www.gov.uk/government/publications/the-green-book-appraisal-and-evaluation-in-central-governent.

Keeler, E. B., and S. Cretin. 1983. Discounting of life-saving and other nonmonetary effects. *Manage Sci* 29 (3):300–306.

National Institute for Health and Care Excellence (NICE). 2004. *Technology Appraisal Guidance [archived].* London: NICE.

National Institute for Health and Care Excellence (NICE). 2013. *Guide to the Methods of Technology Appraisal 2013. NICE article [PMG9].* London: NICE. http://publications.nice.org.uk/pmg9.

Nord, E. 2011. Discounting future health benefits: the poverty of consistency arguments. *Health Econ* 20 (1):16–26.

Paulden, M. 2014. "Time Preference and Discounting." In *Encyclopedia of Health Economics*, edited by A.J. Culyer, 395–403. Waltham, MA: Elsevier.

Paulden, M., and K. Claxton. 2012. Budget allocation and the revealed social rate of time preference for health. *Health Econ* 21 (5):612–618.

Ramsey, F. P. 1928. A mathematical theory of saving. *Econ J (London)* 38 (152):543–559.

Redelmeier, D. A., and D. N. Heller. 1993. Time preference in medical decision making and cost-effectiveness analysis. *Med Decis Making* 13 (3):212–217.

Samuelson, P. A. 1937. A note on measurement of utility. *Rev Econ Stud* 4 (2):155–161.

Solow, R. M. 1974. Intergenerational equity and exhaustible resources. *Rev Econ Stud* 41 (Symposium on the Economics of Exhaustible Resources):29–45.

Thaler, R. 1981. Some empirical evidence on dynamic inconsistency. *Econ Letters* 8:201–207.

Thornburg Investment Management. 2014. A Study of *Real* Real Returns. August 2014. Santa Fe, NM: Thornburg Investment Management, Inc. http://www.thornburginvestments.com/pdfs/th1401.pdf.

Viscusi, W. K. 1995. "Discounting Health Effects for Medical Decisions." In *Valuing Health Care: Costs, Benefits, and Effectiveness of Pharmaceuticals and Other Medical Technologies*, edited by F.A. Sloan, 123–145. New York: Cambridge University Press.

Weinstein, M. C., and W. B. Stason. 1977. Foundations of cost-effectiveness analysis for health and medical practices. *N Engl J Med* 296 (13):716–721.

World Bank. 2014. "Data on Household Final Consumption Expenditure per Capita Growth (Annual %)." http://data.worldbank.org/indicator/NE.CON.PRVT.PC.KD.ZG. Accessed February 24, 2016.

11

Reflecting Uncertainty
in Cost-Effectiveness Analysis

Mark J. Sculpher, Anirban Basu, Karen M. Kuntz,
and David O. Meltzer

11.1 INTRODUCTION

In conducting a cost-effectiveness analysis (CEA) to evaluate the value of a treatment or prevention regimen, the analyst combines evidence, often in the form of parameter values, on the natural course of disease, the clinical effectiveness of the alternative regimens, preferences regarding health outcomes, the costs of interventions and their sequelae, and other aspects of the clinical problem. In addition, analyses usually include a series of structural or model assumptions, which may be expressed as numerical values (parameters) but generally are not. Rather, they represent best judgments about a range of factors included in an analysis, including the most suitable sources of evidence given the decision problem being addressed, the best fitting statistical model with which to estimate one or more parameters, and the ways in which the values of parameters might change beyond the time period for which data are available.

Parameter values used in a CEA are usually derived from sampled data. Even when samples are not the source of the values—for example, in the case of age- and sex-specific mortality risks taken from routine life-tables, which are based on deaths across the entire population over a period of time—they may be considered uncertain for different populations—for example, mortality risks in the whole population in future years or in a given subgroup of the population. Similarly, structural assumptions are inherently uncertain: although they may not be formally parameterized, they generally represent one specific assumption from a large number of possible alternatives.

This chapter builds on concepts presented in Chapter 8 of the original Panel's book (Manning, W.G., D.G. Fryback, and M.C. Weinstein. 1996. "Reflecting Uncertainty in Cost-Effectiveness Analysis." In *Cost-Effectiveness in Health and Medicine*, edited by M.R. Gold, J.E. Siegel, L.B. Russell and M.C. Weinstein, 247–275. New York: Oxford University Press).

An important stage in any CEA is to deal appropriately with this uncertainty, which is unavoidable and relates to each and every study (Drummond et al. 2015). Since the 1996 publication of the original Panel's report, several methods guidelines for CEAs have been developed by countries that routinely use CEA for health technology appraisals; for example, the United Kingdom (National Institute for Health and Care Excellence [NICE] 2013), Canada (Canadian Agency for Drugs and Technologies in Health [CADTH] 2006), and Australia (Australian Government Department of Health 2015). In general these guidelines emphasize the importance of reflecting uncertainty in CEA but are not prescriptive about the methods to be used. The Good Research Practices in Modeling Task Force—a collaboration between the International Society for Pharmacoeconomics and Outcomes Research (ISPOR) and the Society for Medical Decision Making (SMDM)—has published best practice recommendations for conducting uncertainty analysis and provides more detailed guidance on methods and approaches (Briggs et al. 2012). Building on the guidance of the ISPOR-SMDM Task Force and other recent work (Drummond et al. 2015), this chapter describes why uncertainty needs to be considered in CEA if the purpose is to inform policy, what types of assessment need to be made, and what these imply about the methods to be used.

11.2 DEFINITION OF TERMS

The terminology used to describe uncertainty in CEA is evolving and can be a source of confusion. The ISPOR-SMDM Task Force (Briggs et al. 2012) has provided a valuable summary of some of the key terms, which is reproduced in Table 11.1. The table outlines four distinct but related concepts. The first is "stochastic uncertainty"—often referred to as *variability*—which is analogous to the standard deviation associated with a sample mean; that is, it characterizes differences in outcomes between individual patients in a measurement of interest. Stochastic uncertainty is of no direct interest in CEA as it does not directly inform decisions, although, as discussed in Chapter 5, individual-level models use the concept as a way of estimating population means. As such, it is not explored further here.

"Parameter uncertainty" is a second concept and is closely related to the first. The parameters used in CEA are generally estimates of population means based on sampled data. Examples are the costs of being in given health states, the quality of life associated with those states, the rate of clinical events over time, and the relative effectiveness of one intervention versus another. These mean parameter values are estimated with uncertainty reflected, for example, in the standard error and 95% confidence interval associated with an estimated population mean, and these values lie behind measures of parameter uncertainty. Although estimates are ideally taken from primary studies such as clinical trials and observational studies, the absence of such evidence may require the use of formal expert elicitation methods (Soares et al. 2013) (see Chapter 9).

The third concept is "structural uncertainty." As already indicated, this relates to the assumptions made in all CEAs. Although not generally expressed in the form of numerical parameters, the fact that each assumption is chosen from a (potentially

Table 11.1 Defining terms in uncertainty analysis as part of cost-effectiveness analysis (CEA)

Preferred term	Concept	Other terms sometimes employed	Analogous concept in regression
Stochastic uncertainty	Random variability in outcomes between identical patients	Variability; Monte Carlo error; first-order uncertainty	Error term
Parameter uncertainty	The uncertainty in estimation of the parameter of interest	Second-order uncertainty	Standard error of the estimate
Structural uncertainty	The assumptions inherent in the decision model	Model uncertainty	The form of the regression model (e.g., linear, log-linear, etc.)
Heterogeneity	The variability between patients that can be attributed to characteristics of those patients	Variability; observed or explained heterogeneity	Beta coefficients (or the extent to which the dependent variable varies by patient or other characteristics)

Source: Briggs et al. (2012).

large) number of competing alternatives means there is structural or model uncertainty about whether the selected assumption is the only appropriate one.

The final concept is "heterogeneity," which concerns the estimation of parameter values relating to subgroups of the population. The notion of subgroup analysis is based on the process of identifying observed characteristics that provide some level of statistical explanation for the variation (stochastic uncertainty) in a sample. Relevant characteristics are usually those that can be observed when a decision is being made about which of the alternative courses of action is the most cost-effective for specific subgroups of individuals. When heterogeneity is considered to be important and subgroup-specific parameter values are estimated, these form the basis of separate cost-effectiveness estimates of the alternative interventions (i.e., one set of estimates for each relevant subgroup). Heterogeneity often relates to patients or other individuals, but it can also exist when there are systematic differences in parameter values between different jurisdictions (e.g., unit costs and prices, prevalence and baseline risk of clinical events). A failure to reflect the implications of heterogeneity for decision making may risk recommendations that are inconsistent with a cost-effective use of resources (Basu 2011). Although heterogeneity is linked to uncertainty (Espinoza et al. 2014), it is not dealt with further in this chapter. The importance of heterogeneity to CEA is dealt with more fully in Chapter 2. The challenges of identifying and quantifying heterogeneity in available evidence are considered in Chapter 9.

Other analytical concepts are added to these core definitions in this chapter. In particular, those of decision uncertainty (the probability of a decision being wrong, based on available evidence) and value-of-information (VOI) analysis (the expected cost imposed by uncertainty and the value of further research in reducing that cost). The aim of this chapter is to describe how to characterize parameter and structural uncertainty and to consider their implications for decision making regarding the adoption of interventions and generation of additional evidence.

11.3 UNCERTAINTY AND DECISION MAKING

Conducting uncertainty analysis is important for several reasons. One relates to the fact that, in non-linear decision-analytic models such as Markov models, an appropriate estimate of incremental cost-effectiveness requires that the uncertainty in all input parameters be characterized as probability distributions and propagated using simulation (Briggs, Claxton, and Sculpher 2006). In other words, to get the correct results, the model would need to be run probabilistically (i.e., using probabilistic sensitivity analysis—see Section 11.4.2 below) rather than deterministically (i.e., with parameters set at their estimated mean values), even though the differences between these two approaches may be quite small. A second reason for undertaking some forms of uncertainty analysis is to assure the analyst (as well as peer reviewers and, perhaps, decision makers) that the model is working appropriately. That is, by changing the value of individual parameters in deterministic sensitivity analysis, it is possible to check that the model's results are moving in the expected direction and, if not, to assess whether this is due to an error in model structure, parameterization, or coding.

The main purpose of uncertainty analysis, however, is to contribute to better decisions. The purpose of CEA is to inform resource allocation decisions. It follows that the specification of an uncertainty analysis should be guided by the needs of decision making. As discussed in Chapter 2, there are competing normative foundations for economic evaluation in healthcare. The purpose of applied CEA is usually seen as informing decisions aimed at generating the largest benefits (generally with a focus on health outcomes) from available resources. Of course, considerations other than health outcomes are likely to be relevant to decision makers, who may not be focused on benefit maximization because they are risk-averse with respect to costs, health outcomes, or other possible outcomes. In general, however, researchers and decision makers have taken the view that health outcomes (rather than, say, decision makers' preferences) are an appropriate objective to reflect in a CEA. The types of uncertainty analyses to be conducted need to be determined by these decision-making objectives and constraints.

Inferential statistics have a key role in medical research—that is, setting up null and alternative hypotheses and assessing whether the available evidence is sufficiently strong to depart from the null (Armitage, Berry, and Matthews 2002). Despite its widespread use elsewhere, statistical inference is not consistent with the objective of maximizing health outcomes (or any other objective function) subject to resource and other constraints (Claxton 1999). For example, in the context of a comparison of two alternative interventions, a CEA may present an incremental cost-effectiveness ratio (ICER) for the more effective and more costly option based on the expected (estimated mean) differential costs and effects (see Chapter 2). Standard decision rules would suggest that, as long as the estimated ICER is below the relevant cost-effectiveness threshold, the more effective option would also be considered cost-effective. The fact that the expected differences in costs and/or effects (or incremental net benefit—see Chapters 7 and 8) between the two interventions are not formally statistically significantly different from zero would have no relevance given the objective of maximizing benefits from available resources. This is so because the expected (mean) differences in costs and health outcomes represent the best estimate to support decision making on the basis of existing evidence.

In contrast to inferential statistics, the purpose of uncertainty analysis in CEA is to assess whether more appropriate decisions are possible when uncertainty is characterized and quantified, and its implications are assessed. To some extent this depends on the decision maker's responsibilities (Walker et al. 2012). In the context of decisions about the funding of new medical technologies, for example, is there scope for the decision maker to move away from a simple "accept" or "reject" decision at one point in time? If not, then knowing something about uncertainty may not be important, and decisions should simply be based on expected (estimated mean) costs and effects. In most contexts, however, it is possible to broaden the range of decision options. In the United States, for example, where formalized processes for using CEA to support funding decisions are less well established than in some other parts of the world, the analyst should assume that a range of possible decision options is available and be explicit about what has been assumed about those options. Decision options might include one or more of the following (Claxton et al. 2012):

i. Making an "accept" or "reject" decision now, but being able to revisit that decision at some point in the future. The short-term decision may be based on expected cost-effectiveness given existing evidence, but a subsequent review would allow the decision maker to revise the decision if more evidence has emerged (e.g., through further research, a change in prices, or the availability of other interventions).
ii. Funding the interventions only in the context of formal research and having the opportunity to revise the decision when that research reports. As with (i), the decision can be reviewed in the future, but reimbursement/funding during the research period may increase the chances that research of the type required by the decision maker will be undertaken.
iii. Funding the new intervention for general use, but also requiring that further research be undertaken and, again, reviewing the decision in the future. Importantly, this would require the decision maker to take the view, based on existing evidence, that the new technology is expected to be cost-effective but to believe that further research could be successfully undertaken and that a different decision may be required in the future. In the United States, this approach, which has been used in some instances by Medicare, has become known as "coverage with evidence development" (Centers for Medicare & Medicaid Services 2014).
iv. Depending on the nature of the uncertainty (i.e., effectiveness vs cost-effectiveness), a price reduction from the intervention's manufacturer (in the case of a proprietary technology) may change the implications of parameter and structural uncertainty and facilitate, for example, an "accept" or "coverage with evidence development" decision rather than a "reject" decision.

Although the above decision options are couched in terms of new proprietary technologies seeking access to a market, they are also relevant to other types of intervention. For example, public health programs can be evaluated in the same way, and policy options may include, in addition to "accept" and "reject," a decision to review at some future point, fund only in research, and fund generally but include organized research.

The analytical challenge is, therefore, how best to inform the decision-making process regarding which of the available options is best in terms of improving health outcomes from available resources. In this context, decision makers seeking to achieve a cost-effective allocation of resources should consider a series of questions:

- Is the intervention expected to be cost-effective based on existing evidence (i.e., is the ICER expected to be below the cost-effectiveness threshold)?
- Given all sources of parameter and structural uncertainty, what is the likelihood that the intervention is not cost-effective (i.e., the probability that the expected ICER is above the threshold, which is the probability that an "accept" decision would be wrong)? This concept is known as "decision uncertainty." As with the concept of decision rules, this assumes the decision is based on the costs and outcomes included in the CEA.
- What is the expected cost of uncertainty in terms of resources or health outcomes? This is the product of the probability of a wrong decision and the resource/health consequences of that decision. This is also the value of perfect information (Briggs, Claxton, and Sculpher 2006); that is, the maximum value of research that could remove all existing uncertainty.
- What are the expected implications of specific designs of research study in terms of the costs of their conduct and the impact on the cost of uncertainty?
- What is the likelihood of particular research studies being undertaken and of reporting at particular time periods? Inevitably the value of research will depend on whether the study actually takes place and when the results are available to inform a future decision.
- To what extent can "accept" or "reject" decisions be changed in the future in the face of new evidence, and how is this affected by the potentially irreversible effects of the initial decision such as up-front investment in capital equipment and training?

These questions need to be considered by decision makers regardless of the type of formal uncertainty analysis provided. In other words, it is possible to separate the questions that should be addressed in the decision-making process from the uncertainty analysis that informs that process. However, it is clearly preferable that the uncertainty analysis is undertaken in such a way as to inform directly the needs of decision makers and to support the choice of the best policy option. How best to do this is the focus of the rest of this chapter.

11.4 PARAMETER UNCERTAINTY

Once CEA became widely used in health and medicine in the 1970s and 1980s, the field accepted a need for quantitative analysis of the implications of parameter uncertainty for the results of the analysis (Weinstein et al. 1980). Over the subsequent period, methods for conducting such analyses have been developed that can provide a clearer link with the types of decision-making questions outlined above.

11.4.1 Deterministic Sensitivity Analysis

Deterministic sensitivity analysis has been widely used in CEA. The simplest form is *one-way sensitivity analysis*, which involves varying single parameters from their base-case values, one at a time, and reporting the implications for the results. The value of this type of sensitivity analysis is in understanding how changing individual parameter values can influence results. As such, it is of particular value in model checking—i.e., the process of establishing whether changing parameters has predictable effects on results—as mentioned earlier. However, the method is limited in addressing the decision-making questions outlined above. In particular, although one-way sensitivity analysis gives an indication of the *potential* importance of a parameter to the results of an analysis, it provides no quantitative indication of decision uncertainty—the probability that an "accept" decision is wrong based on existing evidence. Furthermore, it cannot show which parameters contribute most to the overall decision uncertainty. This is because, first, decision uncertainty is driven not by changes in the outputs of the model but, rather, by the likelihood that parameter uncertainty will change a decision (i.e., will move the expected ICER to the other side of the cost-effectiveness threshold vis-à-vis the base-case analysis). Second, variation in an input parameter as part of one-way sensitivity analysis is often unrelated to the uncertainty in that parameter. In such circumstances, variation in one parameter may have a pronounced impact on expected costs and effects, whereas variation in another parameter will have much less impact. However, the first parameter may have been estimated with more precision than the second and will consequently have less impact on the ultimate decision.

Guidelines for the use of one-way sensitivity analysis include providing a clear justification for how the upper and lower values of the parameter for the analysis are chosen and how this choice links with available evidence (Briggs et al. 2012). These one-way sensitivity analyses sometimes take "extreme but plausible" values to give the analysis a strong test of robustness. These could, for example, take the values of the bounds of the 95% or 99% confidence interval of the estimated mean, although possible values lie outside these ranges. One-way sensitivity analysis effectively considers three specific values of a parameter (the base-case value, and the upper and lower values), and each of these would have a very small probability of being the "correct" value. The problem is that the analysis does not take into consideration the full range of possible values the parameter could take and the *probability* of each value being the "correct" one.

Multi-way sensitivity analysis is closely related to one-way sensitivity analysis, the difference being that more than one parameter is varied at a time and the impact on outputs is then considered. Results are usually presented graphically, and it is possible to show the implications of variation in two, or perhaps three, parameters. Beyond this number, however, presentation and interpretation becomes a major challenge. As with one-way sensitivity analysis, there is no indication as to the likelihood that parameters take on the particular values they are varied between, as this needs an assessment of any correlation between them.

A variant on deterministic sensitivity analysis is *threshold analysis*, which involves changing the value of one or more parameters until the output of interest crosses some threshold that is considered to have decision relevance. An example would be to vary uncertain parameters until the net cost of an intervention compared to an alternative crosses zero. Another example would be to vary the parameters until the ICER of an intervention crosses a defined cost-effectiveness threshold. In principle, threshold analysis provides useful information because it more closely relates uncertainty in parameters to potential changes in decisions. As with all deterministic sensitivity analyses, however, threshold analysis provides no information on the likelihood that particular parameters will take the values that (singly or jointly) may change decisions.

Although deterministic sensitivity analysis does not provide a full analytical basis for the *uncertainty* assessments outlined above, it can be used as a means of understanding the implications of *heterogeneity*. For example, in the context of potential geographical heterogeneity, an economic evaluation undertaken in the United Kingdom using a given set of unit costs could be applied in the United States by changing the unit costs and other parameters considered to be specific to the United States. Regarding patient-level heterogeneity, a parameter (e.g., the probability of side effects) that is considered suitable for younger patients may need to be changed for older patients. However, when one or more parameters is re-estimated to reflect potential heterogeneity, the relevant parameters are still uncertain, and deterministic sensitivity analysis remains a limited means of assessing the implications of that uncertainty.

11.4.2 Probabilistic Sensitivity Analysis

Given the limitations of deterministic sensitivity analyses in supporting the assessments necessary to make decisions, there has been increasing use of probabilistic sensitivity analysis (PSA) to characterize parameter uncertainty (this is sometimes more generally called probabilistic modeling). This approach is recommended by the ISPOR-SMDM Task Force (Briggs et al. 2012), NICE (National Institute for Health and Care Excellence [NICE] 2013), and CADTH (Canadian Agency for Drugs and Technologies in Health [CADTH] 2006). The key distinctions between PSA and deterministic sensitivity analysis are that PSA characterizes uncertainty in *all* parameters simultaneously, explicitly reflects the *likelihood* that parameters take on particular values, and quantifies *decision uncertainty* on the basis of uncertain parameters.

Probabilistic sensitivity analysis proceeds in two stages. The first involves expressing the uncertainty associated with each parameter. In contrast to deterministic sensitivity analysis, which does this by defining a simple range, PSA defines a probability distribution for each uncertain parameter. This provides an estimate of the full range of values that the parameter can take, together with the probability of each value. The distributions relate to the parameter values (usually estimated population mean values) rather than to variation between patients. This is the important distinction outlined above between parameter uncertainty and stochastic uncertainty (variability). As for any parametric statistical analysis, it is important for the analyst to be transparent regarding the choice and specification of the distribution for each parameter and how this is justified on the basis of the available evidence (Briggs et al. 2012). Table 11.2 summarizes the candidate distributions for common types of parameters in decision-analytic models used for CEA. The choice is constrained by the characteristics of parameters. For example, a probability parameter is constrained between 0 and 1, so the selected distribution should not provide parameter values outside that range. For most types of parameters, there is more than one distribution from which to choose, so clear justification is needed of the selection made, and potentially this choice should be considered as a form of structural uncertainty (see Section 11.5).

Most parameters should be included in a PSA on the basis that they are generally estimated from samples or on the basis of expert elicitation with uncertainty. An exception in the typical cost-effectiveness model is the discount rate, which may be recommended by the decision maker or based on, for example, the rate of return on government bonds (see Chapter 10). The unit cost of resources may also be assumed

Table 11.2 Selecting distributions for uncertain parameters

Parameter	Logical constraint	Form of data	Methods of estimation	Candidate distribution
Probability	$0 \leq \theta \leq 1$	Binomial	Proportion	Beta
		Multinomial	Proportions	Dirichlet
		Time to event	Survival analysis	Lognormal
Relative risk	$\theta > 0$	Binomial	Ratio of proportions	Lognormal
Cost (based on uncertain estimates of resource use)	$\theta \geq 0$	Weighted sum of resource counts	Mean, standard error	Gamma Lognormal
Quality of life weight (utility) decrement including the possibility of health states valued worse than death	$\theta \geq 0$	Continuous	Mean, standard error	Gamma Lognormal
Through central limit theorem, all parameters if sufficient data are available	Any constraint	Any distribution of data	Mean, standard error	Normal

Source: Adapted from Briggs, Claxton, and Sculpher (2006).

to be known with certainty on the basis that, in some situations, this is a specified price paid by a health system (although there may be heterogeneity in prices among systems). However, unit costs of particular types of resource are sometimes estimated from sample data and should consequently be introduced into a model as uncertain variables. Resource use is generally estimated from samples, so a derived estimate of cost (the product of resource use and unit cost) will be an uncertain parameter.

In cost-effectiveness models, parameters are often estimated from secondary sources that present evidence in summary form (e.g., a mean and 95% confidence interval). The way the estimated parameter is presented has implications for the choice of distribution. For example, the beta distribution would be appropriate to express uncertainty in a probability based on a reported proportion, whereas a multivariate normal distribution on the log odds scale would be suitable for a probability estimated from a logistic regression (Briggs, Claxton, and Sculpher 2006).

If parameters are potentially correlated, this needs to be reflected in the PSA, as this can affect the overall estimates of decision uncertainty. Where several parameters have been estimated from individual patient data, estimates of correlation can be readily identified (Briggs, Claxton, and Sculpher 2006). This would be true, for example, if several parameter estimates came from a regression analysis where the variance-covariance matrix provides the basis to estimate their correlations. Indeed, well-reported secondary sources of evidence from statistical models will provide sufficient information to estimate correlations.

In general, when information about a parameter is very limited, this would be reflected in wider, more uncertain distributions. Sometimes the analyst has no information on the uncertainty in a given parameter; for example, a secondary source may only report the estimated mean of a parameter, with insufficient information to characterize its uncertainty. There may also be little or no information on the correlation between parameters. In such cases, explicit assumptions may be needed, which form part of the structural uncertainties in the analysis. These "parameter gaps" may be filled through formal expert elicitation. The latter techniques are discussed more fully below in Section 11.5, and various overviews are available in the literature (O'Hagan et al. 2006; Soares et al. 2011). The absence of information about the uncertainty in a parameter from secondary sources is not a good reason for assuming the parameter is known with certainty and can enter the model as a deterministic parameter.

The second stage of a PSA is based on simulation to propagate uncertain parameters through the decision model. This involves a process of simultaneously selecting a value from each parameter distribution and running the model using the selected vector of values to provide a single estimate of outputs for each option being evaluated. This is then repeated a large number of times (e.g., 10,000), providing a distribution of outputs. Averaging over this distribution provides the overall expected costs, outcomes, and relevant measure of cost-effectiveness (e.g., ICER), but the distribution also provides a means of expressing decision uncertainty (see Section 11.6). The appropriate number of simulations in the PSA will depend on the complexity of the model and the degree of uncertainty in the parameters. The analyst should monitor the overall expected values of the output (the average across all simulations) and assess when these have stabilized.

In some models the use of simulation methods to propagate parameter uncertainty in PSA is challenging. This may be the case, for example, in some individual patient sampling models for which two levels of simulation are needed: one that reflects variability between individual patients (stochastic uncertainty) to calculate one mean cost or outcome, and the other, the PSA, which reflects the distributions of uncertain parameters. These joint simulations can consume a large amount of computation time, a problem that may be mitigated by the use of increasingly powerful computers or clusters. There are also ways of simplifying the computation process using, for example, model emulators or cloning within the patient-level simulation (Stevenson, Oakley, and Chilcott 2004). If a model is so complex as effectively to preclude PSA, a judgment has to be made as to whether the model provides a better guide to decision making than a simpler analysis in which PSA is feasible.

So far this chapter has assumed that a decision-analytic model would be the vehicle for the CEA. Some studies are, however, based on analyses of individual patient data, for example, from randomized controlled trials (RCTs). It is feasible for such analyses to handle parameter uncertainty in a way similar to simulation-based PSA in models. Again, the aim is to generate an expression of the joint uncertainty in the relevant outputs of the analysis based on all sources of parameter uncertainty. This can be achieved using statistical modeling—for example, regression analysis where the estimated coefficients can be interpreted as incremental costs, outcomes, and cost-effectiveness (Willan and Briggs 2006). The standard errors of the estimated coefficients—like PSA based on particular parametric assumptions—can be used to express decision uncertainty, and also provide a way of quantifying the correlation between different parameters. A widely used alternative is non-parametric bootstrapping, which generates a large number of estimates of the expected values of outputs of interest based on a large number of resamples from the data (Briggs, O'Brien, and Blackhouse 2002).

11.5 STRUCTURAL UNCERTAINTY

As described earlier, parameters are not the only source of uncertainty in CEA. Structural (or model) uncertainty also exists in analyses and should be appropriately handled (Bojke et al. 2009). Structural uncertainty can be significant and is often at least as important as parameter uncertainty (Kim and Thompson 2010). What has been termed "structural uncertainty" actually includes a number of different types of uncertainty and might be more accurately termed "unparameterized sources of uncertainty." Although these characteristics of analyses often appear as assumptions or judgments, they represent single possibilities among what may be numerous plausible alternatives. Selecting one assumption from among those many alternatives may affect study results and imply different decisions when compared to other choices. These

unparameterized sources of uncertainty can be of considerable importance in informing decisions. Examples include:

- How to model the effects of an intervention beyond the time horizon of the evidence
  source. This might range from assuming no effect to a continued effect equal to that
  shown by the available evidence to something in between.
- How different states of health and pathways of care are characterized in a model and
  how patients' disease is modeled to progress.
- How disease progression is modeled over time (extrapolated) beyond the follow-up
  period in the study from which the evidence is drawn.
- Assumptions inherent in other forms of extrapolation from available evidence,
  including to other populations and subpopulations and from intermediate outcomes
  to ultimate measures of health.
- The choice of statistical model to estimate a given parameter.
- Judgments about the relevance and appropriateness of different sources of evidence.

Most studies assess the importance of structural uncertainty by varying an assumption
and assessing the impact on model outputs. This is termed *scenario analysis* and can
co-exist with the use of PSA to handle parameter uncertainty, with a new PSA undertaken for each alternative scenario. Scenario analysis is analogous to deterministic
sensitivity analysis for parameter uncertainty, and it suffers from the same limitations.
Specifically, it does not communicate the likelihood of each alternative scenario being
the most appropriate. In effect, scenario analysis can be seen as externalizing the task
of understanding the link between structural uncertainty and decision uncertainty,
placing the burden on decision makers, who are then required to select one scenario
as the most plausible within their context and setting. Although some decision makers
may be willing to take on this responsibility, choosing one scenario effectively implies
that there is a zero chance that the alternatives may be more or most appropriate.

Methods have been developed (and, to a lesser extent, applied) that seek to incorporate structural uncertainty into the PSA and consequently into the presentation of
decision uncertainty (Bojke et al. 2009; Jackson et al. 2011). One approach would be
to parameterize the alternative assumptions with an appropriate probability distribution. To illustrate, assume there are considered to be three alternative assumptions
about long-term treatment effect beyond a trial: it declines to zero, it continues perma-
nently, or it reduces to 50% of its estimated value on a permanent basis. Rather than
simply presenting expected cost-effectiveness and decision uncertainty for three separate scenarios, an uncertainty parameter could be included that weights each scenario
to represent the likelihood that it is the correct assumption. An alternative approach
would be to introduce a single parameter to represent the proportion of the treatment
effect sustained over time. As structural uncertainty has now been parameterized, its
uncertainty can also be characterized as a distribution, and PSA can be undertaken in
the usual way.

Parameterizing structural uncertainty in this way requires an explicit distribution to be assigned to these additional parameters. Expert elicitation methods can

be used to estimate these parameters and to characterize their uncertainty. There are formal methods for this purpose (O'Hagan et al. 2006), which need to be carefully presented and justified. For example, in assessing the cost-effectiveness of alternative treatments for psoriatic arthritis, Bojke et al. (2010) faced uncertainty about disease progression when patients come off a therapy from which they initially benefited. Reflecting a clinical view that there would be some sort of rebound (worsening of outcomes) in this situation, earlier work (Bravo Vergel et al. 2007) had modeled two distinct scenarios: (i) rebound equal to the initial clinical improvement and (ii) rebound equal to the clinical outcome that patients would be experiencing had they never been treated, as defined by the disease's natural history. In subsequent work (Bojke et al. 2010), the authors elicited uncertain quantities relating to the change in outcome from clinical experts, and this was incorporated into the model as a single uncertain parameter. Elicitation methods should be considered as a means of parameterizing structural uncertainties. It is possible, however, that decision makers will take their own views on the elicited values. There may be scope to incorporate these views directly into analyses. For example, Bujkiewicz et al. developed a transparent interactive decision interrogator (TIDI) to allow decision makers to explore the implications of alternative assumptions and scenarios (Bujkiewicz et al. 2011). Where no specific decision maker is associated with a particular analysis, researchers should consider reflecting structural uncertainties using scenario analysis and appropriately elicited quantities.

In some situations structural uncertainty relates to the choice of alternative statistical models to estimate a given (set of) parameter(s). Rather than select one statistical model as the most appropriate and discard the others, a method known as "model averaging" can be used to combine estimates across models, weighting each set of results by a measure of how well each respective model fits the data. For example, Jackson and colleagues' analysis of the cost-effectiveness of implantable cardioverter defibrillators developed a set of statistical models that reflected structural uncertainties in terms of choice of covariates and extrapolation of age effects on survival (Jackson, Thompson, and Sharples 2009). These uncertainties were reflected by averaging the posterior distributions from the alternative models using weights based on the predicted validity of the models.

Despite recent methods developments to parameterize structural uncertainty, these approaches are yet to be widely used in practice. Their advantages mean they should be considered by analysts. In their absence, scenario analysis should be used as the means of presenting the implications of structural uncertainty. A full range of scenarios should be incorporated to reflect the nature of the uncertainty. For each, a PSA should be undertaken.

11.6 DECISION UNCERTAINTY

Probabilistic sensitivity analysis provides stronger analytical support for decision making than deterministic sensitivity analysis, as it provides a means of quantifying *decision* uncertainty. This is particularly the case if relevant structural uncertainties have been parameterized. However, this requires the large number of estimates of relevant model outcomes from the PSA (one for each selected vector of values from parameter distributions) to be communicated in such a way that the implied decision uncertainty is made explicit. This is relatively straightforward when two options are being compared, but it is more difficult when more options are evaluated.

11.6.1 Comparing Two Options

A widely used approach to present PSA is to plot the simulated incremental costs and health effects in the form of a scatterplot on the cost-effectiveness plane. An example is shown in Figure 11.1, which compares two options: a program of community-based pharmaceutical care for elderly patients versus usual care. The simulations from the PSA represent different realizations of uncertain incremental costs and effects. Here they fall in all four quadrants, indicating that there is a non-zero probability of each of the four corresponding CEA results: pharmaceutical care could be dominant (less costly and more effective) in the bottom right quadrant; more effective and more costly (top right); dominated (less effective and more costly) in the top left quadrant; or less costly and less effective in the bottom left. On the basis of a scatterplot, it is possible to report the proportion of PSA iterations that fall, for example, in the bottom two quadrants, showing that an intervention is less costly than its comparator, which is represented as the origin. This can be interpreted as the probability that the intervention is less costly than its comparator. In the case illustrated in Figure 11.1, pharmaceutical care has a 0.10 probability of being less costly than usual care. Similarly, the proportion of iterations to the right of the vertical axis can be interpreted as the probability that an intervention is more effective than the comparator (in this case,

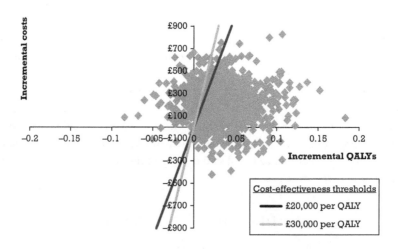

Figure 11.1 Scatterplot of the results of a probabilistic sensitivity analysis (PSA) on the cost-effectiveness plane, showing two cost-effectiveness thresholds. Example is the comparison of pharmaceutical care versus usual care in elderly patients (Respect Trial Team 2010).

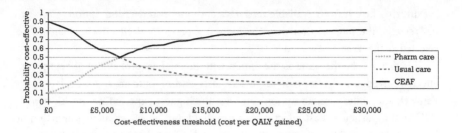

Figure 11.2 Cost-effectiveness acceptability curves showing the probabilities of pharmaceutical care (pharm care) and of usual care being cost-effective in elderly patients as the cost-effectiveness threshold varies; also shown is the cost-effectiveness acceptability frontier (CEAF) indicating the probability of being cost-effective for the option with the highest expected cost-effectiveness. *Source*: Adapted from RESPECT Trial Team (2010).

0.85). The most informative expression of decision uncertainty is the probability that pharmaceutical care is more *cost-effective* than usual care conditional on the model's structural assumptions. This is equivalent to the proportion of the simulations that lie to the southeast of a leading diagonal line going through the origin, the slope of which equals the relevant cost-effectiveness threshold. Figure 11.1 shows two alternative thresholds—£20,000 and £30,000 per QALY gained—representing the NICE threshold range. At these thresholds, pharmaceutical care has probabilities of being cost-effective of 0.775 and 0.812, respectively.

Most decision makers, including those in the United States, do not specify cost-effectiveness thresholds. Although empirical estimates are emerging (Claxton et al. 2015a), it may be necessary to state the probability of an intervention being cost-effective for a range of different cost-effectiveness thresholds. Cost-effectiveness acceptability curves (CEACs) have been developed as a means of communicating this information (Fenwick, O'Brien, and Briggs 2004; van Hout et al. 1994). Examples of two CEACs, shown in Figure 11.2, are based on the same evaluation of pharmaceutical care in the elderly (Respect Trial Team 2010). These show how the probabilities that the intervention and usual care, respectively, are cost-effective vary with the cost-effectiveness threshold. When the cost-effectiveness threshold is very low, much more weight is given to cost differences between the interventions. At one extreme, where the threshold is zero (where there is no value accorded to improving outcomes), the probability that the intervention will be cost-effective is equal to the probability of it being less costly (here, 0.10, as above). When the threshold is very high, much more weight is given to the health outcomes—when the threshold is infinite (no concern for any additional costs), the probability that an intervention is cost-effective is equal to the probability of it being the more effective alternative (here, 0.85, as above). Between these points lies a range of cost-effectiveness threshold values that relate to different probabilities of an intervention being cost-effective.

Clarity is required about how to interpret CEACs, and it is tempting to assume that, for a given cost-effectiveness threshold, the intervention with the highest *probability* of being cost-effective should be preferred. However, as outlined in Chapter 2, it is important to emphasize that, on the basis of existing evidence and assuming an objective of maximizing health from available resources and only two decision options ("accept" or "reject"), the intervention with the highest *expected* cost-effectiveness should be selected as the most cost-effective.

This may not be the same as the option with the highest probability of being cost-effective given the skewness in expected costs and/or outcomes. As explained by Fenwick and colleagues, an option can have the highest expected net health benefit (NHB) at a particular cost-effectiveness threshold, but have a smaller proportion of PSA simulations with the highest NHB (Fenwick, Claxton, and Sculpher 2001) (see Section 11.6.2 for a discussion of how NHBs are calculated). In the case of the program of community-based pharmaceutical care for elderly patients, this happens to the intervention for thresholds between about £6,400 and £6,700 per QALY. Therefore, the decision can be informed by presenting, for a given cost-effectiveness threshold, the probability of cost-effectiveness for the treatment that has the highest expected cost-effectiveness. This is shown in the cost-effectiveness acceptability frontier (CEAF) in Figure 11.2, which presents the probability of cost-effectiveness for the intervention expected to be cost-effective on average for a given cost-effectiveness threshold. In Figure 11.2 the CEAF follows the higher CEAC except between the two threshold values noted above.

It is important to emphasize that the CEAC is unlikely to incorporate all sources of uncertainty in an analysis unless all sources of structural uncertainty have been fully parameterized. If structural uncertainties are left unparameterized, a CEAC needs to be presented for each scenario relating to the structural uncertainty.

11.6.2 Comparing More Than Two Options

Given the principle that all relevant mutually exclusive options need to be considered in a CEA (see Chapter 4), many studies will need to compare more than two alternative options. This is particularly true, for example, of diagnostic studies, which may compare a large number of alternative strategies including combined and sequential tests, and the introduction of different treatments at different points in the patient care pathway. Indeed, even analyses of therapeutic interventions can include a large number of options when the full range of alternatives is considered, which may include sequential treatment strategies and different treatment starting and stopping rules.

Presenting decision uncertainty when more than two options are being compared can be challenging. A scatterplot on the cost-effectiveness plane is presented in Figure 11.3 using the example of alternative testing strategies for coronary heart disease (Walker et al. 2013). The figure shows the iterations from the PSA for each of eight testing strategies. Importantly, iterations no longer represent different realizations from uncertain *differential* expected costs and health outcomes; rather, now these are realizations of uncertain *absolute* values of costs and outcomes for each testing strategy. However, the scatterplot provides a very limited basis for the decision maker to understand decision uncertainty. This is so because there is no information on the inevitable correlation the model induces between the points in the different clusters, so it is not possible to pair relevant iterations for the same run of the model.

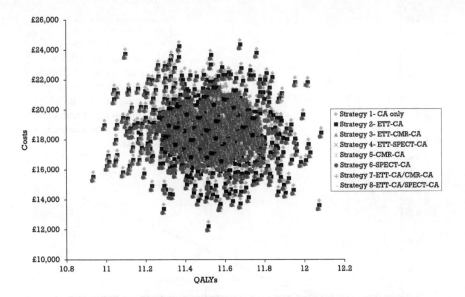

Figure 11.3 Scatterplot showing absolute costs and quality-adjusted life years (QALYs) for eight testing strategies for diagnosing coronary heart disease.
Source: Based on analyses reported in Walker et al. (2013).

Both CEACs and the CEAF can be used to communicate decision uncertainty, as shown in Figure 11.4, which shows, for each of the eight testing options, the probability of being the most cost-effective conditional on the cost-effectiveness threshold—that is, the proportions of the iterations of the PSA for which the given testing strategy is the most effective option with an ICER below the threshold.* The CEAF in Figure 11.4 again shows that the option that is expected to be cost-effective is not always the one with the highest probability of being cost-effective. This applies to Strategy 3 with thresholds between about £8,000 and £12,000. Furthermore, the CEAF in Figure 11.4 shows that, between thresholds of about £65,000 and £100,000 per QALY, Strategy 5 is expected to be cost-effective but has a probability of being cost-effective of less than 0.5.

11.7 ASSESSING THE VALUE OF ADDITIONAL RESEARCH

11.7.1 Rationale

Quantifying decision uncertainty is an important stage in understanding the implications of uncertainty in an analysis. However, as discussed earlier, the use of

---

* This is most easily done by rescaling the ICER to a measure of net benefit conditional on the cost-effectiveness threshold (see Chapter 2), and the option with the highest expected net benefit is the most cost-effective. Net health benefit (NHB) can be expressed in health terms (e.g., QALYs) and is defined as $H - \left(\dfrac{C}{k} \right)$, where H is the expected health outcome associated with an intervention, C is the intervention's expected cost, and k is the cost-effectiveness threshold. The NMB is expressed in monetary terms and is calculated as $\left(H * k \right) - C$.

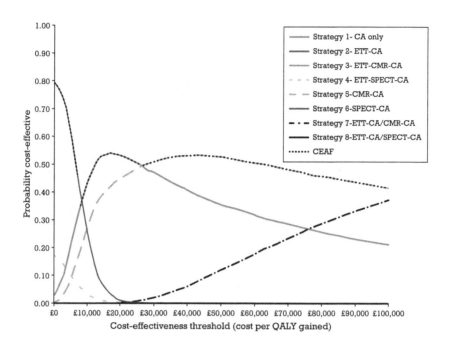

Figure 11.4. Cost-effectiveness acceptability curves and a CEAF for eight testing strategies for diagnosing coronary heart disease.
Source: Based on analyses reported in Walker et al. (2013).

arbitrary error probabilities for inference has no role in decision making, so decision uncertainty in general and CEACs in particular provide no direct indication of the implications of uncertainty for decisions. Rather, it is necessary to consider the implications of wrong decisions and how these can be ameliorated. When making decisions in the context of decision uncertainty, there is a chance that a decision to fund an intervention on the basis of it being *expected* to be cost-effective will be wrong, leading to wasted resources or, equivalently, forgone population health. Similarly, a decision not to fund a technology because its estimated ICER lies above the cost-effectiveness threshold may be incorrect, leading to patients not getting access to a valuable intervention, which will also result in wasted resources or lost health outcomes.

In this context a decision maker needs to consider what options other than "accept" or "reject" may be available. In assessing this wider set of decision options, consideration of whether further research has potential value is important. As for the healthcare interventions themselves, future research provides potential value by reducing decision uncertainty, possibly changing the decision that would be made in its absence and resulting in gains in health outcomes. Of course, a given research activity also consumes resources that could be used to deliver interventions and other types of research, so that the activity can only be considered potentially worth undertaking if its impact on health outcomes justifies its costs.

Assessments about the potential value of additional research should be part of decision making, even in the absence of formal analysis to provide guidance. Value of information analysis, however, provides a set of formal methods to quantify these metrics to support decisions about the funding of healthcare interventions and of specified research activities (Claxton 2014). These methods have a long history in decision theory and risk analysis (Schlaifer 1959), and they have been widely applied in healthcare (Thorn, Coast, and Andronis 2015). Full details of methods to estimate VOI can be found elsewhere (Briggs, Claxton, and Sculpher 2006), but a short overview is provided below.

11.7.2 Quantifying the Maximum Value of Research: Expected Value of Perfect Information

Decision uncertainty quantifies the probability of a wrong decision, but the consequences of incorrect decisions also need to be assessed. The results of a PSA can be used to calculate the *expected cost of uncertainty* given current evidence, and this can be expressed in terms of health outcomes (NHB) or in monetary terms (NMB) (see Section 11.6.2 and footnote in that section). Given that the ideal research would resolve all uncertainty, this expression can also be interpreted as the expected value of perfect information (EVPI). This can be expressed as follows:

- Consider there are j alternative options. For each option, NHB is calculated depending on uncertain parameters θ and a given cost-effectiveness threshold.
- Given existing evidence, the cost-effective option is the one with the highest expected NHB, so the decision would be to $[max_j E_\theta\, NHB(j,\theta)]$.
- The ideal research would resolve all uncertainty, so that the decision maker would know the values of θ before selecting j. They would, therefore, select j to maximize NHB for each particular value of θ. That is, $[max_j\, NHB\,(j,\theta)]$.
- The true values of θ are not known when the decision about whether to fund research is made. So the expected NHB of a decision made when uncertainty has been fully resolved requires averaging these maximum net benefits over all possible results of research—i.e., over the joint distribution of θ. That is, $[E_\theta\, max_j\, NHB(j,\theta)]$.
- Therefore, EVPI is the difference between the expected value of NHB with perfect information about the true values of θ and the expected value of NHB on the basis of existing evidence. That is, $EVPI = [E_\theta\, max_j\, NHB\,(j,\theta)] - [max_j\, E_\theta\, NHB\,(j,\theta)]$.

Expected value of perfect information can be also be understood by showing how it is calculated from the results of the PSA. Table 11.3 shows five iterations ($\theta1$-$\theta5$) from a PSA—that is, each simulation or iteration represents a possible realization of uncertainty relating to the choice between two treatments, A and B (of course there would be more iterations in practice). These iterations show the uncertainty in NHB relating to existing evidence (columns 2 and 3). The more cost-effective treatment, based on current evidence, is the one with the highest expected (average) NHB, namely,

Table 11.3 Using the results of a probabilistic sensitivity analysis (assuming just five iterations) to calculate expected value of perfect information (EVPI)

How things could turn out	Net health benefit (QALYs)			What we could do if we had perfect information
	Treatment A	Treatment B	Best choice	
$\theta 1$	8	12	B	12
$\theta 2$	16	8	A	16
$\theta 3$	9	14	B	14
$\theta 4$	12	10	A	12
$\theta 5$	10	16	B	16
Average	**11**	**12**	-	**14**

Source: Drummond et al. (2015).

Treatment B with 12 QALYs. This is the expression $[max_j \, E_\theta \, NHB \, (j, \theta)]$ above. Ideal research would remove all uncertainty, which is equivalent to the decision maker being able to select the more cost-effective treatment for each iteration of the PSA (column 4, "Best choice"), generating the NHBs shown in column 5 ("What we could do if we had perfect information"). At the point of deciding whether to fund the research, the decision maker does not know which of the iterations is the true one. Therefore, the expectation of the final column (14 QALYs) is the expected value of NHB with perfect information about the true values of θ, $[E_\theta \, max_j \, NHB \, (j, \theta)]$ above. By subtracting the average of column 3 from the average of column 5, the EVPI is calculated (here, $14 - 12 = 2$ QALYs).

This expression calculates EVPI for the average patient. Given that research is a public good, it is of value across all patients with the condition for which the options are being considered, and for as long as the information relating to those options is expected to be of value. The population size can be based on the prevalence and expected future incidence of the condition. The duration of time over which the information is expected to be of value depends on a range of factors, including anticipated changes in the prices of alternative interventions, new interventions becoming available, and research commissioned elsewhere (e.g., in other jurisdictions). However, estimates are possible using information and judgments based on observed developments in similar clinical areas (Philips, Claxton, and Palmer 2008).

Figure 11.5 presents EVPI calculations for the decision relating to the alternative diagnostic strategies for coronary artery disease also considered in Figures 11.3 and 11.4. The calculations relate to the population in the United Kingdom, and they assume 200,000 patients presenting annually. The EVPI is shown in monetary terms based on the relevant cost-effectiveness threshold shown on the horizontal axis and is presented for alternative assumptions regarding the period over which additional research would be useful in guiding decisions about the most cost-effective strategy: 5, 10, and 15 years. The shape of the functions across the range of

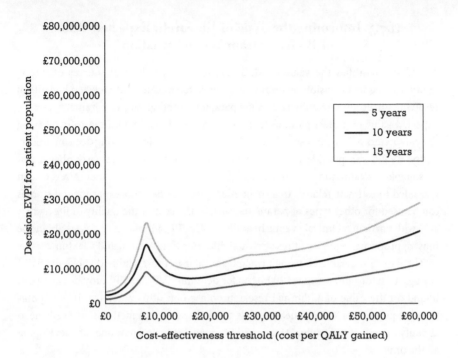

Figure 11.5 Population expected value of perfect information (EVPI) relating to the decision regarding eight testing strategies for diagnosing coronary heart disease. The three functions represent alternative values for the expected useful life of the research.
Source: Based on analyses reported in Walker et al. (2013).

cost-effectiveness thresholds warrants consideration. As the threshold increases from £0, population EVPI increases. It peaks at a cost-effectiveness threshold of about £8,000 per QALY, which is equivalent to the ICER of one of the options, and hence is the point at which the decision about the option is most uncertain because it is the point of indifference between the two options. Beyond this peak, the shape of the EVPI function is determined by the magnitude of two countervailing effects. The first is the fact that, as the cost-effectiveness threshold increases, the value of the gains in population health offered by further research increases. The second is that, as the threshold moves further from the value at which decisions are most uncertain (i.e., an ICER between two options), the value of research is less. The ultimate shape will depend on the relative magnitudes of these two effects; in Figure 11.5, EVPI declines initially but then increases with a smaller peak at a threshold of about £27,000, which is the ICER of another of the options.

The EVPI for a population is the upper bound on the value of research that would resolve all uncertainty. If the EVPI is less than the estimated cost of research, this is a *sufficient* condition for establishing that future research is not of value. If the EVPI is greater than the estimated research cost, this is a *necessary* but not sufficient condition to make that research of value; the costs and benefits of specific research designs need to be considered.

11.7.3 Informing the Type of Research: Expected Value of Perfect Parameter Information

The EVPI quantifies the value of ideal research that resolves all sources of uncertainty relating to a decision. A useful next step is to consider the expected benefits of resolving uncertainty relating to specific parameters and groups of parameters, or the expected value of perfect parameter information (EVPPI). In addition to identifying the parameters for which research would be most valuable in resolving decision uncertainty, EVPPI can provide information on the general types of research that might be suitable for estimating particular parameters—e.g., whether a randomized design is needed to estimate relative treatment effects, or whether non-experimental studies can be used for other types of parameter, such as the cost or the quality of life associated with particular clinical events. In addition, EVPPI can inform decisions about the most appropriate sequence of research activities (Griffin, Welton, and Claxton 2010).

The EVPPI is calculated using principles similar to those outlined above for EVPI (Briggs, Claxton, and Sculpher 2006). As for decision EVPI, EVPPI provides an upper bound on the value of additional research on a group of parameters. The computational requirements for nonlinear models are challenging, but methods are available to simplify this process (Strong, Oakley, and Brennan 2014), and new ones are developing all the time.

11.7.4 Designing Research: Expected Value of Sample Information and Expected Net Benefit of Sample Information

In situations where either the EVPI or the EVPPI is greater than the estimated cost of research, a necessary condition is met for making additional research of value. In such situations methods are available to inform decisions about the value of specific research designs, including efficient sample sizes. The expected value of sample information (EVSI) indicates the value of particular research designs. Detailed methods are available (Ades, Lu, and Claxton 2004; Jalal, Goldhaber-Fiebert, and Kuntz 2015; Strong et al. 2015), but key principles are outlined here. For a sample size n to estimate θ, a sample result of D can be generated. If that sample result was known with certainty, the option with the highest expected NHB based on that sample result could be selected. However, the particular sample result that will be generated is not known at the point of commissioning the research, so the expected value of a sample of n on θ would involve averaging the highest expected NHBs over the range of possible sample results, D. The EVSI is then the difference between the expected NHB based on the sample information and that based on current evidence. Calculating the EVSI can present considerable computational challenge, but methods exist to simplify this process, and more are developing (Kharroubi, Brennan, and Strong 2011; Strong et al. 2015).

To establish the most efficient sample size for a particular study, EVSI calculations are compared for a range of sample sizes. The difference between the EVSI and the estimated costs of generating the sample information is the expected net benefit of sample information (ENBS) or the payoff to research. The most efficient sample size is the one that generates the maximum ENBS. This approach can also be used to establish the efficiency of other aspects of research design, including choice of outcomes, options to compare, length of follow-up, and appropriate combinations of studies (Conti and Claxton 2009; Tuffaha et al. 2014; Welton et al. 2014). The costs of research should also include the expected opportunity costs experienced in the form of health forgone by patients participating in research, some of whom may not receive what is considered the most effective intervention based on existing evidence (McKenna and Claxton 2011). This will depend on whether patients generally get access to treatments while research is being undertaken.

11.7.5 Barriers to Implementing Value of Information Analysis and Potential Solutions

Although there have been a large number of applications of VOI analysis (Thorn, Coast, and Andronis 2015), the uptake of these methods in health and medicine has been slow, and thus resource allocation decisions are not being fully supported by formal analysis. Slow uptake may be due to the difficulty of implementing the methods, particularly for calculating the EVPPI and EVSI in non-linear cohort models and individual simulation models. It should be emphasized that value of information methods provide a framework for thinking about decision uncertainty, the value of additional research, and appropriate decisions. Even if formal analytic implementation is not feasible, decisions can be informed more qualitatively but in a manner consistent with the framework. This would involve a judgment of the magnitude of the decision uncertainty and the likely costs of wrong decisions based on the health/cost impact relating to an individual patient and the size of the patient population.

There have also been proposals for implementing VOI methods more straightforwardly. One suggestion is to recognize that the EVPI and EVPPI bound EVSI, but with lower informational requirements (Meltzer 2001), so that if the EVPI or EVPPI is sufficiently low, then it is not necessary to expend the effort to calculate EVSI. Another response is "minimal modeling," which can be used in some situations to calculate the EVPI directly from clinical studies using individual patient data on costs and outcomes rather than developing a decision model (Meltzer et al. 2011). A more general method has recently emerged to facilitate more efficient computation, particularly for the EVPPI and EVSI (Strong, Oakley, and Brennan 2014; Strong et al. 2015). These methods have been used to provide online access to VOI calculation from the results of PSA (University of Sheffield 2015). VOI methods can also be understood outside formal CEA, as an extension to simple meta-analysis (Claxton et al. 2015b).

11.8 LINKING UNCERTAINTY ANALYSIS TO DECISIONS

In some jurisdictions internationally, CEA is routinely used to guide specific decisions with the active involvement of a group of individuals who are held accountable for those decisions. This is not generally the case in the United States, however, and many CEAs are not aimed at specific decisions at a given point in time. Nonetheless, CEAs should be undertaken and disseminated with a view that decisions by payers, research funders, and other researchers will be guided by the analyses at some point.

Decision makers need to establish the best response to the costs associated with decision uncertainty. For some decision makers who have limited responsibilities, the choice may be between a simple "accept" or "reject" for new interventions, with no scope to review their decisions in the future or to recommend additional research. For such decision makers, there may be little scope to reflect uncertainty in their decisions, and they have to focus on expected cost-effectiveness. However, many decision makers have the scope to widen their decision options to include the request for additional research where the intervention is funded for widespread use or just in the context of research. Assessing the most appropriate decision would need to take into consideration a range of factors. These have been fully discussed elsewhere (Claxton et al. 2012), but are considered briefly below:

- Whether additional research can be expected to reduce the costs of uncertainty sufficiently to justify its cost.
- The uncertainties that should be the focus of the research and the appropriate research designs.
- The likelihood of research being undertaken if an intervention is generally funded (i.e., available for all patients), which may remove the opportunity to undertake research for the benefit of future patients. This will depend, *inter alia*, on patient and clinician willingness to participate in research if the intervention is generally available, which, in turn, may be influenced by the type of research (e.g., randomized versus non-randomized). If research is considered impossible after general funding of the intervention, the expected forgone health benefit associated with a missed opportunity for research needs to be considered alongside the expected benefits to patients of immediate funding (Claxton et al. 2012; Griffin et al. 2011).
- Conversely, if funding of a new intervention is limited to research only, the opportunity costs (in terms of health) of a decision to limit need to be considered. These costs are incurred by patients who are not part of the research and who do not receive the intervention that is (based on current evidence) expected to be cost-effective until publication of the research reports and depending on those results.
- Any likely information that can be expected to come to light and reduce the costs of uncertainty without further research (e.g., changes in the prices of particular interventions, new interventions becoming available).
- The likelihood of research being successfully completed and the expected duration of successful studies.
- Whether implementing a particular intervention on the basis of existing evidence results in irreversible costs which cannot be recovered if research ultimately shows it not to be cost-effective. For example, consider a situation where the purchase of costly capital equipment is necessary before an intervention can be delivered, but there is uncertainty about whether the intervention is cost-effective and future research is

potentially of value. General funding of the intervention may require extensive commitment of resources for equipment, which may have limited value if future research shows the intervention not to be cost-effective. In such circumstances, funding the intervention only in the context of research would limit these irreversible costs.

- Interventions that, although ultimately expected to be cost-effective, offer longer term benefits to patients, but only by incurring short-term intervention costs (e.g., primary prevention initiatives) and result in initial losses in NHB. This result occurs because resources are committed early but improved outcomes are only expected later. Therefore, the initial costs incur negative NHB (in the form of opportunity costs experienced by other patients). This characteristic should factor into decisions about whether patients generally should be given access to a new intervention when there is uncertainty and further research is valuable.

In determining the best approach to undertaking uncertainty analysis, the guiding principle, as with all aspects of economic evaluation, should be how the analysis informs the choice between decision options. Ideally, studies would formally reflect the considerations listed above analytically or by careful interpretation of the implications of the analysis for decision making. In making these analytical choices, however, the researcher is inevitably faced with a set of constraints, particularly the time and other resources available for research. When these constraints require simplification or approximation, the need to support decisions requires that some indication is given of the direction and, ideally, the magnitude of the impact of a constrained analysis compared to a more complete one. This would be required, for example, if resource constraints necessitated the use of a simple decision tree to model expected cost-effectiveness rather than a more detailed state-transition model. The same principle applies to uncertainty analysis. A quantification of decision uncertainty, the potential value of further research, and the implications of the other factors listed above provide the best analytical basis in support of decisions in the context of uncertainty. If research constraints mean that only a deterministic sensitivity analysis is feasible, then the researcher should use that analysis and explicit judgment to provide some indication of the nature of the decision uncertainty and the potential value of different policy responses, including requiring additional research, even if this is more qualitative than quantitative.

A constraint that may preclude a full uncertainty analysis is the use of individual patient simulation, where the size of the computational task just to estimate expected cost-effectiveness may mean that PSA (and formal quantification of decision uncertainty and the value of further research) takes too long to implement. Although ways around this limitation are available, including marshalling greater computing power and developing model emulators (Stevenson, Oakley, and Chilcott 2004), some analysts may decide only to provide deterministic sensitivity analysis. There is, therefore, effectively a trade-off between achieving a more accurate estimate of expected cost-effectiveness (e.g. ICERs) and providing a reliable quantification of decision uncertainty and the value of additional research. In such a situation the analyst should justify the approach adopted and provide an indication of the direction and magnitude of the impact of the omitted analyses on estimated expected cost-effectiveness, decision uncertainty, and the value of further research.

11.9 CONCLUSIONS

The role of CEA is to support resource allocation decisions that aim to maximize benefits (with a general focus on health) subject to resource constraints. Inevitably these decisions are made under (often considerable) uncertainty about the nature and implications of a given disease and the impact of alternative interventions. Accounting for this uncertainty in a manner that is consistent with the objectives and constraints of decision making is an important part of a CEA. A range of analytical methods is now available to guide decisions about the adoption of interventions and the value of additional research. These methods, together with a careful consideration of the context in which an intervention would be used and further research undertaken, provide an appropriate basis to support decisions.

11.10 RECOMMENDATIONS

The following recommendations are based on those of the International Society for Pharmacoeconomics and Outcomes Research (ISPOR) and Society for Medical Decision Making (SMDM) Task Force (Briggs et al. 2012), with some additions and changes as considered appropriate by the Second Panel.

Purpose of Uncertainty Analysis

1. Uncertainty analysis is essential to high-quality cost-effectiveness analysis (CEA). In determining the best approach to uncertainty analysis, the guiding principle should be how the analysis informs the choice among policy options.
2. There should be a clear report regarding what has been assumed about decision makers' policy options, including those relating to decision delay and further research.

Parameter Uncertainty

3. The specifications of all forms of sensitivity analysis require justification on the basis of the available evidence.
4. Deterministic sensitivity analysis can provide useful insights into model behavior and validation. Its role in quantifying decision uncertainty is limited. Probabilistic sensitivity analysis (PSA) provides an analytical basis for estimating decision uncertainty.
5. Where there is very little information on a parameter, this should be reflected in a broad range of possible values in the form of a distribution for PSA and a

range for deterministic sensitivity analysis. Parameters should never be excluded from uncertainty analysis on the grounds that there is insufficient information to estimate uncertainty.

6. For PSA, continuous distributions should generally be used that characterize uncertainty realistically over the theoretical range of the parameter. The analyst should be transparent regarding the choice and specification of the distribution for each parameter.

7. Correlation among parameters should be considered. Jointly estimated parameters, such as those from a regression analysis, will have direct evidence on correlation, which should be reflected in the analysis. Independently estimated parameters will have no such evidence, but this should not necessarily lead to an assumption of independence.

Structural Uncertainty

8. Structural uncertainties should be tested in uncertainty analysis. Consideration should be given to parameterizing these uncertainties for ease of testing. Where this is not considered possible, scenario analysis should be undertaken.

Presenting Decision Uncertainty

9. Decision uncertainty should be presented using probabilities for specified cost-effectiveness thresholds. If structural uncertainties are left unparameterized, these probabilities should be presented for each scenario relating to the structural uncertainty. If cost-effectiveness acceptability curves (CEACs) are used, curves for each option should be plotted on the same graph, together with a cost-effectiveness acceptability frontier (CEAF).

Value of Information Analysis

10. Expected value of information analysis should be used to guide decision making under uncertainty. Other factors with potential relevance to decisions should be considered, including the likelihood that research will be undertaken if an intervention is generally funded compared with being funded only in the context of research; the extent of irreversible costs being incurred in delivering a new intervention; and whether other information of relevance to the decision is likely to emerge over time.

11.11 REFERENCES

Ades, A. E., G. Lu, and K. Claxton. 2004. Expected value of sample information calculations in medical decision modeling. *Med Decis Making* 24 (2):207–227.

Armitage, P., G. Berry, and J. N. S. Matthews. 2002. *Statistical Methods in Medical Research*. 4th ed. Oxford: Blackwell Science Ltd.

Australian Government Department of Health. 2015. *Guidelines for Preparing Submissions to the Pharmaceutical Benefits Advisory Committee.* Version 4.5. Canberra: Commonwealth of Australia. https://pbac.pbs.gov.au/content/information/printable-files/pbacg-book.pdf.

Basu, A. 2011. Economics of individualization in comparative effectiveness research and a basis for a patient-centered health care. *J Health Econ* 30 (3):549–559.

Bojke, L., K. Claxton, Y. Bravo-Vergel, M. Sculpher, S. Palmer, and K. Abrams. 2010. Eliciting distributions to populate decision analytic models. *Value Health* 13 (5):557–564.

Bojke, L., K. Claxton, M. Sculpher, and S. Palmer. 2009. Characterizing structural uncertainty in decision analytic models: a review and application of methods. *Value Health* 12 (5):739–749.

Bravo Vergel, Y., N. S. Hawkins, K. Claxton, C. Asseburg, S. Palmer, N. Woolacott, I. N. Bruce, and M. J. Sculpher. 2007. The cost-effectiveness of etanercept and infliximab for the treatment of patients with psoriatic arthritis. *Rheumatology (Oxford)* 46 (11):1729–1735.

Briggs, A., K. Claxton, and M. Sculpher. 2006. *Decision Modelling for Health Economic Evaluation.* Oxford: Oxford University Press.

Briggs, A. H., B. J. O'Brien, and G. Blackhouse. 2002. Thinking outside the box: recent advances in the analysis and presentation of uncertainty in cost-effectiveness studies. *Annu Rev Public Health* 23:377–401.

Briggs, A. H., M. C. Weinstein, E. A. Fenwick, J. Karnon, M. J. Sculpher, and A. D. Paltiel. 2012. Model parameter estimation and uncertainty analysis: a report of the ISPOR-SMDM Modeling Good Research Practices Task Force Working Group-6. *Med Decis Making* 32 (5):722–732.

Bujkiewicz, S., H. E. Jones, M. C. Lai, N. J. Cooper, N. Hawkins, H. Squires, K. R. Abrams, D. J. Spiegelhalter, and A. J. Sutton. 2011. Development of a transparent interactive decision interrogator to facilitate the decision-making process in health care. *Value Health* 14 (5):768–776.

Canadian Agency for Drugs and Technologies in Health (CADTH). 2006. *Guidelines for the Economic Evaluation of Health Technologies: Canada.* 3rd ed. Ottawa: CADTH. https://www.cadth.ca/media/pdf/186_EconomicGuidelines_e.pdf.

Centers for Medicare & Medicaid Services. 2014. "Coverage with Evidence Development." www.cms.gov/Medicare/Coverage/Coverage-with-Evidence-Development/.

Claxton, K. 1999. The irrelevance of inference: a decision-making approach to the stochastic evaluation of health care technologies. *J Health Econ* 18 (3):341–364.

Claxton, K. 2014. "Value of Information Analysis." In *Encyclopedia of Health Economics*, edited by A.J. Culyer, Vol. 2, 53–60. Waltham, MA: Elsevier.

Claxton K, Griffin S, Koffijberg H, McKenna C. 2015b. How to estimate the health benefits of additional research and changing clinical practice. BMJ 351:h5987. doi: 10.1136/bmj.h5987.

Claxton, K., S. Martin, M. Soares, N. Rice, E. Spackman, S. Hinde, N. Devlin, P. Smith, and M. Sculpher. 2015a. Methods for the estimation of the National Institute for Health and Care Excellence cost-effectiveness threshold. *Health Technol Assess* 19 (14).

Claxton, K., S. Palmer, L. Longworth, L. Bojke, S. Griffin, C. McKenna, M. Soares, E. Spackman, and J. Youn. 2012. Informing a decision framework for when NICE should recommend the use of health technologies only in the context of an appropriately designed programme of evidence development. *Health Technol Assess* 16 (46):1–323.

Conti, S., and K. Claxton. 2009. Dimensions of design space: a decision-theoretic approach to optimal research design. *Med Decis Making* 29 (6):643–660.

Drummond, M. F., M. J. Sculpher, K. Claxton, G. W. Torrance, and G. L. Stoddart. 2015. "Characterising, Reporting, and Interpreting Uncertainty." In *Methods for the Economic Evaluation of Health Care Programmes*, 4th ed, 389–426. Oxford: Oxford University Press.

Espinoza, M. A., A. Manca, K. Claxton, and M. J. Sculpher. 2014. The value of heterogeneity for cost-effectiveness subgroup analysis: conceptual framework and application. *Med Decis Making* 34 (8):951–964.

Fenwick, E., K. Claxton, and M. Sculpher. 2001. Representing uncertainty: the role of cost-effectiveness acceptability curves. *Health Econ* 10 (8):779–787.

Fenwick, E., B. J. O'Brien, and A. Briggs. 2004. Cost-effectiveness acceptability curves—facts, fallacies and frequently asked questions. *Health Econ* 13 (5):405–415.

Griffin, S., N. J. Welton, and K. Claxton. 2010. Exploring the research decision space: the expected value of information for sequential research designs. *Med Decis Making* 30 (2): 155–162.

Griffin, S. C., K. P. Claxton, S. J. Palmer, and M. J. Sculpher. 2011. Dangerous omissions: the consequences of ignoring decision uncertainty. *Health Econ* 20 (2):212–224.

Jackson, C. H., L. Bojke, S. G. Thompson, K. Claxton, and L. D. Sharples. 2011. A framework for addressing structural uncertainty in decision models. *Med Decis Making* 31 (4): 662–674.

Jackson, C. H., S. G. Thompson, and L. D. Sharples. 2009. Accounting for uncertainty in health economic decision models by using model averaging. *J R Stat Soc Ser A Stat Soc* 172 (2):383–404.

Jalal, H., J. D. Goldhaber-Fiebert, and K. M. Kuntz. 2015. Computing expected value of partial sample information from probabilistic sensitivity analysis using linear regression metamodeling. *Med Decis Making* 35 (5):584–595.

Kharroubi, S. A., A. Brennan, and M. Strong. 2011. Estimating expected value of sample information for incomplete data models using Bayesian approximation. *Med Decis Making* 31 (6):839–852.

Kim, L. G., and S. G. Thompson. 2010. Uncertainty and validation of health economic decision models. *Health Econ* 19 (1):43–55.

McKenna, C., and K. Claxton. 2011. Addressing adoption and research design decisions simultaneously: the role of value of sample information analysis. *Med Decis Making* 31 (6): 853–865.

Meltzer, D. 2001. Addressing uncertainty in medical cost-effectiveness analysis implications of expected utility maximization for methods to perform sensitivity analysis and the use of cost-effectiveness analysis to set priorities for medical research. *J Health Econ* 20 (1): 109–129.

Meltzer, D. O., T. Hoomans, J. W. Chung, and A. Basu. 2011. Minimal modeling approaches to value of information analysis for health research. *Med Decis Making* 31 (6):e1-e22.

National Institute for Health and Care Excellence (NICE). 2013. *Guide to the Methods of Technology Appraisal 2013. NICE article [PMG9]*. London: NICE. http://publications.nice.org.uk/pmg9.

O'Hagan, A., C. E. Buck, A. Daneshkhah, J. R. Eiser, P. H. Garthwaite, D. J. Jenkinson, J. E. Oakley, and T. Rakow. 2006. *Uncertain Judgements: Eliciting Experts' Probabilities*. Chichester: John Wiley & Sons Ltd.

Philips, Z., K. Claxton, and S. Palmer. 2008. The half-life of truth: what are appropriate time horizons for research decisions? *Med Decis Making* 28 (3):287–299.

RESPECT Trial Team. 2010. Cost-effectiveness of shared pharmaceutical care for older patients: RESPECT trial findings. *Br J Gen Pract* 60 (570):e20–e27.

Schlaifer, R. 1959. *Probability and Statistics for Business Decisions: An Introduction to Managerial Economics Under Uncertainty.* New York: McGraw-Hill.

Soares, M. O., L. Bojke, J. Dumville, C. Iglesias, N. Cullum, and K. Claxton. 2011. Methods to elicit experts' beliefs over uncertain quantities: application to a cost effectiveness transition model of negative pressure wound therapy for severe pressure ulceration. *Stat Med* 30 (19):2363–2380.

Soares, M. O., J. C. Dumville, R. L. Ashby, C. P. Iglesias, L. Bojke, U. Adderley, E. McGinnis, N. Stubbs, D. J. Torgerson, K. Claxton, and N. Cullum. 2013. Methods to assess cost-effectiveness and value of further research when data are sparse: negative-pressure wound therapy for severe pressure ulcers. *Med Decis Making* 33 (3):415–436.

Stevenson, M. D., J. Oakley, and J. B. Chilcott. 2004. Gaussian process modeling in conjunction with individual patient simulation modeling: a case study describing the calculation of cost-effectiveness ratios for the treatment of established osteoporosis. *Med Decis Making* 24 (1):89–100.

Strong, M., J. E. Oakley, and A. Brennan. 2014. Estimating multiparameter partial expected value of perfect information from a probabilistic sensitivity analysis sample: a nonparametric regression approach. *Med Decis Making* 34 (3):311–326.

Strong, M., J. E. Oakley, A. Brennan, and P. Breeze. 2015. Estimating the expected value of sample information using the probabilistic sensitivity analysis sample: a fast, nonparametric regression-based method *Med Decis Making* 35 (5):570–583.

Thorn, J., J. Coast, and L. Andronis. 2016. Interpretation of the expected value of perfect information and research recommendations: a systematic review and empirical investigation. *Med Decis Making* 36 (3):285–295. doi: 10.1177/0272989X15586552. Epub 2015 May 18

Tuffaha, H. W., H. Reynolds, L. G. Gordon, C. M. Rickard, and P.A. Scuffham. 2014. Value of information analysis optimizing future trial design from a pilot study on catheter securement devices. *Clin Trials* 11 (6):648–656.

University of Sheffield. 2015. "SAVI - Sheffield Accelerated Value of Information." http://savi.shef.ac.uk/SAVI/.

van Hout, B. A., M. J. Al, G. S. Gordon, and F. F. Rutten. 1994. Costs, effects and C/E-ratios alongside a clinical trial. *Health Econ* 3 (5):309–319.

Walker, S., F. Girardin, C. McKenna, S. G. Ball, J. Nixon, S. Plein, J. P. Greenwood, and M. Sculpher. 2013. Cost-effectiveness of cardiovascular magnetic resonance in the diagnosis of coronary heart disease: an economic evaluation using data from the CE-MARC study. *Heart* 99 (12):873–881.

Walker, S., M. Sculpher, K. Claxton, and S. Palmer. 2012. Coverage with evidence development, only in research, risk sharing, or patient access scheme? A framework for coverage decisions. *Value Health* 15 (3):570–579.

Weinstein, M. C., H. V. Fineberg, A. S. Elstein, H. S. Frazier, D. Neuhauser, R. R. Neutra, and B. J. McNeil. 1980. *Clinical Decision Analysis.* Philadelphia: WB Saunders Company.

Welton, N. J., J. J. Madan, D. M. Caldwell, T. J. Peters, and A. E. Ades. 2014. Expected value of sample information for multi-arm cluster randomized trials with binary outcomes. *Med Decis Making* 34 (3):352–365.

Willan, A. R., and A. H. Briggs. 2006. *Statistical Analysis of Cost-Effectiveness Data.* Chichester: John Wiley & Sons Ltd.

12

Ethical and Distributive Considerations

Dan W. Brock, Norman Daniels, Peter J. Neumann,
and Joanna E. Siegel

12.1 INTRODUCTION

Resources to improve health are, have been, and always will be scarce, in the sense that societies—and individuals—must balance investments in health against investments toward other desirable and important goals like education and personal security. It is not possible to provide all the healthcare programs and interventions—including direct healthcare, public health, and healthcare research—that might provide positive health benefits without great and unacceptable sacrifices in other important social goods. Consequently, we cannot maximally provide health benefits to the population without denying healthcare to some individuals. As a result, some form of healthcare prioritization and, essentially, rationing, is unavoidable—that is, we cannot avoid using some means of allocating healthcare resources that denies to some persons some potentially beneficial healthcare.*

In making an explicit decision about the allocation of healthcare resources, it stands to reason that the decision maker would want to know—indeed is responsible for considering—the broader impact of his or her decision. It is the central purpose of CEA to provide information addressing a primary aspect of this impact, namely, the opportunity cost of a given decision (see Chapter 1), that is, the benefit lost when one

This chapter draws heavily on D. Brock, "Ethical Issues in the Use of Cost Effectiveness Analysis for the Prioritization of Health Care Resources," in *Handbook of Bioethics: Taking Stock of the Field from a Philosophical Perspective*, ed. G. Khushf (Dordrecht: Kluwer Academic Publishers, 2004; 353–380). Also in: *Public Health, Ethics, and Equity*, eds. S. Anand, F. Peter, and A. Sen (Oxford: Oxford University Press, 2004; 201–223); and *Making Choices in Health: WHO Guide to Cost-Effectiveness Analysis*, eds. T. Tan-Torres Edejer et. al. (Geneva: World Health Organization, 2003; 289–312).

* Interventions that improve health should be understood broadly and extend substantially beyond direct healthcare interventions. It is widely acknowledged that other factors, such as improved sanitation and economic conditions, have contributed more to the health gains of the past century than has direct healthcare. However, in this chapter we largely confine ourselves to direct healthcare interventions.

alternative is chosen over others. Cost-effectiveness analysis allows the comparison of the aggregate health benefits secured from a given resource expenditure devoted to alternative health interventions and is the standard analytic tool for determining how to maximize the health benefits from limited resources (Gold et al. 1996; Jamison 2002). In thinking of all individuals as "equally" serving as containers of a quantity of health, CEA shares with utilitarianism more generally the idea that everyone counts for one and no more than one, even if this form of equality is not what many insist on, as some individuals have more health than others before or after an intervention. The information provided by a CEA is consistent with a maximization standard, described in Chapter 2, similar to the maximization feature of a utilitarian or consequentialist moral standard that evaluates the justice of actions or practices by the value of the consequences they produce.

Consideration of the opportunity cost of an intervention is ethically justified in that without considering opportunity cost, we would not know if there were a better use of those resources, in terms of the purposes they are intended to serve, than the use under consideration. If the decision maker selects without regard to this information, he or she could easily make choices that provide less overall benefit to a given population than would be possible with such information. An important justification for considering CEA, then, is that it is preferable to the alternative of not considering it when allocating limited resources.

At the same time, however, it is clear that CEA does not provide all the information relevant to a decision. Maximizing the total quantity of health benefits will rarely be the single or even the overriding concern for the decision maker. Who receives the benefits—the distributive concern—also matters. We may have goals, for example, to reduce health inequalities by race or sex or social class. At the same time, however, these goals may conflict with the goal that we may reasonably have to produce as much health benefit as we can in a population given what can be spent on its health. We then may sometimes think that reducing a specific health inequality, even one that an unjust social policy has created, is not worth the loss of health benefit in a population (Daniels 2008). This trade-off can be particularly troubling when there is an imbalance in the size of benefits—when a particularly large total health benefit would be lost in order to reduce health or other inequalities to a much smaller extent. To conduct, report, and use CEA effectively, both the analyst and the decision maker must be aware of the limitations of CEA, the implications of different methodological choices, and what elements can be obscured within the summary information CEA provides.

It is important to note that CEA does not need to be about maximization, within a resource constraint, of health alone. It can be used to maximize any objective function, including one that defines something about distribution. The objective function can include other factors, such as equity considerations (assuming we know how to calculate them), but standard CEA is typically interpreted to aim at health maximization and is generally so understood in this volume. However, it is the objective function, not its maximization, that is ethically controversial in CEA. That is, it is not maximization that is at issue, but rather what considerations are to be maximized. Unfortunately, there may be no social consensus on what should be maximized, and some of the opposition to CEA is based on the fact that in practice it has generally maximized only health.

Many of the ethical concerns raised in what follows could be mitigated by changing the elements of the CEA (again, assuming we know how to calculate and include the modified elements). However, addressing these issues will raise others. Furthermore, many people would argue that it is CEA's role to present information without adjustment, either leaving aside distributive or other troubling issues or relying on decision makers to consider them separately. The point to be emphasized, however, is that although the maximization of health benefits presented in CEA does not necessarily overlook distributive issues, it often does so in practice, and this omission is the basis for many of the ethical objections to CEA.

The literature on ethical issues in CEA is on the whole considerably less well-developed than the literature on many of the methodological issues addressed in this volume (National Institute for Health and Clinical Excellence [NICE] 2008). The latter have benefitted from the attention of practitioners using CEAs in various contexts, as well as the more theoretical attention of health economists. The attention of philosophers, ethicists, and other analysts to the ethical issues in CEA has been much more recent and limited. This is in large part because bioethics has largely focused on ethical issues that are central to clinical interactions, such as informed consent, treatment decision making for incompetent patients, and confidentiality.

By contrast, CEA is employed in various health policy contexts and generally focuses on global or group-level health rather than on individual-level decisions. Many—perhaps most—CEAs are evaluations of alternative interventions for a group of patients with a similar medical condition in need of treatment; they are intended to provide information about the relative benefits and costs of alternative interventions for the same condition and patients. Ethical issues still arise in these contexts, such as whether the different distributional consequences among these patients are justified.

However, most of the difficult issues in the use of CEAs are distributional issues that arise in the course of evaluating alternative interventions that benefit *different* groups of patients. These issues often involve trade-offs between benefits and costs for some patients versus different benefits and costs for other patients. If the decision is which intervention is best for a group of patients, then no one is denied treatment. If the decision is which group of patients should be treated when not all groups can be, the decision is more controversial because some patients will be left without services. There has been considerable reluctance among policymakers, politicians, and other decision makers in the United States, either in private settings but especially in public contexts such as government programs, to use CEA explicitly in making prioritization and coverage decisions for alternative groups of patients. Medicare, the largest public medical program in the United States, is prohibited from denying coverage of an intervention on the basis of its costs (Neumann and Chambers 2012). Denying coverage on the basis of the intervention's cost-effectiveness ratio may violate aspects of the Patient Protection and Affordable Care Act (ACA) of 2010 (42 U.S.C. § 18001 et seq.) as well (see Chapter 1). Nevertheless, as noted above, it would be unethical to neglect considerations of the opportunity costs of different resource uses in making health resource allocation decisions.

Our focus in this chapter is on identifying the ethical issues that can arise in using CEA, and, within the space available, presenting some of the main alternative positions that have been taken on those issues. When possible, we provide brief recommendations for dealing with these issues, although available space is too limited to elaborate in any detail; sometimes the issue is sufficiently controversial that no recommendation is possible.

What, then, are some of the main issues of equity raised by the use of CEA in the allocation of health resources? We begin with some issues that arise when *conducting* a CEA as described in the preceding chapters. We then turn to issues that arise when *using* the results of such analyses to make decisions about health resource prioritization. This is a rough distinction useful here only for exposition; the issues are not listed in order of importance.

12.2 ISSUES IN CONDUCTING A CEA

12.2.1 How Should States of Health and Disability Be Evaluated?

Any CEA in health and medicine requires a summary measure that captures the net health benefits of interventions in a given population (Murray et al. 2002). Early summary measures were often limited in assessing only a single variable, such as life expectancy or mortality, and provided only limited information about that aim. Later developments began to integrate information about quality of life.

Summary measures that combine and assign relative value to morbidity and mortality effects include quality-adjusted life years (QALYs) and disability-adjusted life years (DALYs) (Hausman and McPherson 2009). Although there are several ways to estimate QALYs and DALYs, these methods usually require (1) information on the health status of individuals in different circumstances and at different points in time and (2) a method for converting the health status to numerical values that can be used in the CEA. Methods for both health status assessment and conversion to utilities are discussed in Chapter 7.

The second step—that of assigning relative values or utilities to different health states—is where important ethical concerns are introduced. A fundamental question is whose preferences should be used to determine the relative value of life in different health states. These methods typically use the value judgments of a random sample of ordinary citizens to evaluate different health states. Sometimes, however, the people most affected by a condition cannot be asked about it directly (e.g., children or people who have serious cognitive deficits), and then the random sample of ordinary citizens who are asked about the value of health states contains no one directly affected by the condition.

Whose preferences are to be used is important for a number of reasons. One is that there is often a significant difference between the evaluations of specific limitations of function or health by persons without that limitation versus those with it (Menzel et al. 2002; Salomon and Murray 2002). Why does this difference occur? Part of the answer is that persons who have no experience with a disability often have stereotypes, prejudices, and false beliefs about how the disability affects a person's health-related quality of life.

But there are other reasons for the difference between the evaluations of disabled versus non-disabled people that do not seem to be based on misimpressions or mistakes. Persons who become disabled can usually mobilize specific responses to becoming disabled (Sprangers and Schwartz 1999). These responses include adaptation, coping, adjustment, and other mechanisms, sometimes collectively termed "response shift." Adaptation involves improving one's functional performance through learning and skills development; for example, a right-handed person whose right hand is injured can learn to write with her left hand. Coping involves lowering one's expectations for performance so as to reduce the self-perceived gap between those expectations and one's actual performance; this might include, for example, lowering one's expectations for ability to climb stairs when living with chronic obstructive pulmonary disease. Adjustment involves altering one's life plans to give greater importance to activities in which performance is less diminished by disability; for example, spending less time listening to music and more time reading as a result of severe hearing loss. Disabled persons who have gone through a "response shift" of this sort—and this may be only a subset of the people with disabilities (Daniels, Rose, and Zide 2009)—typically report less distress and limitation of opportunity, and a higher health-related quality of life, with their disability than the non-disabled do in evaluating the same condition.

If the evaluations of disability states are derived from the preferences of non-disabled persons, the disability states will usually be judged more serious—of lower quality—than if the evaluations are derived from preferences of persons who have experienced these states. There will then be stronger reasons to prevent the disability states and to restore function from them. At the same time, however, since the value of extending lives in a CEA is adjusted for the health-related quality of life of those lives, using the preferences of non-disabled persons will result in assigning less value to extending the lives of persons with disabilities. Evaluations obtained in this way will be open to the charge that they reflect ignorance of what it is like to live with the disabilities in question. However if, instead, the preferences of the disabled themselves are used to derive values for states of disability, the values are open to the charge that they reflect a different distortion. The higher values assigned will reduce the value of prevention or rehabilitation as a result of the response shift that the disabled person has undergone.

The goal, then, is to determine an appropriate evaluative standpoint for determining the disutility of different disabilities (Brock 1995). One approach to this issue is to give evaluators from the general population more information about how people typically adjust to disabilities and then have them evaluate this process and its outcome. However, disability measures generally do not do this, and there remains a more fundamental problem. The deeper nature of the problem is that neither the non-disabled nor the disabled need have made any mistake in their different evaluations of quality of life with that disability. They arrive at different evaluations of the quality of life with that disability because they use different evaluative standpoints: the *ex ante* standpoint of the non-disabled person and the disabled person's *ex post* standpoint affected by adaptation, coping, and adjustment. Disabled persons who have undergone response shift can look back and see that before they became disabled they too would have evaluated quality of life as non-disabled people now do; for example, they realize that becoming deaf or blind is not as bad as they formerly thought it would be. But this seems to provide no basis for concluding that their pre-disability evaluation of the quality of life with that disability was mistaken, and so, is no basis for discounting or discarding it because mistaken.

The issue is a perspectives problem: the non-disabled and the disabled evaluate the quality of life with the disability from two different evaluative perspectives, neither of which is mistaken. Neither the *ex ante* nor the *ex post* perspective seems desirable for all cases—it depends on *why* the perspective change has taken place (Menzel et al. 2002). It might seem tempting to use the non-disabled's preferences for assessing the importance of prevention or rehabilitation programs, while using the disabled's preferences for assessing the importance of life-sustaining treatments for the disabled, but this approach would conflict with the necessity of a single unified perspective from which to compare the relative benefits from different health interventions, and to prioritize their full range.

Like the original Panel, the Second Panel recommends the use of community preference weights for health states for CEA to inform resource allocation decisions, concluding that for societal-level decisions, minimizing disability and maximizing full function is the appropriate goal. As a theoretical justification, the Second Panel draws from Rawls's "veil of ignorance," where rational decision makers decide, essentially, from the *ex ante* position (see also Chapter 7). It is important to note that use of community preference weights may have an important impact on the results of a CEA. When this is the case, analysts have the obligation to highlight the implications of their choice.

12.2.2 Age of Beneficiaries

Users of QALYs in CEAs typically assume that a year of life of a given quality has the same social value regardless of the age of the person who receives it. This means that a year of healthy life or life extension for a young child, a forty-year-old, and an eighty-year-old all have the same value in QALYs produced. Age of the beneficiary of the health intervention itself is not the basis for differentiating quality of life, nor is the time of life at which a year of life extension of life occurs. (This approach is, however, compatible with using age-based quality adjustments for interventions affecting groups of patients of varying ages when there are differences in the average quality of life across the different age groups, as is often—or generally—the case. For example, if the average quality of life in a group of patients of average age 85 is less than that of patients of average age 25, then a year of life extension for the 25-year-olds would produce more QALYs than would a year of life extension for the 85-year-olds.)

The disability-adjusted life year (DALY) measure (Murray 1996; World Bank 1993), developed as an alternative approach to measuring the burden of disease in reducing life expectancy and health-related quality of life, did assign different values to a year of life extension based on the age at which an individual receives it. Specifically, a year of life extension for individuals during their adult productive work years was assigned greater value than a year of life extension with the same health-related quality of life for young children or the elderly. The principal justification offered for this feature of DALYs was the different social roles that individuals typically occupy at different ages, and the emotional, physical, and financial dependence of the very young and the elderly on individuals in their productive work years (Murray 1994). (This age weighting was not retained in the 2010 DALYs; we note this age weighting and the criticism of it that follows because of the ethical issue it illustrates.)

The justification given for the DALY's age-based difference in the value of life extension implicitly adopted an ethically controversial social perspective on the value of healthcare interventions that extend life or maintain or restore function—that is, an evaluation of the benefits *to others*. This social perspective is in conflict with the customary focus in clinical decisions and treatment on only the benefits to the individuals who receive the healthcare interventions in question. Typical practice in broader health policy and public health contexts is more ambiguous on this point, because the benefits to others are sometimes given substantial weight in the evaluation and justification of health programs. For example, treatment programs for substance abuse are often argued to merit high priority because of their economic benefits to employers in reductions in lost days of work and in harmful effects on the substance abusers' family members (see the worked example in Appendix A). This social perspective is ethically controversial because it gives weight to differences between individuals—and to efforts to improve their health—based on their social and economic value to others. It discriminates, for example, against persons not in the workforce or with fewer dependencies and social ties, but who have equal health needs. The social perspective justifying the original DALY measure was consequently ethically problematic, if we believe the value of health benefits should focus on the value to the individuals treated. However, incorporating wider social benefits like productivity in a CEA has the same ethical implications as are present in the DALY.

Giving different value to life extension at different ages, however, might be ethically justified for users of either DALYs or QALYs if those values are assigned for different reasons. What Williams called the "fair innings argument" (Williams 1997) holds that individuals deserve the fair innings of a normal life span for their society. For example, if we must distribute scarce life-extending health resources to either 20-year-old patients or to the same number of 50-year-old patients, it would be unfair to give them to the 50-year-olds who have already had more years of life than the younger patients. (The "fair innings" view works best if we consider only "significant" differences in age, not the years that would be lost by 41- vs 42- or 45-year-old people.) Kamm has made a similar argument in terms of the younger patients having a stronger ethical claim to the additional life years (Kamm 2013b). This argument looks back at how many life years the competing patients will have had if they do not get the treatment they need, and so it is different from looking forward at maximizing the benefits or QALYs to be obtained from giving the treatment to either group. It could favor the younger group even if they would get fewer life years than the older patients. Because this argument deals with fairness, it seems not as vulnerable to charges of unfair age discrimination commonly made to favoring younger over older patients.

Moreover, individuals, and in turn their society, might choose to give lesser weight to a year of life extension beyond the normal life span than to a year of life extension before one has reached the normal life span, based on a conception of what equality of opportunity requires, or on the fact that people's plans of life and central long-term projects are usually constructed to fit within the normal life span, so that the completion of these central projects will typically require reaching, but not living beyond, the normal life span (Daniels 1988).

The issue of fairness to different age groups remains a controversial issue in the ethical literature on CEA. The social worth judgments involved in favoring people in the prime of life over the elderly and young children have parallels in many social worth judgments that might be made; favoring those who earn more, for example, might lead to favoring men over women and to favoring dominant groups over racial minorities that earn less in many societies.

12.2.3 What Costs and Benefits Should Count in CEAs of Health Programs?

It is widely agreed that CEAs in health should reflect the direct health benefits for individuals of their medical treatment, such as improving renal function or reducing joint swelling, and of public health programs, such as reducing the incidence of infectious diseases through vaccination programs. The costs of medical treatment and public health programs, such as the costs of healthcare professionals' time and of medical equipment and supplies, should also be reflected. But medical and public health interventions typically also have broader non-health benefits and costs. As described above, for example, some disease and illness principally affects adults during their working years, thereby incurring significant economic costs in lost work days associated with the disease or illness, whereas other conditions principally affect either young children or the elderly, who are not typically employed. Interventions or programs that are given up or not funded (i.e., those that are part of the opportunity costs of decisions) may also have different effects on productivity. It is controversial whether economic burdens of this sort should be given weight in a CEA used to prioritize between different health interventions (Nord et al. 1995).

From an economic perspective, as well as from a broad utilitarian moral perspective, non-health benefits and costs are real benefits and costs of disease and of efforts to treat or prevent it; they should be reflected in the overall cost-effectiveness accounting of how to use scarce health resources to produce the maximum aggregate benefits for society (Sen and Williams 1982) (see Chapter 8). The societal perspective Reference Case analysis recommended here, along with the healthcare sector perspective Reference Case analysis, seeks to identify all consequences of interventions under evaluation, although recognizing the practical limitations of including all such changes in CEAs. There is also a possible moral argument for ignoring such non-health costs and benefits in health resource prioritization grounded in a conception of the moral equality of persons. As mentioned earlier, giving priority to the treatment of one group of patients over another on the grounds that treating the first group would produce non-health benefits for others (e.g., other family members who are dependent on these patients) or would reduce economic costs to others (e.g., the employers of these patients who incur less lost work time) could be seen as failing to treat each group of patients with the equal moral concern and respect that all people deserve. The second group would receive lower priority simply because they are not a means to creating non-health benefits for others, or societal cost savings. Arguably, this violates the Kantian moral injunction against treating people solely as "means" and without their consent for the benefit of others (Kant 2012).

In public policy, a notion of "separate spheres" is sometimes employed, which in this case could be used to argue that the aim of healthcare and of public health interventions is improved health and the reduction of disease, and so only these goals and effects should guide decisions about healthcare and public health programs (Kamm 1993b; Walzer 1983). This view, like the Kantian argument, justifies certain limits to what benefits and costs are included in a CEA. In addition to assuring that the analysis is consistent with the purpose of programs, there are obvious practical grounds for the separate spheres view based on the difficulty of fully determining and calculating non-health benefits and costs. But the Kantian moral argument could serve as a principled moral basis for ignoring non-health benefits and costs to the patients to be treated in a CEA to be used to prioritize health resources and interventions that serve different individuals or groups.

In the norms for clinical medicine, as well, in conditions of scarcity, patients are typically prioritized in terms of their need or urgency, without regard to their social value to others. A notion of the moral equality of persons is sometimes employed as a basis for not distinguishing and prioritizing people's healthcare needs according to differences in their instrumental and economic value to others. But in other cases, distinctions are made. For example, in public health emergencies, healthcare workers are often given priority because they are needed to treat other patients. One ethical issue for the use of CEAs in health policy is whether—or in what cases—these social values should be included in CEAs used to inform health resource prioritization, or alternatively deliberated separately in the prioritization process.

12.3 ISSUES IN THE USE OF THE RESULTS OF CEAS FOR PRIORITIZATION OF HEALTH INTERVENTIONS

12.3.1 Should Priority Be Given to the Sickest or Worst Off?

It is a commonplace that most theories of distributive justice require some special concern for those who are worst off or most disadvantaged (Brock 2002; Nord and

Johansen 2014; Rawls 1971). For example, it is often said that the justness of a society can be measured by how it treats its least well off members. In the context of decisions about healthcare allocation and the prioritization of health interventions, the worst off with regard to need for the good being distributed might reasonably be thought to be the sickest patients. Earlier we saw that giving priority to some age groups over others (young adults over the elderly or young children) means that we would care more about a health benefit at some point in a life than at others; now we are considering whether we should care about the health of some lives more than others. Just as it might matter where a health benefit goes within a life, so to it might matter where it goes between lives.

In conditions of scarcity, clinicians typically prioritize patients in terms of some combination of the severity of their illness and their capacity to benefit—if care is possible and effective, then the sickest patients have the greatest need for care. In many cases, the sickest will also be given priority by a CEA that compares treating them versus less sick patients; the sickest often have greater potential improvement in health-related quality of life because they begin from a lower position; thus, a fully effective treatment will produce greater benefits for the sickest. But in other cases, giving priority to the sickest may require a sacrifice in aggregate health benefits. This occurs when the sickest cannot be helped as much as less sick patients. Examples are patients with severe chronic obstructive pulmonary disease or chronic schizophrenia that is largely resistant to standard treatments. These patients, although sicker, could not benefit as much as, say, patients with milder forms of pulmonary disease or schizophrenia that could be more effectively treated.

Should we give priority to treating the less sick patients because doing so would produce a greater aggregate health benefit at the same cost, as the CEA standard implies, or to treating the patients who are the sickest? In some empirical studies, both ordinary people and health professionals prefer to sacrifice some aggregate health benefits in order to ensure that the sickest patients are treated, although the degree of sacrifice they are prepared to make varies (Nord 1993).

One issue with important implications for healthcare priorities is whether our definition of "worst off" should focus on a person's condition at a specific point in time or over an extended period of time. When choosing among patients to receive a scarce resource, some people defend the idea that the neediest patient is the one whose life as a whole will have been the worst if he or she does not receive the scarce resource (Kamm 1993a). However, some justifications for giving priority to the worst off would suggest that the patient who is sickest here and now is the neediest.

What are the ethical justifications for giving priority to the worst off? One is that we must give priority to the worst off in order to avoid increasing the already unjustified disadvantage or inequality they suffer in comparison to those who are better off (Brock 2002). If most disease and disability is undeserved—for example, a result of bad luck in the genetic or social lottery—then there may be ethical priority to reducing the greater undeserved disadvantage. It is worth noting, however, that this argument is not equivalent to a concern to produce equality in outcomes (Temkin 2003). Equality in outcomes could conceivably be achieved by what Parfit has called "leveling down"—that is, by allowing Group A's health level to deteriorate down to that of Group B, if we cannot raise Group B's level up to that of Group A (Parfit 1991). The fact that no one would defend doing this suggests that this aspect of our notion of equity or justice is better captured by the idea of giving priority to improving the condition of the worst off than by a simple concern for equality in outcomes.

A second possible justification for giving priority to treating the sickest, offered by some participants in Nord's research, is that it may be subjectively more important to the sickest to obtain treatment, even if the health benefits they receive from treatment are less than those for the less sick. This justification might support focusing on those who are worst off at the time the decision is made about whom to treat, rather than on those whose lifetime well-being will be lowest (Nord 1993). But this justification might also imply lower priority to the worst off if they are too sick to appreciate the benefits from the health intervention. The issue then becomes whether to be benefitted they must be able to appreciate or value the benefit.

One final issue concerning giving priority to the worst off should be mentioned. In the context of health resource prioritization it seems natural to consider the sickest as being the worst off, as mentioned earlier. But this may not be correct. At the most fundamental ethical level in general theories of equity and distributive justice, it is plausible that our concern should be for those who are overall or all-things-considered worst off—those who are poorest, or those who have experienced great personal losses—and they will not always be the sickest. A preference for health interventions that raise the level of well-being of those who are worst off in overall well-being, instead of giving priority to the sickest, might be justified so as not to increase the unjustified disadvantage suffered by those with the lowest overall level of well-being. If, instead, the priority to the worst off in health resource prioritization should focus only on health states, a justification for this narrowed focus is needed. A practical consideration is that it may be easier to reach agreement on who are the sickest than on who are the worst off overall—or, alternatively, that we are more likely to be able to improve the lot of the sickest.

Even if we agree that the worst off deserve some priority (and here for convenience we return to our assumption that we are referring to the sickest), there remains the question of how much weight to give to this particular aspect of equity. Virtually no one would give absolute priority to treating the sickest regardless of the cost of their treatment or how small the benefit might be, and regardless of how beneficial and inexpensive treatment for the less sick might be. This absolute priority would have unacceptably high opportunity costs. However, there seems to be no objective, principled basis for determining how much priority to give the sickest, that is, how much aggregate health benefit should be sacrificed in order to ensure their treatment. The most one can say is that most people and most theories of distributive justice have a concern both for maximizing the overall benefits that can be obtained with scarce health resources and for assuring special treatment for the worst off or sickest.

It is important to note that there is a large range of indeterminacy regarding the proper trade-off between these two concerns when they are in conflict. One can elicit public preferences for this trade-off, but that may not be proper way of resolving it;

further, there may be a high degree of heterogeneity in preferences on the matter. Some analysts argue that conflicts between different equity concerns—as well as questions regarding how much weight to give specific concerns—is to be found in person trade-off studies of the conflicting considerations done with actual individuals. However, this position needs more defense than it is usually given, in comparison with normative arguments about appropriate interpretations and weights for concepts like justice, equality, and the like.

12.3.2 When Should Large Benefits to a Small Number of People Receive Priority Over Small, but Greater *Aggregate* Benefits to a Large Number of People?

Cost-effectiveness and utilitarian standards require minimizing the aggregate burden of disease and maximizing the aggregate health of a population without regard to the resulting distribution of disease and health, or who gets what benefits. The issue about priority to the worst off focuses on *who* should receive benefits. A different issue concerns *how much* benefit different individuals receive.

Some people would argue that health benefits are often qualitatively different and so cannot be compared on a single scale like the QALY. The issue here, however, concerns what ethical limits there should be, if any, on aggregating different size benefits for different persons when comparing and prioritizing different health interventions. Cost-effectiveness analysis accepts no such limits—it counts only the aggregate outcomes of the alternatives.

There are many forms in which this issue arises (Kamm 1993d), but the version that has received the most attention—and which Daniels has called the "aggregation problem"—occurs when, if ever, large benefits to a few individuals should take priority over greater aggregate benefits to a different and much larger group of individuals, each of whom receives only a very small benefit (Daniels 1993). This issue arises when costly prevention or treatment targets a debilitating disease or condition experienced by a few people, as compared with an inexpensive intervention that confers a small benefit for many who experience a much more prevalent but also less serious condition. Applying cost-effectiveness, preventing or treating a very prevalent but low-impact disease or condition at a given cost will receive higher priority when doing so produces greater aggregate or total benefits than using the same funds to treat or prevent the disease or condition that affects only a very small number of persons but has a very great impact on each individual affected. The example that received considerable attention in the United States arose in the state of Oregon's revision of its Medicaid priority-setting process, where capping teeth for exposed pulp was initially ranked just above an appendectomy for acute appendicitis, a relatively rare but potentially life-threatening condition (Hadorn 1991). This ranking reflected the calculation that the funds necessary to cover one such appendectomy would cover over 100 tooth cappings, and that the latter would produce greater aggregate benefit. Because Medicaid coverage decisions were to be made according to the list of treatment/condition pairs ranked in terms of their relative cost-effectiveness, it could have turned out, depending on the overall level of resources available, that tooth capping would have been covered while appendectomies were not. (There were problems with Oregon's calculations, but the general problem described here reflects an important concern in using CEA.)

The tooth capping example and similar cases represented unacceptable choices to most people, whose intuitive rankings of the relative importance or priority of health interventions were based on one-to-one comparisons, for example, one tooth capped as opposed to one appendectomy performed. In the face of these results, Oregon made a fundamental change in its prioritization methodology, essentially abandoning the cost-effectiveness standard in favor of a standard that did not account for differences in costs. This fundamental challenge to CEA thus led to abandoning its use in this priority-setting process.

Notwithstanding the counterintuitive results generated by CEA's aggregation of benefits, such aggregation may sometimes be ethically justified. A critical case in the Oregon Medicaid program was that of a 12-year-old boy for whom a bone marrow transplant would provide the only chance to save his life. Oregon denied coverage under its Medicaid program on the grounds that it could do greater good by using its limited resources to improve prenatal care for pregnant women. In this case, the choice to give higher priority to achieving small benefits for many over a potentially much larger but uncertain benefit to one person was felt to be justified.

Sometimes the aggregation of benefits in CEA seems ethically justified and sometimes it does not; the problem is that we do not have an adequate account of the relevant difference. It is worth noting that many public policy choices outside of healthcare choose programs that offer small benefits to many over even life-saving benefits to a few. For example, governments in the United States support public parks used by thousands of persons, each of whom receives only a relatively small benefit, while reducing funding for public hospitals, resulting in quite predictable loss of life for a small number of people.

The cost-effectiveness standard that permits unlimited aggregation of different size benefits to different persons might be defended by distinguishing between the clinical context, in which physicians treat individual patients, and the public health and health policy contexts, in which health resource allocation decisions are made. In emergency settings of extreme scarcity, physicians forced to prioritize between individual patients will typically first treat the patient who will suffer the more serious consequences without treatment, or who will benefit the most from treatment, even if doing so will keep her from treating a larger number of less seriously ill patients. But from a public health or policy perspective, it could be argued that programs improving overall population health should receive much more attention than they do. Despite this argument, the Oregon experience makes clear that even when allocating public resources, it is ethically controversial whether it is always—or even usually—justified to give priority to producing the maximum aggregate benefits when that is achieved by giving small benefits to many at the cost of forgoing very large benefits to a few.

Just as with the problem of what priority to give to the worst off, part of the complexity of the aggregation problem is that for most people and theorists, some but not all cases of aggregation are ethically acceptable. The theoretical problem, then, is to develop a principled account of when, and for what reasons, different forms of aggregation satisfy requirements of equity or justice and when they do not (Kamm 1993b). There is no consensus on this issue within the literature of health policy or ethics and political philosophy more generally—and apparently none among ordinary persons. As with the problem about priority to the worst off, the complexities of this issue have received only limited attention in bioethics, and there is much difficult but important work to be done.

12.3.3 The Conflict Between Fair Chances and Best Outcomes

Another ethical issue in the use of CEA for health resource prioritization has been characterized as the conflict between fair chances and best outcomes (Daniels 1993). The best outcome is assumed to be the alternative that produces the greatest net benefit, whereas fair chances gives all in need of the same or a different intervention that would use the same resources a fair chance of getting what they need. The conflict is most pressing when the health intervention is life-saving and resource scarcity means that not all can receive it. In the context of healthcare, this issue first received attention in organ transplantation, where a scarcity of life-saving organs such as hearts and lungs resulted in thousands of deaths each year among patients on waiting lists for an organ for a transplant (Brock 1988).

However, this conflict has arisen in public health contexts as well. In the World Health Organization's "3 by 5" program, the goal was to get three million HIV patients on anti-retroviral treatment by the end of 2005. However, it was estimated that there were six million patients who could benefit from such treatment. Countries then faced the question of how to prioritize patients for such treatment. Using relatively rough cost-effectiveness calculations, in poor African countries a case could be made for treating only patients in urban areas for at least two reasons: (1) those patients were geographically concentrated and so easier and cheaper to reach and (2) the healthcare facilities needed to treat patients often existed in urban but not rural areas. Concentrating only on urban patients would take countries closest to the goal of treating three million patients. But rural patients could and did argue that it would be unfair to give them no chance to receive this life-saving treatment. Their need for such treatment was just as great as the need of urban patients, and they should receive at least a fair chance of getting it (Daniels 2004). What would constitute a fair chance might be an equal chance, or a proportionally weighted chance, reflecting the fewer patients that could be treated if rural patients were given that chance (Brock 1988; Broome 1984; Kamm 1993e).

Similar conflicts between fair chances and best outcomes can arise when treatments are needed by two groups of patients, available resources are not sufficient to treat both groups, and treatments for one group are slightly cheaper and/or more effective than for the other. This small difference in the costs or effectiveness of treatment between the two groups seems insufficient to justify the big difference in who gets the benefits of treatment. The fair chances issue also arises when the differences are greater between alternatives.

Two considerations will often mitigate the force of the ethical conflict between fair chances and best outcomes. First, allocation of resources in healthcare is typically not an all-or-nothing choice for particular patients but a matter of the relative priority for funding given to different health programs or interventions. If one program offers a slightly larger gain in aggregate health benefits as compared to a competing program, that does not imply that the first would be fully funded and the second not funded at all. Instead, the first would receive higher priority or a higher level of funding. Beneficiaries of the first program would then have a somewhat higher probability of being successfully treated than beneficiaries of the second, but the possibility of treatment would be closer to "fair" for members of each group. When there is significant resource scarcity, funding both programs at some level will involve some sacrifice in aggregate health benefits that might have been produced by always preferring the more cost-effective alternative. But funding both mitigates the complaint by the second group of beneficiaries that the small difference in expected benefits between programs unfairly prevents them from any chance of having their health needs met at all.

The second consideration that may mitigate some of the conflict between fair chances and best outcomes in health resource prioritization is that often the diseases and health problems to be treated or prevented are not directly life-threatening, but instead only affect individuals' health-related quality of life, and often for only a limited time or to a limited degree. In these cases, the difference in health benefits between individuals who receive a needed health intervention that is given a higher priority and individuals who do not receive a needed health intervention because their condition is given lower priority is much less, making the unfairness argument less compelling.

These two considerations may sometimes mitigate, but they do not fully avoid, the conflict between fair chances and best outcomes in prioritization decisions about health interventions compelled by economic scarcity. When a more cost-effective health program is developed for one population instead of a different, slightly less cost-effective health program for a different population, individuals who would have been served by the second program will have a complaint that they did not have a fair chance to have their needs served only because the first program produces slightly greater aggregate benefit. (If the difference is very small it seems inadequate to justify the difference in treatment; if the difference is much greater, then getting the much greater benefit could override the consideration of unfairness.) Because these allocation decisions are not typically all-or-nothing, providing some funding for the less cost-effective program mitigates the conflict, but the issue resurfaces in deciding how much funding to provide for the less cost-effective program. This issue is also relevant to the discrimination issue discussed briefly in the next section, because disabilities often make treating those who have them less cost-effective than treating otherwise similar patients who are not disabled. The fair chances versus best outcome conflict will arise in prioritizing health interventions in health and public health policy; how this conflict can be equitably resolved is complex, controversial, and unclear.

12.3.4 Does Use of CEA to Set Healthcare Priorities Unjustly Discriminate Against Disabled Persons?

In several contexts, using CEA to set healthcare priorities could result in assigning lower priority to both life-extending and quality-of-life-improving treatment for disabled than for non-disabled persons with the same healthcare needs (Brock 1995, 2000). Here are five such contexts. First, because disabled persons may have a lower health-related quality of life than otherwise similar non-disabled persons because of their disability, treatment that extends their life for a given number of years produces fewer QALYs than treatment that extends the life of a non-disabled person for the same number of years. Second, if two groups of patients with the same health-related quality of life have the same need for a life-sustaining or quality-of-life-improving treatment, but one will be restored to full function and the other will be left with a resultant disability, more QALYs will be produced by treating the first group. Third, persons with disabilities often have a lower life expectancy because of their disability than otherwise similar non-disabled persons. As a result, treatments that prevent loss of life or produce lifetime improvements in quality of life will produce fewer QALYs when given to disabled persons than when given to non-disabled persons with the same healthcare needs. Fourth, disabilities often act as comorbid conditions, making a treatment less beneficial in QALYs produced for disabled versus non-disabled persons with the same healthcare needs. Fifth, the presence of a disability can make treatment of disabled persons more difficult and so more costly than treatment of non-disabled persons with the same healthcare needs; the result is a lower cost-effectiveness ratio for treating the disabled persons.

In each of the five cases above, disabled persons have the same medical and healthcare needs as non-disabled persons, and so the same claim to treatment on the basis of their needs. But treating the disabled persons will produce less benefit, that is, fewer QALYs, *because of their disabilities* than treating the non-disabled. Although subgroup analyses are often done in CEAs, they are often not done in cases like these where the subgroups are disabled versus non-disabled patients. The reason this type of subgroup analysis is not done, however, is not that doing so would fail to demonstrate a difference in cost-effectiveness. The reason is instead that it might well result in unjust discrimination against the disabled patients.

This point is relevant in general to objections that, in practice, there is no ethical problem, because no one does CEA in ways that would introduce this type of unjust discrimination. But this reliance on what is done "in practice" does not resolve the general problem regarding CEA. Instead, it highlights the importance of these ethical concerns, as they are recognized by practitioners who adjust their conduct of CEA to avoid uses that would generate the ethical problem. Simply put, analysts do not do a subgroup analysis of disabled versus non-disabled patients for a life-sustaining treatment when the disability would be the only reason for the disabled patients' receiving lower priority for treatment. They avoid subgrouping on the basis of disability, because it would arrguably fail to give equal moral concern to disabled persons' healthcare needs and would be criticized as unjust discrimination on grounds of their disability.

Indeed, United States Health and Human Services Secretary Louis Sullivan denied Oregon's initial request for a waiver of federal regulations for its proposed revisions to its Medicaid plan on the grounds that Oregon's method of prioritization of services was in violation of the Americans With Disabilities Act (ADA) of 1990 (Pub. L. No. 101-336, §2, 104 Stat. 328 [1991]), citing some of the five kinds of cases noted above in support of that position.

Disabled persons have charged that in cases like the first two cited above concerning life-saving treatment, the implication of using CEA to prioritize healthcare is that saving their lives, and so their lives themselves, have less value than non-disabled persons' lives. They quite plausibly find such an implication of CEA threatening and unjust. There are various means of avoiding these problems of discrimination against persons with disabilities, but they generally involve abandoning fundamental features of CEAs (Nord 1999). For example, one response to the first case cited above would be to give equal value to a year of life extension, whatever the quality of that life, so long as it is acceptable to the person whose life it is (Kamm 1993c; Nord et al. 1999). But most people would not accept that a year of extended life has equal value entirely without regard to its quality, rejecting, for example, that a year of life in a persistent vegetative state has equal value to a year of healthy life. There may be a problem for CEA that goes beyond the issue of people with disabilities, however: suppose that people who are interested in health maximization also prefer a system that gives them all the health that they can get from an intervention even if it is less health than others may get from the same intervention (Kamm 2013a; Nord, Daniels, and Kamlet 2009; Nord, Enge, and Gundersen 2010).

The problem of whether CEA unjustly discriminates against the disabled remains a deep and unresolved difficulty for use of CEA and QALYs to prioritize healthcare.

12.3.5 Equity Weights

As noted at the beginning of this chapter, it is theoretically possible to conduct CEAs in such a way as to take account of any of the above ethical issues (Cookson, Drummond, and Weatherly 2009). One strategy is to assign numerical values, commonly called equity weights, to the various ethical considerations, which would then modify the results of the health maximization of CEA by the various ethical considerations. To avoid confusion with CEA, this has been characterized as cost-value analysis (CVA) by Nord (1999). At the time of the original Panel's work, there were insufficient data on which to develop equity weights that could be employed in resource prioritization. Since then, however, a number of population survey studies have measured the weight people give to considerations of severity of illness and potential to benefit, as opposed to QALY maximization. The strategy of assigning equity weights has a definite appeal, for it would modify one quantification by a weighting function and thus yield another quantification that could be used by decision makers. Moreover, those equity weights would almost certainly more closely reflect the combination of health benefits plus at least the two equity concerns for priority to the worst off and persons' potential for benefit that have been most explored by analysts. Nord has summarized these studies and the equity weights they would support (Nord 2015).

There are however, several issues facing this strategy. The first main issue relates to how well population survey results capture the weights people would assign to ethical considerations. Do these results reflect considered, reflective judgments or relatively superficial responses that are significantly shaped by the questions that elicit them? Such framing effects are well known. Second, various ethical considerations—for example, the seriousness of a condition and the potential for benefit from an intervention—interact, and available survey results may not capture all of these interactions. Third, there is likely to be substantial variation in the equity weights different people assign, and consensus is rare. Fourth, the public may not have well-formed or well-considered views about what equity in health it seeks. Survey results may be an attempt to get at beliefs that do not really exist. Fifth, in introducing equity weights, we risk making CEA methodology much less transparent: CEA already encounters the complaint that, for example, weighting life years based on quality of life diminishes the transparency of the method; if we further adjust that result with equity weights, the quantification becomes even less transparent. Sixth, if we do not have a good methodology for establishing equity weights, we cannot calculate the weighting functions the approach presupposes. Seventh, a serious limitation of the equity weights strategy is that sufficient research has not been done across a full range of ethical considerations. In short, we simply do not know how to reliably establish all the equity weights that we would need to address public concerns about equity, so what is theoretically appealing to some falls well below the bar of practical significance.

If we did know how to develop an appropriate set of equity weights, they would provide a clear advance over CEA's usual focus on simple QALY maximization, which captures the concern for efficiency but ignores concern for equity within the analysis. The alternative to incorporating equity weights is to leave CEAs free of the ethical issues we have discussed in this chapter (except for the maximization strategy it shares with utilitarianism). But what is clearly not satisfactory is simply providing decision makers with the results of an "ethics-free" CEA, reminding them only in a general sense that their job in making prioritization decisions is also to take account of the relevant ethical considerations that the CEA leaves out, but with no input on how to do so. This gives them no guidance, with the likely result that the ethics are ignored or dealt with only minimally and arbitrarily, as they generally are now. Work should continue on developing the methodology for a full range of equity weights, making the option of incorporating ethical concerns within a CEA—at a minimum in a sensitivity analysis—a more viable option than at present.

12.3.6 Cost-per-QALY Thresholds

As described in Chapter 1, some countries, most prominently the United Kingdom (at least England and Wales through the National Institute for Health and Clinical Excellence [NICE]), have treated a specific range of cost-per-QALY values (£20,000 to £30,000 per QALY) as a kind of threshold. For cost-per-QALY amounts below

£20,000, NICE will generally recommend coverage; for cost-per-QALY amounts over £30,000, NICE will generally not recommend the intervention be covered. In between those amounts, NICE will more carefully consider coverage decisions. The World Health Organization (WHO) has made a similar recommendation that if the intervention's cost-effectiveness ratio is less than gross domestic product (GDP) per capita, it is considered very cost-effective; if between one and three times GDP per capita, it is considered cost-effective. Above three times GDP per capita, it is considered something to view with caution. In effect, these thresholds demonstrate a resource cap on healthcare interventions (Neumann, Cohen, and Weinstein 2014). Note that as discussed in Chapter 1, the WHO has more recently backed away from this characterization of thresholds and has been reviewing alternative threshold estimation methods.

A question arises about the determination and justification for any threshold or resource cap. One line of argument is simply that resources are limited—by the National Health Service (NHS) budget in the United Kingdom, for example, or by the public health budgets and international donations received by a low-income or middle-income country, and some cutoff for investment is needed to help guide the allocation of those resources to their best uses. It can be argued, however, that what is needed is an argument grounded in justice—rather than just in historical practice— about how much of available resources ought to be provided for health compared with other possible investments, such as education or public safety.

12.4 CONCLUSIONS

Cost-effectiveness analysis is not a tool for deciding an overall budget for expenditures to improve health, and it is not a tool for controlling costs. It is a tool to inform decision makers about the opportunity costs of public health interventions, information that can be helpful in making the best possible use of whatever health resources are available. When, whether, and how to use CEA to set priorities is a normative question. How to factor in the ethical concerns we have described is also a normative question.

We have distinguished above certain distinct issues about equity and justice that arise in the conduct and use of CEA to minimize the burdens of disease and to maximize health benefits. Several of the issues described raise possible criticisms of the health maximization standard embodied in CEA. In each case, the claim is that equity requires attention to the distribution of health benefits and costs to distinct individuals or groups; in each case, some concern for equity seems valid and usually warrants some constraints on a goal of unqualified maximization of health benefits. Most people will favor some departure from the maximization standard of CEA in many of these cases.

There are two broad strategies for responding to concerns about equity in CEA. One strategy is to integrate these concerns into CEA by means of a quantitative tool that measures the specific weight to be given different equity concerns in evaluating interventions that raise issues of distributive justice because they serve different individuals or benefit individuals differently. These weights could be used in a primary analysis, or they could be used in sensitivity analysis to elucidate and highlight equity concerns.

This approach is not widely used for reasons elaborated above; with greater attention, equity weights may be used more widely in the future.

The more common strategy is to present ethical concerns outside of or alongside a CEA. As most analysts argue, CEA is proposed as an aid to decision makers; it is not by itself a sufficient decision-making standard and has not been intended to capture all relevant concerns. That is the position taken by the original Panel on Cost-Effectiveness in Health and Medicine (Gold et al. 1996) and maintained in the present project. Decision makers who must make prioritization and allocation choices in healthcare should have the information a standard CEA provides; they can then be reminded that they must decide whether and how to take account of considerations of equity as well in their decision making. This reminder may be, but usually is not, accompanied by some guidance about alternative substantive positions, and reasons in support of them, on the equity issues.

As we argued above, this is not an entirely satisfactory approach to equity concerns— or, at least, it has not been implemented in a satisfactory way. In many, if not most, uses of CEA in health policy and health program evaluation, important issues of equity often are not raised—for example, in the case of CEA of alternative treatments, each of which has uniform but different benefits for a group of patients with a particular medical condition.

Decision makers should have access to the best possible analyses of the ethical issues relevant to the decisions they are called upon to make. At a minimum, the analysts can then help direct decision makers to the ethical issues they should be addressing that may require deviating from the implications of the CEA. In some cases, there may be opportunities for analysts to work directly with decision makers to expand their treatment of ethical issues, addressing those of greatest concern in a specific decision context. In general, analysts should provide a full explication of the equity concerns raised in a CEA; a full accounting may also involve conducting sensitivity analyses to explore the impact of alternative values, weights, or assumptions within a CEA.

Each of the issues discussed in this chapter is complex, controversial, and important. In each case, there are important ethical and value choices to be made in constructing and using CEA measures; the choices are not merely technical, empirical, or economic, but moral and value choices as well. Each requires explicit attention both by analysts and by decision makers using CEA. The importance of a future agenda for health policy bioethicists should not be ignored.

12.5 RECOMMENDATIONS

1. Where significant accommodation is likely to disability states being evaluated, those accommodations should be reflected in alternative values for relevant health states and examined in sensitivity analysis.
2. When comparing alternative life-extending interventions that would benefit patients of substantially different ages, a decision maker may wish to give greater weight to benefitting the patients who would have had significantly fewer life years

or quality-adjusted life years (QALYs) if they do not receive treatment. Analysts should conduct sensitivity analysis to illustrate the impact.

3. Where the cost-effectiveness analysis (CEA) is of alternatives providing significant benefits to persons in very different initial states of health, the decision maker may wish to consider giving some priority to the worse off potential beneficiaries. Analysts may conduct sensitivity analysis to illustrate the impact of alternative assumptions.

4. When the CEA compares alternatives that provide large benefits to some individuals with other alternatives that provide much smaller benefits to a much larger number of individuals, decision makers may consider giving greater priority to the alternatives that concentrate benefits or disperse burdens. Analysts should highlight this issue when it is important.

5. When the CEA favors one group of beneficiaries over other potential beneficiaries based on a small difference in cost-effectiveness ratios, it is important for decision makers to consider whether mitigating factors cited in Section 12.3.3 reduce the fair chances problem. If not, can the difference be reduced in other ways? Analysts should highlight and discuss this issue when it is important.

6. Users of CEA should assess whether a specific CEA significantly discriminates against disabled patients on the basis of their disabilities and how that discrimination, if present, might be avoided.

7. Whenever recommending departure from the most cost-effective alternative on ethical grounds, decision makers may wish to consider the reduced benefits or increased costs to others of doing so. Sensitivity analyses, which can then be compared with the base-case analysis, do this automatically.

12.6 REFERENCES

Brock, D. W. 1988. "Ethical Issues in Recipient Selection for Organ Transplantation." In *Organ Substitution Technology: Ethical, Legal, and Public Policy Issues*, edited by D. Mathieu, 86–99. Boulder, CO: Westview Press.

Brock, D. W. 1995. Justice and the ADA: does prioritizing and rationing health care discriminate against the disabled? *Soc Philos Policy* 12 (2):159–185.

Brock, D. W. 2000. "Health Care Resource Prioritization and Discrimination against Persons with Disabilities." In *Americans with Disabilities: Exploring Implications of the Law for Individuals and Institutions*, edited by L.P. Francis and A. Silvers, 223–235. New York: Routledge.

Brock, D. W. 2002. "Priority to the Worse Off in Health-Care Resource Prioritization." In *Medicine and Social Justice: Essays in the Distribution of Health Care*, edited by R. Rhodes, M. P. Battin and A. Silvers, 362–372. New York: Oxford University Press.

Broome, J. 1984. Selecting people randomly. *Ethics* 95 (1):38–55.

Cookson, R., M. Drummond, and H. Weatherly. 2009. Explicit incorporation of equity considerations into economic evaluation of public health interventions. *Health Econ Policy Law* 4 (Pt 2):231–245.

Daniels, N. 1988. *Am I My Parents' Keeper? An Essay on Justice Between the Yound and the Old.* New York: Oxford University Press.

Daniels, N. 1993. Rationing fairly: programmatic considerations. *Bioethics* 7 (2-3):224–233.

Daniels, N. 2004. How to Achieve Fair Distribution of ARTs In 3 By 5: Fair Process and Legitimacy in Patient Selection. Background paper for the Consultation on Ethics and Equitable Access to Treatment and Care for HIV/AIDS (co-sponsored by WHO and the Joint UN Programme on HIV/AIDS). Geneva, Switzerland; 26-27 January 2004.

Daniels, N. 2008. *Just Health: Meeting Health Needs Fairly.* New York: Cambridge University Press.

Daniels, N., S. Rose, and E. D. Zide. 2009. "Disability, Adaptation, and Inclusion." In *Disability and Disadvantage*, edited by K. Brownlee and A. Cureton, 54–85. New York: Oxford University Press.

Gold, M. R., J. E. Siegel, L. B. Russell, and M. C. Weinstein, eds. 1996. *Cost-Effectiveness in Health and Medicine.* New York: Oxford University Press.

Hadorn, D. C. 1991. Setting health care priorities in Oregon. Cost-effectiveness meets the rule of rescue. *JAMA* 265 (17):2218–2225.

Hausman, D. M., and M. S. McPherson. 2009. Preference satisfaction and welfare economics. *Econ Philos* 25 (1):1–25.

Jamison, D. T. 2002. "Cost-Effectiveness Analysis: Concepts and Applications." In *Oxford Textbook of Public Health. 4th edition*, 4th ed, edited by R. Detels, J. McEwen, R. Beaglehole and H. Tanaka, 903–919. Oxford: Oxford University Press.

Kamm, F. M. 1993a. "Chapter 8. Are There Irrelevant Utilities?" In *Morality, Mortality. Volume I: Death and Whom to Save from It*, 144–164. New York: Oxford University Press.

Kamm, F. M. 1993b. *Morality, Mortality. Volume I: Death and Whom to Save from It.* New York: Oxford University Press.

Kamm, F. M. 1993c. "Part I. Death: From Bad to Worse." In *Morality, Mortality. Volume I: Death and Whom to Save from It*, 17–71. New York: Oxford University Press.

Kamm, F. M. 1993d. "Part II. Saving Lives: General Issues." In *Morality, Mortality. Volume I: Death and Whom to Save from It*, 75–197. New York: Oxford University Press.

Kamm, F. M. 1993e. "Part III. Scare Resources: Theoretical Issues, Specific Recommendations, and Organ Transplants." In *Morality, Mortality. Volume I: Death and Whom to Save from It*, 201–330. New York: Oxford University Press.

Kamm, F. M. 2013a. "Aggregation, Allocating Scarce Resources, and Discrimination against the Disabled." In *Bioethical Prescriptions: To Create, End, Choose, and Improve Lives*, edited by F.M. Kamm, 425–485. Oxford: Oxford University Press.

Kamm, F. M. 2013b. "Health and Equity." In *Bioethical Prescriptions: To Create, End, Choose, and Improve Lives*, edited by F.M. Kamm, 363–392. Oxford: Oxford University Press.

Kant, I. 2012. *Groundwork of the Metaphysics of Morals.* Cambridge: Cambridge University Press.

Menzel, P., P. Dolan, J. Richardson, and J. A. Olsen. 2002. The role of adaptation to disability and disease in health state valuation: a preliminary normative analysis. *Soc Sci Med* 55 (12):2149–2158.

Murray, C. J. L. 1994. "Quantifying the Burden of Disease: The Technical Basis for Disability-Adjusted Life Years." In *Global Comparative Assessments in the Health Sector: Disease Burden, Expenditures and Intervention Packages*, edited by C. J. L. Murray and A. D. Lopez, 3–19. Geneva: World Health Organization.

Murray, C. J. L. 1996. "Rethinking DALYs." In *The Global Burden of Disease: A Comprehensive Assessment of Mortality and Disability From Disease, Injuries, and Risk Factors in 1990 and Projected to 2020*, edited by C. J. L. Murray and A. D. Lopez, 1–98. Boston: Harvard University Press.

Murray, C. J. L., J. A. Salomon, C. D. Mathers, and A. D. Lopez, eds. 2002. *Summary Measures of Population Health: Concepts, Ethics, Measurement and Applications*. Geneva: World Health Organization. http://whqlibdoc.who.int/publications/2002/9241545518.pdf.

National Institute for Health and Clinical Excellence (NICE). 2008. *Social Value Judgements: Principles for the Development of NICE Guidance*. 2nd ed. London: NICE. www.nice.org.uk/proxy/?sourceurl=http://www.nice.org.uk/aboutnice/howwework/socialvaluejudgements/socialvaluejudgements.jsp.

Neumann, P. J., and J. D. Chambers. 2012. Medicare's enduring struggle to define "reasonable and necessary" care. *N Engl J Med* 367 (19):1775–1777.

Neumann, P. J., J. T. Cohen, and M. C. Weinstein. 2014. Updating cost-effectiveness—the curious resilience of the $50,000-per-QALY threshold. *N Engl J Med* 371 (9):796–797.

Nord, E. 1993. The trade-off between severity of illness and treatment effect in cost-value analysis of health care. *Health Policy* 24 (3):227–238.

Nord, E. 1999. *Cost-Value Analysis in Health Care: Making Sense out of QALYs*. New York: Cambridge University Press.

Nord, E. 2015. Cost-value analysis of health interventions: introduction and update on methods and preference data. *Pharmacoeconomics* 33 (2):89–95.

Nord, E., N. Daniels, and M. Kamlet. 2009. QALYs: some challenges. *Value Health* 12 Suppl 1:S10–S15.

Nord, E., A. U. Enge, and V. Gundersen. 2010. QALYs: is the value of treatment proportional to the size of the health gain? *Health Econ* 19 (5):596–607.

Nord, E., and R. Johansen. 2014. Concerns for severity in priority setting in health care: a review of trade-off data in preference studies and implications for societal willingness to pay for a QALY. *Health Policy* 116 (2-3):281–288.

Nord, E., J. L. Pinto, J. Richardson, P. Menzel, and P. Ubel. 1999. Incorporating societal concerns for fairness in numerical valuations of health programmes. [Erratum appears in Health Econ 1999;8(6):559]. *Health Econ* 8 (1):25–39.

Nord, E., J. Richardson, A. Street, H. Kuhse, and P. Singer. 1995. Who cares about cost? Does economic analysis impose or reflect social values? *Health Policy* 34 (2):79–94.

Parfit, D. 1991. *Equality Or Priority?: The Lindley Lecture, University of Kansas, November 21, 1991*. Lawrence, KS: University of Kansas.

Rawls, J. 1971. *A Theory of Justice*. Cambridge, MA: Harvard University Press.

Salomon, J. A., and C. J. L. Murray. 2002. "A Conceptual Framework for Understanding Adaptation, Coping and Adjustment in Health State Valuations." In *Summary Measures of Population Health: Concepts, Ethics, Measurement and Applications*, edited by C. J. L. Murray, J. A. Salomon, C. D. Mathers and A. D. Lopez, 619–626. Geneva: World Health Organization. http://whqlibdoc.who.int/publications/2002/9241545518.pdf.

Sen, A., and B. Williams, eds. 1982. *Utilitarianism and Beyond*. Cambridge: Cambridge Universtiy Press.

Sprangers, M. A., and C. E. Schwartz. 1999. Integrating response shift into health-related quality of life research: a theoretical model. *Soc Sci Med* 48 (11):1507–1515.

Temkin, L. S. 2003. Equality, priority or what? *Econ Philos* 19 (1):61–87.

Walzer, M. 1983. *Spheres of Justice: A Defense of Pluralism and Equality*. Cambridge, MA: Basic Books.

Williams, A. 1997. Intergenerational equity: an exploration of the "fair innings" argument. *Health Econ* 6 (2):117–132.

World Bank. 1993. *World Development Report 1993: Investing in Health*. New York: Oxford University Press.

13

Reporting Cost-Effectiveness Analyses

Lisa A. Prosser, Peter J. Neumann, Gillian D. Sanders,
and Joanna E. Siegel

13.1 INTRODUCTION

The original Panel on Cost-Effectiveness in Health and Medicine emphasized the importance of appropriately reporting the results of cost-effectiveness analyses (CEAs). The comprehensiveness of a study report affects the degree to which research can be reviewed or extended by other analysts. Its organization and clarity govern its accessibility to an audience, its credibility, and, ultimately, the likelihood that study results will inform clinical or policy decisions. Research has shown that adherence to reporting recommendations in published CEAs has improved over time, and suggests an impact of the original Panel's recommendations (Gold et al. 1996), which have been cited thousands of times (Neumann et al. 2005; Phillips and Chen 2002). A comparison of articles published in 1998–2001 ($n = 305$) with those published in 1976–1997 ($n = 228$), for example, found that studies improved in explicitly identifying the study perspective (73% vs 52%, $p < 0.001$); discounting both costs and quality-adjusted life years (QALYs; 82% vs 73%, $p = 0.0115$); and reporting incremental cost-utility ratios (69% vs 46%, $p < 0.001$) (Neumann et al. 2005).

The Second Panel reiterates this emphasis on the importance of organization and clarity and provides expanded recommendations to improve and standardize reporting. Because CEAs address a wide range of topics and serve multiple purposes, it would be unhelpful and impractical to recommend a strict template for reporting all studies. However, it is important that all the information needed to understand and evaluate CEAs be clearly and readily available. The purpose of this chapter's recommendations is to improve the transparency of CEAs reported in the literature, to aid analysts in assuring the completeness of the CEA report, and to support the presentation of comparable CEA results. More generally, the goal is to help authors communicate

This chapter builds on concepts presented in Chapter 9 of the original Panel's book (Siegel, J. E., M. C. Weinstein, and G. W. Torrance. 1996. "Reporting Cost-Effectiveness Studies and Results." In *Cost-Effectiveness in Health and Medicine*, edited by M. R. Gold, J. E. Siegel, L. B. Russell, and M. C. Weinstein, 276–303. New York: Oxford University Press).

meaningful information about the value of an intervention and where impacts are greatest across sectors and target populations. The chapter highlights several updates to the original Panel's report, such as the reporting of intermediate outcomes and disaggregated results, as well as the addition of an Impact Inventory to better support the use of CEAs.

We recommend that analysts document CEAs in two parts, a *journal article* and a *technical appendix* (see **Recommendation 1** in Section 13.8). These serve complementary purposes. The journal article has been the primary means of communicating CEA results. We use the term "journal article" here to refer to any *summary* manuscript, including book chapters and government reports, intended to communicate the context of the problem and the analysis, its main features, and the results and their interpretation in a relatively brief way.

It is often difficult to describe data and assumptions and to explain and justify methodological decisions in the limited space of a journal article. As a result, reviewers may be unable to determine how the analysis was constructed. Since publication of the original Panel's recommendations, several journals have added requirements for the submission of supplementary material to provide additional transparency on methodological details for submitted CEAs (Annals of Internal Medicine 2015; Journal of the American Medical Association 2015). To support this trend and encourage wider adherence, this chapter aims to provide clarity concerning requirements for such materials. We refer to the recommended set of supplementary materials, which could range from one or more documents to a complete standalone technical manual, as a *technical appendix*.

We recommend that the technical appendix be submitted with the journal article to a peer-reviewed journal, or policy or clinical committee (**Recommendation 2**). It should also be made available at publication, because readers may want to conduct a detailed review of methods and assumptions in order to evaluate the study, improve their understanding of specific data or methods, reproduce the work, or adapt it to local circumstances (**Recommendation 2**). The technical appendix is intended to provide adequate detail for these purposes. Many journals now support online publication of technical appendices. For reports other than peer-reviewed journal articles, such as book chapters, the technical appendix should also be made available online if not included alongside the original print source. Ideally, the level of detail supplied by the combination of the journal article and the technical appendix should enable readers to replicate the analysis, if not exactly, at least in its essential features (**Recommendation 5**).

13.1.1 The Evolution of Reporting Guidelines for CEAs

In the years since the original Panel's report, a number of guidelines for reporting CEAs have been introduced by journals, professional societies, and ad hoc task forces. In 1995, prior to the publication of the original Panel guidelines, the *Annals of Internal Medicine* published the findings of the Task Force on Principles for Economic Analysis of Health Care Technology (1995). This group, comprised of leading researchers and funded by the pharmaceutical industry, recommended that several factors be discussed in economic analyses: "1) the sources of information and methods used to measure and estimate effects; 2) whether an analysis is scientifically sound and relevant to the reader's needs; 3) the validity of conclusions; and 4) the applicability, generalizability, and limits of the reported results" (Task Force on Principles for Economic Analysis of Health Care Technology 1995, 65). The report received wide attention, but met with some criticism because of its funding source (Evans 1995).

In 1996, the original Panel provided specific recommendations on the reporting of data, results, discussion, and technical addenda for CEAs (Siegel et al. 1996). The recommendations emphasized that the reporting of Reference Case results should be standardized to allow for cross-study comparisons (Siegel et al. 1996). That same year, a UK-based group published "Guidelines for authors and peer reviewers of economic submission to the BMJ" (Drummond and Jefferson 1996). That article contained a guide to health-related economic evaluations, as well as checklists for authors and editors evaluating CEAs (Drummond and Jefferson 1996). The guidelines emphasized transparency and requested that disaggregated data, not summary data, be presented to allow the reader to review and critique calculations (Drummond and Jefferson 1996). Other European efforts to review reporting issues, among other topics, included the European Network on Methodology and Application of Economic Evaluation Techniques (EUROMET) in 2000 (Hoffmann and Graf von der Schulenburg 2000). Three years later, in an effort to improve the quality of CEAs, a multidisciplinary team of researchers in the United States created the Quality of Health Economic Studies (QHES) instrument, a 16-question "scorecard" with points (out of 100) earned on the basis of "yes" or "no" answers from the evaluating reader (Ofman et al. 2003). The system, intended to help researchers quickly identify high-quality CEAs, was validated and tested in a pilot-case study (Ofman et al. 2003). The QHES has been cited widely as an available resource, but it does not seem to have been used extensively.

In 2013, a group of researchers convened by the International Society for Pharmacoeconomics and Outcomes Research (ISPOR) published the Consolidated Health Economic Evaluation Reporting Standards (CHEERS) guidelines, intended as a user-friendly framework to facilitate comprehensive and cohesive reporting in health economic evaluations. The group cited a survey of the World Association of Medical Editors, in which 90% of respondents said that they would use such an evaluative tool if it were available and accessible (Husereau et al. 2013a). The CHEERS guidelines, which were published simultaneously in 10 academic journals, include a 24-item comparative checklist for cross-study evaluation (Husereau et al. 2013b). Several other sets of reporting recommendations with similar guidance have also been published (Drummond, Manca, and Sculpher 2005; Hoffmann and Graf von der Schulenburg 2000; Nuijten et al. 1998; Petrou and Gray 2011a, b).

The recommendations in this chapter, based on the original Panel's report and also mindful of other guidelines, differ in several areas of emphasis, specifically the updated Reference Case definition, the newly recommended Impact Inventory, and recommendations to support CEA's role in US decision contexts.

13.2 CHECKLIST FOR REPORTING

The checklist for reporting provided in Table 13.1 is intended to support standardization across analyses and has been updated to capture key changes from the Second Panel. It is recommended for use during the preparation of the journal article and technical appendix to help analysts determine whether all important aspects of a study have been addressed. The checklist can also be used by journals and peer reviewers to ensure completeness in reporting. For publication in journals that require their own checklists, we still recommend that analysts consult the checklist here for items related to the Reference Case, Impact Inventory, and results (intermediate outcomes and disaggregated results).

13.3 CREATING THE JOURNAL ARTICLE AND TECHNICAL APPENDIX

In this section, we outline the essential elements of a CEA study report and make recommendations about which elements should go into the journal article versus the technical appendix. The discussion is organized according to the main headings of a typical journal article: structured abstract; introduction/background; methods and data; results; and discussion.

13.3.1 Structured Abstract

While we recognize that journals may have their own requirements, we recommend that a structured abstract specifically designed for CEAs should be included in the journal article wherever possible (**Recommendation 3**). Table 13.2 provides an example adapted from the requirements of the *Annals of Internal Medicine* (Annals of Internal Medicine 2015). If a journal requires a more generic abstract format (e.g., Objectives, Methods, Results, Conclusions), we recommend that authors incorporate the elements specified in Table 13.2 into the required format as fully as possible.

13.3.2 The Introduction

The introduction of a CEA journal article typically provides contextual background by briefly describing the research question, the significance of the problem under investigation, the decision context and audience, and the intervention(s) being evaluated. Important boundaries to the scope of the study should be highlighted, and the comparator intervention(s) identified.

13.3.3 The Methods and Data Section

13.3.3.1 An Overview of Study Design and Scope

The methods section should begin by describing the overall design and scope of the analysis. This description should identify the target population(s), time horizon,

Table 13.1 Reporting checklist

Element	Journal article	Technical appendix
Introduction		
• Background of the problem	☐	☐
Study design and scope		
• Objectives	☐	☐
• Audience	☐	☐
• Type of analysis	☐	☐
• Target population(s)	☐	☐
• Description of interventions and comparators (including "no intervention," if applicable)	☐	☐
• Other intervention descriptors (e.g., care setting, model of delivery, intensity and timing of intervention)	☐	☐
• Boundaries of the analysis (defining the scope or comprehensiveness of the study)	☐	☐
• Time horizon	☐	☐
• Analytic perspectives (e.g., Reference Case perspectives included [healthcare sector, societal]; other perspectives such as employer or payer)	☐	☐
• Whether this analysis meets the requirements of the Reference Case	☐	☐
• Analysis plan	☐	☐
Methods and data		
• Trial-based analysis or model-based analysis. If model-based:	☐	☐
○ Description of event pathway/model (describe condition or disease and the health states included)	☐	☐
○ Diagram of event pathway/model (depicting the sequencing and possible transitions among the health states included)	☐	☐
○ Description of model used (e.g., decision tree, state transition, microsimulation)	☐	☐
○ Modeling assumptions	☐	☐
○ Software used	☐	☐
• Identification of key outcomes	☐	☐
• Complete information on sources of effectiveness data, cost data, and preference weights	☐	☐
• Methods for obtaining estimates of effectiveness including approach(es) used for evidence synthesis	☐	☐
• Methods for obtaining estimates of costs and preference weights	☐	☐
• Critique of data quality	☐	☐

(continued)

Table 13.1 Continued

Element	Journal article	Technical appendix
• Statement of costing year; this is the year to which all costs have been adjusted for the analysis (e.g., 2016)	☐	☐
• Statement of method used to adjust costs for inflation	☐	☐
• Statement of type of currency	☐	☐
• Source and methods for obtaining expert judgment, if applicable	☐	☐
• Statement of discount rate(s)	☐	☐
Impact Inventory		
• Full accounting of consequences within and outside of the healthcare sector	☐	☐
Results		
• Results of model validation	☐	☐
• Reference Case results (discounted and undiscounted): total costs and effectiveness, incremental costs and effectiveness, incremental cost-effectiveness ratios, measure(s) of uncertainty	☐	☐
• Disaggregated results for important categories of costs, outcomes, or both	☐	☐
• Results of sensitivity analysis	☐	☐
• Other estimates of uncertainty	☐	☐
• Graphical representation of cost-effectiveness results	☐	☐
• Graphical representation of uncertainty analyses	☐	☐
• Aggregate cost and effectiveness information	☐	☐
• Secondary analyses	☐	☐
Disclosures		
• Statement of any potential conflicts of interest relating to funding source, collaborations, or outside interests	☐	☐
Discussion		
• Summary of Reference Case results	☐	☐
• Summary of sensitivity of results to assumptions and uncertainties in the analysis	☐	☐
• Discussion of the study results in the context of results of related CEAs	☐	☐
• Discussion of ethical implications (e.g., distributive implications relating to age, disability, or other characteristics of the population)	☐	☐
• Limitations of the study	☐	☐
• Relevance of study results to specific policy questions or decisions	☐	☐

Table 13.2 Elements recommended for inclusion in a structured abstract for reporting cost-effectiveness analyses

Element	Suggested content
Objective	Succinctly state the research question specific to the analysis.
Interventions	List all interventions included in the analysis, including the comparator(s). Identify the time frame of the interventions.
Target population	Identify the age range(s), clinical characteristics, and other characteristics for all subgroups evaluated in the analysis.
Perspectives	Identify whether the analysis uses the Reference Case perspectives and any alternative perspectives presented.
Time horizon	Specify the time horizon for the analysis. This may differ from the time frame(s) of the intervention(s) and comparator(s).
Discount rate	Specify the discount rate used in the analysis.
Costing year	Specify the costing year used in the analysis.
Study design	Describe whether this is a trial-based or model-based analysis. If model-based, briefly describe the model type (e.g., decision tree, state-transition, microsimulation, discrete event) and the size and characteristics of the simulated population. Indicate whether the analysis meets Reference Case requirements.
Data sources	Describe the types of data used to derive inputs for the analysis (e.g., primary data, secondary data from the published literature, administrative data, unpublished trial data).
Outcome measures	List primary and secondary outcome measures (e.g., ICER in $ per QALY, $ per LY, or $ per clinical endpoint; total costs; total QALYs for a specified cohort; or population-level outcomes).
Results of base-case analysis	Briefly describe results for the primary outcome measure(s), as well as notable results for intermediate outcomes and disaggregated results (e.g., deaths averted, hospitalizations averted, specific subcategories of costs). Identify any substantial changes in non-healthcare-sector consequences.
Results of uncertainty analysis	Briefly describe whether the results are robust to changes explored in the uncertainty analyses.
Limitations	Describe important limitations of the analysis, such as controversial assumptions.
Conclusions	Summarize the key clinical or policy conclusions.

Abbreviations: ICER = incremental cost-effectiveness ratios; LY = life year; QALY = quality-adjusted life year.

perspective(s), interventions and comparators, and other key components of the study design. Characteristics of the intervention(s) to be specified include the care setting (location and type of institution—e.g., hospitals, ambulatory clinics, or primary care practices), the mode of service delivery (equipment, personnel, and other aspects of the strategy used), and details related to timing. Similar care should be devoted to describing the comparator intervention(s). If the study includes one or more perspectives in addition to the Reference Case perspectives, the analyst should identify them. Analysts should carefully describe the scope of the study and boundaries of the analysis. For example, is an analysis of a vaccine-preventable condition limited to transmission to household contacts or extended to the full population? Is the focus a "what-if" scenario analysis intended to demonstrate the impact of the intervention if a certain level of effectiveness is established? The description should be detailed enough to allow readers to determine the appropriateness of generalizing results.

13.3.3.2 *The Definition of the Reference Case*

As described in Chapter 3, the Second Panel recommends that all studies report one Reference Case analysis based on a healthcare sector perspective and another Reference Case analysis based on a societal perspective. These perspectives determine the scope of costs and outcomes included. To clarify the boundaries of the analysis for each Reference Case perspective, we recommend use of an Impact Inventory.

13.3.3.3 *The Impact Inventory*

The Impact Inventory includes costs and effects in the formal healthcare sector and indicates if other sectors are affected and associated sector costs and effects (Table 13.3). For a Reference Case analysis, the Impact Inventory table will identify categories of effects and whether different sectors are included in the analysis. If a sector or consequence within a sector is identified but excluded, analysts should provide a brief account of the rationale in the accompanying text or in the "Notes on Sources of Evidence" section of the Impact Inventory. Some interventions may have impacts limited to the formal healthcare sector. Other interventions, such as public health programs, will have substantive impacts beyond the formal healthcare sector and will require a full enumeration of important categories of benefits, harms, and costs. For example, a public health program to increase physical activity for schoolchildren can affect time requirements for parents. A treatment for autism spectrum disorders could avert costs of special education and also improve school level attainment. Savings on special education costs and potential benefits of improved schooling would be included in the Impact Inventory, whether or not they are quantified and valued in the analysis.

The Impact Inventory may be presented in either the Methods section (in a summarized form) or in the Results. For all analyses, the Impact Inventory should identify the sectors affected and list the specific types of impacts within each sector. If results in a societal Reference Case differ substantially from those in the healthcare sector Reference Case, ideally all identified effects should be quantified, valued, and reported in the results section (see Section 13.3.4.4). Items in categories not estimated

Table 13.3 Impact Inventory template

Sector	Type of impact (list category within each sector with unit of measure if relevant)*	Included in this Reference Case analysis from ... perspective?		Notes on sources of evidence
		Healthcare sector	Societal	
Formal healthcare sector				
Health	*Health outcomes (effects)*			
	Longevity effects	☐	☐	
	Health-related quality-of-life effects	☐	☐	
	Other health effects (e.g., adverse events and secondary transmissions of infections)	☐	☐	
	Medical costs			
	Paid for by third-party payers	☐	☐	
	Paid for by patients out-of-pocket	☐	☐	
	Future related medical costs (payers and patients)	☐	☐	
	Future unrelated medical costs (payers and patients)	☐	☐	
Informal healthcare sector				
Health	Patient time costs	NA	☐	
	Unpaid caregiver time costs	NA	☐	
	Transportation costs	NA	☐	
Non-healthcare sectors (with examples of possible items)				
Productivity	Labor market earnings lost	NA	☐	
	Cost of unpaid lost productivity due to illness	NA	☐	
	Cost of uncompensated household production	NA	☐	
Consumption	Future consumption unrelated to health	NA	☐	
Social services	Cost of social services as part of intervention	NA	☐	
Legal/ criminal justice	Number of crimes related to intervention	NA	☐	
	Cost of crimes related to intervention	NA	☐	

(continued)

Table 13.3 Continued

Sector	Type of impact (list category within each sector with unit of measure if relevant)*	Included in this Reference Case analysis from ... perspective?		Notes on sources of evidence
		Healthcare sector	Societal	
Education	Impact of intervention on educational achievement of population	NA	☐	
Housing	Cost of intervention on home improvements (e.g., removing lead paint)	NA	☐	
Environment	Production of toxic waste or pollution by intervention	NA	☐	
Other (specify)	Other impacts	NA	☐	

* Categories listed are intended as examples for analysts.
Abbreviation: NA = Not Applicable

quantitatively should be addressed in the Discussion section and/or the technical appendix. The Impact Inventory should be completed and reported for all analyses, even those restricted to the healthcare sector, in order to highlight any benefits or costs not fully addressed. We recommend that analysts initially consider the elements of the Impact Inventory as part of the design exercise for an analysis (see Chapter 4) and then include the completed Impact Inventory in the journal article (or the technical appendix, if space limitations preclude inclusion in the journal report) (**Recommendation 4**). We also encourage analysts to include the Impact Inventory as part of the manuscript submission process, even if it is not included in the journal article.

13.3.3.4 *Analytic Approach*

The Methods section should begin by describing the event trajectory for the condition and intervention. The study should trace the sequence of events, describing the links between the intervention, its short-term effects, longer term events, and final outcomes. For example, in a study of an antihypertensive medication, the analyst may relate the short-term effects on lowering blood pressure to a decreased probability of cardiovascular events, and then to reduced cardiovascular mortality, and finally to increased life expectancy. A screening intervention would start with outcomes for the screening algorithm, and condition events would follow. It is important to indicate explicitly the primary and secondary outcomes of interest. For example, the primary outcome may be an improvement in health-related quality of life, and secondary outcomes could include deaths and specific coronary events or screening outcomes. A diagram illustrating the event pathway is recommended (see Chapter 5).

Analysts should specify the type of analysis (trial-based or model-based). If model-based, the type of model employed should be described. Discussion of the modeling strategy should describe the basic conceptualization and elements of the model, including structural assumptions; starting populations and subgroups; whether a cohort or population is being analyzed; and model calibration and validation. Analysts should carefully articulate any special assumptions—for example, detailing any assumptions used to extrapolate intervention effects beyond a study time horizon or to other populations—or structural assumptions if aspects of the condition's natural history are unclear. Analysts should identify the type of software used to conduct the analysis or program the model.

The method of calculating summary measures (e.g., incremental cost-effectiveness ratio [ICER], net monetary benefit [NMB], net health benefit [NHB]) should be identified, as well as the methods and assumptions used to conduct uncertainty analyses, secondary analyses, scenario analyses, and other sensitivity analyses. A table or set of tables should report the quantitative values for the parameter inputs, including any associated distributional assumptions and sources.

The relative balance of material to be included in the main report versus the technical appendix will depend on word limits, journal requirements, and author discretion. The goal should be to communicate the essential elements in the journal article.

13.3.3.5 *Intervention Effectiveness*

An understanding of the evidence for the effectiveness of an intervention is fundamental to assessing the quality and appropriate use of CEAs. A discussion of effectiveness should summarize the body of evidence, describing the direction and magnitude of effect sizes, how the evidence was synthesized, and relevant controversies (see Chapter 9). For example, the analyst may discuss randomization, sample size and representativeness, and other aspects of study design and interpretation, such as the magnitude of effect sizes and confidence intervals for specific study parameters. Analysts should include detail of the evidence synthesis in the technical appendix. If a systematic review was performed specifically for the CEA, then details on the search strategy, inclusion/exclusion criteria, and data analysis methods will be needed (and typically are presented in the technical appendix). If the CEA used findings from an existing systematic review, analysts should discuss the strength of the evidence, the overall quality of the review, and its applicability to the population/interventions of interest. An analysis undertaken before studies of efficacy or effectiveness are completed (a "what-if" scenario analysis) may still be highly useful for guiding policy decisions, but consumers will need to interpret the results in light of heightened uncertainty.

Authors should describe the rationale and assumptions necessary to generalize from primary research or studies in the literature. For example, authors might discuss the extent to which data from a clinical trial reflect patients' adherence outside of the trial setting or for broader populations. The discussion of effectiveness should also include any assumptions required and the methods employed to incorporate other data, such as those to extend the evidence beyond the trial period, which is often required to properly estimate long-term effects.

13.3.3.6 Adjustments for Health-Related Quality of Life

We recommend that analysts include essential descriptors of the preference elicitation used to measure preference weights: direct or indirect (multi-attribute) elicitation method; the elicitation task or measurement system employed; and if the weights reflect community-based preferences or not (**Recommendation 6**) (see Chapter 7). For directly elicited preference weights, the elicitation task (e.g., time trade-off, standard gamble) and the study population should be identified. For indirect methods, analysts should cite the measurement system used (e.g., EQ-5D, HUI). Analysts should indicate whether the preference weights, obtained via direct or indirect elicitation, represent community-based preferences. Any relevant limitations of the weights should be identified. A recent analysis of the Tufts Medical Center Cost-effectiveness Registry found that as many as one-third of published CEAs did not include any details of the preference elicitation technique used (Prosser and Wittenberg 2011). Preference weights for the primary health outcomes should be included in the table reporting parameter inputs. Further details regarding sources of utility weights and a listing of the full set of weights can be reported in the technical appendix.

13.3.3.7 Costs and Resource Use

The journal article should include a complete listing of the resource use associated with the intervention(s), comparator(s), and usual care. Table 13.4 summarizes the cost

Table 13.4 Cost components included in the two Reference Case perspectives

Cost component	Reference Case perspective	
	Healthcare	Societal
Formal healthcare sector:*		
Paid for by third-party payers	✓	✓
Paid for by patients out-of-pocket	✓	✓
Informal healthcare sector:		
Patient time	–	✓
Unpaid caregiver time	–	✓
Transportation costs	–	✓
Non-healthcare sectors:		
Productivity	–	✓
Consumption	–	✓
Social services	–	✓
Legal or criminal justice	–	✓
Education	–	✓
Housing	–	✓
Environment	–	✓
Other (e.g., friction costs)	–	✓

*Includes current and future costs, related and unrelated to the condition under consideration.

components typically included in the two Reference Case perspectives. As described in Chapters 3 and 8, costs included in the numerator of the ICER will include only formal healthcare sector (medical) costs for the healthcare sector Reference Case. For the societal perspective Reference Case, we recommend that the analysis also include time costs of patients in seeking and receiving care, time costs of informal caregivers, transportation costs, effects on future productivity and consumption in added years of life, and other costs and effects outside the healthcare sector.

The general approach used to quantify each type of cost should be identified (e.g., as micro-costing or gross costing). Reasonably detailed information on these types of costs should be provided in the journal article, preferably in tables. If the analyst has separately measured and valued resources using a micro-costing approach, the table should report both the cost per unit of each resource and the number of units consumed. The source of data for each estimate should be described, including the type of study, survey, or database from which data were derived; the characteristics of the source population, such as insurance status (e.g., if data are derived from administrative data); and geographic location. It is important to describe any adjustments made (e.g., use of ratios of cost to charge at a particular institution), and to detail any other methods or models used to estimate unit costs. The author should also specify adjustments for inflation and should state the year and currency in which costs are presented (e.g., 2015 US dollars). As for any category of data input, analysts should comment on the quality and appropriateness of data sources.

The societal perspective Reference Case analysis will include resource use outside of the formal healthcare sector. The same general approach should apply: a table should detail the cost per unit for each resource and the number of units if micro-costing is employed. Chapter 8 includes a more detailed discussion of categories of resource use outside of the formal healthcare sector. For resources not quantified in the analysis, a qualitative description of the type of impact and appropriate sources should be provided in the Impact Inventory.

13.3.3.8 Use of Expert Judgment

If a CEA relies on experts to provide parameter estimates for any category of model inputs, the analysts should describe the basis for selecting the content experts, the number and type of experts, and the process used to elicit their input. Researchers have published best practices for eliciting expert judgment (O'Hagan et al. 2006; Sullivan and Payne 2011), and analysts should describe the extent to which such methods were employed. Authors should also discuss the rationale for using experts (e.g., to reconcile conflicting data, to estimate parameters in an area with little or no available evidence) and provide an assessment of the quality of the approach. Given space limitations, this material may be included in the technical appendix.

13.3.3.9 Discounting

As discussed in Chapter 10, the Second Panel recommends a discount rate of 3% for both costs and health effects in both the healthcare sector and the societal perspective

Reference Case analyses. We recommend an explicit statement of this rate, as well as any alternative rates used for conducting secondary analyses.

13.3.4 The Results Section

13.3.4.1 *Model Calibration and Validation*

As described in Chapter 5, if a model is used, the authors should describe methods and findings for model calibration and validation. The journal article should report that calibration and validation have been conducted. The technical appendix should describe tests performed to demonstrate the accuracy of programming and to establish the face validity of the model calculations and checks for internal and external validity. Appropriate assessments will generally include presentation of intermediate modeling results. For example, in an analysis using QALYs, the author might also describe the model's predictions of the number of episodes of influenza and hospitalized pneumonia occurring with and without an intervention. Appraisals of the model's performance using varying assumptions will demonstrate that the model obtains predictable results. When a previously validated model is used, the authors may choose to cite previous articles that provide evidence of validity.

Analysts are encouraged to provide an electronic copy of the model to peer reviewers, along with the technical appendix, to allow reviewers to test the model and gain an understanding of its dynamics. We encourage researchers to allow use of their models for peer review under the assumption that the same code of conduct applies to models as to data collected in a clinical trial or other study. We encourage analysts to make their models available publicly, though we recognize logistical and practical constraints.

13.3.4.2 *Reference Case Results*

The reporting of the Reference Case for each perspective will require reporting of results from the healthcare sector and the societal perspective (see Chapter 3). Analysts should take care to clearly delineate the results from the two Reference Case perspectives and identify differences. They should consider the decision context when determining if one perspective is to be presented in greater detail.

13.3.4.3 *Base Case Cost-Effectiveness Results*

Reference Case results should generally include tables displaying the costs and effects for each program or intervention (Table 13.5). The suggested accounting of consequences should include totals (total or per capita costs and effects) as well as incremental calculations. Totals allow readers to follow and reproduce computations. We recommend that the tables include discounted total costs and effectiveness estimates.

Table 13.5 Example of Reference Case results: mean costs, QALYs, and ICER per person*

Alternative	Total cost (US $)	Total effectiveness (QALYs)	Incremental cost (US $)	Incremental effectiveness (QALYs)	ICER (incremental costs/ incremental QALYs)
Usual care[+]	11,290	7.926	–	–	
Alternative A	72,356	7.950	–	–	Dominated[‡]
Alternative B	76,959	7.955	65,669	0.029	2,264,448
Alternative C	78,134	7.911	–	–	Dominated

*Confidence intervals should be included for total costs, total QALYs, incremental cost, and incremental QALYs if probability sensitivity analysis has been conducted.

[+]This would be "no intervention" only if that is the standard of care for the condition being studied.

[‡]Extended dominance. ICER compared to Usual Care: $2,544,417.

Abbreviations: ICER = incremental cost-effectiveness ratio; QALYs = quality-adjusted life years.

The main CEA results should include the discounted ICERs for the interventions evaluated. These should be presented in the text of the journal report. Information on incremental costs and incremental effectiveness, as well as the ICERs, are generally presented in an accompanying table (see Table 13.5 for an example).

For further examples of how to report results for the two Reference Case perspectives, see the worked examples in Appendix A and Appendix B.

Many CEAs will include intermediate health outcomes in addition to QALYs: e.g., episodes of illness, hospitalizations, deaths, and other important states of health. The inclusion of disaggregated or intermediate outcomes can help consumers assess the quality and accuracy of a CEA. Intermediate outcomes alongside utility weights for each outcome can allow consumers to assess which outcomes are the largest determinants of QALYs. In addition, this information may also be relevant to researchers or others interested in applying alternative preference weights or calculating alternative ratios, such as cost per case averted.

Incremental cost-effectiveness ratios should be reported as costs per unit of analysis. As described in Chapter 4, analysts should compare each intervention to the next most effective option, after eliminating *dominated* options (i.e., those with higher cost and lower effectiveness than alternatives) to obtain ICERs (**Recommendation 9**). Instead of attempting to calculate ICERs for dominated options, analysts should record in the table that the option is dominated. Similarly, options ruled out by extended dominance should be identified. An example is provided in Table 13.5. For alternatives that generate a cost savings, ratios should not be reported as being negative, as this can lead to ambiguous interpretations. Ratios are not typically reported for dominated strategies. However, if an alternative yields an ICER that is very close to the efficiency frontier, in some cases, it may be useful for decision makers to see results both with and without allowing for extended dominance. This kind of discussion of results is elaborated under the heading "Interpreting Results for Decision Makers" (Section 13.4).

13.3.4.4 *Intermediate Outcomes and Disaggregated Results*

While ICERs provide a concise summary of results, the reporting of intermediate outcomes and disaggregated results can also provide important information. Intermediate outcomes are presented in natural units and can include diagnoses, test outcomes, and health events (either chronic or transient). The reporting of intermediate outcomes, such as number of cases, adverse events, hospitalizations, or deaths, provides readers an opportunity to assess model validity or the magnitude of intervention effectiveness, or to compare results with other analyses that may have utilized intermediate outcomes. Table 13.6 shows an example of intermediate outcomes reported for influenza vaccination for different age and risk subgroups.

The reporting of disaggregated results refers to the attribution of total costs or QALYs to intermediate categories associated with specific cost categories (e.g., intervention-specific or relating to the care of the condition, healthcare sector, or other sector) or intermediate health outcomes. A typical breakdown of costs would report intervention-specific and condition-related costs, along with more detailed categories as relevant (e.g., hospitalizations, outpatient visits). Other categories may be relevant depending on the decision context. Reporting disaggregated results for QALYs can assist decision makers in assessing the magnitude of health benefits. Analysts could present disaggregated results on the contribution of QALYs (gains or losses) from separate categories of health events (see Table 13.7). For example, are QALY gains primarily due to averted deaths or uncomplicated cases of influenza? Or what is the offset in QALYs lost due to side effects or adverse events compared to QALYs gained from an intervention? Examples of intermediate outcomes and disaggregated results are included in the worked examples (see Appendix A, Table 4, and Appendix B, Table 3). We recommend including information on intermediate outcomes and disaggregated results in the journal article and providing more detail in the technical appendix (**Recommendation 7**).

13.3.4.5 *Aggregate Costs and Effectiveness in a Defined Population (Intervention-Specific Costs and Outcomes)*

The aggregate intervention costs implied by a CEA may inform (or constrain) adoption independent of the intervention's cost-effectiveness. Similarly, the total magnitude of benefit (whether to society or an individual) can be a consideration in addition to an intervention's cost-effectiveness. The aggregate cost is the present value of the expected program costs for a decision maker, such as a screening program for a state public health department. Start-up or fixed costs, which may not be included in the primary analysis, may be relevant to the decision context and can be reported as secondary outcomes. Additional tables could include projected results at the population level (e.g., the total US population or for a health system or state, depending on the decision context).

Table 13.6 Example of intermediate outcomes: influenza vaccination compared with no vaccination

Outcome	Most likely estimate	95% CI
Hospitalizations averted (per 1,000 vaccinated)		
Non-high risk		
6–23 months	0.7	0–3.1
2–4 years	0.3	0–1.4
5–11 years	0.5	0.2–1.3
12–17 years	0.1	0–0.4
High risk		
6–23 months	3.0	0.1–12.7
2–4 years	1.5	0.2–5.2
5–11 years	0.9	0.1–4.4
12–17 years	0.5	0–2.3
Deaths averted (per 1,000 vaccinated)		
IIV, Non-high risk		
6–23 months	0.13	0.01–0.37
2-4 years	0.15	0.04–0.34
5–11 years	0.16	0.06–0.34
12–17 years	0.25	0.09–0.53
Adverse events incurred (per 1,000 vaccinated)		
IIV, Non-high risk		
6–23 months	34	15–61
2–4 years	20	8–38
5–11 years	9	4–17
QALYs gained (per 1,000 vaccinated)		
IIV, Non-high risk		
6–23 months	7.5	0.4–23.7
2–4 years	8.3	1.8–21.3
5–11 years	6.7	2.2–15.3
12–17 years	8.0	2.7–17.1
IIV, High risk		
6–23 months	23.6	1.2–65.7
2–4 years	26.6	5.7–59.1
5–11 years	25.7	8.7–54.9
12–17 years	36.0	12.3–76.5

Abbreviations: CI = confidence interval; IIV = inactivated influenza vaccine; QALYs = quality-adjusted life years.

Table 13.7 Example of disaggregated results: QALY gains/losses

Alternative	Total effectiveness (QALYs)	QALY gains attributable to treatment benefits	QALY losses attributable to treatment side effects
Usual care	7.926	–	–
Alternative A	7.950	0.053	(0.029)
Alternative B	7.955	0.080	(0.051)
Alternative C	7.911	0.073	(0.088)

Abbreviation: QALY(s) = quality-adjusted life year(s).

13.3.4.6 Conveying Uncertainty

As described in Chapter 11, two main sources of uncertainty warrant consideration: (1) parameter uncertainty, which arises from uncertainty about the true numerical values of the parameters used as inputs, and (2) model structure uncertainty, which concerns the manner in which elements in the analysis are combined. The journal article should include both deterministic and probabilistic sensitivity analyses when appropriate, as well as key findings from any uncertainty analyses conducted. Any additional secondary or scenario analyses should also be reported. Conveying uncertainty should be part of the Reference Case results. See Chapter 11 for additional details.

Secondary analyses included in a journal article might include:

- *Other perspectives.* Cost-effectiveness analyses are often motivated by policy choices relevant to specific institutions or individuals, such as an employer, state health department, or federal insurance program. Analyses conducted from these or other perspectives should be reported *in addition to* the two Reference Case perspective analyses.
- *Alternative discounting approaches.* In addition to presenting Reference Case results using a 3% discount rate, undiscounted results for disaggregated components of the ICER may be presented and sensitivity analyses conducted using a discount rate other than 3% or alternative approaches (e.g., differential rates for costs and effects, alternative functions).
- *Variations in study design.* Secondary analyses that include alternative target populations, comparator interventions, time horizons, or a change in other scoping parameters that fall outside of the original design of the analysis may be reported.

13.3.4.7 Graphical Representation of Reference Case Results

We recommend that ICERs be presented graphically with a plot of net costs and effectiveness. The resulting illustrations can be placed in the technical appendix if space limitations preclude their inclusion in the journal article. We also recommend visual displays to enhance the user's understanding of key sources of uncertainty. These displays can include tornado diagrams, plots of two- or three-way sensitivity analyses, scatter plots, cost-effectiveness acceptability curves, and other types of displays. For samples of displays of cost-effectiveness results, uncertainty analyses, and sensitivity analyses, see the worked examples in Appendix A (Figures 4–8 and Appendix Figure 2) and Appendix B (Figure 3 and Appendix Figures 4–6).

13.3.5 The Discussion Section

The discussion section provides authors an opportunity to interpret the study findings. It translates quantitative results into a qualitative description, highlights key assumptions, and identifies and considers alternative points of view in interpreting the findings. Generally, the discussion section will address the following: a summary of the results; Reference Case; Impact Inventory; relevance for decision makers; results of other published CEAs; ethical implications; limitations; and overall conclusions.

13.3.5.1 *Summary of Results and their Relevance*

The results of the Reference Case analyses should be highlighted and summarized, including the sensitivity of results to key assumptions and estimates (**Recommendation 8**). The Discussion section allows researchers to place the CEA results in the decision context(s) identified, including the relevance of the results for that decision. Given that many decision makers do not employ strict cost-effectiveness thresholds, the Discussion should explain how the Reference Case results and secondary analyses can support the decisions under consideration. For example, subgroup analysis may inform the development of clinical guidelines. The reporting of disaggregated outcomes could help decision makers understand whether aggregate QALYs gained from an intervention are due to a large number of minor health improvements or a smaller number of large improvements.

13.3.5.2 *Reference Case and Impact Inventory*

The Discussion section should address qualitative and quantitative differences for the two Reference Case perspectives. The analyst can also discuss additional results, such as from additional perspectives, which were included in the technical appendix but not the journal report.

13.3.5.3 *Reporting the Results of Other Published CEAs*

The Discussion section should include a brief review of CEA results of similar or related interventions. For example, a discussion of an analysis of influenza vaccination might describe results of other influenza vaccination CEAs, even if the setting, administration, population, or other aspects differed. Cost-effectiveness results from other analyses should be converted to the currency year in the analyst's study using an appropriate index to facilitate comparisons. If the year is not given in the cited analysis, analysts might plausibly assume the year to be 2 or 3 years prior to the date of publication, reflecting a typical lag between conduct of the CEA and publication. Analysts should discuss important differences across CEAs.

13.3.5.4 *Ethical Implications*

The reporting of ethical concerns in the journal article should relate to the decision context at hand. Chapter 12 discusses a range of ethical issues, including distributive implications relating to age, disability, or other characteristics of the population. The analyst need not include a discussion of universal issues, such as ethical implications of using conventional QALYs. However, the journal article should identify any ethical issues salient for the context (**Recommendation 11**). The analyst should highlight areas where study design decisions, such as the exclusion of patient or caregiver time in the healthcare sector Reference Case, could have ethical implications.

13.3.5.5 *Limitations*

Discussion of study limitations is intended to guide readers in interpreting and generalizing results. For example, if data underlying an analysis are obtained from population subgroups, analysts may recommend caution in generalizing results to other groups. They may also direct readers' attention to assumptions based on expert opinion, theoretical models, or incomplete data. Analysts should be sensitive to lack of consideration of all possible policy options/comparators. Omission of competing choices from the CEA should be discussed together with the possible effect of such an omission on results. If estimates known or suspected to contain bias have been used, authors should explicitly discuss the matter and report results of sensitivity analyses on relevant parameters. Analysts should also discuss any limitations related to utility weight estimation, such as selection of method, measurement technique, or population surveyed. For example, do the domains in the measurement system employed accurately reflect the domains affected by the condition being studied? For a Reference Case CEA, were community-based preferences employed? For directly elicited weights, how well does the study population match the target population being considered? The discussion of limitations should also highlight any specific issues with the data, evidence synthesis, modeling, or analysis. The discussion of limitations should highlight the analyst's efforts to compensate for the study's shortcomings.

13.3.5.6 *The Conclusions*

The conclusions section should provide a succinct summary of the results from the decision maker's context, along with clinical or policy findings. This section should also highlight future areas of research suggested by the analysis.

13.3.5.7 *The Technical Appendix*

The technical appendix should provide enough detail on methods and data sources so that, along with the main journal report, analysts can reasonably replicate the analysis. Additional information in the technical appendix will include detailed descriptions of models, transitions among health states, validation and calibration, micro-costing approaches, elicitation of health utility values, additional sensitivity and scenario analyses, intermediate outcomes, and disaggregated results. Most journals now provide an option to publish such supplementary material online. The length of the technical appendix can vary from a few supplementary tables detailing model parameters or supplementary results to a comprehensive standalone report. The emphasis is on completeness, with the goal of providing sufficient information (when combined with the journal article) for reproducing the analysis.

13.4 INTERPRETING RESULTS FOR DECISION MAKERS

As discussed in Chapter 1, few decision makers in the United States or elsewhere use strict cost-effectiveness thresholds for decision making (Neumann, Cohen, and Weinstein 2014). Consequently, conclusions about the cost-effectiveness of an intervention should be framed with respect to the decision context (e.g., the specific payer or decision maker to whom the results are intended to apply) and how the specific set of results can aid and inform decision making (Russell 2015). Comparisons to a specific threshold should consider a range of possible thresholds (Neumann, Cohen, and Weinstein 2014) and how clinical or policy implications change with consideration of alternative thresholds. If an analyst finds that an intervention results in net economic savings as well as a gain in QALYs, these results are best described as "cost-saving" (Doubilet, Weinstein, and McNeil 1986). The analyst is also encouraged to compare cost-effectiveness results to those of other similar interventions to provide context for decision making (**Recommendation 10**). In general, the analyst is encouraged to provide interpretation of the cost-effectiveness and ancillary results in the frame of the decision context.

Because cost-effectiveness evidence in the United States is unlikely to be used as a sole decision-making criterion, the analyst can and should consider how the vast array of additional information that is generated as part of the CEA can inform decision making. Presenting disaggregated information on costs and results is often crucial to decision makers if they are considering starting a new program or intervention and need information on start-up and implementation costs. Information on intermediate outcomes such as projected cases, deaths, or adverse events for an intervention strategy may also be crucial to informing deliberations on which populations to prioritize in certain situations. Intermediate outcomes can also play a critical role in ensuring transparency, assisting the user in understanding the epidemiology of the condition, and helping the user gain confidence into the structure and assumptions used in the model.

Interpreting results also provides analysts the opportunity and responsibility to discuss differences between the two Reference Case perspectives. It will be critical to highlight the components of the Impact Inventory and categories most affected by the condition under study or that differ between the two perspectives. For interventions that have substantial impacts beyond the formal healthcare sector, such as those that address children's health or public health programs, it will be important to highlight differences between the healthcare sector perspective and the societal perspective.

13.5 REPORTING RESULTS IN NON-PEER-REVIEWED MEDIA

As the number of options available for presenting scientific results outside of peer-reviewed journals increases, it is important to consider how best to use non-peer-reviewed media in describing CEA results. We recommend that authors include all of the key elements from the structured abstract format when presenting results in non-traditional outlets.

13.6 DISCLOSURE OF POTENTIAL CONFLICTS OF INTEREST

Disclosure policy for authors of CEAs should follow the standards formulated by the International Committee of Medical Journal Editors (ICMJE), whether or not the publisher requires their use (**Recommendation 12**). The ICMJE's "Form for Disclosure of Potential Conflicts of Interest" clearly outlines the potential conflicts to be disclosed. These include, but are not limited to, financial and personal relationships of the authors such as employment, stock ownership, consultancy, paid expert testimony, and honoraria (International Committee of Medical Journal Editors 2010), project support (both direct and indirect), and the extent of the authors' access to the study data (International Committee of Medical Journal Editors 2015b). The ICMJE guidelines also include disclosure of intellectual property; financial activities outside of the project that are relevant to the work for 36 months prior to submission; grants received for work outside of the submitted work that could have a financial impact on the outcome (non-public funding); non-financial support (such as equipment provided); and the selection of peer reviewers, editors, and journal staff; among other possible conflicts. For journal manuscripts, the ICMJE requires the disclosure of conflicts of interest both in the manuscript and on the separate notification page or in a cover letter with the submitted materials (International Committee of Medical Journal Editors 2015a).

13.7 CONCLUSIONS

The report of a CEA is designed to communicate all important features of an analysis and to emphasize aspects of the study that are unusual or unexpected. Journal articles provide a concise means of reaching the study's audience, while technical appendices offer a repository for additional information of concern to reviewers, researchers, and those having a particular interest a given study.

Our recommendations for comprehensive reporting of CEAs are summarized below (Section 13.8). Key changes vis-à-vis the original Panel's recommendations include a structured abstract for journal articles and an Impact Inventory to aid analysts in providing a complete and transparent report of the Reference Cases. The overall goals are to provide sufficient detail to enable an appraisal of the quality of the analysis, allow replication and comparison, and contribute to the decision-making process.

13.8 RECOMMENDATIONS

1. Cost-effectiveness analyses (CEAs) should be documented in two parts, a journal article and a comprehensive technical appendix.
2. For peer review, we recommend that editors request and authors submit the technical appendix together with the journal article to assist reviewers in assessing the study's methodology. The technical appendix should also be published along with the journal article, at a minimum in an online format, for the benefit of readers.
3. We recommend use of a structured abstract for the journal article.
4. The Impact Inventory should be reported in the journal article. Any additional perspectives beyond the Reference Case perspectives should be explicitly identified in the journal report.
5. Sufficient detail should be provided on the details of the study design, type of analysis, and modeling approach, inputs, and assumptions to enable replication of the analysis.
6. Analysts should include essential descriptors of the preference elicitation method used to measure preference weights: direct or indirect (multi-attribute) elicitation method; the elicitation task or measurement system employed; and if the weights reflect community-based preferences or not.
7. The following information comprises a basic set of recommended results in the journal article: total costs, total effectiveness, incremental costs, incremental effectiveness, and incremental cost-effectiveness ratios (ICERs). We also recommend reporting intermediate health outcomes and disaggregated results. The basic set of results should also include some measure of the robustness of the results to changes in parameter inputs, model structure, or other sources of uncertainty. The societal perspective Reference Case results will also include potential impacts on non-healthcare sector consequences. A summary of these impacts should be included in the journal article.
8. The report should highlight the Reference Case results. Key sensitivity analyses should be conducted with respect to the Reference Case assumptions.
9. For undominated strategies, ICERs should be reported in increasing order of cost and effectiveness. Incremental cost-effectiveness ratios should not be reported for options ruled out because of dominance or extended dominance.
10. The ICERs for the current analysis should be compared to available ICERs for other interventions that compete for resources with the intervention being considered. These may be drawn from healthcare broadly if the decision context is broad, or from restricted categories, such as a particular condition or type of intervention. The emphasis should be on providing context for the decision maker.

11. The Discussion section of a journal article should include a description of any significant ethical implications of the CEA results.
12. Authors should disclose any potential conflicts of interest relevant to the analysis, including funding source, whether or not this is required by the publisher.

13.9 REFERENCES

Annals of Internal Medicine. 2015. "Information for Authors - Original Research." http://annals.org/SS/authorsinfooriginalresearch.aspx.

Doubilet, P., M. C. Weinstein, and B. J. McNeil. 1986. Use and misuse of the term "cost effective" in medicine. *N Engl J Med* 314 (4):253–256.

Drummond, M., A. Manca, and M. Sculpher. 2005. Increasing the generalizability of economic evaluations: recommendations for the design, analysis, and reporting of studies. *Int J Technol Assess Health Care* 21 (2):165–171.

Drummond, M. F., and T. O. Jefferson. 1996. Guidelines for authors and peer reviewers of economic submissions to the BMJ. The BMJ Economic Evaluation Working Party. *BMJ* 313 (7052):275–283.

Evans, R. G. 1995. Manufacturing consensus, marketing truth: guidelines for economic evaluation. *Ann Intern Med* 123 (1):59–60.

Gold, M. R., J. E. Siegel, L. B. Russell, and M. C. Weinstein, eds. 1996. *Cost-Effectiveness in Health and Medicine*. New York: Oxford University Press.

Hoffmann, C., and J. M. Graf von der Schulenburg. 2000. The influence of economic evaluation studies on decision making. A European survey. The EUROMET group. *Health Policy* 52 (3):179–192.

Husereau, D., M. Drummond, S. Petrou, C. Carswell, D. Moher, D. Greenberg, F. Augustovski, A. H. Briggs, J. Mauskopf, and E. Loder. 2013a. Consolidated Health Economic Evaluation Reporting Standards (CHEERS)—explanation and elaboration: a report of the ISPOR Health Economic Evaluation Publication Guidelines Good Reporting Practices Task Force. *Value Health* 16 (2):231–250.

Husereau, D., M. Drummond, S. Petrou, C. Carswell, D. Moher, D. Greenberg, F. Augustovski, A. H. Briggs, J. Mauskopf, and E. Loder. 2013b. Consolidated Health Economic Evaluation Reporting Standards (CHEERS) statement. *Cost Eff Resour Alloc* 11 (1):6.

International Committee of Medical Journal Editors. 2010. Uniform requirements for manuscripts submitted to biomedical journals: writing and editing for biomedical publication. *J Pharmacol Pharmacother* 1 (1):42–58.

International Committee of Medical Journal Editors. 2015a. "ICMJE Form for Disclosure of Potential Conflicts of Interest." http://www.icmje.org/conflicts-of-interest/.

International Committee of Medical Journal Editors. 2015b. "Recommendations: Author Responsibilities—Conflicts of Interest." http://www.icmje.org/recommendations/browse/roles-and-responsibilities/author-responsibilities--conflicts-of-interest.html.

Journal of the American Medical Association. 2015. "*JAMA* Instructions for Authors." http://jama.jamanetwork.com/public/instructionsForAuthors.aspx.

Neumann, P. J., J. T. Cohen, and M. C. Weinstein. 2014. Updating cost-effectiveness—the curious resilience of the $50,000-per-QALY threshold. *N Engl J Med* 371 (9):796–797.

Neumann, P. J., D. Greenberg, N. V. Olchanski, P. W. Stone, and A. B. Rosen. 2005. Growth and quality of the cost-utility literature, 1976-2001. *Value Health* 8 (1):3–9.

Nuijten, M. J., M. H. Pronk, M. J. Brorens, Y. A. Hekster, J. H. Lockefeer, P. A. de Smet, G. Bonsel, and A. van der Kuy. 1998. Reporting format for economic evaluation. Part II: focus on modelling studies. *Pharmacoeconomics* 14 (3):259–268.

O'Hagan, A., C. E. Buck, A. Daneshkhah, J. R. Eiser, P. H. Garthwaite, D. J. Jenkinson, J. E. Oakley, and T. Rakow. 2006. *Uncertain Judgements: Eliciting Experts' Probabilities*. Chichester: John Wiley & Sons Ltd.

Ofman, J. J., S. D. Sullivan, P. J. Neumann, C. F. Chiou, J. M. Henning, S. W. Wade, and J. W. Hay. 2003. Examining the value and quality of health economic analyses: implications of utilizing the QHES. *J Manag Care Pharm* 9 (1):53–61.

Petrou, S., and A. Gray. 2011a. Economic evaluation alongside randomised controlled trials: design, conduct, analysis, and reporting. *BMJ* 342:d1548.

Petrou, S., and A. Gray. 2011b. Economic evaluation using decision analytical modelling: design, conduct, analysis, and reporting. *BMJ* 342:d1766.

Phillips, K. A., and J. L. Chen. 2002. Impact of the U.S. panel on cost-effectiveness in health and medicine. *Am J Prev Med* 22 (2):98–105.

Prosser, L., and E. Wittenberg. 2011. Trends in utility elicitation methods: is there still a role for direct elicitation? *Med Decis Making* 31 (1):E63–E64.

Russell, L. B. 2015. *The Science of Making Better Decisions About Health: Cost-Effectiveness and Cost-Benefit Analysis*. September 2015. Rockville, MD: Agency for Healthcare Research and Quality. http://www.ahrq.gov/professionals/education/curriculum-tools/population-health/russell.html.

Siegel, J. E., M. C. Weinstein, L. B. Russell, and M. R. Gold. 1996. Recommendations for reporting cost-effectiveness analyses. Panel on Cost-Effectiveness in Health and Medicine. *JAMA* 276 (16):1339–1341.

Sullivan, W., and K. Payne. 2011. The appropriate elicitation of expert opinion in economic models: making expert data fit for purpose. *Pharmacoeconomics* 29 (6):455–459.

Task Force on Principles for Economic Analysis of Health Care Technology. 1995. Economic analysis of health care technology. A report on principles. *Ann Intern Med* 123 (1):61–70.

Summary of Recommendations by Chapter

Peter J. Neumann, Gillian D. Sanders, Anirban Basu,
Dan W. Brock, David Feeny, Murray Krahn, Karen M. Kuntz,
David O. Meltzer, Douglas K. Owens, Lisa A. Prosser,
Joshua A. Salomon, Mark J. Sculpher, Thomas A. Trikalinos,
Louise B. Russell, Joanna E. Siegel, and Theodore G. Ganiats

CHAPTER 3. RECOMMENDATIONS ON PERSPECTIVES FOR THE REFERENCE CASE

Reference Cases and Reference Case Perspectives

1. We recommend that all studies report a Reference Case analysis based on a health-care sector perspective and another Reference Case analysis based on a societal perspective. The Reference Cases are defined by recommendations for components to consider for evaluation, methods to use, and elements for reporting. We recommend that Reference Case analyses measure health effects in terms of quality-adjusted life years (QALYs). Standardizing methods and components within a perspective is intended to enhance consistency and comparability across studies.

Healthcare Sector Reference Case

2. We recommend that the results of the healthcare sector Reference Case analysis be summarized in the conventional form, as an incremental cost-effectiveness ratio (ICER). Net monetary benefit (NMB) or net health benefit (NHB) may also be reported, and a range of cost-effectiveness thresholds should be considered. We recommend that the healthcare sector perspective include formal healthcare sector (medical) costs borne by third-party payers or paid for out-of-pocket by patients. Both types of medical costs include current and future costs, related and unrelated to the condition under consideration.

Societal Reference Case: The Impact Inventory and Summary and Disaggregated Measures

3.A. *Inclusion of an Impact Inventory.* The Second Panel continues to strongly support evaluation of the broader impacts of interventions designed to improve health. We recommend that the societal Reference Case analysis include medical costs (current and future, related and unrelated) borne by third-party payers or paid for out-of-pocket by patients, time costs of patients in seeking and receiving care, time costs of informal (unpaid) caregivers, transportation costs, effects on future productivity and consumption, and other costs and effects outside the healthcare sector. To make this evaluation more explicit and transparent, we recommend inclusion of an "Impact Inventory" that lists the health and non-health impacts of an intervention that should be considered in a societal Reference Case analysis (described in more detail in Chapters 6 and 13). The main purpose of the Impact Inventory is to ensure that all consequences, including those outside the formal healthcare sector, are considered regularly and comprehensively, as they have generally not been to date.

3.B. *Quantifying and valuing non-health components in the Impact Inventory.* We recommend that analysts attempt to quantify and value non-health consequences in the Impact Inventory, unless those consequences are likely to have a negligible effect on the results of the analysis.

3.C. *Summary and disaggregated measures.* The Second Panel agrees that it would be helpful to inform decision makers through the quantification and valuation of all health and non-health impacts of interventions, and to summarize those impacts in a single quantitative measure, such as an ICER, NMB, or NHB. However, there are no widely agreed upon methods for quantifying and valuing some of these broader impacts in cost-effectiveness analysis (CEA). We therefore recommend that analysts present the items listed in the Impact Inventory in the form of disaggregated consequences across different sectors. We also recommend that analysts use one or more summary measures, such as an ICER, NMB, or NHB, that include some or all of the items listed in the Impact Inventory. Analysts should clearly identify which items are included and how they are measured and valued, and provide a rationale for their methodological decisions.

Reporting the Reference Cases and Other Perspectives

4.A. *Stating the perspective.* We recommend that analysts clearly state the perspective of every analysis reported.

4.B. *Presenting other perspectives.* Where specific decision makers have been identified, such as a particular public or private payer, analysts may wish to present results from that decision maker's perspective in addition to the Reference Case perspectives. In such cases, we recommend that analysts clearly state the primary decision maker(s) whose deliberations are intended to be informed by the analysis.

4.C. *The importance of transparency and sensitivity analysis*. The items included in a CEA and the manner in which they are valued involve numerous choices. We recommend that analysts be transparent about how they have conducted analyses, and that they convey how results change with alternative assumptions. Sensitivity analysis should describe as clearly as possible the assumptions to which the results for different perspectives are sensitive.

CHAPTER 4. DESIGNING A COST-EFFECTIVENESS ANALYSIS

1. Cost-effectiveness analysis (CEA), return-on-investment analysis, cost-minimization analysis, cost-consequence analysis, and cost–benefit analysis are alternative forms of analysis. The use of one does not preclude the use of the others.

2. We recommend that all studies report a Reference Case analysis based on a healthcare sector perspective and a Reference Case analysis based on a societal perspective. The Reference Cases include recommended methods, elements for reporting, and recommendations concerning what to include in the healthcare sector and societal perspectives. Inclusion of standardized components and standardization of methods within a perspective are intended to enhance consistency and comparability across studies.

3. We recommend that the results of the healthcare sector Reference Case be summarized in the conventional form, as an incremental cost-effectiveness ratio (ICER). The net monetary benefit (NMB) or net health benefit (NHB) may also be reported, and a range of cost-effectiveness thresholds should be considered. We recommend that the healthcare sector perspective analysis include all formal healthcare (medical) costs—current and future, and related and unrelated—regardless of who bears the costs.

4. The Second Panel strongly supports evaluation of the broader impacts of health interventions. Thus, we recommend that analysts include a societal perspective Reference Case analysis. The societal perspective is essential whenever interventions are likely to have important effects on sectors of the economy outside of healthcare, and when there is a need or desire to understand all costs and effects regardless of to whom they accrue. The societal perspective includes medical costs (current and future, related and unrelated) borne by third-party payers or paid for out-of-pocket by patients, time costs of patients in seeking and receiving care, time costs of informal caregivers, transportation costs, effects on future productivity and consumption in added years of life, and other costs and effects outside the healthcare sector. The Second Panel agrees that it would be helpful to inform decision makers through the quantification and valuation of all health and non-health consequences of interventions, and to summarize those consequences in a single quantitative measure. However, there are no widely agreed upon methods for quantifying and valuing some of these broader impacts in CEA. We therefore

recommend that analysts present the items listed in the Impact Inventory in the form of disaggregated consequences across different sectors. We also recommend that analysts use one or more summary measures, such as an ICER, NMB, or NHB, that include some or all of the items listed in the Impact Inventory. Analysts should clearly identify which items are included and how they are measured, and provide a rationale for their methodological decisions.

5. To help make the evaluation more explicit and transparent, we recommend inclusion of an Impact Inventory in every societal Reference Case analysis, even if the analyst does not quantify or value effects beyond the healthcare sector. The Impact Inventory lists the health and non-health impacts of an intervention that the analyst should consider in a societal Reference Case analysis.

6. All aspects of the interventions that may affect their cost or effectiveness should be defined for the analysis. These will include the target population and features such as the specific technologies used, the type of personnel delivering the intervention, the site of delivery, whether the service is "bundled" with other services, the frequency of the intervention, and its timing.

7. The scope of a study should be defined broadly enough to encompass the full range of groups of people affected by the intervention and all important consequences. For example, if an intervention affects both mother and child, the analyst should include the health impacts and costs to each.

8. When there is heterogeneity in estimates of cost-effectiveness between different subpopulations, the analyst should present these differences as subgroup analyses. The analyst should be aware that subgroup analyses may raise ethical issues and questions of equity as outlined in Chapter 12, which provides a framework for consideration of ethical questions that may be important to the analyst, decision makers, and stakeholders.

9. Both Reference Case analyses should consider the full range of available and feasible options, including existing practice (the status quo) and a do-nothing option, as appropriate.

10. Options being compared may include more than specific interventions, extending, for example, to therapeutic strategies, alternative treatment starting and/ or stopping rules, joint or sequential diagnostic test strategies, alternative levels of intensity of an intervention, and public health interventions. In all cases, these should be specified as mutually exclusive options and be compared using incremental CEA.

11. Costs and outcomes that have little impact on the estimate of cost-effectiveness or the likelihood of an intervention being cost-effective, and therefore little impact on the relevant decisions, can reasonably be excluded from an analysis. Their magnitude should be indicated in the Impact Inventory, clarifying the decision to exclude them.

12. The time horizon adopted in a CEA should be long enough to capture all differences between options in relevant costs and effects.

13. We recommend that analysts develop a written protocol for the design and conduct of the CEA. The protocol should describe, at a minimum, the objectives

of the study, including the research questions; the type of economic evaluation to be conducted; the perspective of the analysis; the intervention and comparators; the population under consideration; the time horizon for the study; sources of data; a list of key assumptions; and an analysis plan, including the outcomes the analysis will assess. The analysts should update the protocol as the study progresses and note any changes from the original protocol.

CHAPTER 5. DECISION MODELS IN COST-EFFECTIVENESS ANALYSIS

1. We recommend that the analyst perform a broad conceptualization of the decision problem with input from clinical and policy experts. The scope of the cost-effectiveness analysis (CEA) for which the model is being used should be clearly defined (see Chapter 4).
2. The initial conceptualization of the model should be independent of the data identification phase. The model should represent the decision problem and be described in a detailed and transparent manner. The model structure should accommodate relevant consequences of the alternatives under consideration. The conceptualization process should be iterative with the model development and parameterization phases.
3. Analysts should consider the following factors, ideally in consultation with the decision maker, to inform the use of a decision model: (1) need for extrapolation (e.g., beyond the time horizon of the available data, beyond intermediate study outcomes, to other populations, to other strategies) and/or (2) need to integrate multiple data sources (e.g., evaluate diagnostic tests, multiple strategies, weighing harms with benefits).
4. Use a model that is appropriate for addressing the study questions. Often more than one model type would work. Factors to consider include (1) short-term fixed time horizon or not; (2) the unit of analysis; (3) interactions between simulated individuals or other model components. Use good practices in modeling guidelines (International Society for Pharmacoeconomics and Outcomes Research [ISPOR] and Society for Medical Decision Making [SMDM] Task Force).
5. Full documentation and justification of structural assumptions should be provided. When there are alternative plausible structural assumptions, appropriate uncertainty analyses to examine their effects on model outputs should be undertaken (see Chapter 11).
6. In developing a model, analysts should specify (1) the starting population(s), including all subgroups, and (2) whether they are analyzing a cohort or a population. Analysts should provide their rationale for analyzing a population instead of defined cohorts.
7. Consider all available evidence for informing model parameters and use a summary of that evidence where appropriate. Identify all data sources within reason and justify the choice of evidence used.

8. The methods used to critically appraise sources of data for cost-effectiveness models should be stated.
9. Use appropriate methods to analyze or combine data from different sources.
10. Calibration is an appropriate way to estimate model parameters. When estimating parameters using a calibration approach the following components should be presented: (1) data sources used for calibration target(s); (2) the goodness-of-fit metric used to determine the degree of fit; (3) the manner in which the parameter space was searched; and (4) the criteria used to determine that the fit was reasonable.
11. The analyst should report how the model results are calculated. If an individual-level simulation is performed, specify and justify the number of iterations per model run. If a probabilistic sensitivity analysis (PSA) is performed, specify the number of simulations per parameter set.
12. Validation of the decision model should occur throughout the conduct of a CEA. The analyst should describe and justify how the model was validated. The types of validation to consider are (1) face validity, (2) internal validity (verification), and (3) external validity.
13. Model descriptions should be detailed enough to allow for reproduction. Model results should be presented in a disaggregated format for purposes of model transparency.

CHAPTER 6. IDENTIFYING AND QUANTIFYING THE CONSEQUENCES OF INTERVENTIONS

1. A cost-effectiveness analysis (CEA) should identify all *types of consequences* affected by the choice of interventions being compared, relating to health (survival and/or health status), resource use in the healthcare sector, and consequences outside the healthcare sector. Both positive consequences (e.g., health benefits, improvements in non-health outcomes such as education, and reductions in resource use) and negative consequences (e.g., health harms, harms in other sectors, and increases in resource use) should be identified.
2. The comprehensive identification of consequences should be summarized in an Impact Inventory, a required part of the Reference Case. The Impact Inventory should organize consequences based on the sector to which they pertain, and it should indicate, for each of the consequences listed, whether the consequence is included in each of the perspectives used in the analysis.
3. Decisions about which of these consequences to *measure and value* in the analysis should, first, be consistent with the specified perspective of the analysis and, second, strike a reasonable balance between expense and difficulty on the one hand, and potential importance in the analysis on the other. Consequences that are deemed likely to be insignificant in the context of the analysis can reasonably be excluded, and this exclusion should be explicitly noted in the Impact Inventory and justified within the supporting information.
4. Estimates of the probabilities or frequencies of health and economic consequences associated with alternative choices should be based on the best available evidence,

in consideration of the full array of available information from either primary or secondary data sources, including corrections for sources of bias to the extent possible, and in recognition of time and resource constraints.

5. Estimates of the probabilities or frequencies of health and economic consequences associated with alternative choices should be specific to the individuals and groups affected by the intervention. Such estimates may have to be transferred to the target setting from other settings, based on credible understanding of pertinent relationships, and with adequate exploration of the invoked assumptions.

CHAPTER 7. VALUING HEALTH OUTCOMES

1. For Reference Case analyses from both the healthcare sector and societal perspectives, the health consequences of changes in morbidity and mortality should be aggregated into a single measure using quality-adjusted life years (QALYs).

2. In general, because people whose lives have been saved or extended by an intervention will not be in perfect health, a saved life year will count as less than 1 full QALY.

3. To satisfy the QALY concept, the quality weights must be preference-based, interval-scaled, and measured or transformed onto an interval scale where the reference point "dead" has a score of 0.0 and the reference point "perfect health" has a score of 1.0.

4. Community preferences for health states are the most appropriate ones for use in the Reference Case analyses. In general, we recommend the use of generic preference-based measures such as the EuroQol 5D (EQ-5D), Health Utilities Index (HUI), Short Form 6D (SF-6D), and Quality of Well-Being (QWB). But we have also noted that there are situations in which using patient preferences would be preferable.

5. When community preferences are used and the program (treatment or prevention) is related to an illness or condition, a sensitivity analysis that furnishes information on preferences of persons with the condition will provide important ancillary information. Such sensitivity analyses may be based on the direct elicitation of preference scores from people with the condition and/or the development of alternative scoring functions based on preference scores from those with the condition.

6. If distinct subgroup preferences are identified that will markedly affect a cost-effectiveness ratio, the Reference Case analyses should provide this information and include separate sensitivity analyses that reflect this difference.

7. The health-related quality of life of those whose lives have been saved or extended by a health intervention may be influenced by characteristics such as the age, sex, race, or socioeconomic status of the population involved. This may affect the Reference Case analyses in ways that are ethically problematic. In these instances, we recommend that sensitivity analysis be conducted to indicate explicitly how the analysis is affected by these characteristics.

8. A cost-effectiveness analysis (CEA) should be based on a health-state classification system that reflects attributes (domains or dimensions) that are important for the particular problem under consideration. If the CEA is intended for use in a Reference Case analysis from either the healthcare sector or societal perspective, the preference measure used should be a generic one or one capable of being compared to a generic system. More fundamentally, a key criterion is empirical evidence on the validity and responsiveness of the instrument in that context.

9. In general, the effects of morbidity on productivity and leisure are probably not adequately reflected in the estimated QALYs and should therefore be estimated in pecuniary terms and included in the numerator in a CEA. This recommendation introduces some risk of double counting. Appropriate sensitivity analyses may be informative. (See Chapter 7, Section 7.7.2 and Chapter 8.)

CHAPTER 8. ESTIMATING COSTS AND VALUATIONS OF NON-HEALTH BENEFITS IN COST-EFFECTIVENESS ANALYSIS

1. In cost-effectiveness analysis (CEA), all resource use should be valued in monetary terms and be included in the numerator of an incremental cost-effectiveness ratio (ICER). The denominator of an ICER should reflect only health as expressed in quality-adjusted life years (QALYs).

2. All resource use that is both germane to the analysis and non-trivial in magnitude should be included in the Reference Case analyses from both the healthcare sector perspective and the societal perspective. Resource use should be reflected regardless of whether a monetary transaction takes place.

3. From a long-term perspective, costs in CEA should reflect the opportunity costs of the resources used, which represent the marginal or incremental costs of resources, rather than average costs. Therefore, attention should be paid to instances in which constant return-to-scale for resources used may not apply when implementing an intervention in a population.

4. In principle, the full three-step approach to determining costs, entailing the identification, measurement (quantification), and valuation of resource use, is preferred. The choice between the mirco-costing and gross-costing approaches should reflect the importance of precise cost estimates, feasibility, and cost.

5. To the extent that prices reflect opportunity costs, they are an appropriate basis for valuing changes in resources. If prices do not adequately reflect opportunity costs because of market distortions, they should be adjusted; when substantial bias is present and adjustment is not feasible, another proxy for opportunity cost should be used. Sometimes the opportunity costs of a resource may be different for the healthcare sector perspective than for the societal perspective.

6. All healthcare resources consumed over the lifetime of the patients as part of, or as a result of, an intervention should be valued in monetary terms and included in the numerator of an ICER.

7. All healthcare costs, related or unrelated, should be considered either when survivals under alternative interventions are not the same or when cost components cannot be readily identified as related to the target condition.

8. Fixed costs for research and development of a healthcare intervention should always be taken into account, unless these fixed costs are similar across all the comparator interventions.

9. In the United States, the Federal Supply Schedule (FSS) for drug prices should be used to reflect the social marginal costs of drugs for Reference Case analyses from both the healthcare sector perspective and the societal perspective. In CEAs conducted from other perspectives, costs should reflect the transaction prices from the perspective of the analysis.

10. In addition to Recommendation 6 for this chapter, for a Reference Case analysis from a societal perspective, all non-healthcare resources consumed over the lifetime of the patients as part of, or as a result of, an intervention should be valued in monetary terms and included in the numerator of an ICER.

11. For a Reference Case analysis from a societal perspective, non-healthcare resources include patients' time costs, caregivers' time costs, productivity benefits, consumption costs, friction/administrative costs, and relevant costs from all other sectors of the economy outside of healthcare. Costs that are transferred from one section of the population to another should not be included.

12. For a Reference Case analysis from a societal perspective, patients' time costs reflect the time spent receiving an intervention. This time resource is assumed to displace leisure time of the patients and is therefore valued at the marginal post-tax wage rate plus fringe benefits. Under compelling evidence that such time spent replaces labor time and not leisure time, it should be valued as productive time as explained in Recommendation 14 for this chapter.

13. For a Reference Case analysis from a societal perspective, if the time spent receiving an intervention has a significant positive or negative impact on health-related quality of life, this impact should be incorporated into the denominator of an ICER, leaving the time component in the numerator.

14. For a Reference Case analysis from a societal perspective, three types of productive time for patients should be considered: (a) time spent in formal labor markets; (b) time spent in informal labor markets; and (c) time spent in household production. Where sufficient data exist, all three types of productive time should be valued with the marginal pre-tax wage rate plus fringe benefits.

15. For a Reference Case analysis from a societal perspective, both formal (paid) and informal (unpaid) caregivers' time should be viewed as productive time and valued with the marginal pre-tax wage rate plus fringe benefits in the formal caregiver market.

16. The degree to which marginal wage rates, tax rates, and fringe benefit rates should be stratified based on age, sex, and/or disease conditions depends on the needs of the decision makers that the analysis aims to inform. If stratified estimates are used, the distributional consequences of such an approach should be discussed.

17. For a Reference Case analysis from a societal perspective, consumption costs should reflect the non-healthcare consumptions. Consumption costs should be considered only where there is differential survival across comparator interventions.

18. As with wage rates, stratification of consumption costs should meet the needs of decision makers. Distributional consequences arising as a result of stratification should be discussed.

19. For a Reference Case analysis from a societal perspective, intrinsic non-healthcare benefits, such as the psychological benefits of a lower crime rate, should be valued in monetary terms and included in the numerator of an ICER. The methods of valuation would depend on the jurisdiction of the analysis. In the United States, willingness-to-pay to value these outcomes would be an acceptable method. Sensitivity analysis should be conducted by presenting the societal ICER with and without these benefits.

20. Cost-effectiveness analyses should be conducted in constant dollars that remove general price inflation. If the prices in question change at a rate different from general price levels, that variation should be reflected in the adjustments used. For example, in the United States, the personal consumption expenditure (PCE) price index and the Personal Health Care (PHC) Expenditure deflator should be used to adjust for inflation in healthcare expenditures. For non-healthcare sector expenditures, the regular Consumer Price Index (CPI) should be used.

21. The costs used in a CEA should reflect the costs in the jurisdiction where the intervention is or will be implemented.

22. Costs should be discounted at the same rate as health effects.

CHAPTER 9. EVIDENCE SYNTHESIS FOR INFORMING COST-EFFECTIVENESS ANALYSIS

1. Follow established guidance on systematic reviews and meta-analyses, modified as per Recommendations 2 through 8, for this chapter.

2. The cost-effectiveness analysis (CEA) team and the evidence synthesis team (if separate) should coordinate to refine the scope and goals of the evidence synthesis.

3. Identify the important model parameters. Important parameters are those that are (i) influential on model results or (ii) critical to the (perceived) validity of the model. Estimates of important parameters should be informed by an evidence synthesis.

4. Provide an analytical description and a critique of the evidence base.

5. Quantitative evidence syntheses should use methods that (i) model statistical variability of data, (ii) allow for between-study heterogeneity, and (iii) yield consistent estimates for all model parameters informed by the synthesis.

6. The evidence synthesis should be explicit about whether and how bias in each study and across studies was handled. The goal of the synthesis should be to produce bias-corrected estimates.

7. The evidence synthesis must be explicit about whether and how estimates were adjusted for transferability. The goal of the synthesis should be to produce estimates applicable to the modeled setting.

8. Enumerate scenarios for sensitivity analyses for (i) structure and (ii) parameter values based on the findings of the qualitative synthesis and assumptions made when accounting for/dealing with biases and transferability of estimates in the quantitative synthesis.

CHAPTER 10. DISCOUNTING IN COST-EFFECTIVENESS ANALYSIS

1. In cost-effectiveness analyses (CEAs) from both the societal and the healthcare sector perspectives, the costs and health effects of all interventions should be expressed in terms of their present value to society, as a prerequisite for generating cost-effectiveness ratios.

2. In the Reference Case analyses from both the societal and healthcare sector perspectives, costs and health effects should be discounted at the same rate.

3.1. The discount rate should be subject to review, and possible revision, over time in light of significant changes in the underlying economic data. However, to retain comparability with existing analyses, we recommend that 3% continue to be used in base-case analyses from both Reference Case perspectives for at least the next 10 years.

3.2. Sensitivity analyses should be conducted on the discount rate used in a CEA.

CHAPTER 11. REFLECTING UNCERTAINTY IN COST-EFFECTIVENESS ANALYSIS

The following recommendations are based on those of the International Society for Pharmacoeconomics and Outcomes Research (ISPOR) and Society for Medical Decision Making (SMDM) Task Force, with some additions and changes as considered appropriate by the Second Panel.

Purpose of Uncertainty Analysis

1. Uncertainty analysis is essential to high-quality cost-effectiveness analysis (CEA). In determining the best approach to uncertainty analysis, the guiding principle should be how the analysis informs the choice among policy options.

2. There should be a clear report regarding what has been assumed about decision makers' policy options, including those relating to decision delay and further research.

Parameter Uncertainty

3. The specifications of all forms of sensitivity analysis require justification on the basis of the available evidence.
4. Deterministic sensitivity analysis can provide useful insights into model behavior and validation. Its role in quantifying decision uncertainty is limited. Probabilistic sensitivity analysis (PSA) provides an analytical basis for estimating decision uncertainty.
5. Where there is very little information on a parameter, this should be reflected in a broad range of possible values in the form of a distribution for PSA and a range for deterministic sensitivity analysis. Parameters should never be excluded from uncertainty analysis on the grounds that there is insufficient information to estimate uncertainty.
6. For PSA, continuous distributions should generally be used that characterize uncertainty realistically over the theoretical range of the parameter. The analyst should be transparent regarding the choice and specification of the distribution for each parameter.
7. Correlation among parameters should be considered. Jointly estimated parameters, such as those from a regression analysis, will have direct evidence on correlation, which should be reflected in the analysis. Independently estimated parameters will have no such evidence, but this should not necessarily lead to an assumption of independence.

Structural Uncertainty

8. Structural uncertainties should be tested in uncertainty analysis. Consideration should be given to parameterizing these uncertainties for ease of testing. Where this is not considered possible, scenario analysis should be undertaken.

Presenting Decision Uncertainty

9. Decision uncertainty should be presented using probabilities for specified cost-effectiveness thresholds. If structural uncertainties are left unparameterized, these probabilities should be presented for each scenario relating to the structural uncertainty. If cost-effectiveness acceptability curves (CEACs) are used, curves for each option should be plotted on the same graph, together with a cost-effectiveness acceptability frontier (CEAF).

Value of Information Analysis

10. Expected value of information analysis should be used to guide decision making under uncertainty. Other factors with potential relevance to decisions should be considered, including the likelihood that research will be undertaken if an intervention is generally funded compared with being funded only in the context of research; the extent of irreversible costs being incurred in delivering a new intervention; and whether other information of relevance to the decision is likely to emerge over time.

CHAPTER 12. ETHICAL AND DISTRIBUTIVE CONSIDERATIONS

1. Where significant accommodation is likely to disability states being evaluated, those accommodations should be reflected in alternative values for relevant health states and examined in sensitivity analysis.

2. When comparing alternative life-extending interventions that would benefit patients of substantially different ages, a decision maker may wish to give greater weight to benefitting the patients who would have had significantly fewer life years or quality-adjusted life years (QALYs) if they do not receive treatment. Analysts should conduct sensitivity analysis to illustrate the impact.

3. Where the cost-effectiveness analysis (CEA) is of alternatives providing significant benefits to persons in very different initial states of health, the decision maker may wish to consider giving some priority to the worse off potential beneficiaries. Analysts may conduct sensitivity analysis to illustrate the impact of alternative assumptions.

4. When the CEA compares alternatives that provide large benefits to some individuals with other alternatives that provide much smaller benefits to a much larger number of individuals, decision makers may consider giving greater priority to the alternatives that concentrate benefits or disperse burdens. Analysts should highlight this issue when it is important.

5. When the CEA favors one group of beneficiaries over other potential beneficiaries based on a small difference in cost-effectiveness ratios, it is important for decision makers to consider whether mitigating factors cited in Chapter 12, Section 12.3.3 reduce the fair chances problem. If not, can the difference be reduced in other ways? Analysts should highlight and discuss this issue when it is important.

6. Users of CEA should assess whether a specific CEA significantly discriminates against disabled patients on the basis of their disabilities and how that discrimination, if present, might be avoided.

7. Whenever recommending departure from the most cost-effective alternative on ethical grounds, decision makers may wish to consider the reduced benefits or increased costs to others of doing so. Sensitivity analyses, which can then be compared with the base-case analysis, do this automatically.

CHAPTER 13. REPORTING COST-EFFECTIVENESS ANALYSES

1. Cost-effectiveness analyses (CEAs) should be documented in two parts, a journal article and a comprehensive technical appendix.
2. For peer review, we recommend that editors request and authors submit the technical appendix together with the journal article to assist reviewers in assessing the study's methodology. The technical appendix should also be published along with the journal article, at a minimum in an online format, for the benefit of readers.
3. We recommend use of a structured abstract for the journal article.
4. The Impact Inventory should be reported in the journal article. Any additional perspectives beyond the Reference Case perspectives should be explicitly identified in the journal report.
5. Sufficient detail should be provided on the details of the study design, type of analysis, and modeling approach, inputs, and assumptions to enable replication of the analysis.
6. Analysts should include essential descriptors of the preference elicitation method used to measure preference weights: direct or indirect (multi-attribute) elicitation method; the elicitation task or measurement system employed; and if the weights reflect community-based preferences or not.
7. The following information comprises a basic set of recommended results in the journal article: total costs, total effectiveness, incremental costs, incremental effectiveness, and incremental cost-effectiveness ratios (ICERs). We also recommend reporting intermediate health outcomes and disaggregated results. The basic set of results should also include some measure of the robustness of the results to changes in parameter inputs, model structure, or other sources of uncertainty. The societal perspective Reference Case results will also include potential impacts on non-healthcare sector consequences. A summary of these impacts should be included in the journal article.
8. The report should highlight the Reference Case results. Key sensitivity analyses should be conducted with respect to the Reference Case assumptions.
9. For undominated strategies, ICERs should be reported in increasing order of cost and effectiveness. Incremental cost-effectiveness ratios should not be reported for options ruled out because of dominance or extended dominance.
10. The ICERs for the current analysis should be compared to available ICERs for other interventions that compete for resources with the intervention being considered. These may be drawn from healthcare broadly if the decision context is broad, or from restricted categories, such as a particular condition or type of intervention. The emphasis should be on providing context for the decision maker.
11. The Discussion section of a journal article should include a description of any significant ethical implications of the CEA results.
12. Authors should disclose any potential conflicts of interest relevant to the analysis, including funding source, whether or not this is required by the publisher.

Overview of Worked Examples

Appendices A and B contain two examples of cost-effectiveness analyses (CEAs). The first assesses treatment strategies for individuals with alcohol use disorders; the second evaluates home palliative care for patients at the end of life.

The two examples illustrate applications of the Second Panel's Reference Case recommendations to specific CEAs. These "worked examples" are not presented as ideal or prototype analyses. Instead, they are intended to demonstrate the types of specific questions and methodological choices that arise in cost-effectiveness research. The studies demonstrate the authors' strategies for confronting data and analytic issues in the context of conducting Reference Case analyses.

In addition to implementing the recommendations for conducting Reference Case analyses, the worked examples also illustrate the recommended format and content for reporting CEAs and the use of the Impact Inventory. Each worked example presents results in two parts: (1) the journal article and (2) the technical appendix. Although the technical appendix would typically be presented in online-only format for a CEA published in an academic journal, it is included here for each worked example to illustrate the content and format of the technical appendix for readers of this book.

Appendix A

Worked Example 1: The Cost-Effectiveness of Treatments for Individuals with Alcohol Use Disorders: A Reference Case Analysis

David D. Kim, Anirban Basu, Sarah Q. Duffy, and Gary A. Zarkin

PART 1: JOURNAL ARTICLE
Structured Abstract

Objective: To evaluate the cost-effectiveness of treatments for individuals with alcohol use disorders (AUDs).

Interventions: Five treatment strategies: 1) combined behavioral intervention alone; 2) medical management alone; 3) medical management + naltrexone; 4) medical management + acamprosate; and 5) medical management + naltrexone + acamprosate.

Target Population: 45-year-old individuals diagnosed with AUDs.

Perspectives: Healthcare sector and societal Reference Case perspectives.

Time Horizon: Lifetime.

Discount Rates: 3% on both costs and health outcomes.

Costing Year: 2014 US dollars.

Study Design: Probabilistic cohort state-transition model.

Data Sources: Initial remission rates of treatment were obtained from the 16-week Combined Pharmacotherapies and Behavioral Interventions (COMBINE) clinical trial. Other relevant information was obtained from published literature, government reports, and administrative data.

Outcome Measures: Incremental cost-effectiveness ratios (ICERs) and net monetary benefits (NMBs) were used as primary outcome measures. For the NMB, we used $100,000 per QALY as a willingness-to-pay (WTP) threshold in the base-case analysis.

Results of Base-Case Analysis: All interventions were dominated by medical management + naltrexone, both from a healthcare sector perspective and a societal perspective. Therapy with medical management + naltrexone was cost-saving and provided the best outcomes in all of the potential consequences, such as shorter time spent in AUD, longer years of employment, higher productivity benefits, as well as reduced numbers of crimes committed, motor vehicle accidents, and associated legal costs.

Results of Uncertainty Analysis: Results were robust across a range of WTP thresholds and across plausible ranges of remission rates and health-related quality of life (HRQoL) in the AUD state. However, substantial uncertainty in final estimates indicates large value of future research on this topic.

Limitations: We excluded some outcomes such as uncompensated household production for a patient, time costs of uncompensated care by caregivers, and spillover effects on HRQoL of caregivers. However, we believe that inclusion of these outcomes would likely not substantially alter the conclusions of our analyses.

Conclusions: From both a healthcare sector perspective and a societal perspective, medical management + naltrexone is cost-saving compared to other standard treatment options. Eliminating decision uncertainty around these results through future research would be valuable.

1 INTRODUCTION

Alcohol use disorders (AUDs) are medical conditions caused by maladaptive patterns of alcohol consumption (American Psychiatric Association 2013). In the United States, AUDs are one of the most prevalent substance abuse disorders and the third leading preventable cause of death, affecting 8.5% of adults in the prior 12 months and 30.3% during their lifetimes (Hasin et al. 2007; Mokdad et al. 2004). A recent study found that AUDs were associated with 65,000 deaths per year, 1,152,000 years of life lost due to premature mortality, and 2,443,000 years of life lost due to disability in the United States in 2005 (Rehm et al. 2014). Alcohol use disorders also have a wide range of other adverse health and social consequences, including relationship troubles, social role failure, financial problems, legal troubles (e.g., crime, driving under the influence, and violence), and an increase in alcohol-related mortality and complications (Caetano and Cunradi 2002; Chou et al. 2006; Ormel et al. 1994; Samokhvalov et al. 2010; World Health Organization 2014; Ye and Kerr 2011). The economic costs attributable to excessive alcohol consumption are significant, estimated at $223.5 billion in 2006 (Bouchery et al. 2011).

To address AUDs, several options have been developed, such as mutual support groups (e.g., Alcohol Anonymous twelve-step program), behavioral interventions (e.g., specialized alcohol counseling conducted by addiction specialists or contingency management), and three medications approved by the US Food and Drug Administration (FDA) (disulfiram, naltrexone, and acamprosate). Although some interventions, especially medications, have shown clinical effectiveness in achieving abstinence (Anton et al. 2006; Bouza et al. 2004; Fleming et al. 2002; Kranzler and Gage 2008; Kranzler and Van Kirk 2001), many individuals with AUDs never receive appropriate treatment. About 85% of individuals who have ever been diagnosed with AUDs never seek any type of treatment (Cohen et al. 2007), and most of those who do use treatment services only at the behest of a court, a family member, or an employer (Parhar et al. 2008). However, some individuals with alcohol dependency (~10%) have been found to return to low-risk drinking or abstinence over a 3-year period without receiving treatment (Dawson et al. 2012).

Considering the significant financial burden of AUDs on society and the potential impacts on reducing alcohol consumption through treatment, policy makers and payers have been interested in economic evaluations of AUD treatments. Previous studies examined the economic impact of AUD treatment on only a selected group of outcomes such as percent days abstinent (Zarkin et al. 2008), reduction in alcohol consumption (Barrett et al. 2006), quality-adjusted life years (QALYs) (UKATT Research Team 2005a), or reductions in disease burden (Smit et al. 2011), and therefore a comprehensive assessment may be important (Zarkin et al. 2010). In addition, most of the clinical trials in AUD treatment evaluated only short-term outcomes, such as abstinence rates, making it difficult to assess the overall effects of treatment in the longer term (Anton et al. 2006; Kranzler and Gage 2008; Kranzler and Van Kirk 2001; UKATT Research Team 2005b).

In this paper, we evaluated the long-term (lifetime) cost-effectiveness of five different treatment strategies for 45-year-old patients with AUDs from the two Reference Case perspectives recommended by the Second Panel on Cost-Effectiveness in Health and Medicine using a probabilistic cohort state-transition model. Key features of our analysis include (1) accounting for multiple outcomes of AUD treatment over a life span based on the effectiveness results of the 16-week Combined Pharmacotherapies and Behavioral Intervention (COMBINE) clinical trial (Anton et al. 2006) and (2) highlighting the consequences of AUD treatment that fall outside of the healthcare sector using an Impact Inventory table.

2 METHODS

2.1 Decision Model

2.1.1 The Conceptual Model

Alcohol use disorders are chronic conditions in which individuals may transition between abstinence, low-risk drinking, and various AUDs, intermittently seeking treatment, over the course of a lifetime. Sustained recovery is often not achieved with a single treatment episode. Accounting for the potentially dynamic and long-term effects of AUDs and treatments is essential in the evaluation of the potential consequences of AUD treatment (Zarkin et al. 2005).

In terms of treatment outcomes, researchers have traditionally used abstinence (no drinking) as a primary outcome in clinical trials of AUD treatments. However, low-risk drinking—defined as non-abstinence but with no days of 5+ alcoholic beverages—has been increasingly considered a reasonable outcome in such trials (US Food and Drug Administration 2013). Recent studies have shown that low-risk drinkers are similar to abstainers in terms of their long-term prognosis, including drinking outcomes, social functioning, and family/social problems, along with healthcare utilization and costs (Dawson and Grant 2011; Kline-Simon et al. 2013; Kline-Simon et al. 2014). Considering that the COMBINE study reported "return to heavy drinking" as an outcome measure (Anton et al. 2006), we combined *Abstinence/Low-Risk Drinking*,

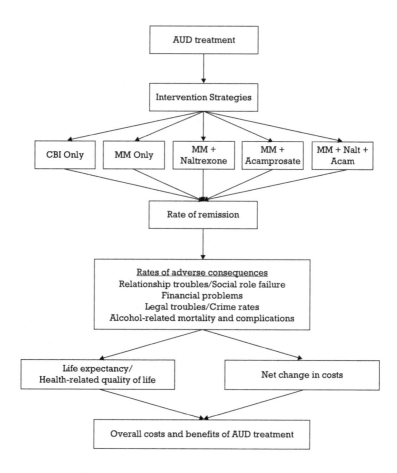

Figure 1 Overview of long-term effects of alcohol use disorders (AUD) treatment.
Abbreviations: AUD = alcohol use disorders; CBI = combined behavioral intervention; MM = medical management.

denoted as the *LRD* state, as a stage of remission from AUDs. The goal of our analysis was to evaluate the long-term effects of initial treatment choices for individuals diagnosed with AUDs.

Figure 1 provides an overview of the way in which the long-term effects of AUD treatments are realized. The AUD treatment alternatives estabilsh the initial rates of remission from the *AUD* state and the transition into the *LRD* state at the end of AUD treatment (Anton et al. 2006; Mann, Lehert, and Morgan 2004; Mason 2003). These transitions determine key outcomes over the lifetime of the subjects, including life expectancy, health-related quality of life (HRQoL), and societal costs through modifying rates of possible adverse health and social consequences.

2.1.2 *Perspectives of the Analysis*

From an economic point of view, AUDs impose consequences from a wide range of perspectives, including patient, payer (private and government), and societal perspectives.

From a patient perspective, potential consequences of AUDs include diminished HRQoL due to symptoms of AUDs and alcohol-related complications, as well as out-of-pocket costs for alcohol consumption and healthcare utilization. During treatment, patients are responsible for cost-sharing of treatment options, and they incur time costs associated with traveling and treatment. Payers commonly account for most AUD treatment costs, which include the sum of facilities, labor, medication, laboratory costs for each intervention healthcare utilization attributable to AUDs, and current and future healthcare costs. In addition to patients and payers, AUDs impose significant costs on society by adversely affecting broader social outcomes, including productivity, property damage due to alcohol-related crimes, motor vehicle accidents, and criminal justice system costs, including police protection, the court system, and arrests. Therefore, we conducted Reference Case analyses from both the healthcare sector and societal perspectives as prescribed by the Second Panel. In addition, we also presented results from the patient's perspective.

2.1.3 Treatment Strategies

The COMBINE study was a multicenter randomized controlled trial that evaluated whether various combinations of three treatment modalities—including two medications (naltrexone and acamprosate) and/or a behavioral intervention—can improve outcomes over a 16-week course of treatment. Results from the trial are available in Anton et al. (2006). There were nine intervention arms in the trial (i.e., one control arm and eight experimental arms). Patients assigned to the control arm received a combined behavioral intervention alone without any medication (CBI Only). The CBI Only intervention provided intensive counseling delivered by alcoholism treatment specialists. Patients in the eight experimental groups received one of the following medications: a placebo pill, naltrexone, acamprosate, or both naltrexone and acamprosate, along with a complementary component, called "medical management" (MM), which provided support for compliance to medications and reduction in drinking. Half of the experimental groups received CBI in addition to assigned medications and MM.

Of the nine interventions evaluated in the COMBINE trial, we selected five to form the comparators in our analysis: CBI Only, MM Only (i.e., MM + placebo in the actual trial), MM + naltrexone, MM + acamprosate, and MM + naltrexone + acamprosate. The selection of five comparators was based on separately conducted cost-effectiveness analyses (CEAs) to estimate cost-effectiveness of the interventions evaluated in the COMBINE trial from a provider perspective (Zarkin et al. 2008; Zarkin et al. 2005), as well as from a patient perspective (Dunlap et al. 2010). These studies found that three interventions (e.g., MM Only, MM + naltrexone, and MM + naltrexone + acamprosate) were potentially cost-effective, whereas other treatment modalities were dominated by those interventions. However, even though MM + acamprosate was more costly and less effective than MM + naltrexone in the original CEA of the COMBINE trial (Zarkin et al. 2008), CEAs based on other trials have shown that adjuvant acamprosate therapy is cost-effective compared to standard counseling therapy (Palmer et al. 2000; Schadlich and Brecht 1998). Finally, we included the CBI Only group without additional medications or MM as standard of care. Although one could argue that a "do-nothing" strategy is most prevalent in AUD cases, we did not consider a "do-nothing" strategy to be an appropriate intervention for AUD patients.

2.1.4 The Cohort State-Transition Model

In order to translate the conceptual model into a mathematical framework, we developed a simplified probabilistic cohort state-transition simulation model to represent a typical individual's natural history of AUDs. Figure 2 illustrates treatment choices in the decision-analytic model, followed by a simplified state-transition model to represent the natural history of AUDs. We implemented an annual time period as cycle length.

In the model, individual subjects could make transitions between two mutually exclusive health states at any given time: *Abstinence/Low-Risk Drinking (LRD)* and *Alcohol Use Disorders (AUD)*. At the initial time period, t_0, non-institutionalized individuals are assigned to one of the five treatment strategies (CBI Only, MM Only, MM + naltrexone, MM + acamprosate, or MM + naltrexone + acamprosate); these strategies then determine transitions to the *AUD* or *LRD* states based on initial remission rates from the end of the 16-week treatment period in the COMBINE trial. In the subsequent period, t_1, we applied treatment-specific rates of relapse from the *LRD* state to the *AUD* state based on 1-year post-treatment follow-up results from the COMBINE trial (Anton et al. 2006). During the first year, we assumed that treated patients did not have access to another treatment in order to match with the 1-year post-treatment results. After the first year, individual subjects could make transitions based on rates of natural history for relapse (i.e., from the *LRD* state to the *AUD* state) or recovery (i.e., from the *AUD* state to the *LRD* state without receiving additional future treatment), and patients could seek further AUD treatment while in the *AUD* state over their lifetimes. For the sake of simplicity with the lack of appropriate data, we did not allow the initial treatment choice to alter the propensity to seek additional treatment in the future conditional on being in the *AUD* state. Therefore, the effect of the initial treatment choice is mediated solely through the initial remission rates of the treatment and the first-year rates of relapse (Appendix Figure 1).

Individuals in the model are subject to *AUD*- and *LRD*-specific model parameters, including transition probabilities, HRQoL, and associated costs. We assumed that individuals convicted of a criminal offense would be incarcerated for at least 1 year, with a 43% chance of being released in the next year, based on data from government reports (Carson and Golinelli 2013; Glaze and Herberman 2013). We also assumed that incarcerated individuals could not be employed and would not have access to AUD treatment, because we focus on clinically based AUD treatment. Further, we assumed that incarcerated individuals follow the rates of natural recovery from the *AUD* state to the *LRD* state, but we assumed no relapse from the *LRD* state back to the *AUD* state because there was no access to alcohol while being incarcerated. Details are provided below, under the headings "State-dependent model parameters" (Section 2.3.1) and "State-independent model parameters" (Section 2.3.2).

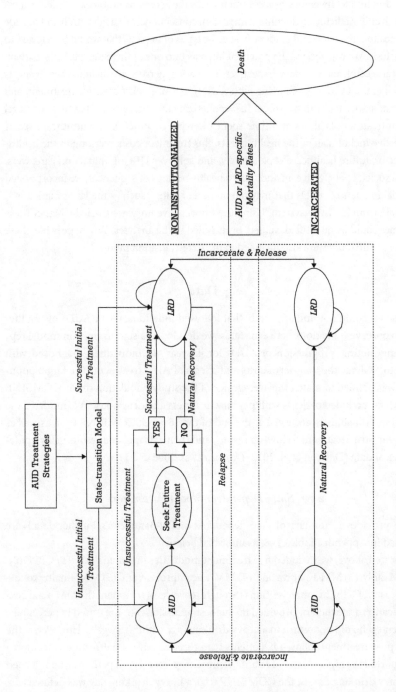

Figure 2 Schematic diagram for state-transition models.

Abbreviations: AUD = alcohol use disorders; LRD = low-risk drinking or abstinence.

2.2 Impact Inventory

We used an Impact Inventory, as recommended by the Second Panel on Cost-Effectiveness in Health and Medicine, to document important consequences that fall within and outside of the healthcare sector, and to identify specific types of impacts that would be relevant to our analysis. We categorized the potential impacts into one of three perspectives: patient, healthcare sector, and societal perspectives. The patient perspective included health effects (e.g., life years, QALYs, years living with AUDs), out-of-pocket costs for treatment, and time costs associated with treatment (i.e., monetizing the average reported time for travel to/from treatment facilities and time spent receiving treatment). The healthcare sector perspective includes all of the health effects plus treatment costs accruing to the healthcare sector, future healthcare expenditures, and spillover HRQoL impact on caregivers. From a societal perspective, in addition to health-related consequences, we incorporated potential impacts of AUDs that may fall on other sectors, such as the labor market and the legal/criminal justice system. Using the Impact Inventory, we labeled whether these outcomes could be quantified, valued, or included in the analyses. Where possible, these additional outcomes were also included in the state-transition model.

2.3 Data

Because we could not find any study that followed individuals with AUDs over a lifetime to observe transitions between states, we developed a state-transition model representing lifetime progression of AUDs for 45-year-old individuals diagnosed with AUDs to evaluate the long-term costs and effects of AUD treatment. The target population was defined to match the average age of the study population in the COMBINE trial, which excluded patients with psychiatric illness and drug abuse. We modeled the transition probabilities observed at the end of the 16-week COMBINE trial, as well as the 1-year post-treatment follow-up results, and then extrapolated results using epidemiological data (Dawson et al. 2012; Dawson et al. 2008).

2.3.1 State-Dependent Model Parameters

Table 1 provides a summary of state-dependent model parameters. Further details are provided in Appendix Tables 1–8, as indicated below.

As stated above, we included five treatment modalities in our analysis: (1) CBI Only, (2) MM Only, (3) MM + naltrexone, (4) MM + acamprosate, and (5) MM + naltrexone + acamprosate. Of the five interventions through 16 weeks of treatment the MM + naltrexone + acamprosate therapy provided the highest remission rate, measured in percentage of patients who did not return to a heavy drinking day within 16 weeks. However, at the 1-year post-treatment follow-up, patients who received MM + naltrexone + acamprosate reported the highest rates of relapse, defined as percentage of patients who returned to a heavy drinking day. In the COMBINE trial, a heavy drinking day was defined as ≥ 4 drinks/day for women and ≥ 5 drinks/day for men (Anton et al. 2006).

With regard to the natural history of AUD patients, an epidemiological study reported a 3% probability of natural relapse (i.e., transitions from *LRD* to *AUD*)

Table 1 Summary of state-dependent model parameters

Annual parameters	States		References
	Alcohol use disorder (AUD) Mean (SE)	Low risk drinking (LRD) Mean (SE)	
Costs (2014 USD)			
Costs of intervention and delivery[A]			
Combined behavioral intervention (CBI) Only	$640 (18.1)	–	Zarkin et al. (2008)
		–	
Medical management (MM) Only	$474 (7.52)	–	
MM + Naltrexone	$777 (19.5)	–	
MM + Acamprosate	$866 (22.4)	–	
MM + Naltrexone + Acamprosate	$1,162 (36.7)		
Time costs associated with treatment[B]			
CBI Only	$1,164 (102)	–	Dunlap et al. (2010)
MM Only	$1,014 (86.9)	–	
MM + Naltrexone	$1,090 (111)	–	
MM + Acamprosate	$1,128 (143)	–	
MM + Naltrexone + Acamprosate	$1,046 (101)	–	
Annual healthcare expenditure	See Appendix Table 7	See Appendix Table 6	Author's calculation
Quality-of-life valuations			
State-specific health-utility weight	0.76 (0.06)	0.81 (0.02)	Petrie et al. (2008)
Probabilities			
Initial treatment remission rates[C]			
CBI Only	0.21 (0.04)	–	Anton et al. (2006); Zarkin et al. (2008)
MM Only	0.248 (0.03)	–	
MM + Naltrexone	0.325 (0.04)	–	
MM + Acamprosate	0.289 (0.04)	–	
MM + Naltrexone + Acamprosate	0.351 (0.04)	–	
Prob (Relapse, 1 year after initial treatment)			
CBI Only	–	0.076 (0.008)	Anton et al. (2006)
MM Only	–	0.091 (0.009)	
MM + Naltrexone	–	0.111 (0.011)	
MM + Acamprosate	–	0.098 (0.010)	
MM + Naltrexone + Acamprosate	–	0.175 (0.017)	
Pr (seeking future treatment)[D]	0.051 (0.005)	–	Hasin et al. (2007)

(continued)

Table 1 Continued

Annual parameters	States		References
	Alcohol use disorder (AUD) Mean (SE)	Low risk drinking (LRD) Mean (SE)	
Pr (remission from future treatment)[E]	0.314 (0.046)	–	Author's calculation
Pr (natural recovery from AUD)[F]	0.036 (0.004)	–	Dawson et al. (2012)
Pr (relapse from LRD, atural history)[G]	–	0.027 (0.001)	Dawson et al. (2008)
Relative risk of mortality among AUD patients	See Appendix Table 2	–	Roerecke and Rehm (2013)
Labor market participation rates	See Appendix Table 3	See Appendix Table 3	Mullahy and Sindelar (1991)
Pr (any crime)[H]	0.177 (0.038)	0.032 (0.018)	Bray et al. (2007); Federal Bureau of Investigation (2013)
Pr (motor vehicle accident)	0.052 (0.022)	0.0126 (0.006)	(Bray et al. 2007)

[A]For more details on the micro-costing approach to estimate costs of intervention and delivery, see Appendix Table 5.

[B]The patient's time costs were estimated by multiplying the average reported time for treatment and travel with the average hourly wage ($24.4/hour) (wage) after adjusting individual effective income tax rates (T) and the average rates of fringe benefits (B).

[C]Remission rates are defined as a proportion of patients who didn't return to heavy drinking after the end of the 16-week treatment.

[D]After the initial treatment, those who moved back to AUD or relapse from LRD may choose to receive additional treatment. However, since we do not know which treatment the patient will receive in the future, we just applied average remission rates of all five treatment strategies.

[E]The probability of remission from future treatment was the average of the initial remission rates among all treatment options

[F]Natural recovery rates from AUD represented an annualized transition probability to abstinent or non-abstinent recovery from patient with alcohol dependency and no history of previous treatment based on the 3-year follow-up study.

[G]Due to the lack of follow-up data on the long-term rates of relapse among treated individuals with AUD, we used an annualized transition probability of developing alcohol abuse and/or alcohol dependency from drinkers without an AUD at baseline based on the 3-year follow-up study.

[H]The estimate is defined as the probability of involvement with criminal justice system. The Criminal-justice domain includes the number of arrests, number of court appearances, visits to parole/probation officer, and nights in jail.

(Dawson et al. 2008) and a 10.3% probability of natural recovery from *AUD* without benefit of AUD treatment over the 3-year follow-up period (Dawson et al. 2012). We converted these 3-year rates into 1-year transition probabilities and incorporated these into the model parameters (Fleurence and Hollenbeak 2007).

We also accommodated the possibility of receiving treatment in the future, and the remission rates from future treatment were assumed to be the average of the initial remission rates among the five treatment options. Individuals in the *LRD* state, are assumed to follow annual mortality rates from the general population, whereas we captured the age-specific relative risk of mortality among AUD patients from a previous meta-analysis – 1.7 to 4.7 times higher risks of mortality in AUD patients as in the general population (Roerecke and Rehm 2013) (Appendix Tables 1 and 2). We also included state-specific rates of committing any crime and of motor vehicle accidents because patients with AUDs experience much higher rates of both.

Regarding labor outcomes, we included health state-specific labor participation rates for non-institutionalized individuals. Based on the previous literature, we assumed that individuals in the *LRD* state follow the same labor force participation rates as individuals who were diagnosed with AUD at any point in the past, whereas those in the *AUD* state follow the same rates as individuals who were diagnosed with AUD in the past year (Mullahy and Sindelar 1991) (Appendix Tables 3 and 4).

Any patient who is prescribed to AUD treatment incurs the costs of that treatment, along with the patient time costs associated with treatment and travel time (Dunlap et al. 2010; Zarkin et al. 2008). More details on micro-costing methodology for estimating costs of intervention and delivery are presented in Appendix Table 5. Patient time costs were estimated by multiplying the average travel time for receiving treatment by the average hourly wage (wage) after adjusting for individual effective income tax rates (T) and the average rates of fringe benefits (B)—i.e., time costs = time*wage*$(1-T+B)$. In addition, age-specific annual healthcare expenditures among AUD patients and the general population were directly estimated using 2003–2012 Medical Expenditure Panel Survey to account for unrelated future healthcare costs. (Appendix Tables 6 and 7).

State-dependent HRQoL measures were based on health states defined by the Alcohol Use Disorders Identification Test (AUDIT) and state-specific utilities measured by the EuroQol-5D (EQ-5D), which is a preference-based, multi-attribute utility instrument that provides utilities measured on an interval scale, where the value of being dead represents a score of 0 and the value of being in perfect health has a value of 1 (Petrie et al. 2008). The study reported EQ-5D scores of 0.757 (standard error: 0.06) among very high-risk individuals, and 0.814 (0.02) among low-risk individuals with past alcohol problems. Previous literature that evaluated HRQoL among patients with alcohol dependence using the Short Form 36 Health Survey (SF-36) supports that patients with alcohol dependence reported lower HRQoL (Morgan et al. 2004; Volk et al. 1997). However, another study, focused on older Canadians, reported higher HRQoL measured by the Health Utilities Index Mark 3 (HUI3) among heavy drinkers than in past drinkers (Kaplan et al. 2014). Unmeasured confounding factors that force patients to refrain from drinking during their early years (e.g., alcohol-related health problems) may explain the higher HRQoL among older heavy drinkers. To address uncertainty around these state-specific HRQoL estimates from a single study, we placed a probabilistic distribution around each of the state-specific HRQoL estimates; we also conducted uncertainty analyses to examine the impact of changes in the estimates.

The COMBINE trial reported no significant differences in overall rates of serious adverse events across treatment groups. However, there were significant differences in rates of some types of minor adverse events, including nausea, vomiting, diarrhea, and the like (Anton et al. 2006). To accommodate the impact of adverse events from AUD treatment on overall HRQoL, we incorporated disutility associated with these adverse events into health utility. Using the EQ-5D, we derived the disutility estimates based on a previous study that examined the disutility of adverse events in patients with type 2 diabetes mellitus to quantify tolerability issues with oral antidiabetic medications (Pollack et al. 2010) (Appendix Table 8).

2.3.2 State-Independent Model Parameters

Table 2 provides a summary of state-independent model parameters. Further details are provided in Appendix Tables 9 and 10, as indicated below.

Because of uncertainty surrounding the future treatment choice, costs of future treatment were estimated through the average costs of all treatment modalities. Also, we applied end-of-life costs for all individuals who died in the specific year, instead of annual state-specific future healthcare expenditures. From a societal perspective, to capture effects on employment by returning to LRD from AUD, productivity benefits were estimated by multiplying the average annual earnings after accounting for the value of fringe benefits with age-specific labor force participating rates for each state (Appendix Table 9). Because of the lack of data on uncompensated work, we assumed that there is no productivity benefit to individuals who do not work. Annual non-healthcare consumption costs over a lifetime were also included to capture net future resources use explicitly. The annual average consumption costs represent average annual expenditures that each person is expected to spend on food, housing, transportation, education, personal insurance, and so on, excluding annual healthcare expenditures (Appendix Table 10).

For legal costs, we aggregated the associated costs of crime (tangible costs and quality of life), the criminal justice system, motor vehicle accidents, and incarceration. Tangible costs of crime include costs related to medical and mental healthcare, public programs, and property damage losses caused by alcohol or any other drug-related crime (Miller et al. 2006). The costs of crime related to the loss of quality of life represent monetary values on the pain, suffering, and lost quality of life that victims and their families experience due to injury and death (Miller et al. 2006). The details of these valuations are reported in Miller et al. (2006). Other probabilities, such as probability of being arrested conditional on committing a crime, probability of being convicted given arrest, and so on were included in the model. We assume that there is no additional hazard in mortality for incarcerated individuals because death rates in jails and prisons are broadly comparable to those in the general population (McCarthy 2013; Noonan and Ginder 2014).

Table 2 Summary of state-independent model parameters

Parameters	Mean (SE)	References
	Costs (2014 USD)	
Costs of future treatment[A]	$1,872 (252)	Author's calculation
End-of-life costs[B]	$37,421 (4,857)	Christensen and Callahan (2013)
Average earnings[C]	See Appendix Table 9	Author's calculation
Average rates of fringe benefits[D]	46.2%	Bureau of Labor Statistics (2015)
Individual effective income tax rates[E]	9.2%	Tax Policy Center (2013)
Average consumption costs[F]	See Appendix Table 10	Author's calculation
Costs of crimes—cangible[G]	$1,568 (314)	Miller et al. (2006)
Costs of crimes—quality of life[H]	$14,245 (2,849)	Miller et al. (2006)
Costs of criminal justice system[I]	$1,445 (270)	US Census Bureau (2012)
Costs of motor vehicle accidents[J]	$8,581(1,716)	Blincoe et al. (2015)
Costs of incarceration	$34,710 (9,235)	Henrichson and Delaney (2012)
	Quality-of-life valuations	
Disutility of adverse events during treatment	See Appendix Table 8	Anton et al. (2006); Pollack et al. (2010)
Disutility of being incarcerated[K]	−0.075 (0.004)	Lee et al. (2008); Chong et al. (2009)
	Probabilities	
Pr (death—general mortality)	See Appendix Table 1	Arias (2014)
Pr (arrested | crime)[L]	0.213 (0.123)	Bray et al. (2007); Federal Bureau of Investigation (2013)
Pr (conviction | arrest)[M]	0.338 (0.143)	US Department of Justice (2014)
Pr (release from jail or prison)[N]	0.430 (0.149)	Carson and Golinelli (2013); Glaze and Herberman (2013)

[A] Future treatment costs were estimated through the average costs of all treatment options, $783.8 (51.2) plus the average time costs associated with all treatment, $1,088 (247).

[B] End-of-life costs represent the average spending per chronically ill Medicare patient in the last year of life.

[C] The annual average earnings were calculated by annualizing weekly earnings of wage and salary workers.

Table 2 Continued

ᴰ Productivity costs were estimated by multiplying the annual average earnings with (1 + average rates of fringe benefits).

ᴱ Average individual effective income tax rates were estimated across all income percentiles based on expanded cash income. Individual income taxes were based on after-tax credits, including refundable portion of earned income and child tax credits.

ᶠ The annual average consumption costs represent average annual expenditures that each person is expected to spend on food, alcoholic beverages, housing, transportation, entertainment, education, personal insurance, etc., excluding annual healthcare expenditures.

ᴳ This estimate represents costs per alcohol or any other drug involved crime, including violent crimes (rape, robbery, assault, murder, and child abuse) and property crimes (larceny, burglary, motor vehicle theft). The estimate only includes tangible costs, such as medical and mental healthcare, public programs, and property damage losses.

ᴴ Costs of crime related to quality of life places a dollar value on the pain, suffering, and lost quality of life that victims and their families experience due to injury and death.

ᴵ The estimate represents average costs of criminal justice system per person, including justice system, police protection, judicial and legal costs, and corrections.

ᴶ The estimate represents the economic costs per motor vehicle accident (MVA), calculated by dividing total economic costs of MVA by the incidence of MVA in 2010. The estimate only includes tangible costs, such as medical costs and property damage losses.

ᴷ The study reported decrements of 0.075 in the mean SF-6D utility among Australian prisoners (e.g., mean: 0.725, SE: 0.004) relative to the average Australian population (e.g., mean: 0.80, SE: 0.001)

ᴸ The estimate was calculated by dividing the number of people arrested for violent and property crime by the total number of violent and property crimes.

ᴹ Probability of conviction among arrested individuals was estimated by [(# of cases presented/# of arrests reviewed)*conviction rates among dispositions].

ᴺ The estimate was calculated by dividing # of sentenced state federal prison releases by the total # of persons incarcerated in prison in 2012.

2.4 Analyses

2.4.1 Cost-Effectiveness Analysis

We estimated the lifetime cost-effectiveness of five treatment modalities for AUD patients and present the results from a healthcare sector perspective and a societal perspective, as included in the Second Panel's Reference Case recommendations. Following the Panel's further recommendations, we converted all cost estimates to 2014 US dollars (USD), using the general Consumer Price Index (CPI) for earnings, patients' out-of-pocket costs, and legal costs, while applying the Personal Health Care (PHC) and medical CPI for treatment costs and healthcare expenditures (Agency for Healthcare Research and Quality 2015; Bureau of Labor Statistics 2015). We measured health outcomes in QALYs and applied a 3% annual discount rate to both costs and effects to convert future dollars and future health outcomes to their present values.

We calculated and report two summary measures: incremental cost-effectiveness ratios (ICERs) and incremental net monetary benefits (NMBs). The ICER is defined as the difference in costs between two alternatives (net costs) divided by the difference in health outcomes (net effectiveness) and shows how much it costs to buy one more unit of health.

Typically, ICERs are presented as $/QALY or as "Dominated," which indicates a strategy that is less effective and more costly than another alternative. "Cost-saving" represents a strategy that costs less with better health outcomes (e.g., QALYs gained) compared to another alternative. Net monetary benefit is defined as the difference between monetized benefits and costs for a single intervention, expressed in dollar terms. In our base case, we monetized clinical benefits, measured in QALYs, using a $100,000/QALY threshold, while also examining a range of thresholds from $50,000/QALY to $200,000/QALY. Incremental NMB represents the difference in NMB between two interventions.

In addition to those primary summary measures, we also report projected clinical outcomes and disaggregated costs to allow readers to assess the potential magnitude of health outcomes and the breakdown of cost components.

We developed the main model and conducted all analyses using the MATA programming language available in STATA 13 (StataCorp. 2013. Stata: Release 13. Statistical Software. College Station, TX: StataCorp LP).

2.4.2 *Uncertainty Analyses*

We addressed parameter uncertainty using probabilistic sensitivity analysis (PSA), which allowed us to vary all of the parameters in the model simultaneously. In PSA, we used the beta distribution for probability and health utility parameters, and applied the normal distribution to cost parameters because of small standard errors relative to the mean values (i.e., the normal distribution is very unlikely to generate negative cost estimates). From the parametric distributions, we drew 10,000 samples to estimate standard errors of summary measures. Further details of the parametric distributions are presented in Appendix Table 11. Based on the Monte Carlo simulations that derived joint distributions of costs and effects, we generated a cost-effectiveness acceptability curve (CEAC) for the choice of AUD treatment to summarize the uncertainty in the model. The CEAC illustrates the probability of an intervention being the most cost-effective strategy for a range of different cost-effectiveness thresholds. We provide two CEACs, one for the healthcare sector perspective and the other for the societal perspective.

Because we incorporated parametric distributions for every parameter in the model, instead of setting deterministic values, we were unable to perform a traditional deterministic one-way sensitivity analysis that examines the impact on results of changes in a single parameter. However, we addressed this issue by conducting conditional PSA. The conditional PSA provides a CEAC (or NMB) based on deterministic changes in a single parameter while maintaining parametric distributions for all of the other parameters. In this analysis, we considered treatment remission rates, state-specific HRQoL weights, 1-year post-treatment rates of relapse, rates of natural recovery, and rates of natural relapse as important parameters in the sense that variation of these parameters might significantly influence the results. For treatment remission rates, we varied the remission rates of one treatment strategy at a time from 0 to 0.6, with a 0.05 increment, and reported CEACs for a range of different remission rates of each intervention. For state-specific HRQoL weights, we changed both *AUD*- and *LRD*-specific HRQoL weights from 0.5 to 1.0, with a 0.05 increment. In addition, we examined a range of 1-year post-treatment rates of relapse from 0.0 to 0.25, with a 0.025 increment. Finally, we varied rates of natural recovery and rates of natural relapse from 0 to 0.1, with a 0.01 increment.

2.4.3 Value of Information Analysis

Based on the 10,000 samples estimated from PSA, we conducted value of information analysis to quantify treatment decision uncertainty. Value of information analysis is used to estimate the loss of the opportunity costs due to suboptimal decisions caused by existing uncertainty (Briggs, Claxton, and Sculpher 2006). The more uncertain a decision, the more expected loss there could be. Using this framework, we estimated the expected value of perfect information (EVPI), which represents the hypothetical value of new information obtained from a trial with an infinite number of subjects (i.e., no uncertainty exists). The EVPI is considered as an upper bound on the returns from future research. Population EVPIs evaluate the value of new information to the potentially affected population with AUDs. We estimated population EVPIs by multiplying per subject EVPI by age-specific 12-month prevalence of AUDs in the US adult population aged 45 to 64. We also assumed, based on a previous epidemiological study, that only 14.6% of the AUD population seeks treatment (Cohen et al. 2007) (Appendix Table 12).

3 RESULTS

3.1 Model Calibration and Validation

We incorporated two important parameters from the COMBINE trial: the initial rates of remission and the 1-year post-treatment rates of relapse, which correspond to the initial distributions of the *AUD* and *LRD* states at the initial period, t_0, and at the subsequent period, t_1, respectively. We calibrated our model to match with observed distributions of the *AUD* and *LRD* state in each of those time periods.

For validation, we verified that our model behaved as intended through multiple simulations and testing processes. Also, we ensured that model assumptions and parameter information corresponded to current science and information, as judged by co-authors with expertise in the AUD field. However, because of the lack of long-term follow-up data on AUD patients who receive AUD treatment, we were unable to provide external validation. Nevertheless, we reported changes in distribution of *LRD/AUD/Death* over the lifetime horizon for selected treatment modalities in Figure 3.

3.2 Impact Inventory

The Impact Inventory (Table 3) identifies relevant outcomes across all sectors, including the healthcare, labor market, and legal/criminal justice sectors. We quantified and valued each outcome for the purpose of incorporating into our analysis. However,

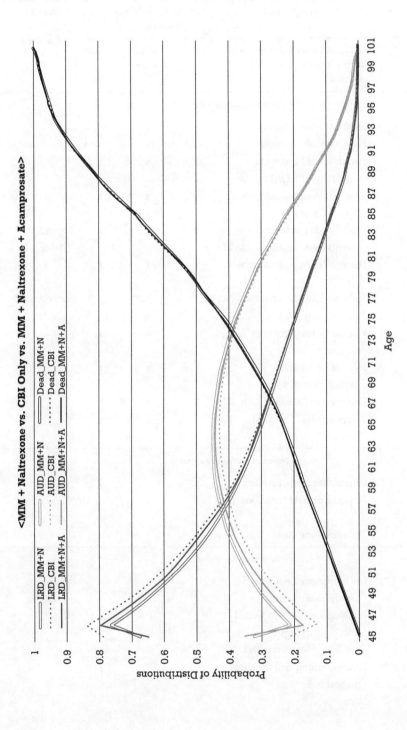

Figure 3 Distribution of LRD/AUD/dead over the lifetime horizon.

Abbreviations: AUD = alcohol-use disorders; LRD = low-risk drinking or abstinence; MM = medical management; CBI = combined behavioral intervention; MM + N, MM + Naltrexone; MM + N + A, MM + Naltrexone + Acamprosate.

Table 3 Impact Inventory

Sector	Type of impact	Included in analysis from the following perspective?			Notes on sources of evidence
	(Categories impacted within each sector with unit of measure if relevant)	Patient	Healthcare sector	Societal	
	Formal healthcare sector				
Health	*Health outcomes (effects):*				
	Longevity effects, years	x	x	x	
	Health-related quality of life (HRQoL), QALYs	x	x	x	
	Years in alcohol use disorders (AUD), Years	x	x	x	
	Disutility due to adverse events from treatment, QALYs	x	x	x	Appendix Table 8
	Disutility of being incarcerated, QALYs	x	x	x	
	Spillover HRQoL, caregiver				See Footnote^
	Medicalc costs				
	Paid for by third-party payers, $		x	x	
	Paid for by patients out-of-pocket, $	x	x	x	
	Future related medical costs, $		x	x	
	Future unrelated medical costs, $		x	x	
	Informal healthcare sector				
HEALTH	Patient time costs, earnings $	x		x	
	Unpaid caregiver time costs				No data available
	Transportation costs				
	Non-healthcare sector				
PRODUCTIVITY	Uncompensated household production, patient				No data available
	Productivity effects in formal market, earnings $			x	
	Years in employment, years			x	
CONSUMPTION	Future consumption unrelated to health, $			x	
SOCIAL SERVICES	None			-	

(continued)

Table 3 Continued

Sector	Type of impact	Included in analysis from the following perspective?			Notes on sources of evidence
	(Categories impacted within each sector with unit of measure if relevant)	Patient	Healthcare sector	Societal	
LEGAL/ CRIMINAL JUSTICE	Costs of AUD-related crimes—tangible, $			x	
	Costs of AUD-related crimes—QoL, $			x	
	Costs related to criminal justice system, $			x	
	# of AUD-related crimes, # of crimes			x	
	Years in incarceration, years			x	
	# of AUD-related motor vehicle accident (MVA), # of MVA			x	
EDUCATION	None			–	
HOUSING	None			–	
ENVIRONMENT	None			–	

A Caregivers for individuals with current or previous alcohol problem reported significant higher caregiver distress, compared to those for individuals with no previous alcohol problem. The caregiver burden was measured by the Neuropsychiatric Inventory Caregiver Distress Scale (NPI-D) and the Family Burden Scale (FBS) in the original study, and we were unable to convert the estimate of the caregiver burden into the health utility weight.

we were unable to quantify some health and productivity outcomes due to a lack of appropriate data, such as uncompensated household production by patients, spillover effects on HRQoL of caregivers, and time costs of uncompensated care. A previous study found that caregivers for individuals with a current or previous alcohol problem reported significantly higher caregiver distress compared to caregivers for individuals with no previous alcohol problem (Sattar et al. 2007). However, the caregiver burden was measured using the Neuropsychiatric Inventory Caregiver Distress Scale and the Family Burden Scale, and we were unable to convert the estimate of the caregiver burden into the health utility weights. Finally, we were unable to locate appropriate data sources for quantifying uncompensated household production by patients and time spent by caregivers. All of the other relevant impacts of AUD treatment were identified and incorporated into the model as parameters.

3.3 Projected Intermediate (Clinical) Outcomes and Costs

In order to evaluate a wide range of consequences of an initial AUD treatment episode over a lifetime time horizon, we report disaggregated results in Table 4, which is categorized by three different perspectives: patient, healthcare sector, and societal. Of the five interventions evaluated, MM + naltrexone achieved the best results for all outcomes assessed. Over a lifetime, an individual patient who received the MM + naltrexone therapy lived 19.22 years and gained 15.01 QALYs on average (3% discounted). The patient spent 13.68 years in the *AUD* state, compared to 14.41 years for a patient who received CBI Only. None of the differences in consequences between MM + naltrexone and other treatments was statistically significant due to minor differences in initial remission rates reported in the COMBINE trial and dynamic transitions under the natural history. However, MM + naltrexone was associated with longer years of employment, higher productivity benefits, smaller number of crimes committed, reduced number of motor vehicle accidents, and lower legal costs than the alternative interventions.

3.4 Main Results

3.4.1 Cost-Effectiveness Analysis Results

3.4.1.1 Healthcare sector perspective

We provide the conventional cost-effectiveness plane in Figure 4 and summary cost-effectiveness results in Table 5 to highlight overall costs and QALYs gained from all five AUD treatment interventions from both the healthcare sector perspective and the societal perspective. From a healthcare sector perspective, the four intervention strategies CBI Only, MM Only, MM + acamprosate, and MM + naltrexone + acamprosate were all dominated because they were more costly and less effective than MM + naltrexone. Based on $100,000/QALY as a WTP threshold, the MM + naltrexone therapy reported the largest NMB of $1,250,239 per patient, followed by MM + acamprosate at $1,244,704 per patient.

3.4.1.2 Societal perspective

After accounting for costs and effects in non-healthcare sectors, the total societal costs of all five AUD treatment interventions became negative (i.e., cost-saving), highlighting the fact that productivity benefits outweigh the sum of the healthcare costs, consumption costs, and legal costs for all five treatments. From a societal perspective, the other four intervention strategies were dominated by MM + naltrexone as well, and the overall NMB of the MM + naltrexone therapy increased to $1,556,178 per patient versus $1,250,239 per patient in the healthcare sector perspective analysis (i.e., increased by $305,939 per patient) (Figure 4, Table 5).

3.4.1.3 Patient perspective

From a patient perspective, potential health effects were compared to the out-of-pocket costs for treatment and time costs associated with AUD treatment strategies. Although the result is not presented in Table 5, the MM + naltrexone therapy reported the largest NMB of $1,499,695 based on $100,000/QALY as a WTP threshold, and all

Table 4 Projected health outcomes, non-healthcare sector outcomes, and costs (time horizon: lifetime)

	CBI only Mean (SE)	MM only Mean (SE)	MM + Naltrexone + Acamprosate Mean (SE)	MM + Acamprosate Mean (SE)	MM + Naltrexone Mean (SE)
	Patient perspective				
Life years	19.07 (0.13)	19.11 (0.12)	19.15 (0.13)	19.18 (0.13)	19.22 (0.13)
QALYs	14.89 (0.67)	14.91 (0.66)	14.93 (0.65)	14.97 (0.64)	15.01 (0.64)
Years in AUD	14.41 (0.80)	14.21 (0.75)	14.03 (0.79)	13.89 (0.77)	13.68 (0.76)
Out-of-pocket (OOP) costs*	$222 (8.87)	$173 (3.82)	$307 (7.00)	$263 (5.70)	$214 (4.84)
Time costs for treatment	$1,162 (102)	$1,014 (86)	$1,046 (102)	$1,126 (143)	$1,091 (112)
	Healthcare sector perspective				
Treatment costs (including OOP costs)	$640 (18)	$474 (7)	$1,162 (37)	$866 (22)	$777 (20)
Healthcare expenditure†	$253,445 (6,371)	$252,464 (6,248)	$251,640 (6,331)	$250,952 (6,244)	$249,968 (6,189)
	Societal perspective				
Years employed	13.85 (0.30)	13.86 (0.29)	13.88 (0.29)	13.89 (0.29)	13.90 (0.29)
Years in jail	0.55 (0.51)	0.55 (0.50)	0.54 (0.50)	0.54 (0.49)	0.53 (0.49)
Number of crimes	3.03 (0.61)	3.00 (0.60)	2.98 (0.60)	2.96 (0.60)	2.93 (0.59)
Number of motor vehicle accidents	0.94 (0.33)	0.93 (0.33)	0.93 (0.33)	0.92 (0.32)	0.92 (0.32)
Productivity benefits	$768,162 (14,314)	$768,450 (14,212)	$768,694 (14,131)	$768,905 (14,058)	$769,195 (13,967)
Consumption costs	$412,161 (5,820)	$413,103 (5,706)	$413,898 (5,795)	$414,561 (5,731)	$415,508 (5,714)
Legal costs‡	$48,535 (16,382)	$48,022 (16,261)	$47,568 (16110)	$47,187 (16,001)	$46,657 (15,850)

*Out-of-pocket costs were estimated from the sum of expected prescription copayments for medication and expected office visit copayments for session visits.

†Healthcare expenditure includes costs of future treatment, future unrelated healthcare expenditure, and end-of-life costs.

‡Legal costs comprise all costs associated with the legal/criminal justice sector, including tangible costs of crime, costs of crime related to quality of life, costs of criminal justice system, costs of motor vehicle accidents, and costs of incarceration.

Abbreviations: CBI = combined behavioral intervention; MM = medical management; QALYs = quality-adjusted life years; AUD = alcohol use disorders.

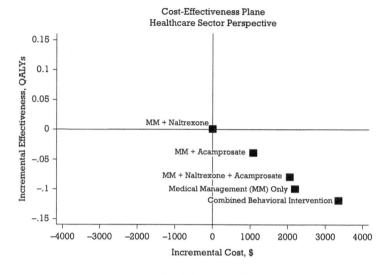

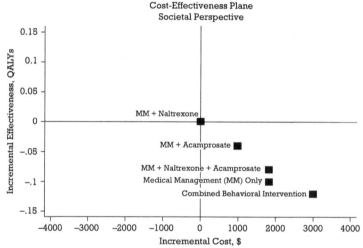

Figure 4. Cost-effectiveness ratios for intervention strategies displayed in the cost-effectiveness plane.

Notes: All treatment strategies were compared to the most cost-effective intervention, Medical Management + Naltrexone. Abbreviation: QALY = quality-adjusted life years.

other strategies were dominated by the MM + naltrexone therapy. Appendix Figure 2 shows changes in incremental NMB of four interventions versus CBI Only from three different perspectives (i.e., patient perspective, healthcare sector perspective, and societal perspective) in a single triangular spider chart.

3.4.2 Uncertainty Analyses

To evaluate significant uncertainty presented in the model, we provide CEACs in Figure 5. We found that MM + naltrexone was the most cost-effective strategy across

Table 5 Reference Case cost-effectiveness results (time horizon: lifetime; costs and health effects discounted at 3%)

Alternative	Total costs* Mean (SE)	Total QALYs Mean (SE)	Incremental cost**	Incremental effectiveness† (QALYs)	NMB* Mean (SE)	Incremental NMB†	ICER† (Incr. Cost/ Incr. QALY)
			Healthcare sector perspective				
MM + Naltrexone	$250,745 (6,191)	15.01 (0.64)	–	–	$1,250,239 (66,599)	–	–
MM + Acamprosate	$251,817 (6,246)	14.97 (0.65)	$1,072	–0.04	$1,244,704 (65,876)	–$5,535	Dominated‡
MM + Naltrexone + Acamprosate	$252,802 (6,335)	14.93 (0.65)	$985	–0.04	$1,240,052 (64,972)	–$4,652	Dominated‡
MM Only	$252,938 (6,246)	14.91 (0.66)	$136	–0.02	$1,238,119 (66,963)	–$1,933	Dominated‡
CBI Only	$254,085 (6,380)	14.89 (0.67)	$1,147	–0.02	$1,234,822 (68,308)	–$3,297	Dominated‡
			Societal perspective				
MM + Naltrexone	–$55,195 (20,181)	15.01 (0.64)	–	–	$1,556,178 (68,324)	–	–
MM + Acamprosate	–$54,213 (20,382)	14.97 (0.65)	$982	–0.04	$1,550,734 (69,208)	–$5,444	Dominated‡

(continued)

Table 5 Continued

Alternative	Total costs* Mean (SE)	Total QALYs Mean (SE)	Incremental cost**	Incremental effectiveness[†] (QALYs)	NMB* Mean (SE)	Incremental NMB[†]	ICER[†] (Incr. Cost/ Incr. QALY)
MM + Naltrexone + Acamprosate	-$53,379 (20,564)	14.93 (0.65)	$834	-0.04	$1,546,233 (69,984)	-$4,501	Dominated[‡]
MM Only	-$53,373 (20,747)	14.91 (0.66)	$6	-0.02	$1,544,430 (70,410)	-$1,803	Dominated[‡]
CBI Only	-$52,219 (20,956)	14.89 (0.67)	$1,164	-0.02	$1,541,126 (71,617)	-$3,304	Dominated[‡]

*Negative values indicate that all of the AUD treatments are cost-saving to society, mainly owing to the larger productivity benefits relative to other associated costs

**Net monetary benefits (NMB) were based on $100,000/QALY; NMB = (QALY * $100,000/QALY) – Costs

[†]The incremental cost, incremental effectiveness, incremental NMB and ICER of an alternative strategy were estimated in relation to the next best strategy.

[‡]Dominated: an alternative strategy is dominated if it is less effective and more costly than another alternative.

Abbreviations: CBI = combined behavioral intervention; MM = medical management; QALY = quality-adjusted life years; ICER = incremental cost-effectiveness ratio.

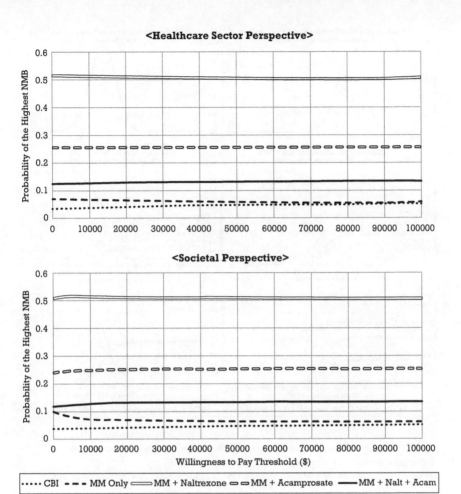

Figure 5 Cost-effectiveness acceptability curve for the choice of AUD treatment.
Abbreviations: AUD = alcohol use disorder; NMB = net monetary benefit; CBI = combined behavioral intervention;
MM = medical management.

all WTP thresholds regardless of perspective, with an approximately 50% probability of being the most cost-effective strategy. The results were most sensitive to changes in the remission rates, state-specific HRQoL, and 1-year post-treatment rates of relapse.

Also, although the results are not shown here, we examined the effects of different time horizons on the incremental NMB (3 years vs 20 years vs lifetime). Compared to the shorter (3-year) time horizon, we found that the longer time horizons (20 years and lifetime) provided higher incremental NMB because many of spillover effects were not captured in the shorter time horizon.

The results of our conditional PSA are shown in Figures 6–8. The top panel in each of those figures represents the initial probabilistic distributions of each parameter in the base case, corresponding to the likelihood of the parameter. We then plotted a CEAC at a given WTP threshold with a plausible range of a single parameter that we

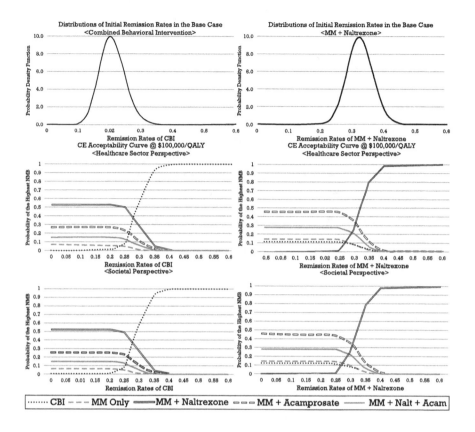

Figure 6 Conditional sensitivity analysis on treatment remission rates in a base case probabilistic model.

Abbreviations: CE = cost-effectiveness; CBI = combined behavioral intervention; MM = medical management.

deterministically varied (e.g., the left middle panel in Figure 5 represents a CEAC from the healthcare sector perspective with a WTP threshold of $100,000/QALY when we varied the remission rates of CBI Only from 0 to 0.6, holding other parameter distributions constant).

Figure 6 shows that changes in remission rates from treatment significantly influenced the CEA results. Holding other parameter distributions constant, if remission rates with CBI Only become higher than 30% (note: 21% in the base case), CBI Only has a probability of 58% or more of being the most cost-effective intervention, and that probability rises to 99.7% with remission rates of 40% or higher. In varying remission rates with MM + naltrexone, if these reduce to 30% (note: 32.5% in the base case), MM + acamprosate becomes the most cost-effective intervention, with a probability of 36%, followed by MM + naltrexone, with a 24.8% chance. If remission rates with MM + naltrexone fall below 25%, then there is almost no chance that the MM + naltrexone therapy will be the most cost-effective intervention, and consequently, MM + acamprosate becomes the most cost-effective strategy (~45.7%), followed by MM + naltrexone + acamprosate (~27.5%). However, based on the primary distributions of

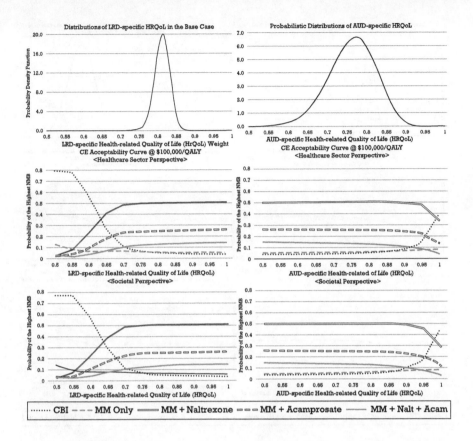

Figure 7 Conditional sensitivity analysis on state-specific health-related quality of life (HRQoL) in a base case probabilistic model.

Abbreviations: CE = cost-effectiveness; CBI = combined behavioral intervention; MM = medical management; LRD = low-risk drinking or abstinence; AUD = alcohol use disorders.

remission rates for CBI Only and MM + naltrexone, those scenarios are very unlikely to happen, and MM + naltrexone is the most cost-effective strategy in most of the plausible scenarios. The results of this conditional PSA on remission rates did not vary by the perspective used (healthcare sector vs societal).

Figure 7 shows that changes in the *LRD-/AUD*-specific HRQoL also significantly affected the results across all three perspectives. Holding other parameter distributions constant (note: HRQoL for the *AUD* state was 0.76), the lower the *LRD*-specific HRQoL was (e.g., < 0.65), the more likely it was that CBI Only and MM Only would be the most cost-effective interventions. Also, with unchanged other parameter distributions (note: HRQoL for the *LRD* state was 0.81), if the *AUD*-specific HRQoL is higher than 0.98, CBI Only becomes the most cost-effective intervention, with ~40% chance. However, the primary distributions of the state-specific HRQoL showed that MM + naltrexone is the most cost-effective strategy in most scenarios.

Figure 8 shows the conditional PSA of varying the 1-year post-treatment rates of relapse after the initial treatment. In the COMBINE trial, the MM + naltrexone +

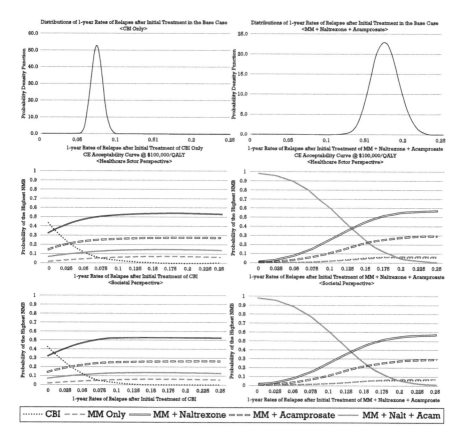

Figure 8 Conditional sensitivity analysis on 1-year rates of relapse after initial treatment in a base case probabilistic model.

Abbreviations: CE = cost-effectiveness; CBI = combined behavioral intervention; MM = medical management; LRD = low-risk drinking; AUD = alcohol use disorder.

acamprosate therapy had the highest initial remission rate at the end of the 16-week treatment period (35.1%, followed by 32.5% for MM + naltrexone), but it also had the highest rate of relapse at the 1-year post-treatment follow-up (17.5%, followed by 11.1% of MM + naltrexone) (Anton et al. 2006). Therefore, it would be important to evaluate what would happen if the 1-year rates of relapse were different. Holding other parameter distributions constant, (note: 1-year rates of relapse of MM + naltrexone were 11.1%), if the 1-year rates of relapse of MM + naltrexone + acamprosate were 12.5%, versus 17.5% in the base case, the MM + naltrexone + acamprosate therapy would become the most cost-effective strategy, with a 40% chance. We also found that the lower the 1-year rates of relapse for the MM + naltrexone + acamprosate were, the higher its chances were of being the most cost-effective strategy. In order for CBI Only to be the most cost-effective strategy over MM + naltrexone, the 1-year relapse rate would have to be lower than 1%, which is very unlikely. We also examined how

Table 6 Value of information
estimates: expected value of perfect
information (EVPI; time horizon: lifetime)

EVPI	Perspectives	
	Health sector	Societal
Per subject EVPI	$2,800	$2,701
Population EVPI*	$1.79B	$1.73B

*Population EVPIs were estimated by multiplying
per subject EVPI with age-specific prevalence of 12-
month AUD in the US adult population aged 45–64.
We assume that only 14.6% of the AUD population
seeks treatment. The number of population that
would seek treatment among AUD patients aged 45–
65 would be 0.64 million (see Appendix Table 10).
Notes: All estimates are expressed in 2014 US$;
discount rate 3%.

changes in the rates of natural recovery and rates of natural relapse would affect the
CEAC, and we found that our results were robust to changes in those parameters.

3.4.3 *Value of Information Analysis*

Results from the value of information analysis are presented in Table 6. A healthcare
sector perspective provided the largest per subject EVPI, at $2,800, and the per subject
EVPI from a societal perspective was almost identical, at $2,701. These findings high-
lighted the presence of large uncertainty in making decisions based on the most cost-
effective strategy on average (MM + naltrexone) and underscore the need for future
research to reduce parameter uncertainty in the model. Population EVPI estimates
showed that if we had perfect information to guide every individual patient to choose
"optimal" treatment that provides the highest NMB on average, the value of information would be $1.73 billion for the population with AUDs aged 45 to 64.

4 DISCUSSION

We found that all interventions were dominated by MM + naltrexone in analyses from
both a healthcare sector perspective and a societal perspective. However, in the presence
of minor differences in initial remission rates and 1-year rates of relapse after initial treatment, probabilistic sensitivity analyses showed a moderate possibility that other interventions, such as CBI only or MM + naltrexone + acamprosate, could be the most cost-effective
intervention.

Compared to the healthcare sector perspective, the societal perspective analysis provided much larger NMBs for all five AUD treatment strategies. These findings reflect significant impacts on outside of the healthcare sector, including increased labor force participation, and reduced crime rates, arrests, incarcerations, and motor vehicle accidents. With regard to incremental NMBs of the four other treatment options relative to CBI Only, estimates from a societal perspective were slightly smaller than those from a healthcare sector perspective. This is because the additional consumption costs from the longevity effects were almost equivalent to the benefits of reducing healthcare expenditures, increased productivity through labor participation, and decreased legal/crime costs from AUD treatment.

We also found that there were no statistically significant differences in incremental NMBs among interventions. We conjectured a few possible explanations: (1) no significant difference in the initial remission rates among the five interventions; (2) dynamic transitions between the *AUD* and *LRD* state (i.e., very high rates of relapse during 1-year post-treatment and higher rates of natural recovery than rates of natural relapse); and (3) no significant difference in state-specific HRQoL (i.e., 0.76 [standard error: 0.06] for the *AUD* state vs. 0.81 [0.02] for the *LRD* state).

Another contributing factor to the lack of statistically significant differences among interventions was the large standard error of some parameters, especially cost parameters, which was caused by the expensive, but rare occurrences of hospital stays, arrests, and motor vehicle accidents. We examined the potential impact of changes in these parameters in conditional PSA and found that the results were sensitive to treatment remission rates, state-specific HRQoL weights, and 1-year post-treatment rates of relapse. Although MM + naltrexone is the most cost-effective strategy under most of the plausible scenarios, clinical and/or policy decision makers should acknowledge that this group of interventions may be perceived as roughly equivalent based on current information with considerable uncertainty. The presence of significant uncertainty in some of the parameters underscores the importance of future research that would provide valuable information to reduce decision uncertainty. From the value of information analysis, the EVPI at the population level was $1.73 billion from a societal perspective. Although it is conditional on the perfect implementation of research findings in practice, this issue signifies that the expected value of future research remains very large for potential consequences of AUD.

Lastly, we compared the long-term costs and effectiveness of three medication options (i.e, MM + naltrexone and/or acamprosate) and a MM only option with CBI Only in this analysis. Since CBI Only is not a "do-nothing" strategy, but rather a treatment strategy, the CBI Only intervention still provided some clinical benefits of remission to low-risk drinking or abstinence. Also, because the COMBINE trial offered patients in the MM Only group placebo medications, additional placebo effects might exist. Although we did not consider "do-nothing" to be an appropriate treatment strategy for AUD patients and did not include it as a comparator, if the interventions evaluated were directly compared to a "do-nothing" strategy, more apparent changes in the initial remission rates would be expected, considering that the rates of natural recovery among AUD patients who did not receive any treatment were about 3.6% annually.

There are some limitations of this study. One of the main limitations is that we extrapolated clinical results (i.e., the age group and remission rates) from a single clinical trial (Anton et al. 2006). This is a trial-based analysis and so the analysis was restricted to the average age of the trial population (age 45). Although the COMBINE study did not provide age-specific subgroup results, a previous study found that compared with younger adults, older adults had greater attendance at therapy sessions and greater adherence to the medication in a randomized controlled trial of naltrexone for the treatment of alcohol dependence (Oslin, Pettinati, and Volpicelli 2002). If so, the AUD treatment may be more cost-effective for the older population than the younger group, but further study on heterogeneous effects of AUD treatment on age groups is needed.

In addition, the initial remission rate is the primary determinant of the proportion of patients transitioning into the *AUD* state, which is intrinsically associated with higher mortality rates, lower labor force participation rates, and higher probabilities of committing crimes and having motor vehicle accidents than the *LRD* state. Therefore, the variability in the initial remission rates could significantly change our results. For example, if there are other combinations of medication and behavioral therapy that could significantly increase remission rates, the cost-effectiveness of the interventions would also significantly increase. Also, in the COMBINE trial, AUD patients with substantial concurrent psychiatric illness and drug abuse were excluded. However, a substantial proportion of AUD patients also experience psychiatric illness and drug abuse, limiting generalizability of this study to the entire population of AUD patients. The potential effects on CEA results of excluding AUD patients with comorbid conditions remain unclear. Despite having more room for improved outcomes due to initially severe health conditions, AUD patients with more comorbidities might improve less with AUD treatment than AUD patients without comorbid conditions.

Another limitation rests on the nature of the "memorylessness" property of state-transition models, that is, that state-transition models assume that the transition probabilities to the next state depend only on the current state, regardless of the individual's prior state. For example, we assume that every individual in the *LRD* state shares the same transition probabilities regardless of previous history of successful treatment. In reality, individuals who become low-risk drinkers or become abstinent after successful AUD treatment may have a different propensity to relapse compared to an individual who happens to be in the *LRD* state after natural recovery. If individuals who returned to the *LRD* state after receiving treatment are more likely to relapse than those who volitionally became low-risk drinkers, the assumption of the "memorylessness" property would result in positive bias (i.e., more cost-effective) toward AUD treatment strategies with higher initial remission rates.

Also, we were unable to include some outcomes, such as uncompensated household production, time costs of uncompensated care for caregivers, and spillover effects on HRQoL of caregivers due to the lack of ability to incorporate existing information into the model parameters and the absence of available data sources. Considering that those missing factors are associated with positive benefits of AUD treatment—that is, AUD treatment with higher remission rates would increase uncompensated household productivity (e.g., nurturing children), increase HRQoL of caregivers, and reduce time for caregivers to take care of AUD patients—we believe that incorporating these factors would support our findings more strongly.

Despite some limitations, this study makes important contributions to the economic evaluation literature by conducting and reporting the Reference Case CEAs as recommended by the Second Panel on Cost-Effectiveness in Health and Medicine. In this analysis, we have estimated the overall cost-effectiveness of AUD treatment and highlighted the importance of presenting multiple outcomes and incorporating the spillovers of consequences of AUD treatment that fall outside of the healthcare sector.

PART 2: TECHNICAL APPENDIX

Appendix Table 1 Life table for the total population: United States, 2009

Age group	Probability of dying
41–45	0.0021
46–50	0.0033
51–55	0.0051
56–60	0.0073
61–65	0.0105
66–70	0.0158
71–75	0.0240
76–80	0.0379
81–85	0.0618
86–90	0.1050
91–95	0.1709
96–100	0.2589
100+	1.0000

Source: CDC/NCHS, National Vital Statistics System
http://www.cdc.gov/nchs/data/nvsr/nvsr62/nvsr62_07.pdf

Appendix Table 2 Age-specific relative risk for mortality among AUD patients

Age	N	Mean	SE
40–49	1,894	4.70	0.62
50–59	2,155	3.21	0.36
60+	2,221	1.74	0.22

Notes: Because the original data provided the age- and gender-specific relative risk (RR) for mortality among non-veteran clinical samples, I estimated the weighted average of men and women based on the sample size, and then converted to RRs for mortality for the general population based on differences between pooled RRs from all-study and pooled-RRs from clinical studies; Also, in the original systematic review and meta-analysis, the authors assumed that "standardized mortality ratios (i.e., comparisons of mortality risks of people with AUD with the age-specific general population), hazard ratios, odds ratios and RRs were treated as equivalent measures of risk."
Source: Roerecke and Rehm (2013).

Appendix Table 3 Labor force participation rates as full-time workers

Age group	Total	AUD-ever		AUD-year	
		No	Yes	No	Yes
All ages	0.764	0.775	0.719	0.776	0.663
22 ≤ age ≤ 29	0.675	0.652	0.738	0.678	0.657
30 ≤ age ≤ 44	0.845	0.875	0.733	0.873	0.643
45 ≤ age ≤ 59	0.826	0.858	0.684	0.829	0.786
60 ≤ age ≤ 64	0.566	0.565	0.571	0.568	0.500

Notes: We assume that individuals who moved to low-risk drinking (LRD) after treatment just follow labor force participation rates as individuals who were ever diagnosed with AUD (AUD-ever: Yes), and those who remain in AUD follow the rates as individuals who were diagnosed with AUD in the past year. (AUD-year: Yes).

Source: Mullahy and Sindelar (1991).

Appendix Table 4 Labor force participation rates at age 65 and over (full-time workers)

Age group	General population	AUD population[†]
65 ≤ Age ≤ 69	0.321	0.274
70 ≤ Age ≤ 74	0.195	0.167
75 ≤ Age	0.076	0.065

Source: Civilian labor force participation rates by age, sex, race, and ethnicity (2012 Data) http://www.bls.gov/emp/ep_table_303.htm

[†] AUD-specific rates over age 65 were estimated, assuming that compared to the general population, only 85.5% of individuals with AUD participate in the labor force based on Appendix Table 6.

Appendix Table 5 Detailed information on micro-costing approach of costs of intervention and delivery

Treatment strategy	No. of patients	Mean cost, $ (2014 USD)					
		Medication[A]	Labor[B]		Assessment[C]		Total cost of treatment
			MM	CBI	Non-laboratory	Laboratory	
CBI Only	153	–	–	$391.7	$126.7	$121.5	**$640**
MM Only	157	–	$193.8	–	$153.2	$126.9	**$474**
MM + Naltrexone[D]	154	$310.9	$188.3	–	$152.0	$126.1	**$777**
MM + Acamprosate[E]	152	$400.8	$188.9	–	$152.0	$124.1	**$866**
MM + Naltrexone + Acamprosate	148	$700.5	$184.4	–	$151.7	$124.9	**$1,162**

Note: The information and explanations presented in this table are excerpted from previously published literature: (1) Cost-methodology of COMBINE (Zarkin G. A. et al., *J Stud Alcohol Suppl.* July 2005;(15):50-55) and (2) Cost and cost-effectiveness of the COMBINE Study in Alcohol-Dependent Patients (Zarkin G. A. et al., *Arch Gen Psychiatry.* 2008; 65(10):1214-1221). More details on costing methodology are available in those studies.

[A] Pharmaceutical costs of acamprosate and naltrexone were based on the Federal Supply Schedule, representing the price negotiated by Veterans Affairs and publicly available.

[B] Labor costs for MM or CBI were based on the actual clinician time spent on MM or CBI estimated from the data, which were collected prospectively as a part of the COMBINE study.

[C] Assessment cost is the sum of the labor costs associated with assessment or intervention, the space used in conducting that activity, such as the room and building, and all supplies and materials used. Laboratory costs specifically cover the cost of collecting, processing, and testing biological samples and providing laboratory reports.

[D] From the COMBINE protocol, the dosage for naltrexone was titrated as 25 mg for days 1–4, 50 mg for days 4–7 and 100 mg thereafter. Based on the original cost-effectiveness study conducted by Zarkin et al., the federal supply schedule price of naltrexone was $1.37 per 50 mg tablet, and this translated to a daily cost of $2.74 for naltrexone in 2007 USD. We converted this cost to 2014 USD.

[E] From the COMBINE protocol the dosage for acamprosate was 3 g (or 3000 mg) per day. Based on the original cost-effectiveness study conducted by Zarkin et al., the federal supply schedule price of acamprosate was $0.64 per 333 mg tablet, and this translated to a daily cost of $5.76 for acamprosate in 2007 USD. We converted this cost to 2014 USD.

Abbreviations: CBI = combined behavioral intervention; MM = medical management.

Appendix Table 6 Annual healthcare costs among the general population (2014 USD)

Age group	Mean	SE
All ages	$4,455	$48
Age < 25	$1,828	$40
25 ≤ Age < 35	$2,728	$60
35 ≤ Age < 45	$3,457	$125
45 ≤ Age < 55	$5,039	$91
55 ≤ Age < 65	$7,780	$188
65 ≤ Age < 75	$9,814	$183
75 ≤ Age	$12,037	$191

Note: Population estimates were calculated using survey weight adjustment.
Source: Authors' calculation based on the Medical Expenditure Panel Survey (MEPS) 2003-2012.

Appendix Table 7 Annual healthcare costs among individuals with AUD (2014 USD)

Age group	N	Mean	SE
All ages	632	$10,987	$1,093
Age < 25	108	$6,261	$1,498
25 ≤ age < 45	246	$8,038	$1,135
45 ≤ age < 65	228	$12,230	$1,420
65 ≤ age	50	$31,196	$8,944

Notes: The estimates were calculated using survey weight adjustment. Patients with alcohol-related disorders were identified using clinical classification code (660) available in MEPS—Medical condition database.
Source: Authors' calculation based on the Medical Expenditure Panel Survey (MEPS) 2003-2012.

Appendix Table 8 Disutility of adverse events during treatment

Event	Disutility[++] Mean (SE)	Placebo (n = 309)	Naltrexone (n = 309)	Acamprosate (n = 303)	Acamprosate + naltrexone (n = 305)
Nausea	-.02 (0.01)	65 (21%)	101 (34%)	72 (24%)	125 (42%)
	Beta	Binomial	Binomial	Binomial	Binomial
	a = 3.9, b = 191.2	N = 309, p = 0.21	N = 309, p = 0.34	N = 303, p = 0.24	N = 305, p = 0.42
Vomiting	-0.02 (0.01)	26 (9%)	45 (15%)	27 (9%)	52 (18%)
	Beta	Binomial	Binomial	Binomial	Binomial
	a = 3.9, b = 191.2	N = 309, p = 0.09	N = 309, p = 0.15	N = 303, p = 0.09	N = 305, p = 0.18
Diarrhea	-0.02 (0.01)	108 (35%)	92 (31%)	193 (65%)	165 (56%)
	Beta	Binomial	Binomial	Binomial	Binomial
	a = 3.9, b = 191.2	N = 309, p = 0.35	N = 309, p = 0.31	N = 303, p = 0.65	N = 305, p = 0.56
Decreased appetite	-0.06 (0.015)	41 (13%)	63 (21%)	57 (19%)	75 (25%)
	Beta	Binomial	Binomial	Binomial	Binomial
	a = 15.0, b = 235	N = 309, p = 0.13	N = 309, p = 0.21	N = 303, p = 0.19	N = 305, p = 0.25
Somnolence	N/A	72 (24%)	112 (37%)	94 (31%)	91 (31%)
AST or ALT 5 times upper limit normal	N/A	0 (0%)	6 (2%)	1 (0%)	5 (2%)
Sources	Pollack et al. (2010)		Anton et al. (2006)		

Note: Because of the lack of available data, we were not able to incorporate disutility of having somnolence and AST or ALT 5 times the upper limit of normal, as well as other adverse events that were not statistically significant across medication groups, such as alcohol detoxification and other serious adverse events.

[++]The original study examined disutility of adverse events in patients with type 2 diabetes mellitus to quantify tolerability issues with oral antidiabetic medications, and health-related quality of life of specific adverse events among those patients was measured by the EQ-5D index. To account for uncertainty around the disutility estimate, we drew 10,000 samples from a specified beta distribution, then multiplied by negative one (−1).

Abbreviations: AST = aspartate aminotransferase; ALT = alanine aminotransferase.

Appendix Table 9 Average annual earnings per person (2014 USD)

Age group	Mean	SE
All ages	$44,245	$316
Age < 25	$20,398	$462
25 ≤ age ≤ 34	$39,907	$537
35 ≤ age ≤ 44	$51,366	$733
45 ≤ age ≤ 54	$52,749	$721
55 ≤ age ≤ 64	$53,329	$825
65 ≤ age ≤ 74	$41,317	$1,568
75 ≤ age	$37,300	$3,432

Source: Author's calculation using the Current Population Survey 2014 July data set Data Available at: http://thedataweb. rm.census.gov/ ftp/cps_ftp.html#cpsbasic

Appendix Table 10 Average annual expenditures per person (i.e., consumption costs) (2014 USD)

Age group	Total expenditures		Healthcare expenditures		Net expenditures	
	Mean	SE	Mean	SE	Mean	SE
All ages	$20,440	$329	$1,452	$34	$18,988	$330
Age < 25	$15,187	$688	$472	$53	$14,715	$691
25 ≤ age ≤ 34	$17,174	$574	$782	$48	$16,392	$576
35 ≤ age ≤ 44	$17,289	$516	$938	$73	$16,352	$521
45 ≤ age ≤ 54	$22,416	$680	$1,408	$70	$21,009	$683
55 ≤ age ≤ 64	$26,615	$702	$2,085	$86	$24,530	$707
65 ≤ age ≤ 74	$24,609	$897	$2,731	$79	$21,878	$901
75 ≤ age	$21,489	$908	$3,069	$104	$18,420	$914

Note: The original table provided annual expenditures per consumer units. To estimate annual expenditures per person, we divided the annual expenditures by the average number of people in consumer unit that was provided in the same table.

Source: Bureau of Labor Statistics. Consumer Expenditure Survey. Washington DC: US Dept of Labor Statistics, 2014. http://www.bls.gov/cex/2013/combined/age.pdf

Appendix Table 11 Parameters and distributions used in probabilistic sensitivity analyses

State-dependent parameters	Baseline value		Distribution	Parameters
	AUD mean (SE)	LRD mean (SE)		normal: μ = mean, s = SE Beta: a = shape, b = shape
Costs (2014 USD)				
Costs of intervention and delivery				
CBI Only	$640 (18.1)	–	Normal	μ = 640, s = 18.1
MM Only	$474 (7.52)	–	Normal	μ = 474, s = 7.52
MM + Naltrexone	$777 (19.5)	–	Normal	μ = 777, s = 19.5
MM + Acamprosate	$866 (22.4)	–	Normal	μ = 866, s = 22.4
MM + Naltrexone + Acamprosate	$1,162 (36.7)	–	Normal	μ = 1162, s = 36.7
Patient's time costs for treatment				
CBI Only	$1,164 (102)	–	Normal	μ = 1164, s = 102
MM Only	$1,014 (86.9)	–	Normal	μ = 1014, s = 86.9
MM + Naltrexone	$1,090 (111)	–	Normal	μ = 1090, s = 111
MM + Acamprosate	$1,128 (143)	–	Normal	μ = 1128, s = 143
MM + Naltrexone + Acamprosate	$1,046 (101)	–	Normal	μ = 1046, s = 101
Quality-of-life valuations				
State-specific health-utility weight	0.76 (0.06)	0.81 (0.02)	Beta	a = 37.7, b = 11.9 [AUD] a = 310.8, b = 72.9 [LRD]
Probabilities				
Initial treatment remission rates				
CBI Only	0.21 (0.04)	–	Beta	a = 21.6, b = 81.1
MM Only	0.248 (0.03)	–	Beta	a = 51.1, b = 155.1
MM + Naltrexone	0.325 (0.04)	–	Beta	a = 44.2, b = 91.9
MM + Acamprosate	0.289 (0.04)	–	Beta	a = 36.8, b = 90.6
MM + Naltrexone + Acamprosate	0.351 (0.04)	–	Beta	a = 49.6, b = 91.8
Relapse, 1 year after initial treatment				
CBI Only	–	0.076 (0.008)	Beta	a = 92.3, b = 1122
MM Only	–	0.091 (0.009)	Beta	a = 90.8, b = 907.1
MM + Naltrexone	–	0.111 (0.011)	Beta	a = 88.8, b = 711.1
MM + Acamprosate	–	0.098 (0.010)	Beta	a = 90.1, b = 829.3
MM + Naltrexone + Acamprosate	–	0.175 (0.017)	Beta	a = 82.3, b = 388.1

State-dependent parameters	Baseline value		Distribution	Parameters normal: μ = mean, s = SE Beta: a = shape, b = shape
	AUD mean (SE)	LRD mean (SE)		
Pr (seeking future treatment)	0.051 (0.005)	–	Beta	a = 98.7, b = 1836
Pr (remission from future treatment)	0.314 (0.046)	–	Beta	a = 31.4, b = 68.6
Pr (natural recovery from AUD)	0.036 (0.004)	–	Beta	a = 78.0, b = 2090
Pr (relapse from LRD, natural history)	–	0.027 (0.001)	Beta	a = 709.3, b = 25561
Pr (any crime)	0.177 (0.038)	0.032 (0.018)	Beta	a = 17.7, b = 82.3 [AUD] a = 3.2, b = 96.8 [LRD]
Pr (motor vehicle accident)	0.052 (0.022)	0.013 (0.006)	Beta	a = 5.2, b = 94.8 [AUD] a = 3.78, b = 296.2 [LRD]

State-independent Parameters	Mean (SE)	Distribution	Parameters
	Costs (2014 USD)		
Costs of future treatment	$1,872 (252)	Normal	μ =1872, s = 252
End-of-life costs	$37,421 (4,857)	Normal	μ = 37421, s = 4857
Costs of crimes—tangible	$1,568 (314)	Normal	μ = 1568, s = 314
Costs of crimes— quality of life	$14,245 (2,849)	Normal	μ = 14245, s = 2849
Costs of criminal justice system	$1,445 (270)	Normal	μ = 1445, s = 270
Costs of motor vehicle accidents	$8,581 (1,716)	Normal	μ = 8581, s = 1716
Costs of incarceration	$34,710 (9,235)	Normal	μ = 34710, s = 9235
	Quality-of-life valuations		
Disutility of adverse events	See Appendix Table 8		
Disutility of being incarcerated	−0.075 (0.004)	Beta	a = 325, b = 4010
	Probabilities		
Pr (arrested | crime)	0.213 (0.123)	Beta	a = 2.13, b = 7.87
Pr (conviction | arrest)	0.338 (0.143)	Beta	a = 3.38, b = 6.62
Pr (release from jail or prison)	0.430 (0.149)	Beta	a = 4.3, b = 5.7

(continued)

Appendix Table 12 Age-specific prevalence of 12-months AUD and the number of the affected population

Age group	Prevalence of 12 months AUD	US population (millions)	Number of the affected population (millions)	Number of the population that seeks treatment* (millions)
20 ≤ age ≤ 29	16.2%	42.7	6.92	1.01
30 ≤ age ≤ 44	9.7%	61.0	5.92	0.86
45 ≤ age ≤ 64	5.4%	81.5	4.40	0.64
65 ≤ age	1.4%	40.3	0.56	0.08
Total	–	–	17.8	2.59

*Estimated based on a previous study that reported only 14.6% of individuals who met lifetime criteria for an AUD reported ever having received alcohol treatment (Cohen et al. 2007).

Source: Hasin et al. (2007); Age and Sex Composition: 2010. US Census Bureau, 2010 Census. http://www.census.gov/prod/cen2010/briefs/c2010br-03.pdf

The State-transition Model

(i.e., Using remission rates at the end of 16 weeks treatment to specify initial distributions of the AUD/LRD states, then use the treatment group-specific relapse rates for the 1-year post-treatment, then follow the natural history model)

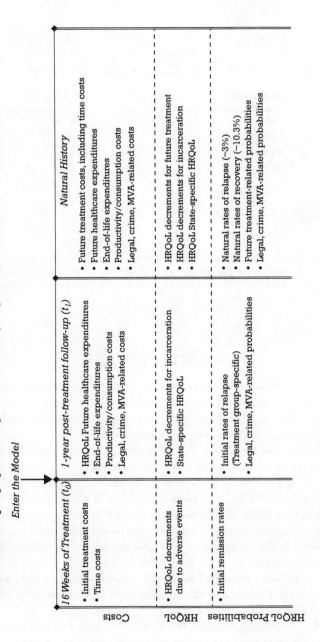

Appendix Figure 1 Relevant model parameters based on the time horizon.
Abbreviations: AUD = alcohol use disorder; LRD = low-risk drinking or abstinence; MVA = motor vehicle accident; HRQoL = health-related quality of life.

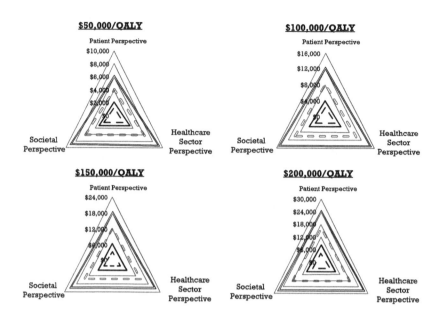

Appendix Figure 2 Incremental net monetary benefit (NMB) of AUD treatment.

Notes: Each treatment strategy was directly compared to "CBI Only" at a range of various willingness-to-pay thresholds. Abbreviations: QALY = quality-adjusted life years; CBI = combined behavioral intervention; MM = medical management.

5 REFERENCES

Agency for Healthcare Research and Quality. 2015. "Medical Expenditure Panel Survey (MEPS). Using Appropriate Price Indices for Analyses of Health Care Expenditures or Income Across Multiple Years." Last Modified April 3, 2015. Accessed March 4, 2016. http://meps.ahrq.gov/about_meps/Price_Index.shtml.

American Psychiatric Association. 2013. *Diagnostic and Statistical Manual of Mental Disorders*. 5th ed. Arlington, VA: American Psychiatric Publishing.

Anton, R. F., S. S. O'Malley, D. A. Ciraulo, R. A. Cisler, D. Couper, D. M. Donovan, D. R. Gastfriend, J. D. Hosking, B. A. Johnson, J. S. LoCastro, R. Longabaugh, B. J. Mason, M. E. Mattson, W. R. Miller, H. M. Pettinati, C. L. Randall, R. Swift, R. D. Weiss, L. D. Williams, A. Zweben, and the COMBINE Study Research Group. 2006. Combined pharmacotherapies and behavioral interventions for alcohol dependence: the COMBINE study: a randomized controlled trial. *JAMA* 295 (17):2003–2017.

Arias, E. 2014. "United States Life Tables, 2009." In *Natl Vital Stat Rep*. vol 62 no 7. Hyattsville, MD: National Center for Health Statistics. http://www.cdc.gov/nchs/data/nvsr/nvsr62/nvsr62_07.pdf.

Barrett, B., S. Byford, M. J. Crawford, R. Patton, C. Drummond, J. A. Henry, and R. Touquet. 2006. Cost-effectiveness of screening and referral to an alcohol health worker in alcohol misusing patients attending an accident and emergency department: a decision-making approach. *Drug Alcohol Depend* 81 (1):47–54.

Blincoe, L. J., T. R. Miller, E. Zaloshnja, and B. A. Lawrence. 2015. *The Economic and Societal Impact of Motor Vehicle Crashes, 2010. (Revised).* (Report No. DOT HS 812 013).

Washington, DC: National Highway Traffic Safety Administration. www-nrd.nhtsa.dot. gov/Pubs/812013.pdf.

Bouchery, E. E., H. J. Harwood, J. J. Sacks, C. J. Simon, and R. D. Brewer. 2011. Economic costs of excessive alcohol consumption in the U.S., 2006. *Am J Prev Med* 41 (5):516–524.

Bouza, C., M. Angeles, A. Munoz, and J. M. Amate. 2004. Efficacy and safety of naltrexone and acamprosate in the treatment of alcohol dependence: a systematic review. *Addiction* 99 (7):811–828.

Bray, J. W., G. A. Zarkin, W. R. Miller, D. Mitra, D. R. Kivlahan, D. J. Martin, D. J. Couper, and R. A. Cisler. 2007. Measuring economic outcomes of alcohol treatment using the Economic Form 90. *J Stud Alcohol Drugs* 68 (2):248–255.

Briggs, A., K. Claxton, and M. Sculpher. 2006. *Decision Modelling for Health Economic Evaluation.* Oxford: Oxford University Press.

Bureau of Labor Statistics. 2015. *Employer Costs for Employee Compensation Historical Listing: March 2004-March 2015.* Washington, DC: Bureau of Labor Statistics. National Compensation Survey. www.bls.gov/ncs/ect/sp/ececqrtn.pdf.

Caetano, R., and C. Cunradi. 2002. Alcohol dependence: a public health perspective. *Addiction* 97 (6):633–645.

Carson, E. A., and D. Golinelli. 2013. *Prisoners in 2012: Trends in Admissions and Releases, 1991-2012.* Washington, DC: US Department of Justice. www.bjs.gov/content/pub/pdf/p12tar9112.pdf.

Chong, C. A., S. Li, G. C. Nguyen, A. Sutton, M. H. Levy, T. Butler, M. D. Krahn, and H. H. Thein. 2009. Health-state utilities in a prisoner population: a cross-sectional survey. *Health Qual Life Outcomes* 7:78.

Chou, S. P., D. A. Dawson, F. S. Stinson, B. Huang, R. P. Pickering, Y. Zhou, and B. F. Grant. 2006. The prevalence of drinking and driving in the United States, 2001-2002: results from the National Epidemiological Survey on Alcohol and Related Conditions. *Drug Alcohol Depend* 83 (2):137–146.

Christensen, A., and A. Callahan. 2013. Medicare Spending and Care Intensity at the End of Life Increases, While Time in the Hospital Declines: New Findings Show Longitudinal Change for Care Provided to Chronically Ill Medicare Patients. Lebanon, NH: The Dartmouth Institute for Health Policy & Clinical Practice. www.dartmouthatlas.org/downloads/press/EOL_release_061213.pdf.

Cohen, E., R. Feinn, A. Arias, and H. R. Kranzler. 2007. Alcohol treatment utilization: findings from the National Epidemiologic Survey on Alcohol and Related Conditions. *Drug Alcohol Depend* 86 (2-3):214–221.

Dawson, D. A., R. B. Goldstein, W. J. Ruan, and B. F. Grant. 2012. Correlates of recovery from alcohol dependence: a prospective study over a 3-year follow-up interval. *Alcohol Clin Exp Res* 36 (7):1268–1277.

Dawson, D. A., and B. F. Grant. 2011. The "gray area" of consumption between moderate and risk drinking. *J Stud Alcohol Drugs* 72 (3):453–458.

Dawson, D. A., F. S. Stinson, S. P. Chou, and B. F. Grant. 2008. Three-year changes in adult risk drinking behavior in relation to the course of alcohol-use disorders. *J Stud Alcohol Drugs* 69 (6):866–877.

Dunlap, L. J., G. A. Zarkin, J. W. Bray, M. Mills, D. R. Kivlahan, J. R. McKay, P. Latham, and J. S. Tonigan. 2010. Revisiting the cost-effectiveness of the COMBINE study for alcohol dependent patients: the patient perspective. *Med Care* 48 (4):306–313.

Federal Bureau of Investigation. 2013. Crime in the United States, 2012. US Department of Justice. www.fbi.gov/about-us/cjis/ucr/crime-in-the-u.s/2012/crime-in-the-u.s.-2012.

Fleming, M. F., M. P. Mundt, M. T. French, L. B. Manwell, E. A. Stauffacher, and K. L. Barry. 2002. Brief physician advice for problem drinkers: long-term efficacy and benefit-cost analysis. *Alcohol Clin Exp Res* 26 (1):36–43.

Fleurence, R. L., and C. S. Hollenbeak. 2007. Rates and probabilities in economic modelling: transformation, translation and appropriate application. *Pharmacoeconomics* 25 (1):3–6.

Glaze, L. E., and E. J. Herberman. 2013. *Correctional Populations in the United States, 2012.* Washington, DC: US Department of Justice. www.bjs.gov/content/pub/pdf/cpus12.pdf.

Hasin, D. S., F. S. Stinson, E. Ogburn, and B. F. Grant. 2007. Prevalence, correlates, disability, and comorbidity of DSM-IV alcohol abuse and dependence in the United States: results from the National Epidemiologic Survey on Alcohol and Related Conditions. *Arch Gen Psychiatry* 64 (7):830–842.

Henrichson, C., and R. Delaney. 2012. *The Price of Prisons: What Incarceration Costs Taxpayers.* New York: Vera Institute of Justice. vera.org/sites/default/files/resources/downloads/price-of-prisons-updated-version-021914.pdf.

Kaplan, M. S., N. Huguet, D. Feeny, B. H. McFarland, R. Caetano, J. Bernier, N. Giesbrecht, L. Oliver, P. Ramage-Morin, and N. A. Ross. 2014. The association between alcohol use and long-term care placement among older Canadians: a 14-year population-based study. *Addict Behav* 39 (1):219–224.

Kline-Simon, A. H., D. E. Falk, R. Z. Litten, J. R. Mertens, J. Fertig, M. Ryan, and C. M. Weisner. 2013. Posttreatment low-risk drinking as a predictor of future drinking and problem outcomes among individuals with alcohol use disorders. *Alcohol Clin Exp Res* 37 Suppl 1:E373–E380.

Kline-Simon, A. H., C. M. Weisner, S. Parthasarathy, D. E. Falk, R. Z. Litten, and J. R. Mertens. 2014. Five-year healthcare utilization and costs among lower-risk drinkers following alcohol treatment. *Alcohol Clin Exp Res* 38 (2):579–586.

Kranzler, H. R., and A. Gage. 2008. Acamprosate efficacy in alcohol-dependent patients: summary of results from three pivotal trials. *Am J Addict* 17 (1):70–76.

Kranzler, H. R., and J. Van Kirk. 2001. Efficacy of naltrexone and acamprosate for alcoholism treatment: a meta-analysis. *Alcohol Clin Exp Res* 25 (9):1335–1341.

Lee, B. B., M. T. King, J. M. Simpson, M. J. Haran, M. R. Stockler, O. Marial, and G. Salkeld. 2008. Validity, responsiveness, and minimal important difference for the SF-6D health utility scale in a spinal cord injured population. *Value Health* 11 (4):680–688.

Mann, K., P. Lehert, and M. Y. Morgan. 2004. The efficacy of acamprosate in the maintenance of abstinence in alcohol-dependent individuals: results of a meta-analysis. *Alcohol Clin Exp Res* 28 (1):51–63.

Mason, B. J. 2003. Acamprosate and naltrexone treatment for alcohol dependence: an evidence-based risk-benefits assessment. *Eur Neuropsychopharmacol* 13 (6):469–475.

McCarthy, K. 2013. Number of Jail Deaths at Lowest Recorded Level During 2011. Washington, DC: Bureau of Justice Statistics. www.bjs.gov/content/pub/press/mljsp0011pr.cfm.

Miller, T. R., D. T. Levy, M. A. Cohen, and K. L. Cox. 2006. Costs of alcohol and drug-involved crime. *Prev Sci* 7 (4):333–342.

Mokdad, A. H., J. S. Marks, D. F. Stroup, and J. L. Gerberding. 2004. Actual causes of death in the United States, 2000. *JAMA* 291 (10):1238–1245.

Morgan, M. Y., F. Landron, P. Lehert, and the New European Alcoholism Treatment Study Group. 2004. Improvement in quality of life after treatment for alcohol dependence with acamprosate and psychosocial support. *Alcohol Clin Exp Res* 28 (1):64–77.

Mullahy, J., and J. L. Sindelar. 1991. *Alcoholism, Work, and Income Over the Life Cycle: Working Paper No. 3909, NBER Working Papers Series*. Cambridge, MA: National Bureau of Economic Research. www.nber.org/papers/w3909.pdf.

Noonan, M. E., and S. Ginder. 2014. *Mortality in Local Jails and State Prisons, 2000-2012: Statistical Tables*. Washington, DC: US Department of Justice. Bureau of Justice Statistics. www.bjs.gov/content/pub/pdf/mljsp0012st.pdf.

Ormel, J., M. VonKorff, T. B. Ustun, S. Pini, A. Korten, and T. Oldehinkel. 1994. Common mental disorders and disability across cultures. Results from the WHO Collaborative Study on Psychological Problems in General Health Care. *JAMA* 272 (22):1741–1748.

Oslin, D. W., H. Pettinati, and J. R. Volpicelli. 2002. Alcoholism treatment adherence: older age predicts better adherence and drinking outcomes. *Am J Geriatr Psychiatry* 10 (6):740–747.

Palmer, A. J., K. Neeser, C. Weiss, A. Brandt, S. Comte, and M. Fox. 2000. The long-term cost-effectiveness of improving alcohol abstinence with adjuvant acamprosate. *Alcohol Alcohol* 35 (5):478–492.

Parhar, K. K., J. S. Wormith, D. M. Derkzen, and A. M. Beauregard. 2008. Offender coercion in treatment: a meta-analysis of effectiveness. *Criminal Justice and Behavior* 35 (9):1109–1135.

Petrie, D., C. Doran, A. Shakeshaft, and R. Sanson-Fisher. 2008. The relationship between alcohol consumption and self-reported health status using the EQ5D: evidence from rural Australia. *Soc Sci Med* 67 (11):1717–1726.

Pollack, M. F., F. W. Purayidathil, S. C. Bolge, and S. A. Williams. 2010. Patient-reported tolerability issues with oral antidiabetic agents: Associations with adherence; treatment satisfaction and health-related quality of life. *Diabetes Res Clin Pract* 87 (2):204–210.

Rehm, J., D. Dawson, U. Frick, G. Gmel, M. Roerecke, K. D. Shield, and B. Grant. 2014. Burden of disease associated with alcohol use disorders in the United States. *Alcohol Clin Exp Res* 38 (4):1068–1077.

Roerecke, M., and J. Rehm. 2013. Alcohol use disorders and mortality: a systematic review and meta-analysis. *Addiction* 108 (9):1562–1578.

Samokhvalov, A. V., S. Popova, R. Room, M. Ramonas, and J. Rehm. 2010. Disability associated with alcohol abuse and dependence. *Alcohol Clin Exp Res* 34 (11):1871–1878.

Sattar, S. P., P. R. Padala, D. McArthur-Miller, W. H. Roccaforte, S. P. Wengel, and W. J. Burke. 2007. Impact of problem alcohol use on patient behavior and caregiver burden in a geriatric assessment clinic. *J Geriatr Psychiatry Neurol* 20 (2):120–127.

Schadlich, P. K., and J. G. Brecht. 1998. The cost effectiveness of acamprosate in the treatment of alcoholism in Germany. Economic evaluation of the Prevention of Relapse with Acamprosate in the Management of Alcoholism (PRAMA) Study. *Pharmacoeconomics* 13 (6):719–730.

Smit, F., J. Lokkerbol, H. Riper, M. C. Majo, B. Boon, and M. Blankers. 2011. Modeling the cost-effectiveness of health care systems for alcohol use disorders: how implementation of eHealth interventions improves cost-effectiveness. *J Med Internet Res* 13 (3):e56.

Tax Policy Center. 2013. "Table T13-0174. Average Effective Federal Tax Rates by Filing Status; by Expanded Cash Income Percentile, 2014" http://www.taxpolicycenter.org/numbers/displayatab.cfm?DocID=3933.

UKATT Research Team. 2005a. Cost effectiveness of treatment for alcohol problems: findings of the randomised UK alcohol treatment trial (UKATT). *BMJ* 331 (7516):544.

UKATT Research Team. 2005b. Effectiveness of treatment for alcohol problems: findings of the randomised UK alcohol treatment trial (UKATT). *BMJ* 331 (7516):541.

US Census Bureau. 2012. "Table 345. State and Local Government Expenditures Per Capita by Criminal Justice Function and State: 2007." In *Statistical Abstract of the United States*. www.census.gov/compendia/statab/2012/tables/12s0345.pdf.

US Department of Justice. 2014. *United States Attorneys' Annual Statistical Report: Fiscal Year 2013*. US Department of Justice. www.justice.gov/usao/reading_room/reports/asr2013/13statrpt.pdf.

US Food and Drug Administration. 2013. FDA Statement on Clinical Trials for Drugs to Potentially Treat Alcoholism. US Food and Drug Administration. www.fda.gov/Drugs/DrugSafety/ucm369499.htm.

Volk, R. J., S. B. Cantor, J. R. Steinbauer, and A. R. Cass. 1997. Alcohol use disorders, consumption patterns, and health-related quality of life of primary care patients. *Alcohol Clin Exp Res* 21 (5):899–905.

World Health Organization. 2014. *Global Status Report on Alcohol and Health*. Geneva: World Health Organization. www.who.int/substance_abuse/publications/global_alcohol_report/msb_gsr_2014_1.pdf.

Ye, Y., and W. C. Kerr. 2011. Alcohol and liver cirrhosis mortality in the United States: comparison of methods for the analyses of time-series panel data models. *Alcohol Clin Exp Res* 35 (1):108–115.

Zarkin, G. A., J. W. Bray, A. Aldridge, M. Mills, R. A. Cisler, D. Couper, J. R. McKay, and S. O'Malley. 2010. The effect of alcohol treatment on social costs of alcohol dependence: results from the COMBINE study. *Med Care* 48 (5):396–401.

Zarkin, G. A., J. W. Bray, A. Aldridge, D. Mitra, M. J. Mills, D. J. Couper, R. A. Cisler, and the COMBINE Cost-Effectiveness Research Group. 2008. Cost and cost-effectiveness of the COMBINE study in alcohol-dependent patients. *Arch Gen Psychiatry* 65 (10):1214–1221.

Zarkin, G. A., L. J. Dunlap, K. A. Hicks, and D. Mamo. 2005. Benefits and costs of methadone treatment: results from a lifetime simulation model. *Health Econ* 14 (11):1133–1150.

Appendix B

Worked Example 2: The Cost-Effectiveness of Home Palliative Care for Patients at the End of Life

Ba' Pham and Murray Krahn

PART 1: JOURNAL ARTICLE

Structured Abstract

Objective: To evaluate the cost-effectiveness of home palliative care (HPC) for end-of-life (EOL) patients.

Interventions: In the usual care (UC) strategy, patients receive acute and palliative care from primary care physicians and community-based services. In the combined HPC+UC strategy, patients identified with an EOL prognosis in their last year of life received additional palliative services by an interdisciplinary team, coordinated by a palliative advanced practice nurse and delivered to the patient's home.

Target Population: Patients approaching EOL following characteristic trajectories of clinical and functional decline due to terminal illness, organ failure, and frailty (average 76 years of age), and their primary family caregivers (average 56 years of age).

Perspectives: Payer (Ontario Ministry of Health and Long-Term Care), healthcare sector, and societal perspectives.

Time Horizon: The last year of life of the target population.

Discount Rates: Costs and health outcomes were not discounted, as the analysis was limited to 1 year.

Costing Year: 2014 Canadian dollars (C$).

Study Design: Cost-utility analysis using a state-transition microsimulation model.

Data Sources: Systematic reviews evaluating the effectiveness of HPC for patients with advanced illnesses, population-based data from linked health administrative databases, and additional literature searches.

Outcome Measures: Mean costs, mean quality-adjusted life years (QALYs), incremental costs, incremental QALYs, and incremental cost per QALY. Health outcomes included dying at home, days at home, and health-related quality of life (HRQoL) spillover effects on the family primary caregivers.

Results of Base-Case Analysis: The mean duration of HPC services was 239 days for HPC patients, with a mean cost of C$4,430 per patient. The model predicted that HPC patients were 5% more likely than UC patients to die at home; stayed on average 6 more days at home; and experienced fewer emergency department (ED) visits, fewer hospitalizations, and shorter intensive care unit (ICU) length of stay (LOS). The model also predicted that the time costs of unpaid caregiving and non-medical household spending increased when patients spent more time at home.

From the payer perspective, the predicted mean cost for the UC strategy was approximately C$49,000, and the predicted mean health outcome was 0.60 QALYs. The HPC+UC strategy was a dominant strategy, with an incremental cost saving of C$2,275 and an incremental health gain of 0.002 QALYs. The probability that the HPC+UC strategy was cost-effective was 64% (65%) at a cost-effectiveness threshold of C$50k (C$100k) per QALY. The cost-effectiveness analysis (CEA) results from the healthcare sector perspective were similar to those from the payer perspective.

From the societal perspective, the mean cost was approximately C$107,000 for the UC strategy. The HPC+UC strategy was a dominant strategy, with an incremental cost saving of C$1,054. The probability that the HPC+UC strategy was cost-effective was 59% (60%) at a cost-effectiveness threshold of C$50k (C$100k) per QALY.

Results of Uncertainty Analyses: The CEA results were sensitive to the HPC effects on survival time, ED visits, and hospital LOS. The results were also sensitive to the daily cost of HPC services, and to estimates of acute care resource utilization according to the UC strategy, including daily costs of hospital stays, ICU LOS, and hospital LOS.

Given the clinical evidence from a recent systematic review evaluating the HPC effects in patients with advanced illnesses, the HPC+UC strategy was likely to be cost-effective if the HPC program was associated with the reported average reduction in the use of acute care resources, including fewer ED visits and hospitalizations and shorter hospital and ICU LOS.

Limitations: The decision model was structured according to EOL patterns from a retrospective cohort of decedents in Ontario. Health utility estimates were based on multi-attribute instruments that inadequately assess domains relevant to the EOL experience, including domains pertaining to quality of life, quality of care, and quality of dying. Improving QALYs may not be fully consistent with the intended aim of palliative care interventions, which tend to focus on comfort care and quality of death rather than prolonging life.

Conclusions: Our results suggest that a policy of providing comprehensive HPC services by an interdisciplinary team to patients identified with an EOL prognosis in current practice is likely to be cost-effective. The results also indicate the potential to increase the caregiving burden to the family, as patients are likely to remain longer at home. EOL program development should consider and potentially mitigate caregiver effects, in addition to considering the resource and health effects associated with patient care.

1 Introduction

Providing high-quality, compassionate, and affordable care at the end of life (EOL) is growing internationally in importance as a health policy priority. The EOL is the time when individuals live with an advanced illness from which they will not stabilize or recover, and from which they will eventually die (Lorenz et al. 2008). It is not limited to the period immediately before death, and it may encompass the months leading up to death.

With the population aging, the number of people requiring EOL care is expected to grow. Most dying people are old and suffer from cardiovascular diseases, cancers, chronic respiratory diseases, dementia, diabetes, and chronic renal disease, among other conditions (GBD 2013 Mortality and Causes of Death Collaborators 2015). While these chronic debilitating conditions may impose several years of intensive treatment and functional limitation, patients' care preferences significantly change from aggressive approaches toward more holistic approaches at the EOL. Palliative care at the EOL focuses on improving comfort and quality of life for the patient and caregivers. Multiple services are required to support EOL patients and their families. Managing the balance between acute and palliative care during EOL in a way that is consistent with the wishes and preferences of the patient is challenging.

"Dying in a favorite place" is one of the important aspects that define a good death (Miyashita et al. 2007). The majority of people prefer to die at home, but most ended up dying in hospital (Gomes et al. 2013b; Gomes et al. 2011; Gomes et al. 2012). Illness-related factors (e.g., longer survival, less complex care needs), individual factors (e.g., personal preferences, cultural factors), and environmental factors (e.g., caregiver support, financial support) are possible determinants influencing the preference for home as the place of death (Murray et al. 2009). Family members report that quality of life is significantly better for patients who die at home compared to those who die in hospitals (Kinoshita et al. 2015; Wright et al. 2010). In addition, patients who die in hospitals are more likely to undergo aggressive, costly, and often unnecessary diagnostic tests and interventions (Goodman et al. 2011; Ho et al. 2011).

The societal cost for providing EOL care is substantial. For example, approximately 25% of all Medicare payments in the United States are directed to care in the last year of life of beneficiaries (Riley and Lubitz 2010). In Ontario, the estimated annual healthcare cost of EOL care for cancer patients was C$544 million in 2002 and 2003 (Walker et al. 2011). Family members also experience substantial out-of-pocket (OOP) expenses and productivity loss due to caregiving time (Pivodic et al. 2014). In the mid-2000s, the annual economic contribution of unpaid caregivers of EOL patients was estimated to be approximately C$26 billion in Canada, US$354 billion in the United States, and £87 billion in the UK (Hollander, Liu, and Chappell 2009).

Various palliative care models have been developed and tested for acute, home, and residential care settings (Luckett et al. 2014). Home palliative care (HPC) is a model that considers the patient and family preferences for the place of dying; timely assessment of physical, psychosocial, and spiritual needs of the patient; and adequate provision of care to the home. Key components of the HPC model include the delivery of specialized palliative care by an interdisciplinary team, communication and coordination of care by a single team member in charge of the care for the patient, advance care planning, and training and education for the patient and family (Luckett et al. 2014).

A recent systematic review by Gomes et al. (2013a) compares a combination of HPC plus usual care (UC) with UC alone (e.g., including primary or specialist care at home, hospital care, and in some instances palliative or hospice care). According to the results, HPC doubles the odds of dying at home. It reduces patients' symptom burden and has no negative effect on caregiver grief (Gomes et al. 2013a; Gomes, Calanzani, and Higginson 2014). Results concerning the effects of HPC on patients' pain, physical function, and quality of life were inconclusive (Gomes et al. 2013a). In addition, the evidence on the cost-effectiveness of HPC was inconclusive.

The aim of the present study was to evaluate the cost-effectiveness of HPC by an interdisciplinary team to improve EOL care for patients and their families. This work was commissioned by Health Quality Ontario in support of policy development to improve EOL care in Ontario, and was conducted with the support and guidance of the Health Quality Ontario End-of-Life Expert Panel (OHTAC End-of-Life Collaborative 2014).

2 METHODS

2.1 Study Design

We conducted a cost-utility analysis using a state-transition, microsimulation model. The analysis considered quality-adjusted life years (QALYs) of the patient, as well as a "spillover" measurement that captured the collateral effects of the patient's illness on the health-related quality of life (HRQoL) of the family primary caregiver (hereafter the "family HRQoL spillover effect"). It was conducted according to the recommendations of the Second Panel on Cost-Effectiveness in Health and Medicine, including Reference Case analyses based on a healthcare sector perspective and a societal perspective. The analysis was also conducted from the perspective of the Ontario Ministry of Health and Long-Term Care (payer perspective), which follows current Canadian guidelines on cost-effectiveness analysis (Canadian Agency for Drugs and Technologies in Health [CADTH] 2006).

The healthcare sector perspective considered medical costs covered by the public health insurance in Ontario (including those unrelated to EOL care) and OOP costs related to medical care incurred by the patient and family (e.g., care-related travel expenses, insurance payments). The societal perspective additionally valued the time costs of caregiving by family members, and non-medical household spending when the patient was cared for at home. Costs are expressed in 2014 Canadian dollars (C$) and were inflated to 2014 values using the health component of the Statistics Canada Consumer Price Index for Health and Personal Care (Chai et al. 2014).

2.2 Target Population

The target population is EOL patients and their families (Qaseem et al. 2008). We included patients who tend to follow characteristic patterns of clinical and functional decline as they approach the EOL, including the following trajectories: terminal illness, organ failure, and illnesses associated with frailty (ICD-10 codes for grouping assignment of EOL trajectories are given in Appendix Table 1) (Lunney, Lynn, and Hogan 2002). Patients with terminal illness (e.g., cancer) often die after a steep functional decline in the last weeks or months (Teno et al. 2001). Patients with organ failure (e.g., heart and lung) tend to become weak, with intermittent serious exacerbations, making the timing of their death unpredictable (Fox et al. 1999). Patients with frailty and dementia usually decline slowly (Knaus et al. 1995).

Our analysis took into account the uncertainties regarding how to define the EOL and how to identify EOL patients. In practice, EOL can be defined as having a fatal condition, risking death with the next exacerbation, or patients beginning to acknowledge the risk of death (Lorenz et al. 2008). Waiting for near-certainty would fail to identify most dying people (Selby et al. 2011). Various approaches are used to identify EOL patients. For example, prognostic tools usefully characterize subpopulations (e.g., heart failure), but many patients with fatal conditions have substantial probabilities for 2- or 6-month survival, even in their last week of life (Fox et al. 1999). The "surprise" question ("Would I be surprised if this patient died in the next year?") is widely used as a screening tool, albeit with limited testing (Della Penna 2001; Moss et al. 2008; Moss et al. 2010; You et al. 2014). In our cost-effectiveness analysis (CEA), we dealt with these uncertainties by characterizing the target population using population-based data.

We selected a target population of patients who died due to terminal illness, organ failure, and frailty from linked health administrative databases at the Ontario Institute for Clinical Evaluation Sciences (ICES) (Tanuseputro et al. 2015). The last year of life was defined as a reasonable time horizon that is likely to capture the consequences of EOL interventions (Gomes et al. 2009). Under the UC setting, we defined an identifiable EOL patient as a decedent who had received one or more palliative services during their last year of life. We assumed that identifiable EOL patients could be considered as candidates for the HPC program. The EOL phase was defined from the time when these patients received the first palliative service up until death. The start of the EOL phase was therefore stochastic and empirically determined (below).

2.3 Intervention Strategies

- *UC strategy:* UC consisted of standard services to meet the needs of patients and followed Ontario Community Care Access Centre guidelines for home care criteria (Seow et al. 2010). These services included various amounts and levels of home, acute, primary, and palliative care services according to the population-based patterns observed in the ICES data (Tanuseputro et al. 2015). Home care generally includes nursing, personal support, and homemaking services. Access to palliative care is through family physicians, although referral generally occurs in the last few months of life or not at all (Klinger et al. 2013). Palliative care services are provided in hospitals, complex continuing care facilities, residential hospices, or are delivered to the home, with considerable variation in available services by care settings (Johnson et al. 2009; Towns et al. 2012).

- *HPC+UC strategy:* Patients in the HPC+UC strategy receive HPC services in addition to UC. The HPC program we evaluated is a home-based program designed to provide services with the primary intent of enhancing comfort, managing symptoms, and improving quality of life (Klinger et al. 2013). It offers pain management and other comfort care in the patient's home, and it is designed with features intended to increase timely referral and access to the program, including systematic and timely identification of EOL patients, needs assessment, coordinated care by a palliative advanced practice nurse (APN), 24/7 access to a palliative care consultation for symptom management, and psycho-spiritual and bereavement care.

The HPC program uses an interdisciplinary team approach, with the core team consisting of the patient, family, APN, a physician, and a social worker, all with expertise in palliative care (Klinger et al. 2013). Additional team members (e.g. a spiritual counselor, chaplain, or bereavement coordinator) join the core team in service provision as needed. The team is responsible for coordinating and managing care across all settings. They assess the physical, medical, psychological, social, and spiritual needs of the patient and family. Advanced care planning is provided, with an emphasis on involving patients and family in making informed decisions and choices about goals of care. Patients and families are trained in the use of medications, self-management skills, and crisis intervention in the home, with the goal of stabilizing the patient and minimizing excessive emergency department (ED) visits and acute care admissions.

Identifiable EOL patients (i.e., those who received palliative care services under UC) were considered for additional HPC services. Other EOL patients received UC. In other words, the scope of the CEA was to assess the cost-effectiveness of providing additional HPC services to identifiable EOL patients under UC, and not to estimate the impact of expanding HPC to the broader population of all patients in the target population.

2.4 Impact Inventory

As recommended by the Second Panel on Cost-Effectiveness in Health and Medicine, we used an Impact Inventory to consider the potential impacts of the HPC program in terms of consequences that fall within and outside of the healthcare sector (Table 1). Within the formal healthcare sector, we quantified the HPC impacts on health (e.g., increase in patient's time at home and QALYs), family HRQoL spillover effect, and medical costs (including costs of HPC services, acute care utilization, and care-related OOP expenses). For the societal perspective, which includes other sectors in addition to the healthcare sector, we estimated the costs of additional time lost from paid work, household work, and leisure by family caregivers (Chai et al. 2014), and the non-medical household spending when the patient stayed longer at home (Stajduhar 2013). We also considered the opportunity costs of time lost to illness (and traveling

Table 1 Impact Inventory

Sector	Type of impact (list category within each sector with unit of measure if relevant)	Included in this analysis from … perspective?			Notes on sources of evidence
		Payer	Healthcare sector	Societal	
	Formal healthcare sector				
Health	*Health outcomes (effects)*				
	Longevity effects, days	✓	✓	✓	See Methods
	Health-related quality of life effects, QALYs	✓	✓	✓	
	Chance of dying at home, % dying at home	✓	✓	✓	
	Time at home, days at home	✓	✓	✓	
	HRQoL spillover effect,[†] QALYs	✓	✓	✓	
	Quality of death	✗	✗	✗	See Discussion
	Satisfaction with care received	✗	✗	✗	See Discussion
	Medical costs				
	Paid for by third-party payers, $	✓	✓	✓	Covered by Ontario Ministry of Health and Long-Term Care (OMHLTC)*
	Paid for by patients out-of-pocket		✓	✓	
	Future related medical costs (payers and patients)	✗	✗	✗	Not applicable to EOL population
	Future unrelated medical costs (payers and patients)	✗	✗	✗	Not applicable to EOL population
	Informal healthcare sector				
HEALTH	Patient time costs			✗	See Methods
	Unpaid caregiver time costs, $			✓	
	Transportation costs, $			✓	

(continued)

Table 1 Continued

Sector	Type of impact (list category within each sector with unit of measure if relevant)	Included in this analysis from . . . perspective?			Notes on sources of evidence
		Payer	Healthcare sector	Societal	
Non-healthcare sectors (with examples of possible items)					
PRODUCTIVITY	Labor market earnings/ productivity, $			✓	
	Cost of lost productivity due to illness and to seeking and receiving care			✗	See Discussion
CONSUMPTION	Cost of non-medical household expenses for the patient, $			✓	
SOCIAL SERVICES	Cost of social services as part of HPC‡			✗	See Methods
LEGAL/ CRIMINAL JUSTICE	None				
EDUCATION	None				
HOUSING	None				
ENVIRONMENT	None				

*Including costs of primary care, ED visits, hospitalization, outpatient visits, complex continuing care, long-term care, home care, palliative care, physician services, diagnostic and laboratory tests, prescription drugs, and medical devices, among others.

†A disutility associated with the collateral effects of the patient's illness on the quality of life of the primary family caregiver to be combined with the patient's utility as an additional component of the total QALYs.

‡Only included costs of social services provided on an as-needed basis as part of the services provided by the interdisciplinary HPC team (see Section 2.3 under Intervention Strategies).

to, seeking, and waiting for care), quality of death, and satisfaction with care. Because of a lack of supporting data, we were not able to quantify these impacts; they are qualitatively assessed in the Discussion (see Section 4).

2.5 Model Structure

Figure 1 outlines the model structure, with a set of health states that are defined by the physical location of the patients and the healthcare they received. The locations included in the model are home, nursing home, hospital ward, and residential hospice. As needed, patients may receive home, nursing home, and acute care. Patients could start out at home, with or without home care, or in a nursing home. They could visit an ED and could be admitted to a hospital and an intensive care unit (ICU). Identifiable EOL patients were transitioned to corresponding health states in which they received a combination

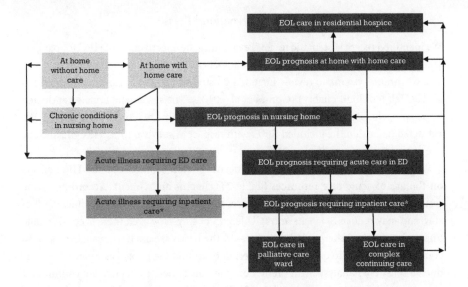

Figure 1 Structure of the state-transition model for end of life (EOL) patients.

* Simulated events related to inpatient care included time spent in general wards and intensive care units (ICUs), with different implications in costs and health utility (e.g., higher costs and lower health utility for ICU time compared to ward time).

Notes: Dark boxes represent health states for patients identified with a palliative prognosis. Light boxes represent health states in which patients are at home or in a long-term care facility. The remaining boxes represent patients receiving ED or hospital care for acute conditions. Possible transitions are denoted by arrows and no transitions occur otherwise. At the start of the last year of life, patients were distributed into the health states according to an observed population-based distribution (see Table 2). Abbreviation: ED = emergency department.

of curative and palliative care. In the weeks prior to death, they might get transferred to palliative care wards, complex continuing care facilities, or residential hospices.

At the beginning of the last year of life, simulated patients were distributed among the health states according to a distribution that was observed for a cohort of decedents in Ontario, including patients who started out with an EOL prognosis. Those without an EOL prognosis might eventually be identified with such a prognosis according to a distribution of how decedents in the cohort had received palliative care services. The timing of an EOL prognosis depends on the care setting (i.e., home, nursing home, and acute care) and the time to death (e.g., in the last 3 months of life). In the HPC+UC strategy, only identifiable EOL patients in the target population received additional HPC services; those without an identifiable EOL prognosis received UC.

The model simulated an event pathway for each individual patient through a series of transitions across health states, with a cycle length of 1 day. Model transitions were assumed to depend on care setting and the number of days prior to the date of death. Simulated patients were assumed to die at the last day in the last year of life. The decision model was implemented in TreeAge Pro 2015 (TreeAge Software Inc.).

2.6 Model Inputs

We derived model inputs from systematic reviews evaluating the effectiveness of HPC, linked health administrative databases, and additional literature searches.

2.6.1 Intervention Effects

We identified recent systematic reviews evaluating the effectiveness of HPC for patients with advanced illness (Gomes et al. 2013a; OHTAC End-of-Life Collaborative 2014). The Cochrane systematic review included 23 studies (16 randomized controlled trials [RCTs], 6 of high quality) (Gomes et al. 2013a). The systematic review conducted by Health Quality Ontario included 10 RCTs (Health Quality Ontario 2014). We extracted data from the included RCTs with respect to survival time, HRQoL, and the use of acute care resources.

We used a random-effects model to derive pooled estimates of the HPC effects on the use of acute care resources (Table 2) (Higgins and Green). According to the results in Table 2, HPC significantly reduces hospital admission and hospital length of stay, and may reduce ED visits and ICU length of stay. However, there is considerable uncertainty around the pooled estimates. In the base case analysis, we used the 95% confidence intervals to quantify the uncertainty around the pooled estimates. We conducted sensitivity analysis with prediction intervals to better quantify the within- and between-study variation (Dias et al. 2013; Higgins, Thompson, and Spiegelhalter 2009)

We could not derive a pooled estimate of the HPC effect on survival time, because of the variation in how the related data were reported in the included RCTs (Gomes et al. 2013a). Because the aim of the HPC program is to improve symptom management and quality of life, and not to prolong life, we assumed that the program has no effect on survival time. Sensitivity analysis was conducted to assess the impact of this assumption on the CEA results. Similarly, we could not estimate the HPC effect on patients' HRQoL from the reported data.

2.6.2 Population-Based Model Inputs

Linked health administrative databases maintained at ICES were used to estimate rates and conditional probabilities of transitions between health states from the final 12 months of data on a cohort of 256,284 Ontarians who were ≥18 years of age and died between April 1, 2009, and March 31, 2012. The average age of the target population was 76 years. The average age for the primary family caregiver was estimated to be 56 years.

Table 2 displays the initial distribution of patients into the health states, including 17% who were identifiable EOL patients because they had received one or more palliative services before the last year of life. Figure 2 summarizes the patterns of palliative care services. Between 26% and 52% of decedents did not receive any palliative care services in the last year of life. Among those who did receive those services, they were likely to receive them in the last few months prior to death. Based on these patterns, we estimated the probability that a simulated patient was identified with an EOL prognosis according to care setting and time to death.

Table 2 also displays estimates of transition rates (e.g., ED visits per 1,000 person-months), conditional probabilities (e.g., inpatient care admission from EDs, ICU admission from general wards), and hospital and ICU LOS in the 12 months before

Table 2 Model input estimates

Parameter	Base-case value (range or standard error)	Distribution	Sources
HPC effects on acute care utilization	**HPC versus UC**		
ED visit—Pooled rate ratio estimate (95% CI)	0.87 (0.70, 1.08)	Log normal	Aiken et al. (2006); Brumley et al. (2007); Hughes et al. (1992); Zimmer, Groth-Juncker, and McCusker (1985)
ED visit—95% predicted interval of rate ratio estimate	(0.27, 2.73)	Log normal	Hughes et al. (1992); Jordhoy et al. (2000); McCorkle et al. (2000); Rabow et al. (2004); Zimmer, Groth-Juncker, and McCusker (1985)
Hospital admission—Pooled relative risk estimate (95% CI)	0.81 (0.67, 0.98)	Log normal	
Hospital admission – 95% predicted interval of relative risk estimate	(0.45, 1.45)	Log normal	
Hospital LOS (days)—Pooled difference estimate (95% CI)	−2.88 (−5.24, −0.52)	Normal	Hughes et al. (1992); Jordhoy et al. (2000); McCorkle et al. (2000); Rabow et al. (2004); Zimmer, Groth-Juncker, and McCusker (1985)
Hospital LOS (days) - 95% predicted interval of LOS difference	(−11.89, 6.13)	Normal	Hughes et al. (1992)
ICU LOS (days)—LOS difference estimate (95% CI)	−0.32 (−0.83, 1.01)	Normal	
Initial distribution of patients to health states	**Percent estimate**	Fixed	ICES data*
At home without home care	51.07%		
At home with home care	17.34%		
EOL prognosis at home with home care	9.41%		
Chronic conditions in nursing home	13.91%		
EOL prognosis in nursing home	6.66%		

(continued)

Table 2 Continued

Parameter	Base-case value (range or standard error)	Distribution	Sources
Acute illness requiring ED care	0.22%		
EOL prognosis requiring acute care in ED	0.04%		
Acute illness requiring inpatient care	0.15%		
EOL prognosis requiring inpatient care	0.03%		
EOL care in complex continuing care (CCC)	1.17%		
Transition from home at 12 months before death[§]	*Mean (standard error)*		
Daily rate of ED visits per 1,000 person-days	3.69 (0.70)	Gamma	ICES data*
Probability of inpatient admission from ED	0.46 (0.08)	Beta	ICES data*
Probability of ICU admission from general ward	0.15 (0.02)	Beta	ICES data*
Daily rate of home care admission per 1,000 person-days	7.96 (2.63)	Gamma	ICES data*
Daily rate of nursing home admission per 1,000 person-days	0.10 (0.06)	Gamma	ICES data*
Transition from nursing home in the 12 months before death[§]			
Daily rate of ED visits per 1,000 person-days	1.99 (0.47)	Gamma	ICES data*
Probability of inpatient admission from ED	0.43 (0.03)	Beta	ICES data*
Probability of ICU admission from general ward	0.07 (0.05)	Beta	ICES data*
Hospital length of stay (LOS) for patients admitted from home			
Hospital LOS (days)	14.16 (26.35)	Gamma	ICES data*
ICU LOS (days)	7.31 (19.40)	Gamma	ICES data*

Hospital LOS for patients admitted from a nursing home			
Hospital LOS (days)	9.35 (16.07)	Gamma	ICES data*
ICU LOS (days)	5.36 (4.37)	Gamma	ICES data*
Transition involving patients with EOL prognosis[§]			
Probability of transferring from general ward to palliative care ward (PCW)	0.52 (0.08)	Beta	Estimated (Towns et al. 2012)
Probability of transferring from general ward to CCC	0.05 (0.04)	Beta	Estimated (Towns et al. 2012)
Probability of transferring from general ward to residential hospice	0.09 (0.03)	Gamma	Estimated (Towns et al. 2012)
LOS (days) in PCW, CCC or residential hospice	21.8 (24.0)	Gamma	Local CCC[†]
Health utility			
Base health utility for patients with palliative prognosis	Profile over time	Fixed	Van den Hout (2006); van den Hout et al. (2006); van den Hout et al. (2003)
Health utility for patients at home without home care	0.68 (0.20)	Log normal	Wodchis, Hirdes, and Feeny (2003)
Health utility for patients at home with home care	0.55 (0.23)	Log normal	Wodchis, Hirdes, and Feeny (2003)
Health utility for patients in a nursing home	0.37 (0.17)	Log normal	Thein et al. (2010)
Health disutility of recurrent events involving acute care			
Disutility associated with an ED visit	−0.014 (0.0015)	Normal	Church et al. (2012)
Disutility associated with a hospital stay	−0.06 (0.085)	Normal	Ghatnekar et al. (2013)
Disutility associated with an ICU stay	−0.108 (0.022)	Normal	Dinglas et al. (2013)

(continued)

Table 2 Continued

Parameter	Base-case value (range or standard error)	Distribution	Sources
	Health disutility for family HRQoL spillover effect[‡]		
Base case estimate	−0.056 (0.02)	Normal	Davidson, Krevers, and Levin (2008)
Alternative estimate	−0.104 (n/a)	Normal	Prosser et al. (2015)
Alternative estimate (positive spillover)	0.015 (0.007)	Normal	Wittenberg, Ritter, and Prosser (2013)
	Direct medical costs at 12 months before death		
Daily cost of HPC services	18.47 (25.86)	Gamma	Klinger et al. (2013)
Cost of ED visit	520 (388)	Gamma	ICES data[*]
Cost of a hospital day	846 (1,201)	Gamma	ICES data[*]
Cost of an ICU day	644 (223)	Gamma	ICES data[*]
Cost of a CCC day	560 (722)	Gamma	Local CCC[†]
Cost of a day in a residential hospice	376 (484)	Gamma	Stukel et al. (2012)
Cost of a day in a palliative care ward	592 (841)	Gamma	ICES data[*]
Home care cost per day[**]	34 (36)	Gamma	ICES data[*]
Long-term care cost per day[**]	91 (11)	Gamma	ICES data[*]
Cost of rehabilitation per day[**]	3.09 (0.95)	Gamma	ICES data[*]
Cost of outpatient visit per day[**]	8.67 (0.99)	Gamma	ICES data[*]
Cost of primary care physician per day[**]	14.05 (14.37)	Gamma	ICES data[*]
Cost of drugs or medical devices per day[**]	9.58 (0.36)	Gamma	ICES data[*]
Other cost per day[††]	1.38 (0.08)	Gamma	ICES data[*]
Health-related out-of-pocket expenses[#]	2.47 (1.61)	Gamma	Chai et al. (2014); Guerriere et al. (2010)

Costs of caregiving by family at 12 months before death			
Daily cost of time lost from housework & leisure	195.37 (46.01)	Gamma	Chai et al. (2014); Guerriere et al. (2010)
Daily costs of time lost from paid work	8.54 (2.01)	Gamma	Chai et al. (2014); Guerriere et al. (2010)
Ratio of costs of caregiving when a patient was at home relative to when patient was in a hospital or nursing home	0.5 (0.10)	Beta	Alzheimer Society of Ontario (2005)
Non-medical household (NMHH) expenses			
Average annual NMHH expense	$21,363 (1,199)	Gamma	Government of Canada. 2016a; 2016b
Ratio of NMHH expenses when a patient was in a hospital or nursing home relative to when patient was at home	0.5 (0.10)	Beta	Assumption

*Population-based estimates from linked health administrative databases at the Institute for Clinical Evaluation Sciences in Toronto for a cohort of 256,284 Ontarians who were ≥ 18 years of age and who died between April 1 2009 and March 31 2012.

§In the state-transition model, transition rates were assumed to be a function of time to death and to be the same for patients with or without EOL prognosis. Daily transition rate estimates for each of the 12 months in the last year of life were used in the model.

†Bridgepoint Active Healthcare facility (a complex continuing care facility) in Toronto (personal communication, Mr. Michael Gekas, Director of Ambulatory Care and Business Operations, December 16, 2013).

‡The family HRQoL spillover effect was assumed to apply to the primary family caregiver.

#The OOP expenses included care-related travel expenses, payments for household help, healthcare consultations, health insurance payments, payments for medications, and the costs of care-related supplies and equipment.

††Including the costs of laboratory billings and non-physician billings covered by the Ontario Health Insurance Plan. Daily estimates were derived by taking the average other costs of all decedents.

**Daily cost estimates were derived by taking the average cost of all decedents.

Abbreviations: UC = usual care; HPC = home palliative care; ED = emergency department; ICES = Institute for Clinical Evaluative Sciences; ICU = intensive care unit; CCC = complex continuing care; PCW = palliative care ward; HRQoL = health-related quality-of-life.

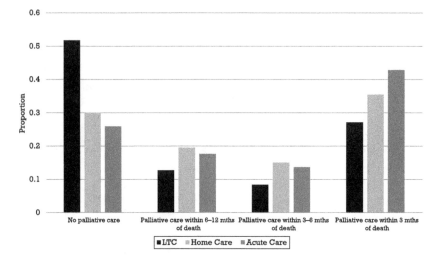

Figure 2 Patterns of palliative care services in the last year of life.
Notes: The patterns were derived from linked health administrative databases at the Institute for Clinical Evaluation Sciences for a cohort of 256,284 Ontarians ≥18 years of age who died between April 1 2009 and March 31 2012. The data were used to estimate the time-dependent probability that a patient was identified with an EOL prognosis.

the date of death. These estimates differed between patients admitted to inpatient care from home versus those admitted from a nursing home. Appendix Table 2 displays corresponding estimates at selected months in the last year of life, illustrating the increasing trend in some of these estimates in the months prior to death (e.g., rates of ED visit and admission to home care and long-term care). In the model we used time-dependent daily estimates for each of the 12 months prior to death.

2.6.3 Adjustments for HRQoL

We conducted literature searches to obtain health utility estimates. For patients with an EOL prognosis, average health utility decreases as the date of death approaches (Appendix Figure 1). This profile was constructed using data from a study including 1,454 cancer participants with a median life expectancy of 6 months who filled out the EQ-5D questionnaire weekly for 12 weeks and biweekly for another 28 weeks (van den Hout et al. 2006; van den Hout et al. 2003). The study authors derived the EQ-5D health utility estimates using community-based preferences representative of the general populations of the United States, UK, and Netherlands (personal communication, Dr. van den Hout, Leiden University Medical Centre, the Netherlands, March 2, 2015) (Van den Hout 2006). Health utility estimates were also derived using a power transformation of the EQ-5D visual analogue scores (VAS) (Stiggelbout et al. 1996). We used estimates for the US population in the CEA and conducted a sensitivity analysis with estimates from the transformed EQ-5D VAS scores.

Average health utility estimates for patients with chronic conditions prior to an EOL prognosis were obtained from a survey of utility scores in a community-dwelling population with chronic conditions. The survey used the Health Utility Index Mark 3 (HUI3) questionnaire for data collection and Canadian community-based preferences for deriving health utility estimates (Table 2) (Tam et al. 2013).

From the base health utility profile described above, we assumed that recurrent events in the model (including ED visits [average LOS of approximately 1 day], hospitalizations [average LOS of 21 days for hospitalizations that occurred in the 3 months prior to death], and ICU admission [average LOS of 12 days]) were associated with short-term disutility, calculated as 1 minus the health utility of the health state being valued (Table 2). Disutility estimates associated with time spent in these locations were obtained from studies that used the EQ-5D questionnaire in hospitalized patients (not specific to EOL conditions) and UK community-based preferences, including disutility associated with ED visit (−0.01), hospital stay (−0.06), and ICU stay (−0.11) (Church et al. 2012; Dinglas et al. 2013; Ghatnekar et al. 2013).

2.6.4 Family HRQoL Spillover Effects

Terminal illnesses may have large spillover effects on family members' health and well-being. Family members may experience a sense of helplessness and vulnerability, anxiety, and depression (Boyd et al. 2012; Tanuseputro et al. 2015). According to a systematic review of spillover effects, there is limited guidance regarding how to incorporate spillover effects into CEA (Wittenberg and Prosser 2013). Starting from the premise that illness affects more than just the patient, analyses can be framed on a multiple individual basis, including the patient plus an "other," and both individuals' costs and benefits. Alternately, an individual-based analysis would require the measurement of spillover alone, as an isolated quantity to be combined with the patient's health as an additional component of total QALYs. We used the latter approach in our analysis.

Within the individual-based analysis, the spillover effect could be negative if the family member's health utility is negatively affected by the ill patient, zero if no effect exists, and positive if there is an altruistic effect of providing care to an ill family member (Brouwer et al. 2005; Wittenberg, Ritter, and Prosser 2013). We used an estimate of −0.056, derived by assessing the EQ-5D health utility of relatives and comparing it to the health utility assessed using a hypothetical scenario in which the elderly patient was healthy and caregiving was not required (Table 2) (Davidson, Krevers, and Levin 2008). We conducted sensitivity analyses with an estimate of −0.10, derived from a national sample of US adults with direct health utility assessment (Prosser et al. 2015), and a positive spillover of 0.015, estimated using EQ-5D health utility scores from a US sample (Wittenberg, Ritter, and Prosser 2013).

2.6.5 Intervention Costs

Costs of HPC services were estimated from a micro-costing study of 95 palliative patients enrolled in a HPC program in Ontario over 15 months (Klinger et al. 2013). Averaged over the study period, HPC services cost approximately C$19 per patient per day, of which 61% was allocated for additional nursing services, 22% for medications, transportation, and equipment, and 6% for palliative care physician consultations.

2.6.6 Payer Medical Costs

Medical costs falling directly on the payer include costs of primary care, inpatient care, ED visits, outpatient visits, complex continuing care, nursing home care, home care, palliative care, physician services, diagnostic and laboratory tests, prescription drugs and medical devices, and non-physician services. Costs were obtained from an analysis of data from linked health administrative databases at ICES, which was conducted according to established guidelines on person-level costing using health administrative databases in Ontario (Tanuseputro et al. 2013; Tanuseputro et al. 2015).

Table 2 displays the cost estimates of direct medical care at the start of the last year of life. Appendix Table 3 displays cost estimates at selected months in the last year, illustrating the increasing trend in some of these estimates in the months preceding death. In the CEA, we used time-dependent daily cost estimates for each of the 12 months prior to death.

2.6.7 OOP Expenses and Costs of Unpaid Caregiving

Care provided by the family generally includes domestic chores and household tasks, personal care, help with activities of daily living, symptom management, and emotional and social support (Table 2). Estimates of unpaid care cost and OOP expenses were obtained from a Canadian study involving 169 caregivers of palliative cancer patients (Chai et al. 2014; Guerriere et al. 2010). The OOP expenses included care-related travel expenses, payments for household help, healthcare consultations, health insurance payments, payments for medications, and the costs of care-related supplies and equipment (Chai et al. 2014). Time lost from paid work was valued using average earnings matched by age and sex. Time lost from household work and leisure was valued according to estimated earnings of a homemaker. Estimated costs of time lost included estimates of employer-paid benefits, vacation days, and holidays. We used daily cost estimates derived from the monthly averages in Appendix Table 3.

Unpaid caregiving time has been reported to be almost double when patients are cared for at home rather than in other settings (Alzheimer Society of Ontario 2005). A 1:2 cost ratio of caregiving when patients were institutionalized in a hospital or nursing home relative to when they were at home was used in the base-case analysis (Table 2).

2.6.8 Non-Medical Household Expenses

There are limited data on household expenses to cover non-medical needs of an EOL patient, which may be substantial (Stajduhar 2013; Stajduhar et al. 2008). We used data from the 2013 Canadian Survey of Household Spending to estimate non-medical household expenses (Table 16.2). We assumed that non-medical household expenses were twice as high when patients were cared for at home as when they were in other care settings (e.g., nursing home, hospital).

2.6.9 Discounting

Cost and effectiveness outcomes were not discounted, as the analysis was limited to 1 year. For simplicity, discounting was not used in sensitivity analyses assessing differential survival time between strategies, which ran slightly more than 1 year.

2.7 Model Verification and Calibration

We verified modeled predictions against observed targets from the ICES data. The first targets were proportions of patients with at least one use of healthcare resources over the last year of life (e.g., emergency, home, hospital, long-term, and hospice care) (Tanuseputro et al. 2015). The second target was the physical location of death (i.e., home, hospital, nursing home, ED, or residential hospice). Model calibration was necessary to reduce discrepancies between the observed and predicted targets. The calibration varied the rates of ED visit, home care admission, nursing home admission, and the conditional probability of hospital admission from the ED. Calibration was conducted by applying a scaling factor to the monthly profile of each model input that was allowed to vary during the calibration process (Delorme et al. 2003). For example, the daily rates of ED visit (Appendix Table 3) were adjusted upward by 1.45 so that the predicted proportion of patients with at least one ED visit approached the observed proportion. We used one-way sensitivity analysis to derive the good-fit estimates of the scaling factors. Good-fit estimates were selected by visual inspection of the distance between the predicted and observed targets. Calibrated estimates of the scaling factors are summarized in Appendix Table 4.

2.8 Cost-Effectiveness Analysis

The projected health outcomes included the probability of dying at home, number of days at home, and QALYs. The projected economic outcomes included incremental costs, incremental QALYs, incremental cost per QALY, and incremental net monetary benefits (NMB) of the HPC+UC strategy relative to the UC strategy at a cost-effectiveness threshold of C$50k or C$100k per QALY.

2.9 Sensitivity Analysis

Results of the CEA were subjected to one-way sensitivity analysis (SA) and probabilistic sensitivity analysis (PSA). One-way SA was conducted to assess the impact of key assumptions and to verify the impact of varying model inputs across their plausible ranges (Table 2). The PSA was conducted with 10,000 random samples from input distributions, and the microsimulation model evaluated with 3,000 simulated patients.

3 RESULTS

3.1 Model Verification and Calibration

Results of the model verification are displayed in Appendix Figure 2 and Appendix Figure 3. Under UC and according to population-based data, approximately 80% of patients used emergency care in the last year of life, 60% used home care, 75% used hospital care, and 20% used nursing-home care (Appendix Figure 2). Approximately 46% of patients died at home (or in a nursing home), and 48% died in the hospital (Appendix Figure 3). In both figures, the predicted values from the model were close to the observed values from the population-based data.

3.2 Disaggregated Results

Home palliative care patients were 5% more likely than UC patients to die at home and stayed on average 6 more days at home (Table 3). The expected family HRQoL spillover effect was small and virtually the same for both strategies. The expected quality-adjusted life expectancy was 0.60 QALYs for UC patients and was slightly larger for HPC patients (an increase of 0.002 QALYs).

The expected per-patient cost of the HPC program was C$4,430 (Table 3). The program reduced ED visits (a reduction of 0.13 visits, at an expected saving of C$279 in ED visit costs), hospitalizations (a reduction of 0.21 hospital admissions and a reduction of 0.45 ICU admissions, at an expected saving of C$6,426 in hospital costs). From the payer perspective, the expected direct medical cost was C$49,467 for UC patients, and it was C$2,275 lower for HPC patients. From the healthcare sector perspective, the corresponding costs remained virtually unchanged because the expected OOP expenses were relatively small and were similar for UC and HPC patients.

Relative to the healthcare sector perspective, the expected cost from the societal perspective for UC patients was twice as large because the cost of unpaid caregiving was almost as large as the direct medical cost, and the non-medical household expense was also substantial (Table 3). The expected cost savings associated with the reduction in acute care resources with HPC services were offset by the increased costs of caregiving time and the additional non-medical household expenses incurred when patients stayed longer at home. The expected cost from the societal perspective was C$107,405 for UC patients, and it was C$1,054 less for HPC patients.

3.3 CEA Results

From the payer perspective and in the base case analysis, the HPC+UC strategy was associated with an incremental cost reduction of C$2,275 and very small incremental

Table 3 Disaggregated results

	UC Mean	HPC+UC Mean	Difference
Health outcomes (effects)			
Chance of dying at home	47%	52%	5%
Time spent at home in the last year of life (days)	337	343	6
Patient's QALYs	0.6142	0.6162	0.0020
Family HRQoL spillover effect—Change in QALYs	−0.0146	−0.0147	−0.0001
Total QALYs	0.5996	0.6015	0.0018
Costs—payer perspective			
Resources and costs that are affected by the HPC program			
Cost of HPC services	$0	$4,430	$4,430
ED visit (number of ED visits)	3.39	3.25	−0.13
ED cost	$1,111	$832	−$279
Hospitalization (number of hospitalizations)	2.96	2.75	−0.21
ICU admission (number of ICU admissions)	2.26	1.81	−0.45
Hospital cost	$26,577	$20,152	−$6,426
ICU cost[‡]	$6,583	$4,659	−$1,924
Other medical costs that are not affected by the HPC program	$21,778	$21,778	$0
Payer cost	$49,467	$47,192	−$2,275
Costs—healthcare sector perspective (additional costs)			
Out-of-pocket (OOP) expense	$539	$545	$6
Healthcare sector cost	$50,006	$47,737	−$2,269
Costs—societal perspective (additional costs)			
Family—Time lost from paid work due to caregiving	$1,887	$1,972	$85
Family—Time lost from leisure and household work due to caregiving	$42,631	$43,505	$874
Patients—Non-medical household expenses	$12,882	$13,138	$256
Societal cost	$107,405	$106,351	−$1,054

[‡] Estimated ICU cost as part of hospital cost.

Abbreviations: UC = usual care; HPC = home palliative care; QALY = quality-adjusted life year; HRQoL = health-related quality of life; ED = emergency department; ICU = intensive care unit; OOP = out-of-pocket.

QALYs gained per patient (Table 4). It was a dominant strategy, with an incremental NMB of C$2,366 (C$2,457) at a cost-effectiveness threshold of C$50k (C$100k) per QALY. At the C$50k (C$100k) threshold, the HPC+UC strategy was 64% (65%) likely to be more cost-effective than the UC strategy. Results from the healthcare sector perspective were virtually identical to those of the payer perspective. From the societal perspective, the HPC+UC strategy was again a dominant strategy, with an incremental NMB of C$1,145 (C$1,236). It was 59% (60%) likely to be more cost-effective than the UC strategy.

3.4 Results of Sensitivity Analyses

Home palliative care patients required services over a duration of 239 days, at a cost of C$4,430 per patient. From the societal perspective, the HPC+UC strategy remained a cost-effective strategy at a threshold of C$50k (C$100k) per QALY if the HPC daily cost per patient increased from the value of C$18.5 used in the base case analysis to C$23.1 (C$24.3) per patient. At the upper threshold cost of C$23.1 (C$24.3) per patient per day, the average cost per patient was C$5,521 (C$5,796). From the healthcare sector perspective, the corresponding upper threshold cost was C$25.4 (C$26.6) per patient per day, and the expected cost was C$6,071 (C$6,620) per patient.

From the societal perspective, the results were sensitive to the differential survival time between the strategies. Given a cost-effectiveness threshold of C$50k (C$100k) per QALY, if the survival time for HPC patients increased by ≤ 8.9 (12.2) days, the HPC+UC strategy was cost-effective; if the increase was > 8.9 (12.2) days, the HPC+UC strategy was not cost-effective. Conversely, if the survival time decreased for HPC patients (e.g., –5 days), the HPC+UC strategy was generally not cost-effective because the incremental QALYs were negative. From the healthcare sector perspective, the corresponding threshold for increasing survival time was 18.1 (19.3) days. Again, the HPC+UC strategy was generally not cost-effective if the HPC program was associated with a decrease in survival time.

The CEA results were not sensitive to different estimates of the health utility profile of patients nearing EOL or to family HRQoL spillover effects.

Figure 3 displays one-way sensitivity analyses from the societal perspective in the form of variation in the incremental NMB (at C$50k per QALY) of the HPC+UC strategy. Relative to the UC strategy and base-case values, the HPC+UC strategy was cost-effective if hospital cost was ≥ $832 per day, ICU length of stay was ≥ 6.0 days, hospital LOS was ≥ 12.3 days, the rate ratio of ED visit associated with HPC was ≤ 0.98, the reduction in hospital days associated with the HPC program was ≥ 0.7 days, and the ICU admission rate was ≥ 12.5%. The results were not sensitive to variation in other model inputs. The corresponding results when the incremental NMB was evaluated at a threshold of C$100k per QALY were similar (data not shown).

Appendix Figure 4 displays results of one-way sensitivity analyses from the healthcare sector perspective. Relative to the societal perspective, results from the healthcare sector perspective were less sensitive to variation in model inputs (base-case values in Table 2). Specifically, the HPC+UC strategy was cost-effective if the hospital cost was

Table 4 Cost-effectiveness analysis results

Perspective	UC		HPC+UC			HPC+UC vs UC			
	Cost♦	QALY	Cost*	QALY	ΔC	ΔQALY	ICER	INMB*	Acceptability†
Payer	$49,467	0.5996	$47,192	0.6015	−$2,275	0.0018	Dominant	$2,366/$2,457	0.64/0.65
Healthcare sector	$50,006	0.5996	$47,737	0.6015	−$2,269	0.0018	Dominant	$2,360/$2,451	0.64/0.65
Societal	$107,405	0.5996	$106,351	0.6015	−$1,054	0.0018	Dominant	$1,145/$1,236	0.59/0.60

*Incremental net monetary benefit was calculated at cost-effectiveness threshold of C$50k and C$100k per QALY, respectively.

†Probability that the HPC+UC strategy is more cost-effective than the UC strategy at thresholds of C$50k and C$100k per QALY.

♦Mean cost per patient.

Abbreviations: UC = usual care; HPC = home palliative care; QALY = quality-adjusted life year; ΔC = difference in the mean costs of the HPC+UC strategy relative to the UC strategy; ΔQALY = the respective difference in the mean QALYs; ICER = incremental cost-effectiveness ratio; INMB = incremental net monetary benefit.

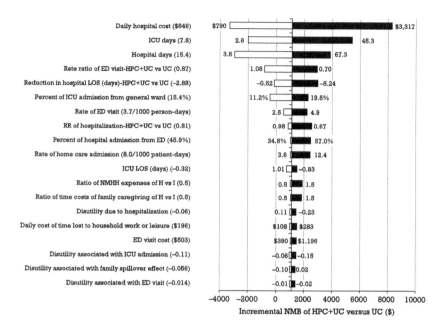

Figure 3 Results of one-way sensitivity analysis from the societal perspective.

Notes: The vertical axis displays individual variables included in the one-way sensitivity analysis, with the value used in the base case analysis displayed in parentheses. The horizontal axis displays variation in the incremental net monetary benefits (at a cost-effectiveness threshold of $50k per QALY) when an individual variable was varied from its lower to its upper values: the lower value is displayed to the left and the upper value to the right of the horizontal bar. Abbreviations: NMB = net monetary benefit; HPC = home palliative care; UC = usual care; ED = emergency department; ICU = intensive care unit; LOS = length of stay; H. vs I = home versus institutional setting (e.g., hospital, long-term care facility); NMHH expense = non-medical household expense.

≥ $823 per day, the ICU length of stay was ≥ 4.5 days, and the hospital length of stay was ≥ 7.3 days. The CEA results were not sensitive to the variation in other model inputs.

Appendix Figure 5 and Appendix Figure 6 display the cost-effectiveness plane from the probabilistic sensitivity analysis of the base case, which varied slightly whether confidence intervals (base case analysis) or prediction intervals (sensitivity analysis) were used to characterize the distributions of pooled estimates of the HPC effects on ED visits, hospital admission, hospital days, and ICU length of stay (Table 2). At a threshold of C$50k (100k) per QALY and with prediction intervals, the HPC+UC strategy was 53% (55%) likely to be more cost-effective than the UC strategy from the societal perspective. The corresponding value was 59% (61%) from the healthcare sector perspective.

4 DISCUSSION

The clinical evidence from recent systematic reviews indicates that for patients with advanced illness, HPC is associated with an increased chance of dying at home, fewer symptoms, and no change in caregiver grief (Gomes, Calanzani, and Higginson 2014; Health Quality Ontario 2014). Results from our CEA suggest that compared to the UC strategy, the HPC+UC strategy is likely to be a dominant strategy, with a very small improvement in the total QALYs of patients and their families, and a saving in costs from the societal, healthcare sector, and healthcare payer perspectives.

Our findings provide supporting economic evidence for a policy of increasing HPC services for EOL patients. For example, of the 87,000 patients who died every year in Ontario, approximately 45,000 patients could have been identified as candidates to receive additional HPC services in their last year of life. Those patients could have benefited from a comprehensive HPC program, including palliative care services that are co-ordinated and delivered to the home by a multidisciplinary team. Increasing access to this HPC program among patients who could be identified as approaching their EOL under current practice could improve their quality of life, free up acute care resources for other patients, and address the preferences of patients who wish to die at home (Gomes et al. 2013b).

4.1 Impact Inventory

We used the Impact Inventory (Table 1) recommended by the Second Panel on Cost-Effectiveness in Health and Medicine to consider all consequences that were deemed to be important regarding the impacts of the HPC program, especially impacts such as family caregiving time, non-medical household spending for the patient, and the family HRQoL spillover effect. Below, we discuss the impacts that could be quantified and other impacts that we could not quantify due to limited supporting data.

First, our CEA results were sensitive to the assumption that the HPC program has no effects on the survival time of EOL patients. The plausibility of this assumption rests on the observation that the HPC program is designed to provide services for pain management and symptom control, not to prolong life. There has been contrary evidence regarding the unintended effects of palliative care. In patients with metastatic non–small-cell lung cancer, for example, those receiving early palliative care integrated with standard oncology care, as compared with standard oncology care alone, had less aggressive care at the EOL phase and longer survival (11.6 months for early palliative care vs 8.9 months for usual care) (Temel et al. 2010). Similar effects have not, however, been reported for HPC for patients with advanced illness (Gomes et al. 2013a; Gomes, Calanzani, and Higginson 2014; Health Quality Ontario 2014). Among the 16 included RCTs in a recent systematic review, 7 reported survival data but none reported any significant survival differences between the interventions (Gomes et al. 2013a; Gomes, Calanzani, and Higginson 2014). We believe that large differences in survival time attributable to the HPC program we evaluated are unlikely.

According to the clinical evidence, HPC patients have fewer symptoms than UC patients (Gomes et al. 2013a; Gomes, Calanzani, and Higginson 2014). According to our modeled predictions, HPC patients are likely to stay longer at home. In the program we evaluated, HPC services are centrally coordinated and delivered directly to the patient's home. These aspects of the HPC program suggest that HPC services are likely to reduce the time spent seeking and receiving care. Because valuation of the time when patients are nearing their EOL is challenging, we could not quantify the impact of this time reduction in the disaggregated results of the CEA.

We derived health utility estimates using data obtained from multi-attribute instruments (i.e., EQ-5D and HUI3) assessing HRQoL domains that are generic to most diseases and conditions. It has been suggested that domains included in such generic multi-attribute health utility instruments are not sufficiently specific to capture aspects of the EOL experience, which generally involves subjective evaluation of the quality of life, quality of care, and quality of dying (Lo et al. 2009). In the EOL context, the quality of life construct generally encompasses domains related to the physical, psychological, social, spiritual, and existential experience. Quality of care incorporates all of the domains of the EOL experience, but it is focused on the extent to which healthcare structures and processes affect outcomes pertaining to these domains. Quality of dying incorporates these domains and also includes the nature of healthcare, life closure and death preparation, and the circumstances of death. For example, common aspects of a good death include freedom from pain and suffering, preferences about death preparation (e.g., death expected or not), and circumstances of death (e.g., home-death or in-hospital death). We postulate that some aspects of a good death are likely to be influenced by the HPC program, as the associated services increase the chance of dying at home (Gomes et al. 2013b; Gomes et al. 2012). Owing to a lack of supporting data, we were unable to quantify other impacts of the HPC program on the quality of dying and death.

The HPC effect on satisfaction with care is uncertain (Gomes et al. 2013a). Among the five RCTs included in a recent systematic review, two reported no statistically significant differences and three found significantly positive effects. Positive effects were reported for a hospital-based specialist HPC service in Norway (Jordhoy et al. 2000), and two HPC services in the United States (Brumley et al. 2007; Hughes et al. 1992). The HPC program we evaluated is structured similarly to one of the latter services (Brumley et al. 2007), including an interdisciplinary team, care co-ordination and management across all settings, training and education for patients and family, and as-needed additional support from social services. It is likely that the HPC program we evaluated has a positive effect on satisfaction with care for patients and families.

In terms of the burden to the family, we found that, compared to the UC strategy, the HPC+UC strategy was associated with increases in care-related OOP expenses, unpaid caregiving time by the family, non-medical household spending for the patient, and a slightly higher family HRQoL spillover effect. To assess the impact of the HPC program on the family HRQoL spillover effect in the CEA, we used an individual-based approach instead of a multiple-individual approach. The latter approach would have allowed us to explicitly incorporate the effects of the patient's illness on the health of family members. It has been reported that family caregivers experience a level of anxiety that is higher than the level of the dying patients (Grunfeld et al. 2004), and a level of depression that is much higher than that of the general population (Burge et al. 2008; Grunfeld et al. 2004). We believe that the impact of the HPC program on the health of the family could be larger than we were able to quantify. We therefore suggest that a policy of extending HPC services to EOL patients would need to provide additional support to the family.

4.2 Limitations

First, we assumed that an EOL prognosis was identified by the first palliative care service documented in the health administrative databases in the last year of life. However, the reliability of the procedure for identifying EOL patients through health administrative databases at ICES is still under evaluation (Tanuseputro P et al. 2013). We used QALYs to capture the effects of the HPC program on the combined outcome of HRQoL and survival time (Drummond et al. 2005). Improving QALYs, however, may not be fully consistent with the intended aim of palliative care interventions, which tend to focus on providing comfort care rather than prolonging life (Trotta 2007). The health utility estimates we used were derived using different instruments (i.e., EQ-5D and HUI3) and different community-based preferences (i.e., Canadian, United States, and UK). The health disutility estimates we used for health states related to ED visits, hospitalization, and ICU stay were derived for hospitalized patients but were not specific to EOL patients.

The retrospective cohort we used in the simulation model corresponds to a cohort of decedents in the linked health administrative databases. A prospective cohort approach, which better approximates real life, requires identifying patients with a palliative diagnosis and then following them forward until EOL. In analyses using health administrative databases, this relies on physician billing to identify patients with a palliative diagnosis, which is unlikely to be accurate (Tanuseputro P et al. 2013). A previous study examined both approaches and recommended the retrospective cohort approach for estimating patterns of care and healthcare costs for EOL patients (Tanuseputro P et al. 2013). Because most of the palliative care costs for EOL patients tend to occur in a few months prior to death, we believe that our findings are likely to be valid despite the limitations with the retrospective cohort approach.

4.3 Summary

The evidence supporting the cost-effectiveness of HPC in the literature is uncertain (Gomes et al. 2013a). Our findings are also not definitive, as the probability that the HPC+UC strategy was more cost-effective than the UC strategy varied around 60%. Nevertheless, we have shown that the HPC program is likely to be a dominant strategy resulting in cost savings from the payer, healthcare sector, and societal perspectives. Our results suggest that a policy of providing comprehensive HPC services by an interdisciplinary team to EOL patients is likely to be economically attractive. The results also indicate an increase in the caregiving burden when patients remain longer at home with the support of the HPC team, suggesting that the HPC program should include provision of services to support the family. The economic evidence from this study contributed to a recent policy recommendation by Health Quality Ontario that all patients approaching EOL have access to home palliative team care across multiple care settings (Seow et al. 2014).

PART 2: TECHNICAL APPENDIX

Appendix Table 1 ICD-10-CA codes used for Trajectory Group Assignment (Canadian Institute for Health Information 2011)

Trajectory group	Underlying cause of death code (ICD10CA)
Frailty	A02^, A03^, A04^, A08^, A09^, A37^, A48^, A49^, B01^, B02^, B37^, B95^, B96^, E4^, E5^, E60^, E61^, E62^, E63^, E64^, E86^, E87^, E97^, F00^, F01^, F02^, F03^, G20^, G21^, G22^, G23^, G24^, G25^, G26^, G30^, G31^, G32^, G35^, G36^, G37^, G81^, G82^, I21^, I25.0, I25.3, I25.4, I25.5, I25.6, I25.8, I25.9, I25I^, I69^, J00^, J01^, J02^, J03^, J04^, J05^, J06^, J10^, J11^, J12^, J13^, J14^, J15^, J16^, J18^, J20^, J21^, J22^, J69^, J80^, K59^, L89^, M00^, M01^, M02^, M03^, M05^, M06^, M07^, M08^, M09^, M11^, M12^, M13^, M14^, M15^, M16^, M17^, M18^, M19^, M32^, M33^, M34^, M35^, M36^, M41^, M42^, M43^, M45^, M46^, M80^, M81^, M82^, M83^, M84^, M85^, M91^, M92^, N30^, R54^, R63.3, R63.4
Terminal illness	B24^, C^, D1^, D2^, D3^, D40^, D41^, D42^, D43^, D44^, D45^, D46^, D47^, D48^, N18^
Organ failure	A15^, A16^, A17^, A18^, A19^, A50^, A51^, A52^, A53^, A80^, A81^, A86^, A87^, A88^, A89^, B15^, B16^, B17^, B18^, B19^, B90^, B91^, B92^, B93^, B94^, D5^, D6^, D70^, D71^, D72^, D73^, D74^, D75^, D76^, D77^, D80^, D81^, D82^, D83^, D84^, D86^, D89^, E00^, E01^, E02^, E03^, E04^, E05^, E06^, E07^, E10^, E11^, E12^, E13^, E14^, E15^, E16^, E2^, E30^, E31^, E32^, E33^, E34^, E35^, E65^, E66^, E67^, E68^, E70^, E71^, E72^, E73^, E74^, E75.0, E75.1, E75.2, E75.3, E75.4, E75.5, E75.6, E76^, E77^, E78^, E79^, E80^, E83^, E84^, E85^, E88^, F1^, G0^, G10^, G11^, G12^, G13^, G40^, G41^, G45^, G46^, G47^, G5^, G60^, G61^, G62^, G63^, G64^, G70^, G71^, G72^, G73^, G80^, G90^, G91^, G92^, G93^, G94^, G95^, H0^, H1^, H2^, H3^, H4^, H5^, H6^, H7^, H8^, H91^, H92^, H93^, H94^, H95^, I01^, I05^, I06^, I07^, I08^, I09^, I10^, I11^, I12^, I13^, I15^, I20^, I22^, I23^, I24^, I25.2, I26^, I27^, I28^, I3^, I4^, I50^, I51^, I52^, I60^, I61^, I62^, I63^, I64^, I65^, I66^, I67^, I68^, I70^, I71^, I72^, I73^, I74^, I77^, I78^, I79^, I8^, I95^, I97^, I98^, I99^, J30.0, J30.1, J30.2, J30.3, J30.4, J31.0, J31.1, J31.2, J32^, J33^, J34^, J35^, J36^, J37^, J38^, J40^, J41^, J42^, J43^, J44^, J45^, J47^, J60^, J61^, J62^, J63^, J64^, J65^, J66^, J67^, J68^, J70^, J81^, J82^, J84^, J85^, J86^, J90^, J91^, J92^, J93^, J94^, J96^, J98^, J99^, K0^, K10^, K11^, K12^, K13^, K14^, K20^, K21^, K22^, K23^, K25^, K26^, K27^, K28^, K29^, K30^, K31^, K35^, K36^, K37^, K38^, K40^, K41^, K42^, K43^, K44^, K45^, K46^, K50^, K51^, K52^, K55^, K56^, K57^, K58^, K60.0, K60.1, K60.2, K60.3, K60.4, K60.5, K61.0, K61.1, K61.2, K61.3, K61.4, K62^, K63^, K65^, K66^, K67^, K70^, K71^, K72^, K73^, K74.0, K74.1, K74.2, K74.3, K74.4, K74.5, K74.6, K75^, K76^, K77^, K80^, K81^, K82^, K83^, K85^, K86^, K90^, K92^, K93^, L00^, L01.0, L01.1, L02^, L03^, L04^, L05^, L08^, L10^, L11^, L12^, L13^, L14^, L20^, L21^, L22^, L23^, L24^, L25^, L26^, L27^, L28.0, L28.1, L28.2, L29^, L30^, L40^, L41^, L42^, L43^, L44^,

(continued)

Appendix Table 1 Continued

Trajectory group	Underlying cause of death code (ICD10CA)
	L45^, L50^, L51^, L52^, L53^, L54^, L70^, L71^, L72^, L73^, L74^, L93.0, L93.1, L93.2, L94^, L95.0, L97^, L98^, L99^, M10^, M22^, M23^, M24^, M25^, M30^, M31^, M47^, M48^, M49^, M51^, M73^, M79^, M86^, M87^, M88^, M89^, M90^, M93^, M94^, N00^, N01^, N02^, N03^, N04^, N05^, N06^, N07^, N08^, N10^, N11^, N12^, N13^, N14.0, N14.1, N14.2, N14.3, N14.4, N15^, N16^, N17^, N19^, N20^, N21^, N22^, N25^, N26^, N27^, N28^, N29^, N31^, N32^, N33^, N34.0, N34.1, N34.2, N34.3, N35^, N36^, N37^, N39^, N40^, N41^, N42^, N43^, N44^, N45^, N47^, N48^, N49^, N50^, N51^, N60^, N61^, N62^, N63^, N64^, N70^, N71^, N72^, N73^, N74^, N75^, N76^, N77^, N8^, N90^, N91^, N92^, N93^, N94^, N95^, N96^, Q00^, Q01^, Q02^, Q03^, Q04^, Q05^, Q06^, Q07^, Q10^, Q11^, Q12^, Q13^, Q14^, Q15^, Q16^, Q17^, Q18^, Q20^, Q21^, Q22^, Q23^, Q24^, Q25^, Q26^, Q27^, Q28^, Q3^, Q40^, Q41^, Q42^, Q43^, Q44^, Q45^, Q50^, Q51^, Q52^, Q53^, Q54^, Q55^, Q56^, Q6^, Q7^, Q8^, Q9^
Other	A00^, A01^, A05^, A06^, A07^, A20^, A21^, A22^, A23^, A24^, A25^, A26^, A27^, A28^, A30^, A31^, A32^, A33^, A34^, A35^, A36^, A38^, A39^, A40^, A41^, A42^, A43^, A44^, A46^, A54^, A55^, A56^, A57^, A58^, A59^, A60^, A63^, A64^, A65^, A66^, A67^, A68^, A69^, A70^, A71^, A74^, A75^, A76^, A77^, A78^, A79^, A82^, A85^, A91^, A92^, A93^, A94^, A95^, A96^, A97^, A98^, A99^, B00^, B03^, B04^, B05^, B06^, B07^, B08^, B09^, B25^, B26^, B27^, B30^, B33^, B34^, B35^, B36^, B38^, B39^, B4^, B5^, B6^, B7^, B80^, B81^, B82^, B83^, B85^, B86^, B87^, B88^, B89^, B97^, B99^, F04^, F05^, F06^, F07^, F09^, F20^, F21^, F22^, F23^, F24^, F25^, F28^, F29^, F30^, F31^, F32^, F33^, F34^, F38^, F39^, F40^, F41^, F42^, F43^, F44^, F45^, F48^, F50^, F51^, F52^, F53^, F54^, F55^, F59^, F6^, F7^, F8^, F9^, G43^, G83^, G96^, G97^, G98^, G99^, I00^, I02^, J17^, J39^, J95^, K91^, L55^, L56^, L57^, L58^, L59^, L60^, L61^, L62^, L63^, L64^, L65^, L66^, L67^, L68^, L80^, L81^, L82^, L83^, L84^, L85^, L86^, L87^, L88^, L90^, L91^, L92^, M20^, M21^, M40^, M50^, M53^, M54^, M60^, M61^, M62^, M63^, M65^, M66^, M67^, M68^, M70^, M71^, M72^, M75^, M76^, M77^, M95^, M96^, M99^, N46^, N97^, N98^, N99^, O00^, O01^, O02^, O03^, O04^, O05^, O06^, O07^, O08^, O10^, O11^, O12^, O13^, O14^, O15^, O16^, O21^, O22^, O23^, O24^, O25^, O26^, O28^, O29^, O30^, O31^, O32^, O33^, O34^, O35^, O36^, O40^, O41^, O42^, O43^, O44^, O45^, O46^, O47^, O48^, O6^, O70^, O71^, O72^, O73^, O74^, O75^, O8^, O90^, O91^, O92^, O95^, O96^, O97^, O98^, O99^, P00^, P01^, P02^, P03^, P04^, P05^, P06^, P07^, P08^, P10^, P11^, P12^, P13^, P14^, P15^, P2^, F35^, P36^, P37^, P38^, P39^, P5^, P60^, P61^, P70^, P71^, P72^, P73^, P74^, P75^, P76^, P77^, P78^, P80^, P81^, P82^, P83^, P90^, P91^, P92^, P93^, P94^, P95^, P96^, R0^, R1^, R20^, R21^, R22^, R23^, R25^, R26^, R27^, R28^, R29^, R3^, R4^, R50^, R51^, R52^, R53^, R55^, R56^, R57^, R58^, R59^, R60^, R61^, R62^, R63^, R64^, R65^, R66^, R67^, R68^, R69^, R7^, R8^, R90^, R91^, R92^, R93^, R94^, R98^, R99^, W00^, W01^, W02^, W04^, W05^, W06^, W07^, W08^, W09^, W10^, W18^, W19, Y4^, Y5^, Y6^, Y7^, Y8^, Y9^

Appendix Table 2 Transition rate estimates and hospital length of stay at selected months in the last year of life

| | Time to death | | | | | Distribution |
| | 12 months | 6 months | 3 months | 2 months | 1 month | |
	Mean (SE)	Mean (SE)	Mean (SE)	Mean (SE)	Mean (SE)	
Transitions from home						
Daily rate of ED visits per 1,000 person-days	3.69 (0.70)	4.98 (1.13)	9.56 (3.33)	14.04 (5.34)	37.26 (12.87)	Gamma
Probability of inpatient admission from ED	0.46 (0.08)	0.49 (0.08)	0.57 (0.09)	0.65 (0.09)	0.85 (0.06)	Beta
Probability of ICU admission from general ward	0.15 (0.02)	0.16 (0.03)	0.16 (0.05)	0.18 (0.07)	0.29 (0.15)	Beta
Daily rate of home care admission per 1,000 person-days	7.96 (2.63)	9.86 (3.18)	13.73 (4.98)	16.34 (6.54)	22.33 (10.97)	Gamma
Daily rate of nursing home admission per 1,000 person-days	0.10 (0.06)	0.13 (0.08)	0.19 (0.10)	0.25 (0.14)	0.29 (0.15)	Gamma
Transitions from nursing home						
Daily rate of ED visits per 1,000 person-days	1.99 (0.47)	2.36 (0.42)	3.84 (0.80)	5.67 (1.15)	15.39 (5.81)	Gamma
Probability of inpatient admission from ED	0.43 (0.03)	0.44 (0.05)	0.50 (0.05)	0.58 (0.05)	0.66 (0.02)	Beta
Probability of ICU admission from general ward	0.07 (0.05)	0.07 (0.05)	0.08 (0.04)	0.09 (0.01)	0.11 (0.01)	Beta
Hospital LOS for patients admitted from home						
Hospital LOS (days)	14.16 (26.35)	16.44 (27.38)	20.71 (22.63)	20.16 (15.96)	9.07 (7.19)	Gamma
ICU LOS (days)	7.31 (19.40)	8.60 (18.91)	11.83 (17.00)	11.73 (12.53)	5.54 (5.16)	Gamma
Hospital LOS for patients admitted from nursing homes						
Hospital LOS (days)	9.35 (16.07)	9.02 (11.39)	10.31 (10.62)	11.55 (9.83)	7.76 (5.51)	Gamma
ICU LOS (days)	5.36 (4.37)	4.93 (7.05)	6.68 (10.22)	7.21 (8.32)	4.98 (4.17)	Gamma

Note: All estimates were derived using summary data from the ICES data analysis. Daily transition rate estimates for each of the 12 months in the last year of life were used in the decision model.

Abbreviations: ED = emergency department; ICU = intensive care unit; LOS = length of stay; SE = standard error.

Appendix Table 3 Cost estimates at selected months in the last year of life

Type of care	Mean daily cost, C$ (SE)						Distribution
	12 months	6 months	3 months	2 months	1 Month		
Healthcare							
ED visit	520 (388)	554 (404)	630 (425)	684 (432)	807 (432)		Gamma
Hospital stay	846 (1,201)	803 (927)	829 (1,046)	824 (1,023)	820 (996)		Gamma
Home care (per day)*	34 (36)	37 (39)	45 (49)	49 (56)	63 (76)		Gamma
Long-term care (per day)*	91 (11)	92 (14)	94 (18)	94 (19)	107 (20)		Gamma
Rehabilitation (per day)*	3.09 (0.95)	0.49 (0.05)	0.49 (0.05)	0.49 (0.06)	0.38 (0.06)		Gamma
Outpatient visit (per day)*	8.67 (0.99)	10.21 (0.39)	9.44 (0.39)	8.72 (0.32)	8.40 (0.32)		Gamma
Physician visit (per day)*	14.05 (14.37)	9.37 (0.52)	7.95 (0.31)	7.66 (0.31)	7.34 (0.31)		Gamma
Drugs/devices (per day)*	9.58 (0.36)	8.62 (0.08)	8.46 (0.08)	8.19 (0.10)	8.17 (0.10)		Gamma
Other† (per day)*	1.38 (0.08)	1.42 (0.03)	1.37 (0.03)	1.32 (0.02)	1.30 (0.02)		Gamma
Unpaid caregiving by family members							
Out-of-pocket expenses#	2.47 (1.61)	26.59 (9.50)	25.82 (12.38)	20.36 (13.99)	24.70 (13.18)		Gamma
Time lost from paid work	8.54 (2.01)	14.42 (1.86)	20.06 (6.04)	20.87 (7.60)	30.91 (8.77)		Gamma
Time lost from housework & leisure	195.37 (46.01)	329.73 (42.57)	458.90 (138.20)	477.34 (184.21)	706.95 (226.77)		Gamma

Note: All estimates were derived using summary data from the ICES data analysis. Cost estimates for each of the 12 months in the last year of life were used in the state-transition model.

* Average daily cost across all decedents

† Including the costs of laboratory billings and non-physician billings covered by the Ontario Health Insurance Plan.

The OOP expenses included care-related travel expenses, payments for household help, healthcare consultations, health insurance payments, payments for medications, and the costs of care-related supplies and equipment.

Abbreviations: ED = emergency department; ICU = intensive care unit; LOS = length of stay; SE = standard error.

Appendix Table 4 Estimates of multiplying factors in the model calibration

Adjusting inputs	Factor estimate
Daily rate of ED visit	1.45
Probability of hospital admission from ED	1.67
Daily rate of home care admission	0.90
Daily rate of nursing home admission	1.55

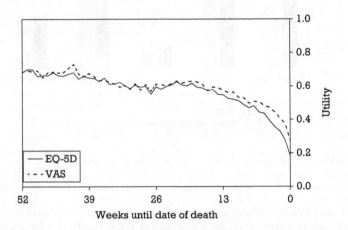

Appendix Figure 1 Mean EQ-5D health utility estimates and visual analog score (VAS)-transformed health utility scores among end of life patients as a function of time to date of death.
Notes: The mean health utility profile was constructed using data from a study including 1,454 cancer patients with a median life expectancy of 6 months who filled out the EQ-5D questionnaire weekly for 12 weeks and biweekly for another 28 weeks (van den Hout et al. 2006; van den Hout et al. 2003). The EQ-5D health utility estimates were derived using community-based preferences that are representative of the general populations of the United States (personal communication, Dr. van den Hout, Leiden University Medical Centre, the Netherlands, March 2, 2015; Van den Hout [2006]). The EQ-5D VAS-based health utility estimates were derived using a power transformation of the EQ-5D VAS (Stiggelbout et al. 1996).
Sources: Van den Hout (2006); van den Hout et al. (2006); van den Hout et al. (2003).

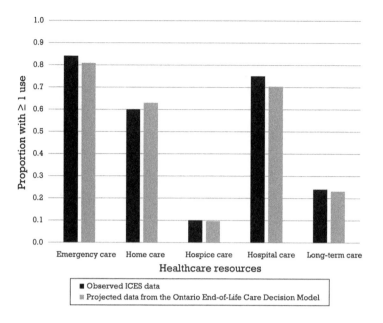

Appendix Figure 2 Observed and predicted use of healthcare resources.

Notes: Observed data were derived from linked health administrative databases at the Institute for Clinical Evaluation Sciences in Toronto for a cohort of 256,284 Ontarians who were ≥ 18 years of age and who died between April 1 2009 and March 31 2012.

Projected data were derived from the state-transition model. Hospice care includes ≥ 1 use of complex continuing care, palliative care wards, and residential hospice care. Abbreviation: ICES = Institute for Clinical Evaluative Sciences.

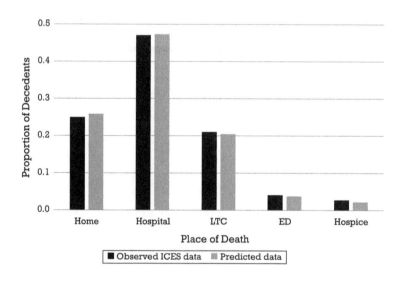

Appendix Figure 3 Observed and predicted place of death.

Notes: Observed data were derived from linked health administrative databases at the Institute for Clinical Evaluation Sciences in Toronto for a cohort of 256,284 Ontarians who were ≥ 18 years of age and who died between April 1 2009 and March 31 2012. Projected data were derived from the state-transition model. Abbreviation: ICES = Institute for Clinical Evaluative Sciences.

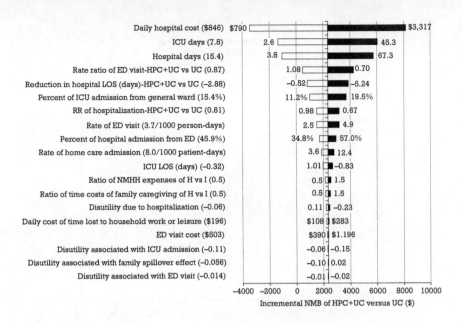

Appendix Figure 4. Results of one-way sensitivity analysis from the healthcare sector perspective
Notes: The vertical axis displays individual variables included in the one-way sensitivity analysis, with the value used in the base case analysis displayed in parentheses. The horizontal axis displays variation in the incremental net monetary benefits (at a cost-effectiveness threshold of $50k per QALY) when an individual variable was varied from its lower to its upper values: the lower value is displayed to the left and the upper value to the right of the horizontal bar. Abbreviations: NMB = net monetary benefit; HPC = home palliative care; UC = usual care; ED = emergency department; ICU = intensive care unit; LOS = length of stay; H. vs I = home versus institutional setting (e.g., hospital, long-term care facility); NMHH expense = non-medical household expense.

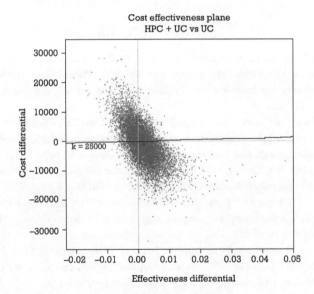

Appendix Figure 5 Cost-effectiveness plane from the societal perspective.
Notes: The horizontal axis displays the incremental QALYs and the vertical axis the incremental costs. Plotted data were from the probabilistic sensitivity analysis with 10,000 random samples from model input distributions (Table 2). For each of the random samples, the microsimulation model was evaluated with 3,000 simulated patients. Approximately 59% of the random samples fall below the cost-effectiveness threshold of C$50k per QALY.

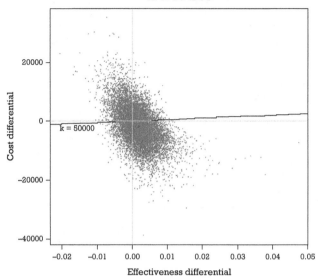

Cost effectiveness plane
HPC+UC vs UC

Appendix Figure 6 Cost-effectiveness plane from the health sector perspective.

Notes: The horizontal axis displays the incremental QALYs and the vertical axis the incremental costs. Plotted data were from the probabilistic sensitivity analysis with 10,000 random samples from model input distributions (Table 2). For each of the random samples, the microsimulation model was evaluated with 3,000 simulated patients. Approximately 64% of the random samples fall below the cost-effectiveness threshold of C$50k per QALY.

5 REFERENCES

Aiken, L. S., J. Butner, C. A. Lockhart, B. E. Volk-Craft, G. Hamilton, and F. G. Williams. 2006. Outcome evaluation of a randomized trial of the PhoenixCare intervention: program of case management and coordinated care for the seriously chronically ill. *J Palliat Med 9* (1):111–126.

Alzheimer Society of Ontario. 2005. A Profile of Ontario's Home Care Clients with Alzheimer's Disease or Other Dementias. http://www.alzheimer.ca/niagara/~/media/Files/on/PPPI%20Documents/Profile-of-Home-Care-Clients-April-2007.pdf.

Boyd, K., B. Kimbell, S. Murray, and J. Iredale. 2012. Living and dying well with end-stage liver disease: time for palliative care? *Hepatology 55* (6):1650–1651.

Brouwer, W. B., N. J. van Exel, B. van den Berg, G. A. van den Bos, and M. A. Koopmanschap. 2005. Process utility from providing informal care: the benefit of caring. *Health Policy 74* (1):85–99.

Brumley, R., S. Enguidanos, P. Jamison, R. Seitz, N. Morgenstern, S. Saito, J. McIlwane, K. Hillary, and J. Gonzalez. 2007. Increased satisfaction with care and lower costs: results of a randomized trial of in-home palliative care. *J Am Geriatr Soc 55* (7):993–1000.

Burge, F. I., B. J. Lawson, G. M. Johnston, and E. Grunfeld. 2008. A population-based study of age inequalities in access to palliative care among cancer patients. *Med Care 46* (12):1203–1211.

Canadian Agency for Drugs and Technologies in Health (CADTH). 2006. *Guidelines for the Economic Evaluation of Health Technologies: Canada.* 3rd ed. Ottawa: CADTH. https://www.cadth.ca/media/pdf/186_EconomicGuidelines_e.pdf.

Canadian Institute for Health Information. 2011. Health Care Use at the End of Life in Atlantic Canada. Ottawa: CIHI. Available from: https://secure.cihi.ca/estore/product-Series.htm?pc=PCC569.

Chai, H., D. N. Guerriere, B. Zagorski, and P. C. Coyte. 2014. The magnitude, share and determinants of unpaid care costs for home-based palliative care service provision in Toronto, Canada. *Health Soc Care Community 22* (1):30–39.

Church, J., S. Goodall, R. Norman, and M. Haas. 2012. The cost-effectiveness of falls prevention interventions for older community-dwelling Australians. *Aust N Z J Public Health 36* (3):241–248.

Davidson, T., B. Krevers, and L. A. Levin. 2008. In pursuit of QALY weights for relatives: empirical estimates in relatives caring for older people. *Eur J Health Econ 9* (3):285–292.

Della Penna, R. 2001. Asking the right question. *J Palliat Med 4* (2):245–248.

Delorme, J., S. Badin, A. G. Le Corroller, A. A. Auvrignon, M. F. Auclerc, V. Gandemer, P. Bordigoni, J. P. Lamagnere, F. Demeocq, Y. Perel, C. Berthou, F. Bauduer, B. Pautard, J. P. Vannier, D. Braguer, T. Leblanc, G. Leverger, A. Baruchel, and G. Michel. 2003. Economic evaluation of recombinant human granulocyte colony-stimulating factor in very high-risk childhood acute lymphoblastic leukemia. *J Pediatr Hematol Oncol 25* (6):441–447.

Dias, S., N. J. Welton, A. J. Sutton, and A. E. Ades. 2013. Evidence synthesis for decision making 5: the baseline natural history model. *Med Decis Making 33* (5):657–670.

Dinglas, V. D., J. M. Gifford, N. Husain, E. Colantuoni, and D. M. Needham. 2013. Quality of life before intensive care using EQ-5D: patient versus proxy responses. *Crit Care Med 41* (1):9–14.

Drummond, M. F., M. J. Sculpher, G. W. Torrance, B. J. O'Brien, and G. L. Stoddart. 2005. *Methods for the Economic Evaluation of Health Care Programmes.* 3rd ed. Oxford: Oxford University Press.

Fox, E., K. Landrum-McNiff, Z. Zhong, N. V. Dawson, A. W. Wu, and J. Lynn. 1999. Evaluation of prognostic criteria for determining hospice eligibility in patients with advanced lung, heart, or liver disease. SUPPORT Investigators. Study to Understand Prognoses and Preferences for Outcomes and Risks of Treatments. *JAMA 282* (17):1638–1645.

GBD 2013 Mortality and Causes of Death Collaborators. 2015. Global, regional, and national age-sex specific all-cause and cause-specific mortality for 240 causes of death, 1990-2013: a systematic analysis for the Global Burden of Disease Study 2013. *Lancet 385* (9963):117–171.

Ghatnekar, O., A. Bondesson, U. Persson, and T. Eriksson. 2013. Health economic evaluation of the Lund Integrated Medicines Management Model (LIMM) in elderly patients admitted to hospital. *BMJ Open 3* (1):e001563. doi:10.1136/bmjopen-2012-001563

Gomes, B., N. Calanzani, V. Curiale, P. McCrone, and I. J. Higginson. 2013a. Effectiveness and cost-effectiveness of home palliative care services for adults with advanced illness and their caregivers. *Cochrane Database Syst Rev 6*:CD007760.

Gomes, B., N. Calanzani, M. Gysels, S. Hall, and I. J. Higginson. 2013b. Heterogeneity and changes in preferences for dying at home: a systematic review. *BMC Palliat Care 12*:7.

Gomes, B., N. Calanzani, and I. J. Higginson. 2014. Benefits and costs of home palliative care compared with usual care for patients with advanced illness and their family caregivers. *JAMA 311* (10):1060–1061.

Gomes, B., J. Cohen, L. Deliens, and I. J. Higginson. 2011. "International Trends in Circumstances of Death and Dying Amongst Older People." In *Living with Ageing and Dying: Palliative and End of Life Care for Older People*, edited by M. Gott and C. Ingleton, 3–18. Oxford: Oxford University Press.

Gomes, B., R. Harding, K. M. Foley, and I. J. Higginson. 2009. Optimal approaches to the health economics of palliative care: report of an international think tank. *J Pain Symptom Manage 38* (1):4–10.

Gomes, B., I. J. Higginson, N. Calanzani, J. Cohen, L. Deliens, B. A. Daveson, D. Bechinger-English, C. Bausewein, P. L. Ferreira, F. Toscani, A. Menaca, M. Gysels, L. Ceulemans, S. T. Simon, H. R. Pasman, G. Albers, S. Hall, F. E. Murtagh, D. F. Haugen, J. Downing, J. Koffman, F. Pettenati, S. Finetti, B. Antunes, R. Harding, and Prisma. 2012. Preferences for place of death if faced with advanced cancer: a population survey in England, Flanders, Germany, Italy, the Netherlands, Portugal and Spain. *Ann Oncol 23* (8):2006–2015.

Goodman, D. C., A. R. Esty, E. S. Fisher, and C.- H. Chang. 2011. Trends and Variation in End-of-Life Care for Medicare Beneficiaries with Severe Chronic Illness. April 12, 2011. Lebanon (NH): The Dartmouth Institute for Health Policy & Clinical Practice. www.dartmouthatlas.org/downloads/reports/EOL_Trend_Report_0411.pdf.

Government of Canada. 2016a. Statistics Canada. Table 203-0026: Survey of household spending (SHS), household spending, by age of reference person. CANSIM (database). Available from: http://www5.statcan.gc.ca/cansim/a26?lang=eng&id=2030026.

Government of Canada. 2016b. Statistics Canada. Table 282-0002: Labour force survey estimates (LFS), by sex and detailed age group. CANSIM (database). Available from: http://www5.statcan.gc.ca/cansim/a26?lang=eng&id=2820002.

Grunfeld, E., D. Coyle, J. Whelan, J. Clinch, L. Reyno, C. C. Earle, A. Willan, R. Viola, M. Coristine, T. Janz, and R. Glossop. 2004. Family caregiver burden: results of a longitudinal study of breast cancer patients and their principal caregivers. *CMAJ 170* (12):1795–1801.

Guerriere, D. N., B. Zagorski, K. Fassbender, L. Masucci, L. Librach, and P. C. Coyte. 2010. Cost variations in ambulatory and home-based palliative care. *Palliat Med 24* (5):523–532.

Health Quality Ontario. 2014. Team-based models for end-of-life care: an evidence-based analysis. *Ont Health Technol Assess Ser [Internet] 14* (20):1–49. Available from: http://www.hqontario.ca/evidence/publications-and-ohtac-recommendations/ontario-health-technology-assessment-series/eol-team-based-models.

Higgins, J. P., S. G. Thompson, and D. J. Spiegelhalter. 2009. A re-evaluation of random-effects meta-analysis. *J R Stat Soc Ser A Stat Soc 172* (1):137–159.

Higgins, J. P. T., and S. Green, eds. 2011. *Cochrane Handbook for Systematic Reviews of Interventions*: Version 5.1.0 [updated March 2011]. The Cochrane Collaboration. Available from: www.cochrane-handbook.org.

Ho, T. H., L. Barbera, R. Saskin, H. Lu, B. A. Neville, and C. C. Earle. 2011. Trends in the aggressiveness of end-of-life cancer care in the universal health care system of Ontario, Canada. *J Clin Oncol 29* (12):1587–1591.

Hollander, M. J., G. Liu, and N. L. Chappell. 2009. Who cares and how much? The imputed economic contribution to the Canadian healthcare system of middle-aged and older unpaid caregivers providing care to the elderly. *Healthc Q 12* (2):42–49.

Hughes, S. L., J. Cummings, F. Weaver, L. Manheim, B. Braun, and K. Conrad. 1992. A randomized trial of the cost effectiveness of VA hospital-based home care for the terminally ill. *Health Serv Res 26* (6):801–817.

Johnson, A. P., T. Abernathy, D. Howell, K. Brazil, and S. Scott. 2009. Resource utilisation and costs of palliative cancer care in an interdisciplinary health care model. *Palliat Med 23* (5):448–459.

Jordhoy, M. S., P. Fayers, T. Saltnes, M. Ahlner-Elmqvist, M. Jannert, and S. Kaasa. 2000. A palliative-care intervention and death at home: a cluster randomised trial. *Lancet 356* (9233):888–893.

Kinoshita, H., I. Maeda, T. Morita, M. Miyashita, A. Yamagishi, Y. Shirahige, T. Takebayashi, T. Yamaguchi, A. Igarashi, and K. Eguchi. 2015. Place of death and the differences in patient quality of death and dying and caregiver burden. *J Clin Oncol 33* (4):357–363.

Klinger, C. A., D. Howell, D. Marshall, D. Zakus, K. Brazil, and R. B. Deber. 2013. Resource utilization and cost analyses of home-based palliative care service provision: the Niagara West End-of-Life Shared-Care Project. *Palliat Med 27* (2):115–122.

Knaus, W. A., F. E. Harrell, Jr., J. Lynn, L. Goldman, R. S. Phillips, A. F. Connors, Jr., N. V. Dawson, W. J. Fulkerson, Jr., R. M. Califf, N. Desbiens, P. Layde, R. K. Oye, P. E. Bellamy, R. B. Hakim, and D. P. Wagner. 1995. The SUPPORT prognostic model. Objective estimates of survival for seriously ill hospitalized adults. Study to Understand Prognoses and Preferences for Outcomes and Risks of Treatments. *Ann Intern Med 122* (3):191–203.

Lo, C., D. Burman, S. Hales, N. Swami, G. Rodin, and C. Zimmermann. 2009. The FAMCARE-Patient scale: measuring satisfaction with care of outpatients with advanced cancer. *Eur J Cancer 45* (18):3182–3188.

Lorenz, K. A., J. Lynn, S. M. Dy, L. R. Shugarman, A. Wilkinson, R. A. Mularski, S. C. Morton, R. G. Hughes, L. K. Hilton, M. Maglione, S. L. Rhodes, C. Rolon, V. C. Sun, and P. G. Shekelle. 2008. Evidence for improving palliative care at the end of life: a systematic review. *Ann Intern Med 148* (2):147–159.

Luckett, T., J. Phillips, M. Agar, C. Virdun, A. Green, and P. M. Davidson. 2014. Elements of effective palliative care models: a rapid review. *BMC Health Serv Res 14*:136.

Lunney, J. R., J. Lynn, and C. Hogan. 2002. Profiles of older Medicare decedents. *J Am Geriatr Soc 50* (6):1108–1112.

McCorkle, R., N. E. Strumpf, I. F. Nuamah, D. C. Adler, M. E. Cooley, C. Jepson, E. J. Lusk, and M. Torosian. 2000. A specialized home care intervention improves survival among older post-surgical cancer patients. *J Am Geriatr Soc 48* (12):1707–1713.

Miyashita, M., M. Sanjo, T. Morita, K. Hirai, and Y. Uchitomi. 2007. Good death in cancer care: a nationwide quantitative study. *Ann Oncol 18* (6):1090–1097.

Moss, A. H., J. Ganjoo, S. Sharma, J. Gansor, S. Senft, B. Weaner, C. Dalton, K. MacKay, B. Pellegrino, P. Anantharaman, and R. Schmidt. 2008. Utility of the "surprise" question to identify dialysis patients with high mortality. *Clin J Am Soc Nephrol 3* (5):1379–1384.

Moss, A. H., J. R. Lunney, S. Culp, M. Auber, S. Kurian, J. Rogers, J. Dower, and J. Abraham. 2010. Prognostic significance of the "surprise" question in cancer patients. *J Palliat Med 13* (7):837–840.

Murray, M. A., V. Fiset, S. Young, and J. Kryworuchko. 2009. Where the dying live: a systematic review of determinants of place of end-of-life cancer care. *Oncol Nurs Forum 36* (1):69–77.

OHTAC End-of-Life Collaborative. 2014. Health care for people approaching the end of life: an evidentiary framework. *Ont Health Technol Assess Ser [Internet] 14* (14):1–45. Available from: http://www.hqontario.ca/evidence/publications-and-ohtac-recommendations/ontario-health-technology-assessment-series/eol-evidentiary-framework.

Pivodic, L., L. Van den Block, K. Pardon, G. Miccinesi, T. Vega Alonso, N. Boffin, G. A. Donker, M. Cancian, A. Lopez-Maside, B. D. Onwuteaka-Philipsen, L. Deliens, and I. Euro. 2014.

Burden on family carers and care-related financial strain at the end of life: a cross-national population-based study. *Eur J Public Health 24* (5):819–826.

Prosser, L. A., K. Lamarand, A. Gebremariam, and E. Wittenberg. 2015. Measuring family HRQoL spillover effects using direct health utility assessment. *Med Decis Making 35* (1):81–93.

Qaseem, A., V. Snow, P. Shekelle, D. E. Casey, Jr., J. T. Cross, Jr., D. K. Owens, Clinical Efficacy Assessment Subcommittee of the American College of Physicians, P. Dallas, N. C. Dolan, M. A. Forciea, L. Halasyamani, R. H. Hopkins, Jr., and P. Shekelle. 2008. Evidence-based interventions to improve the palliative care of pain, dyspnea, and depression at the end of life: a clinical practice guideline from the American College of Physicians. *Ann Intern Med 148* (2):141–146.

Rabow, M. W., S. L. Dibble, S. Z. Pantilat, and S. J. McPhee. 2004. The comprehensive care team: a controlled trial of outpatient palliative medicine consultation. *Arch Intern Med 164* (1):83–91.

Riley, G. F., and J. D. Lubitz. 2010. Long-term trends in Medicare payments in the last year of life. *Health Serv Res 45* (2):565–576.

Selby, D., A. Chakraborty, T. Lilien, E. Stacey, L. Zhang, and J. Myers. 2011. Clinician accuracy when estimating survival duration: the role of the patient's performance status and time-based prognostic categories. *J Pain Symptom Manage 42* (4):578–588.

Seow, H., L. Barbera, D. Howell, and S. M. Dy. 2010. Using more end-of-life homecare services is associated with using fewer acute care services: a population-based cohort study. *Med Care 48* (2):118–124.

Seow, H., K. Brazil, J. Sussman, J. Pereira, D. Marshall, P. C. Austin, A. Husain, J. Rangrej, and L. Barbera. 2014. Impact of community based, specialist palliative care teams on hospitalisations and emergency department visits late in life and hospital deaths: a pooled analysis. *BMJ 348*:g3496.

Stajduhar, K. I. 2013. Burdens of family caregiving at the end of life. *Clin Invest Med 36* (3):E121–E126.

Stajduhar, K. I., D. E. Allan, S. R. Cohen, and D. K. Heyland. 2008. Preferences for location of death of seriously ill hospitalized patients: perspectives from Canadian patients and their family caregivers. *Palliat Med 22* (1):85–88.

Stiggelbout, A. M., M. J. Eijkemans, G. M. Kiebert, J. Kievit, J. W. Leer, and H. J. De Haes. 1996. The 'utility' of the visual analog scale in medical decision making and technology assessment. Is it an alternative to the time trade-off? *Int J Technol Assess Health Care 12* (2):291–298.

Stukel, T. A., E. S. Fisher, D. A. Alter, A. Guttmann, D. T. Ko, K. Fung, W. P. Wodchis, N. N. Baxter, C. C. Earle, and D. S. Lee. 2012. Association of hospital spending intensity with mortality and readmission rates in Ontario hospitals. *JAMA 307* (10):1037–1045.

Tam, V. C., Y.J. Ko, N. Mittmann, M. C. Cheung, K. Kumar, S. Hassan, and K. K. Chan. 2013. Cost-effectiveness of systemic therapies for metastatic pancreatic cancer. *Current Oncology 20* (2):e90–e106.

Tanuseputro, P, S. Budhwani,. Y. Q. Bai,., and W. P. Wodchis. 2013. Palliative care applied health research question: results for Central East Local Health Integration Network. Palliative Care Applied Health Research (AHRQ) 2013 [Internet]. Toronto (ON): Health System Performance Research Network; 2013 June. Available from: http://www.hsprn.ca/uploads/files/HSPRN_EoL%20AHRQ%201%20Evidence%20Brief%20June%202013%20%289-5-2014%29.pdf.

Tanuseputro, P., W. P. Wodchis, R. Fowler, P. Walker, Y. Q. Bai, S. E. Bronskill, and D. Manuel. 2015. The health care cost of dying: a population-based retrospective cohort study of the last year of life in Ontario, Canada. *PLoS ONE [Electronic Resource] 10* (3):e0121759.

Temel, J. S., J. A. Greer, A. Muzikansky, E. R. Gallagher, S. Admane, V. A. Jackson, C. M. Dahlin, C. D. Blinderman, J. Jacobsen, W. F. Pirl, J. A. Billings, and T. J. Lynch. 2010. Early palliative care for patients with metastatic non-small-cell lung cancer. *N Engl J Med 363* (8):733–742.

Teno, J. M., S. Weitzen, M. L. Fennell, and V. Mor. 2001. Dying trajectory in the last year of life: does cancer trajectory fit other diseases? *J Palliat Med 4* (4):457–464.

Thein, H. H., T. Gomes, M. D. Krahn, and W. P. Wodchis. 2010. Health status utilities and the impact of pressure ulcers in long-term care residents in Ontario. *Qual Life Res 19* (1):81–89.

Towns, K., E. Dougherty, N. Kevork, D. Wiljer, D. Seccareccia, G. Rodin, L. W. Le, and C. Zimmermann. 2012. Availability of services in Ontario hospices and hospitals providing inpatient palliative care. *J Palliat Med 15* (5):527–534.

Trotta, R. L. 2007. Quality of death: a dimensional analysis of palliative care in the nursing home. *J Palliat Med 10* (5):1116–1127.

Van den Hout, W. B. 2006. EuroQol data in terminally-ill cancer patients. Poster presentation to the 28th Annual Meeting of the Society for Medical Decision Making (October 15-18, 2006) Boston, MA. https://smdm.confex.com/smdm/2006ma/techprogram/P2931.HTM.

van den Hout, W. B., G. W. Kramer, E. M. Noordijk, and J. W. Leer. 2006. Cost-utility analysis of short- versus long-course palliative radiotherapy in patients with non-small-cell lung cancer. *J Natl Cancer Inst 98* (24):1786–1794.

van den Hout, W. B., Y. M. van der Linden, E. Steenland, R. G. Wiggenraad, J. Kievit, H. de Haes, and J. W. Leer. 2003. Single- versus multiple-fraction radiotherapy in patients with painful bone metastases: cost-utility analysis based on a randomized trial. *J Natl Cancer Inst 95* (3):222–229.

Walker, H., M. Anderson, F. Farahati, D. Howell, S. L. Librach, A. Husain, J. Sussman, R. Viola, R. Sutradhar, and L. Barbera. 2011. Resource use and costs of end-of-life/palliative care: Ontario adult cancer patients dying during 2002 and 2003. *J Palliat Care 27* (2):79–88.

Wittenberg, E., and L. A. Prosser. 2013. Disutility of illness for caregivers and families: a systematic review of the literature. *Pharmacoeconomics 31* (6):489–500.

Wittenberg, E., G. A. Ritter, and L. A. Prosser. 2013. Evidence of spillover of illness among household members: EQ-5D scores from a US sample. *Med Decis Making 33* (2):235–243.

Wodchis, W. P., J. P. Hirdes, and D. H. Feeny. 2003. Health-related quality of life measure based on the minimum data set. *Int J Technol Assess Health Care 19* (3):490–506.

Wright, A. A., N. L. Keating, T. A. Balboni, U. A. Matulonis, S. D. Block, and H. G. Prigerson. 2010. Place of death: correlations with quality of life of patients with cancer and predictors of bereaved caregivers' mental health. *J Clin Oncol 28* (29):4457–4464.

You, J. J., R. A. Fowler, D. K. Heyland, and Canadian Researchers at the End of Life Network. 2014. Just ask: discussing goals of care with patients in hospital with serious illness. *CMAJ 186* (6):425–432.

Zimmer, J. G., A. Groth-Juncker, and J. McCusker. 1985. A randomized controlled study of a home health care team. *Am J Public Health 75* (2):134–141.

Index

Page numbers followed by *f* indicate figures; *t*, tables; *b*, boxes.

Public Health Service, U.S. (*cont.*)
  Second Panel on Cost-Effectiveness
    in Health and Medicine, xviii–xix,
    67–73, 100*b*
PubMed/MEDLINE, 251
PyscINFO. *See* Psychological Information
  Database

QALY(s). *See* quality-adjusted life year(s)
QHES. *See* Quality of Health Economic
  Studies
qualitative bias analysis, 159
qualitative synthesis, 253–54
quality-adjusted life year(s) (QALY[s]), 14,
  400–401
  ACA and, 16
  age and, 44
  alternatives to, 45
  calculation of, 24–25, 52, 96, 127
  conventional approach, 362
  definition of, 6–7, 52, 80
  effectiveness measured by, 80
  estimation of, 53, 167, 169, 174, 179, 180,
    185, 190, 213, 322
  example, 2*t*
  gained from intervention, 171–72, 171*f*
  health outcomes measured by, xxvii, 7, 19,
    44, 52, 69, 92, 171–73, 184–85, 279*t*
  health state and, 52, 205, 209
  intrinsic and instrumental values
    measured by, 204
  maximizing, 46, 54, 62, 204, 213,
    325, 335–36
  PCORI prohibition of, xxiii, 16
  problems with, 185
  productivity effects, xxvii, 209–10
  reductions in, 88
  theoretical foundations in, xxiv, 52–54
  time value through, 58, 61,
    110–11, 112*t*
  U.S. $50,000 benchmark, 10, 23–24,
    467*f*, 468*f*
  utility measure, 45, 52–53, 61–62, 80,
    167, 204
  valuation of, 184–85, 205, 324–25
  as welfare measure, 44, 52, 204, 213
Quality of Health Economic Studies (QHES)
  instrument, 345

quality of life, 92
  economic costs and, 210
  non-preference-based approaches to, xxvi
  preference-based approaches, xxvi, 168–
    69, 172–73, 177–78
  QALYs for measurement of, 45
quantification, of non-health
  consequences, 70
quantitative bias analysis, 148, 158, 159, 239,
  252, 264
quantitative synthesis, 258, 263
  data on costs or utilization rates, 261–62
  intervention effects, 259–60
  test performance measures, 261

random-effects model, 255–56, 256*f*, 257
randomized controlled trials (RCTs), 98, 99,
  105, 107, 147, 251
  effectiveness of interventions and, 115
  efficacy *vs.* effectiveness, 115
  patient selection in, 148
  testing arm in, 153
  time horizon limits, 108
rating scales, 174
  category scaling, 175
  visual analog scales, 175, 179, 180
Rawlsian principles, 55, 182
RCTs. *See* randomized controlled trials
R&D. *See* research and development
receiver operating characteristic (ROC)
  curve, 152
recommendations
  on cost estimated and valuations of non-
    health benefits, 228–30, 376–78
  on decision models, 130–31, 373–74
  on disaggregated measures, 370
  on discounting, 286, 379
  on ethical and distribution
    considerations, 338–39, 381
  on evidence synthesis, 269, 378–79
  on healthcare sector Reference Case,
    69–70, 369
  on Impact Inventory, 370
  on interventions, 161–62, 374–75
  on Reference Case perspectives, 67–73, 369
  on reporting, of CEA, 365–66, 381–82
  on reporting Reference Case, 370–71
  on societal Reference Case, 370

retirement, time valuation in, 224
return-on-investment (ROI) analyses, 79, 213
returns to scale, 228
risk, attitudes toward, 60
Robert Wood Johnson Foundation, xix
robustness analysis, 268
ROC. *See* receiver operating characteristic
ROI. *See* return-on-investment
rule of reason, 144, 212

Scandinavian Simvastatin Survival Study, 113
scenario analysis, 82, 300
scope of study, 91–93, 346, 348–49
scoring systems
  CHU-9D, 187
  EQ-5D, 186, 187, 263
  HUI3, 187
  indirect utility measures, 178
screening. *See also* cancer screening
  HIV, 5t, 14, 87
secondary data, 97
Second Panel on Cost-Effectiveness in Health and Medicine, xviii
  Bill and Melinda Gates Foundation funding, xix
  members and leaders of, xiii
  perspective considerations, 68–69
  potential analyst burden, 100b
  Reference Case perspective recommendations, 67–73
  Robert Wood Johnson Foundation funding, xix
selection bias, 146, 148, 149, 154, 158–59, 221, 251, 265
selective analysis bias, 265, 266
selective outcome reporting bias, 265, 266
sensitivity analysis, xxvii, xxviii, 71, 98, 268, 371. *See also* deterministic sensitivity analysis; probabilistic sensitivity analysis
  on AUD, 412f, 413f, 414f
  on HPC and EOL, 452, 453t, 454, 454f, 455–56
  multi-way, 296
  one-way, 295
  structural, 121–22

sensitivity estimates, 153
shadow price, of constraint, 46
short-term time horizon, 111, 117
simulation
  discrete event models, 120
  dynamic models, 118t, 120
  microsimulation models, 118t, 119
  population, for infectious disease models, 125
  populations *vs.* cohort, 122, 125
single-age cohort analyses, 125
single test performance measurements, 152
SMDM. *See* Society for Medical Decision Making
smoking cessation programs, 4, 5t
  boundaries of, 91–92
  characteristics of, 93
  conceptual model of, 87, 96
  time horizons for, 93–94
social contract principle, 182
social discount rates, 282
social effects, of direct testing, 151
social welfare, 46
societal perspective, xxiv, 370
  AUD Reference Case, 406, 408f, 411f
  for CEA, 7, 41, 42, 67, 68
  constraints and, 58
  consumption and transportation costs, xxvii, 72, 84
  costs, xxvii, 7, 47–48, 72, 84
  cross-sector consequences in, 83–84
  definition, 83
  discount rates from, 283–84
  health outcomes in, 6–7
  patient and caregivers time costs, xxvii, 72, 84
  practicality concerns, 68
  productivity benefits, xxvii, 72, 84
  Reference Case perspectives recommendations, 70
  since original Panel, 67–68
  supply side cost-effectiveness thresholds, 24, 25
  welfare and, 205
Society for Medical Decision Making (SMDM), 106, 290
software, meta-analysis, 268–69
special populations, 186–87

decisions linked to, 311–14
in health states, 53
from individual to population level, 60
purpose of, 314
uses of, 292
what is and what if studies, 77
United Kingdom (UK)
NICE of, xviii, 16, 19–20, 27, 125–27,
129–30, 214
opportunity costs thresholds in, 24–25
United States (U.S.)
CEA in, 13–17
EPA, 24, 161
$50,000 per QALY cost-effective
threshold, 10, 23–24, 467f, 468f
Public Health Service, xvii–xix,
67–73, 100b
United States Preventive Services Task Force
(USPSTF), 15
on breast and colorectal cancer
screening, 17, 76
unrelated healthcare costs, 206–8
U.S. See United States
USPSTF. See United States Preventive
Services Task Force
utilitarianism
costs value, 281
welfare maximization, 54
utility
individual, xxiv, 44, 53–58
lifetime, 60–61
marginal of income, 280–81, 281t
scores content and meaning,
179–80
utility maximization, 49–50, 53
utility measurements
direct, 174–76
indirect, 177–78
of morbidity, 180
overview, 173–74
QALY as, 45, 52–53, 61–62,
80, 167, 204
utility of consumption
marginal, 280–82, 281t, 284
over time, 61–62
utility scores
interpretation of, 179
productivity effects in, 179–80

utility theory, expected, 44, 52, 53, 60
utility weights, 188–89
utilization information, 98

VA. See Department of Veterans Affairs
vaccinations, 13
validation, xxix
cross, 130
of decision models, 129–30
in journal article results section, 356
validity
construct, 172–73
content, 172
cross-section construct, 172
in evidence synthesis pre-analytical
phase, 246
external, 149–50, 155–56, 160
face, 129, 251
internal, 149, 154–55, 158
of preference measurement, xxvi, 172–73
valuation
contingent, 81
of costs, 58–59
of effectiveness, 52–53
of health states, 52
of QALY, 184–85, 205, 324–25
of resources, 202, 218–27
of time, 55, 58–59
value judgments, 17, 44, 45, 84
value of additional research
barriers to implementation, 311
decision making and, 305–11, 306f
EVPI and, 306f, 307–9, 308t, 402, 415f
EVSI and ENBS of sample
information, 310–11
value of information (VOI)
analysis, 315, 380–81, 402, 415
estimates, 19, 63, 77, 292, 311
values
absolute, of costs, 304–5, 305f
of health evidence, 24
intrinsic and instrumental, in QALY, 204
leisure time, 56, 59
parameter, 289, 291
positive predictive, 154
probability of, 52, 295, 297
time, through QALY, 58, 61,
110–11, 112t